DATE DUE

NOV 1 1 2011			

Demco

D1441881

Globalization and Health

GLOBALIZATION AND HEALTH

Edited by
Ichiro Kawachi
Sarah Wamala

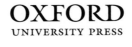
OXFORD
UNIVERSITY PRESS
2007

OXFORD
UNIVERSITY PRESS

Oxford University Press, Inc., publishes works that further
Oxford University's objective of excellence
in research, scholarship, and education.

Oxford   New York
Auckland   Cape Town   Dar es Salaam   Hong Kong   Karachi
Kuala Lumpur   Madrid   Melbourne   Mexico City   Nairobi
New Delhi   Shanghai   Taipei   Toronto

With offices in
Argentina   Austria   Brazil   Chile   Czech Republic   France   Greece
Guatemala   Hungary   Italy   Japan   Poland   Portugal   Singapore
South Korea   Switzerland   Thailand   Turkey   Ukraine   Vietnam

Copyright © 2007 by Oxford University Press

Published by Oxford University Press, Inc.
198 Madison Avenue, New York, New York 10016

www.oup.com

Library of Congress Cataloging-in-Publication Data
Globalization and health / [edited by] Ichiro Kawachi, Sarah Wamala.
p. cm.
Includes bibliographical references and index.
ISBN-13 978-0-19-517299-7
ISBN 0-19-517299-X
1. Globalization—Health aspects.   2. World health.
[DNLM: 1. World Health.
2. Population Dynamics.   3. Socioeconomic Factors. WA 530.1 G564 2006]
I. Kawachi, Ichiro.   II. Wamala, Sarah P.
RA441.G5852 2006
362.1'042—dc22   2005026737

1 3 5 7 9 8 6 4 2

Printed in the United States of America
on acid-free paper

Foreword

Ilona Kickbusch

One of the fundamental consequences of modernity is globalization.
—A. *Giddens*, The Consequences of Modernity

Globalization greatly affects the socioeconomic-political context of health. Experts disagree about the overall impact of globalization on health—whether, on the whole, globalization is a positive or negative force. One fact, however, is clear: the political challenge is to take control of the effects of globalization rather than continue to consider them a force of nature (Messner, 1999). In order to develop a sound strategy, the global public health community must better understand the impacts of globalization on health and vice versa.

Kawachi and Wamala's *Globalization and Health* analyzes the current and emerging threats to health in a systematic way that takes into account the contextual changes occurring in the global health arena. In recent years, the territory of health has rapidly expanded. In 1978 the Declaration of Alma-Ata on primary health care and the subsequent health-for-all strategy of the World Health Organization (WHO) opened the door to understanding health in the context of development and reinforced a classic public

health dictum that the most influential actions to create health are found in sectors other than health. Research on the determinants of health has shown that the health care sector is only one of many sectors—including transportation, housing, education, and environment—that both affect and are affected by health. But the force and dynamic of globalization are themselves determinants of the health of nations. The report of the Commission on Macroeconomics and Health entitled *Macroeconomics and Health: Investing in Health for Economic Development* underlined that health is a central component to poverty reduction and economic development of nations (WHO, 2001). It brought the health agenda firmly into the economic development agenda and closer to the agenda of ministries of finance. This was reinforced further by the prominence given to health in the Millennium Development Goals. But the shift to a public health model based on determinants of health requires a perception of policies that takes into account the structural causes many of which are no longer amenable to a response solely at the level of the nation-state. The classic dictum by Geoffrey Rose (1992), "the primary determinants of disease are mainly economic and social, therefore its remedies must also be economic and social" (p. 129), now needs to be understood at a global level.

Part I of *Globalization and Health* addresses the expanding territory of health by examining threats to health beyond the medical system. Tord Kjellstrom and colleagues, for instance, examine the health effects of the globalizing car culture and transport policy in chapter 6, while Kawachi and Wamala analyze the impact of economic inequality in chapter 7. In doing so, contributing authors address what Kimmo Leppo (1998, p. 3) calls "one of the great paradoxes in the history of health policy . . . that despite all the evidence and understanding that has accrued about determinants of health and the means available to tackle them, the national and international policy arenas are filled with something quite different" (p. 3). In addition to describing the global threats to health, the authors in part II (Reidpath, O'Keefe, and Scott-Samuel) provide a toolkit for evaluating the impact of economic globalization on the world's health. These tools, which can be useful in forecasting future impacts of globalization, include key indicators of population health status, summary measures of population health, and health impact assessment as a tool for evaluation.

Concurrent with the expansion of the territory of health has been the proliferation of global health actors. This is evidenced by the growth of civil society organizations and collaborative arrangements for health as well as the increasing health mandate of organizations such as the World Bank, regional development banks, and regional organizations such as the European Union. New organizations and initiatives, such as UNAIDS; the Global Fund to Fight AIDS, Tuberculosis, and Malaria; and the "3 by 5" Initiative, are continually formed to take on health matters. While this growth has helped to save lives across the globe, the role of key institutions in protecting and promoting health is becoming more complex. The increased interconnectedness between health and nonhealth actors is blurring their traditional boundaries and raising questions as to whether they are indeed protecting or threatening the public's health. The proliferation of global health actors and partnerships has reduced transparency and accountability, and the permeability of national borders has diminished governmental control over a growing number of health determinants. It

is apparent that new interactions among global health players are transforming the global playing field in health—its norms, rules, practices, and, especially, its power politics (Kickbusch, 2003).

The contributing authors in part III respond to these challenges by analyzing the global politics and some of the key institutions and policies that shape global public health. In chapter 13, Breman and Shelton, for instance, assess the World Bank and International Monetary Fund's structural adjustment policies that have been harshly critiqued by many in global public health. The authors provide a theoretical framework by which to measure the impact of structural adjustment policies on health outcomes. The role of the World Trade Organization in protecting health has been another source for fiery debate in the global health field. Gregg Bloche and Elizabeth Jungman, in chapter 15, analyze the organization's influence on national health polices through the General Agreement on Tariffs and Trade (GATT) as well as the Agreement on Trade-Related Aspects of Intellectual Property Rights (TRIPS) and the Agreement on Sanitary and Phytosanitary Measures (SPS). These types of objective assessments are crucial in order to address the global governance challenges that have emerged in the health field.

FUTURE ACTION AREAS

Studying the relationship between health and globalization brings to light a number of key action areas for the future of global health. A new dynamics emerges as to what needs to be resolved at national and global levels, what is public versus private or proprietary, and how health is valued in our globalizing world. Five key areas of focus emerge for this new historical phase of public health: (1) responding to health as a global public good, (2) regarding health as a key component of global human security, (3) strengthening global health governance for interdependence, (4) accepting health as a key factor of sound business practice and social responsibility, and (5) recognizing the ethical principle of health as a right of global citizenship.

Responding to Health as a Global Public Good

Health must principally be considered a global public good. Such an approach is built on the premise that not only does globalization affect health, but also health is a major force within globalization. It is key to the global marketplace and central to world economic growth. The recent outbreaks of SARS have illustrated that health cannot be reduced to a commodity and that health at all levels of governance must be supported by governance infrastructure with public financing mechanisms. Society must ensure the value of health and keep it high on the global political agenda. This requires international collective action such as defining common agendas, increasing the importance of global health treaties, and pooling of sovereignty by nation-states in the area of health.

Regarding Health as a Key Component of Global Human Security

The spread of communicable diseases due to global integration is forcing health onto the security agenda of modern nation-states. Disease outbreaks are a threat to global and human security. Increased human mobility, whether voluntary or involuntary, is affecting health and disease patterns across the world, as described by Pascale Allotey and Anthony Zwi in chapter 9. New prominence will need to be given to the mandate of the WHO in global health surveillance role and its interventionist power in the international health regulations. Other security concerns that affect health and need to be addressed at the national and global levels include the health threats posed by military spending (as assessed by Ray Hyatt in chapter 18) and criminal activities such as tobacco smuggling, the global arms trade, biological weapons terrorist activities, and trafficking of illicit drugs.

Increasingly, it is acknowledged that "a fairer world is a safer world," as is frequently stated by Secretary General of the United Nations, Kofi Annan. Globalization, some critics argue, is concentrating political, economic, and cultural resources into a handful of developed countries, which could potentially be creating a security risk. The poorest countries are presently feeling the devastating effects of global health disparities, but there are mounting signals that a new health divide is in the making in the developed world, as well. Social and economic inequities—both within and between nations—must be rigorously analyzed and addressed at the global level. Continued action on Millennium Development Goal 8 on partnerships can help to achieve this. Rich nations must increase their foreign aid to the minimum 0.7% gross national product and also aim to reduce poverty via trade, investment, migration, environment, security, and technology.

Strengthening Global Health Governance for Interdependence

Strong governance must accompany the changes occurring among global health actors. Expansion in the territory of health and growth in the health actors have profound implications for the governance of global health. Strengthening global health governance for interdependence requires understanding the role of global politics in shaping global health in our interdependent world. It is important to examine the impact of global strategies and policies on health, such as poverty reduction strategies. In chapter 14, Wamala, Kawachi, and Mpepo assess the empirical evidence that links poverty reduction strategies to health outcomes in sub-Saharan Africa, Asia, and Latin America.

Health professionals must pay particular attention to the role of WHO as a key player in promoting global health. It is important to examine how the constitutional role of WHO could be adapted, as well as how its functions could be applied more fully to the global international environment while maintaining its legitimacy. In chapter 16, Bonita, Irwin, and Beaglehole explain the need to expand the scope of public health and to strengthen the global public health workforce and infrastructure. Nation-states should support WHO in developing a global approach rather than obstruct the road to agreements on global access to safe consumer products. They also need to realize the importance of global health governance and solidarity and help build stronger international institutions and policy networks.

Accepting Health as a Key Factor of Sound Business Practice and Social Responsibility

As globalization alters the balance of power among public and private sector actors in health, businesses are playing an increasingly predominant role in the global health arena. More and more, sound business practice is being understood in terms of corporate citizenship, which makes companies more accountable for public goods—in particular, those that improve health.

Accepting health as a key factor of sound business practice means that businesses must invest in health at the workplace, marketplace, community, and policy levels. In the workplace, companies provide safe working conditions for their employees. But as explained by Hogstedt, Wegman, and Kjellstrom in chapter 8, the globalized, neo-liberal economic system has resulted in the reduction of wage controls, union protections, and workplace standards. Also, large transnational corporations need to be held more accountable for the effects of their marketing strategies, particularly the tobacco and fast food industries. While this is occurring more and more in developed nations, globalization has provided companies with access to new, less regulated markets in developing countries. Providing inducements for corporate action on health can also help to increase sound business practice for health.

Recognizing the Ethical Principle of Health as a Right of Global Citizenship

The understanding of health as a right of global citizenship is essential. It requires challenging the dominant neo-liberal paradigm in the world today. A key responsibility of the public health community is to advance this principle of social justice. Ethical norms must also apply to international relations. As inequities in health become increasingly prominent, the notion of health as a human right is gaining support. Nigel Dower (2003) points out, "If citizens are increasingly motivated by global concerns then cosmopolitan goals enter domestic policy in that way and people can be effective global citizens by being effective global oriented citizens of their own states" (p. 132). In particular, this implies a common notion of social justice and a system of international law where human rights constitute a legal claim. Health is central in advancing this principle of social justice.

CONCLUSION

The effects of globalization on health are vast. The positioning of health lies not in instruments of technical assistance but in policies of interdependence. The global health community must, on the one hand, strengthen international organizations in a way that that allows them to fulfill new functions in an inter-dependent world and, on the other hand, develop efficient forms of network governance for health. Both strategies must intersect in forms of global accountability and financing that need to be developed and institutionalized.

The key aim of the global public health community must be to establish health as a right of global citizens and promote global public goods for health. Health is not an afterthought to globalization but lies at its core. Together with a strategy of empowerment and community involvement, such a global health approach also acts as a spearhead to enable and support individual health behaviors. This has become obvious in the response to the obesity and tobacco epidemics: the globalization of food markets and the global marketing of tobacco make it necessary to find common global response mechanisms, such as the International Framework Convention on Tobacco Control.

Rudolf Virchow, the great public health pioneer of the nineteenth century, underlined that health and disease always have two key determining factors: one pathological and one political. This book shows clearly that the public health community is making strides in both arenas: we can show with more clarity and confidence the evidence at the interface between globalization and health in its pathological and its political dimensions. Indeed, as the forces of globalization restructure the world, the politics of health need to change. This book is an excellent guide for the priorities that must be addressed.

References

Dower, N. (2003). *An Introduction to Global Citizenship.* Edinburgh University Press, Edinburgh.

Kickbusch, I. (2003). Global Health Governance: Some Theoretical Considerations in a New Political Space. In Lee, K. (ed.), *Health Impacts of Globalization* (pp. 192–203). Palgrave MacMillian, Hampshire, UK.

Leppo K. (1998). Introduction. In: Koivisalo M, Ollila E. (eds.), *Making a Healthy World.* Zed Books, London.

Messner, D. (1999). Globalisierung, Global Governance und Entwicklungspolitik. *Internationale Politik*, 1, S.5–S.18.

Rose, G. (1992). *The Strategy of Preventive Medicine.* Oxford University Press, Oxford.

WHO. (2001). *Macroeconomics and Health: Investing in Health for Economic Development.* World Health Organization Commission on Macroeconomics and Health, Geneva.

Acknowledgments

The editors, Ichiro Kawachi and Sarah Wamala, are grateful for the generous support of the Swedish National Institute of Public Health (Statens folkhälsoinstitut). The backing of the institute and its director general, Dr. Gunnar Ågren, as well as the director of research, Professor Christer Hogstedt, made possible the collaboration between the editors that led to the production of the book.

The authors of chapter 4 (Barry Popkin and Michelle Mendez) thank the National Institutes of Health (R01-HD30880 and R01-HD38700) for financial support for the analysis. They also thank Ms. Frances L. Dancy for administrative assistance, Mr. Tom Swasey for graphics support, and Mr. Lu Bing for research assistance.

The author of chapter 11 (Daniel Reidpath) thanks Pascale Allotey, Kit Yee Chan, and Rebecca Marsh for the opportunities to discuss the ideas, for their input, and for their judicious editing.

The authors of chapter 15 (Gregg Bloche and Elizabeth Jungman) thank Audrey Chapman, Steve Charnovitz, Victoria Espinel, John Jackson, Daniel Tarullo, and Daniel Wueger for their suggestions. Their chapter is an adaptation of articles previously published in the *Journal of International Economic Law* and the *Journal of Law, Medicine, and Ethics*.

The authors of chapter 16 (Ruth Bonita, Alec Irwin, and Robert Beaglehole) are grateful for comments and input on an earlier draft from colleagues at the World Health Organization, in particular, Desmond Avery; and from the editors of the volume.

The authors of chapter 17 (Ted Schrecker and Ronald Labonte) are grateful for the research assistance of Madeline Johnson and Jenifer Rodenbush. Their initial research on the G8 and global health was supported by the International Development Research Centre (Canada). All views expressed are exclusively theirs.

Contents

Contributors

Pascale Allotey, PhD
School of Health Sciences and Social Care
Brunel University
Uxbridge, UK

Robert Beaglehole, DSc, FRS (NZ)
Department of Chronic Diseases and Health
    Promotion
World Health Organization
Geneva, Switzerland

M. Gregg Bloche, MD, JD
Georgetown University Law Center–Johns
    Hopkins University Bloomberg School of Public
    Health Joint Program in Law and Public Health
Washington, DC, USA

Ruth Bonita, MPH, PhD, MD(hc)
Evidence and Information for Policy
World Health Organization
Geneva, Switzerland

Anna Breman, PhD
Stockholm School of Economics
Stockholm, Sweden

Barbara Cannito, MSc
Centre on Global Change and Health
London School of Hygiene and Tropical Medicine
London, UK

Stanton Glantz, PhD
University of California, San Francisco
San Francisco, CA, USA

Ross Hammond, MA
Campaign for Tobacco Free Kids
San Francisco, CA, USA

Sarah Hinde, BSc, GDPH
National Centre for Epidemiology and Population
    Health
Australian National University
Canberra, Australia

CHRISTER HOGSTEDT, MD
National Institute of Public Health
Stockholm, Sweden

RAYMOND R. HYATT, JR., PHD
Friedman School of Nutrition Science and Policy
Tufts University
Boston, MA, USA

ALEC IRWIN, PHD
Evidence and Information for Policy
World Health Organization
Geneva, Switzerland

ELIZABETH R. JUNGMAN
Georgetown University Law Center and the Johns
   Hopkins University Bloomberg School of Public
   Health
Washington, DC, USA

ICHIRO KAWACHI, MD, PHD
Harvard Center for Society and Health
Harvard School of Public Health
Boston, MA, USA

ILONA KICKBUSCH, PHD
Swiss Federal Office for Health
Bern, Switzerland

TORD KJELLSTROM, MED DR, MME
National Institute of Public Health, Stockholm,
   Sweden; and
National Centre for Epidemiology and Population
   Health,
Australian National University, Canberra, Australia

RONALD LABONTE, PHD
Institute for Population Health
University of Ottawa
Ottawa, Ontario, Canada

KELLEY LEE, MPA, MA, DPHIL
Centre on Global Change and Health
London School of Hygiene and Tropical Medicine
London, UK

A.J. MCMICHAEL, MBBS, PHD, FAFPHM, FTSE
National Centre for Epidemiology and Population
   Health
The Australian National University
Canberra, Australia

MICHELLE MENDEZ, PHD
Dept of Nutrition, School of Public Health

University of North Carolina at Chapel Hill
Chapel Hill, NC, USA

BESINATI PHIRI MPEPO, MA
Civil Society for Poverty Reduction
Lusaka, Zambia

EILEEN O'KEEFE, BA
Department of Applied Social Science
London Metropolitan University
London, UK

BARRY M. POPKIN, PHD
Dept of Nutrition, School of Public Health
University of North Carolina at Chapel Hill
Chapel Hill, NC, USA

G. RANMUTHUGALA, MBBS, PHD
National Centre for Epidemiology and Population
   Health
The Australian National University
Canberra, Australia

DANIEL D. REIDPATH, PHD
School of Health Sciences and Social Care
Brunel University
Uxbridge, UK

LANCE SAKER, MSc MRCP
Centre on Global Change and Health
London School of Hygiene and Tropical Medicine
London, UK

TED SCHRECKER, MA
Institute for Population Health
University of Ottawa
Ottawa, Ontario, Canada

ALEX SCOTT-SAMUEL, MBCHB, MCOMMH, FFPH
International Health Impact Assessment Consortium
Division of Public Health
University of Liverpool, UK

CAROLYN SHELTON, MPH
Pan American Health Organization/World Health
   Organization
Washington, DC, USA

SARAH WAMALA, MSc, PHD
Swedish National Institute of Public Health; and
   Karolinska Institute
Stockholm, Sweden

DAVID H. WEGMAN, MD, MSc
University of Massachusetts
Lowell, MA, USA

HEATHER WIPFLI, MA
Institute for Global Tobacco Control
Johns Hopkins Bloomberg School of Public Health
Baltimore, MD, USA

DEREK YACH, MBChB, MPH
The Rockefeller Foundation
New York, NY, USA

ANTHONY ZWI, MBBCh, PhD
School of Public Health and Community Medicine
University of New South Wales
Sydney, Australia

Globalization and Health

Chapter 1

Globalization and Health: Challenges and Prospects

Ichiro Kawachi and Sarah Wamala

"Globalization" is hardly a new phenomenon. Past world leaders from Churchill to Bismarck each insisted in their time that their countries were living through unparalleled transformations stemming from technological change, industrialization, and global commerce (Hutton and Giddens 2000). However, a distinctive characteristic of the current era of globalization is the intensity of the debate concerning its benefits versus adverse impacts. This debate has been carried out in academic journals, the mass media, the Internet, and even in the streets of Seattle and Genoa, where antiglobalization protestors clashed with local police.

According to Stanley Fischer, the former deputy director of the International Monetary Fund (IMF), the word "globalization" was never even mentioned in the pages of the *New York Times* during the 1970s. In the 1980s the word appeared less than once a week, and in the latter half of the 1990s no more than three times a week. However, by 2002, there were 393 references, or more than one mention per

day (Fischer 2003). Even the concept of being "antiglobalization" did not exist prior to about 1999. Using the Google search engine, Fischer (2003) estimated that the key word "globalization" yielded 1.6 million links.

Despite the skepticism evinced by the overuse of the term, almost everyone—both the cheerleaders (Friedman 1999) and the street protestors—agrees that the present era of globalization seems distinct from previous episodes. Globalization in the twenty-first century is breaking down economic, political, cultural, social, demographic, and symbolic barriers across the world at a pace hitherto unseen in the history of civilization.

Every day, more than $2 trillion is exchanged in the world's currency markets. Yet globalization in the present day represents much more than the free flow of money and commodities across national borders. The new globalization is marked by new actors (e.g., the World Trade Organization [WTO] with authority over national governments, multinational corporations with more economic power than many states, as well as the global networks of nongovernmental organizations), new rules of governance (e.g., multilateral agreements on trade and intellectual property), new forms of communication (e.g., the Internet, satellite television), and the global movements of populations (whether as economic migrants, refugees, or trafficked individuals).

Each manifestation of globalization poses new challenges and opportunities to the health of nations. Opening up to international trade and foreign investment has helped many poor countries to grow faster and to lift people out of poverty. At the same time, it has exposed many countries to financial volatility and repeated currency crises. Global competition has opened up job opportunities in poor countries and lowered the cost of consumer goods in rich countries. On the other hand, the pressures of global competition have resulted in more "flexible" work arrangements in both rich and poor countries (translation: fewer institutional protections and greater job insecurity). Growing travel and global media communications have reduced the sense of isolation among many parts of the developing world and provided people with access to knowledge well beyond the reach of even the wealthiest in any country a century ago (Stiglitz 2002). At the same time, both travel and migration have helped to spread contagious diseases such as HIV/AIDS and SARS, while the Internet has provided a convenient vehicle for the global illicit traffic in laundered money, drugs, women, and weapons (United Nations Development Programme 1999).

Finally, the globalization of markets, governance, and knowledge has been accompanied by mounting frustration about the pace of benefits that it is supposed to deliver to the world's poor. Despite the promise of raising living standards, globalization has actually widened the gap between the haves and have-nots of the world. Worldwide, the number of people subsisting on less than $2 per day increased by 85 million over the last decade of the twentieth century, even as total world income rose by an average of 2.5% annually. In sub-Saharan Africa the number of extreme poor increased from 164 million to 316 million (Dollar 2004). The growing inequality spawns environmental degradation from both ends. Poor people, having little choice, are putting pressure on the environment, while many of those in the wealthiest parts of the world drive around in sport utility vehicles.

The aim of this book is to provide a survey of current and emerging global threats to health and to analyze the collective and institutional responses to globalization. The book also addresses the role of key intergovernmental institutions (the World Bank, the IMF, the WTO, the World Health Organization [WHO], and the Group of Eight Nations [G8]) in protecting—or, some claim, threatening—the health of the global public.

WHAT IS "GLOBALIZATION"?

The passion with which the globalization debate has been carried out in recent times seems all the more remarkable given that there is no single agreed-upon definition of "globalization." As remarked by the New Zealand economist Brian Easton:

> The definition of globalisation is problematic. Many writers avoid defining it analytically, instead characterizing it by a series of particular phenomena such as increasing trade, or capital flows, or logos, or international inequality; or to particular international institutions such as the World Trade Organization or the International Monetary Fund and the World Bank or the European Union, or multinational corporations; or to particular policies such as free trade, liberalised capital movements, and so on. The London *Economist* described globalisation as "international capitalism"; many anti-globalisers might agree, perhaps adding "together with U.S. hegemony." (Easton 2004, p. 2)

Absent universal agreement about its definition, we should not be surprised that the globalization debate often sounds like two groups of people talking past each other. For example, some writers blame globalization for the homogenization of world culture. That is, they view the progressive "Coca-Colaization" of the globe as a *consequence* of globalization. Yet others view cultural homogenization as partly a *mechanism* of globalization, or they view the process as *intrinsic* to the definition of globalization. Obviously, we would not get very far in analyzing the connections between globalization and health without a definition. In preparing this book, we encouraged the authors of individual chapters to think about globalization as simply the "closer integration of economies and societies." An example of a more comprehensive attempt at definition comes from the International Labour Office (2003) (see box 1.1).

Box 1.1 – The Challenges of the Social Dimension of Globalization

"Globalization" is a term that is used in many ways, but the principal underlying idea is the progressive integration of economies and societies. It is driven by new technologies, new economic relationships, and the national and international policies of a wide range of actors, including governments, international organizations, business, labor, and civil society.

Broadly speaking, the process of globalization has two aspects. The first refers to those factors—such as trade, investment, technology, cross-border production systems, flows of information, and communication—that bring societies and citizens closer together.

The second refers to policies and institutions, such as trade and capital market liberalization, international standards for labor, the environment, corporate behavior and other issues, agreements on intellectual property rights, and other policies pursued at both the national and international level, that support the integration of economies and countries. In terms of the latter aspect, the existing pattern of globalization is not an inevitable trend—it is at least in part the product of policy choices. While technological change is irreversible, policies can be changed. Technological advances have also widened the policy choices available.

The social dimension of globalization refers to the impact of globalization on the life and work of people, their families, and their societies. Concerns and issues are often raised about the impact of globalization on employment, working conditions, income, and social protection. Beyond the world of work, the social dimension encompasses security, culture and identity, inclusion or exclusion, and the cohesiveness of families and communities.

Source: International Labour Office (2003).

Notwithstanding the appealing simplicity of defining globalization as "the closer integration of economies and societies," it is not sufficient for analytical purposes. As Easton (2004) has argued, any definition of globalization must be also based upon a theory of causal mechanism underlying the process. What is driving the closer integration of economies and societies? The most convincing mechanism, Easton (2004) suggests, is that globalization is driven by the *decreasing cost of distance*.

In the first wave of modern globalization, which ran from about 1870 to 1914 (more about this later), the main impetus for global integration came about because of the development of railways, steam shipping, and the telegraph, all of which reduced the costs of distance. The more recent period of globalization (from about 1980 to the present) seems to have been spurred again by dramatic declines in the costs of distance, this time via air transport and telecommunications.

As Jared Diamond pointed out in a *Guardian* column:

> We are accustomed to thinking of globalization in terms of us rich advanced first worlders sending our good things, such as the Internet and Coca-Cola, to those poor backward third worlders. But globalization means nothing more than improved worldwide communications, which can convey many things in either direction; globalization is not restricted to good things carried only from the first to the third world. (Diamond 2005)

That said, many people on the planet have still not caught up with telephones and roads, let alone air travel or the Internet. That is to say, the cost of distance is falling at different rates for people in different parts of the world. One tiny example of globalization in action can be seen in the village of Hurufa in central Ethiopia. Until recently, the village was a six-hour walk along a dirt path to the nearest small city of Awasa. A serious medical emergency in this situation was akin to a death sentence. Then the Ethiopian government built a dirt-and-gravel road, connecting Hurufa to Awasa, partly financed by the World Bank. According to a dispatch filed by the *New York Times*, the villagers divide their history into two periods: Before the Road and After the Road (Dugger 2004). Now that the road is built, a patient with cerebral malaria can reach medical treatment within a one-hour truck ride to town. The dramatically decreased cost of distance has also allowed local farmers to fetch better prices at market, children to attend distant schools, and women to decrease the time they spend gathering water. Closer connection to the outside world has also meant that government health workers can more easily reach the village to deliver childhood immunizations and to educate women about birth control.

GLOBALIZATION THROUGH HISTORY

By viewing globalization through the lens of declining costs of distance, it is possible to reinterpret previous episodes in history. According to most conventional accounts, the first great wave of globalization ran from about 1870 to the outbreak of the First World War (1914), aided by steam shipping, telegraph cables, and rail roads (Dollar 2004). For instance, British ocean freight rates were relatively constant between 1740 and 1840, before plunging by about 70% between 1840 and 1910 (Bourguignon et al. 2002). This drop in the cost of distance was accompanied by a near doubling of world trade volume that occurred during the same period (Dollar 2004). And it was not just commodities that were shipped across the globe, but also people. Nearly 10% of the world's population migrated during this era, 60 million alone from poor countries of Europe to the United States. Reflecting on the comparative openness of international borders at the time, the economist John Maynard Keynes remarked that a Londoner prior to the Great War

> could order by telephone, sipping his morning tea in bed, the various products of the whole earth, in such quantity as he might see fit, and reasonably expect their early delivery upon his doorstep. . . . He could secure forthwith, if he wished it, cheap and comfortable means of transit to any country or climate without passport or other formality, could dispatch his servant to the neighbouring office of a bank for such supply of the precious metals as might seem convenient, and could then proceed abroad to foreign quarters, without knowledge of their religion, language, or customs. (Keynes 1918, pp. 11–12, as quoted in Sachs 2005)

Admittedly, Keynes wrote from a position of considerable privilege. As Milanovic (2003) reminds us, globalization in the late nineteenth century was also accomplished "at the point of a gun" in many parts of the world, and through the institutions of colonialism that benefited rich countries at the expense of poor ones.

Global integration suffered a major set back during the next period, spanning the two World Wars and the Great Depression. Trade as well as migration was set back to pre–turn-of-the-century levels by a combined backlash of protectionist policies adopted by nations as well as restrictions imposed on immigration. These setbacks were only gradually and selectively reversed over the four decades from the end of the Second World War to about 1980. David Dollar (2004) estimates that capital flows and foreign direct investment returned to 1914 levels only by about 1980.

The most recent episode of globalization began some time in the mid-1970s and continues to the present day. The stimulus for the current wave can be traced to dramatic declines in the cost of air transport and telecommunications in combination with outward-oriented domestic and international policies. In contrast to the late nineteenth-century wave of globalization, the present wave is characterized by much larger short-term capital flows, much greater involvement of multinational firms in cross-border acquisitions ("foreign direct investment"), as well as the greater flow of technology and ideas across borders (Bourguignon et al. 2002). Global economic integration is also governed by new institutions such as the WTO, which came into existence on January 1, 1995, and whose mandate is to remove international trade barriers. A further driving force behind the late twentieth-century wave of globalization has been the so-called Washington Consensus forged by the international financial institutions (the IMF and the World Bank) and the U.S. Treasury during the 1980s (Fischer 2003). The three pillars of the Washington Consensus advice—market liberalization, privatization, and fiscal austerity—were often thrust upon developing countries throughout the 1980s and 1990s as an integral part of the package of "structural adjustment loans" made by the IMF and World Bank (Stiglitz 2002).

The question addressed by this book is: What does globalization have to do with health? Should public health professionals care about the closer integration of the world? In some instances, the connections to health are obvious. For example, falling transport costs have resulted in more temporary movement of people, including tourism. More than two million travelers are estimated to cross international borders on a daily basis. A traveler infected with SARS could circumnavigate the globe six times within the incubation period of this deadly disease (Alleyne 2003). In other instances, closer global integration achieved through policies can have a direct impact on health. For example, the multilateral Agreement on Trade-Related Aspects of Intellectual Property Rights (TRIPS), administered by the WTO, ostensibly exists to protect patents and copyrights. However, the agreement has also been blamed for denying access to life-saving drugs for people living in the poorest countries of the world. The aim of this book is to examine the variety of impacts of globalization—both positive and negative—on the health of the world's people.

STRUCTURE OF THE BOOK

This book is organized into three parts. Part I provides a survey of current as well as emerging global threats to health. Individual chapters deal with communicable diseases, lifestyle behaviors (tobacco, obesity), environmental threats (global climate change and car culture), the economic consequences of globalization (poverty, inequality, and working conditions), and vulnerable populations (women and displaced populations). Part II presents methods and tools for monitoring the impacts of globalization on population health, including summary measures of population health status and health impact assessment. Finally, part III turns to the international institutional responses to globalization—that is, the roles of the World Bank, the IMF, the WTO, and the WHO, as well as the roles of national governments.

PART I. THE HEALTH CONSEQUENCES OF GLOBALIZATION

Communicable Diseases

The decline in the cost of distance has both beneficial and adverse consequences (Easton 2004). On the negative side of the balance sheet, being more closely integrated with the rest of the world can facilitate the spread of infectious diseases. In the past, this proved

calamitous to some populations, as demonstrated by the "fatal impact" wrought by smallpox and measles on native people who came into contact with European explorers and colonizers between 1500 and 1800 (Moorehead 1966; Diamond 1997). Communicable diseases are the quintessential example of a health threat that respects no borders (i.e., unless the potential victims are kept apart by long distances).

Chapter 2 by Lance Saker, Kelley Lee, and Barbara Cannito provides an overview of the evolving relationship between globalization and the burden of communicable diseases. They point out that globalization has potentially both beneficial and harmful consequences for infectious disease burden. For example, the rising demand in rich countries for the year-round availability of fresh fruits and vegetables has led to the occasional outbreaks of serious infectious illness among consumers of contaminated Mexican scallions and Guatemalan raspberries. On the other hand, globalization, particularly in the form of transfer of knowledge and technology, has also contributed to the control of infectious diseases through vaccinations and antibiotic/antiparasitic therapy. However, contrary to classical epidemiological transition theory (Omran 1971), infectious diseases are far from being conquered. Saker and colleagues also draw attention to the distributional consequences of globalization on infectious disease burden. There is mounting evidence that infectious diseases affect the poor disproportionately because of inequities in living conditions and lack of access to health care.

Globalization and Lifestyle Behaviors

Besides communicable diseases, globalization is increasingly implicated in the spread of noncommunicable diseases. In the twenty-first century, the rising global burden of noncommunicable diseases such as cardiovascular disease, cancer, and diabetes will primarily occur through changes in population *behavior* (cigarette smoking, diet, sedentarism).

The globalized manufacture and marketing of cigarettes represents a well-understood health threat that is nevertheless still far from solved. Despite more than four decades of understanding about the hazards of tobacco smoking, the burden of premature mortality and morbidity caused by cigarettes shows no sign of abating, particularly in developing countries. In 1995, cigarettes caused 3 million deaths worldwide, of which 2 million occurred in rich countries and 1 million in developing countries. By 2025, the annual death toll is projected to rise to 10 million, of which developing countries will account for 7 million (Peto et al. 1994).

Some skeptics might question the role of the transnational tobacco trade in boosting cigarette consumption around the world. After all, the bulk of cigarettes consumed in countries targeted by transnational tobacco companies are manufactured locally. In other words, it is argued that the same number of cigarettes is consumed whether American cigarettes are present or not. This argument is belied by the aggressive marketing tactics of transnational companies in the parts of the world where they have exported their product (Honjo and Kawachi 2000), as well as the results of econometric analyses demonstrating that opening domestic markets to foreign cigarettes leads to an overall increase in per capita cigarette consumption (Jha and Chaloupka 2000). As Derek Yach, Heather Wipfli, Ross Hammond, and Stanton Glantz argue in chapter 3, the global control of tobacco will require global collective action, of which WHO's Framework Convention on Tobacco Control represents a first step.

Obesity is another rapidly rising epidemic within both rich countries and poor ones. The causes of the epidemic are multifactorial, but high on the list of suspects are the marketing and increased consumption of diets high in refined carbohydrates combined with a shift toward more sedentary lifestyles (e.g., greater reliance on automobiles). Barry M. Popkin and Michelle Mendez in chapter 4 show that obesity and overweight can no longer be considered afflictions of affluence. The burden of obesity (and its health consequences) has been shifting toward lower socioeconomic groups, even in developing countries. As in the case of tobacco, control of the worldwide obesity epidemic will require global collective action, of which the Global Strategy on Diet, Physical Activity and Health, adopted by the World Health Assembly in May 2004, represents an initial significant step.

Globalization and Environmental Threats

The next two chapters in part I address emerging environmental threats to global health, namely, climate change (A. J. McMichael and G. Ranmuthugala, chapter 5) and the spread of "car culture" (Tord Kjellstrom and Sarah Hinde, chapter 6). There is no evidence, in general, that globalization is bad for the environment (Bourguignon et al. 2002), although one can identify harmful consequences in some specific instances.[1] Instead, major threats to the planetary environment, such as greenhouse gas emissions or the clearing for forests for farming and habitation, seem to be driven by additional factors besides globalization such as industrialization, urbanization, population pressure, consumption patterns, and even rising living standards. Globalization may speed up these other processes, but a more direct causal connection to environmental degradation remains elusive. Some have linked the recent Asian tsunami catastrophe with the effects of globalization on the environment. There has been large-scale destruction of mangrove swamps[2] to make way for shrimp farming in Southeast Asia. Shrimp consumption in North America, Japan, and Western Europe increased by 300% during the last ten years. In Canada, the consumption of shrimp went up by 200% between 1990 and 1995, turning shrimp farming into a billion dollar industry and changing it from a small-scale activity to a major commercial industrial operation. In 1991, thousands of people were killed when a tsunami hit the coast in an area of Bangladesh where shrimp farms had destroyed all the mangrove swamps. By contrast, when a tsunami of similar magnitude hit the same area back in 1960, there was not a single fatality (Goldsmith 1996).

One thing is abundantly clear: global climate change, like communicable diseases, respects no national borders. Consequently, environmental spillovers between nations cannot be solved by individual countries acting alone.

"Car culture" is the term used by Kjellstrom and Hinde to describe the increasing reliance of the world's people on automotive means of transport. By accelerating the conquest of distance (as in the example of the village of Hurufa described above), vehicular transport represents an important cog in the engine of globalization. At the same time, it poses major public health challenges, not simply on account of the spread of sedentary lifestyles and the rising toll of traffic injuries, but also because cars are a major source of greenhouse gases and hence of global climate change. As Kjellstrom and Hinde argue, managing the adverse environmental impacts of car culture poses a classic public goods problem. There are many private benefits of car ownership, as many drivers in developed countries can attest. Unfortunately, the negative environmental externalities stemming from automotive transport are not fully borne by their owners.

The Economic Consequences of Globalization

Chapters 7 and 8 deal with topics that are often at the core of accusations leveled against globalization by street protesters. Globalization has been blamed for an unprecedented rise in inequality around the world, as well as the impoverishment of millions in poor countries. These charges have been rebutted by the equally dramatic counterclaims of pro-globalizers (some of them employed by the IMF and the World Bank), who contend that globalization, particularly in the form of trade openness, is responsible for spectacular improvements in the standard of living that lifted millions out of poverty (Dollar and Kraay 2001). The seemingly contradictory statements made by the opposing camps mark one facet of the lively contemporary "globalization debate."

In chapter 7, Ichiro Kawachi and Sarah Wamala sift through the evidence and attempt to reconcile the contesting claims that have been made about the impacts of globalization on poverty and inequality. They conclude that both camps in the debate are telling parts of the truth. On the one hand, there has been a dramatic reduction in extreme poverty (people subsisting on less than US$1 per day) during the most recent period of globalization (1980 to the present). On the other hand, the pattern of poverty reduction has been decidedly uneven across the globe. The accomplishments of just two countries, China and India, make up the bulk of poverty reduction during the past two decades. Their gains have been offset by stagnation or marked increases in poverty elsewhere, notably in sub-Saharan Africa. Inequalities within and between countries (though not between persons) also seem to have risen. In turn, persistent poverty and inequality pose major obstacles to human development, and together contribute to many of the global health threats discussed in this book, including environmental degradation, the spread of communicable diseases, civil conflict, and population displacement. To the extent that these problems spill over to the rest of the world, poverty constitutes a global health threat, and accordingly, poverty reduction must be seen as a *global public good* (Bettcher and Lee 2002).

Chapter 8 by Christer Hogstedt, David H. Wegman, and Tord Kjellstrom focuses on the other economic dimension of the globalization debate, namely, whether the closer integration of nations can be held accountable for the decline in labor standards and working conditions around the globe. Through outsourcing, competition, and insistence on "labor flexibility," protesters contend that globalization has resulted in a "race to the bottom" in global labor standards, job insecurity, and the exploitation of sweatshop workers, including child labor.

The reality is that it is hard to pinpoint evidence that implicates globalization per se in declining labor or environmental standards. Indeed, some evidence suggests that multinationals set higher environmental standards than do local counterparts, and they pay higher wages than do local employers. In the words of Joseph Stiglitz (who is not noted for being an uncritical advocate of globalization), while "people in the West may regard low-paying jobs at Nike as exploitation . . . for many people in the developing world, working in a factory is a far better option than staying down on the farm and growing rice" (Stiglitz 2002, p. 4).

That is not to deny that egregious working conditions persist in much of the world (as carefully documented by Hogstedt and colleagues) or that outsourcing has resulted in the loss of jobs in high-wage countries.[3] The important point to recall is that globalization and the insistence on higher labor standards are not zero sum (Elliott and Freeman 2003). By improving the prospects for economic growth, globalization can (and does) improve the prospects for raising labor standards.

Globalization and Vulnerable Populations

Part I concludes with two chapters dealing with populations that are especially vulnerable to the forces of globalization: women and displaced populations.

If the nineteenth-century wave of globalization was marked by the voluntary migration of millions, Pascale Allotey and Anthony Zwi argue in chapter 9 that the present wave is increasingly characterized by the forced migration of populations fleeing disasters, conflict, and violence. Migration, both voluntary and forced, has strained the capacity of host nations, resulting in a widespread backlash of discrimination, xenophobia, and intolerance. At the same time, Allotey and Zwi express cautious optimism over the "globalization of human rights" and the potential for globally coordinated actions to mount humanitarian responses to population displacement.

In chapter 10, Sarah Wamala and Ichiro Kawachi trace the impacts of globalization on the health of women around the world. Feminist scholars have long contended that the globalization debate has been carried out in the absence of gender analyses. Yet it is evident that women bear the brunt of many adverse health impacts linked to globalization, whether in the form of sexually transmitted diseases, human trafficking, or their restricted access to basic health care and education brought about by the imposition of "user charges" for these services at the insistence of international lending institutions. International migration has become progressively "feminized" to the extent that half of the world's 120 million legal and illegal migrants are now believed to be women (Ehrenreich and Russell Hochschild 2002). While economic migration enables women from the developing world to earn higher wages, many are also at risk of being abused or exploited as maids, nannies, and service workers. As Allotey and Zwi note, women are also at greatest risk of sexual violence among displaced persons.

Seventy percent of the people living in extreme poverty are women (Jaggar 2002), leaving them (and their children) vulnerable to economic slowdowns. Yet, feminist scholars contend that the conventional economic approaches to evaluating globalization policies are gender-blind. Despite the fact that women perform two-thirds of productive labor around the globe, their contribution remains invisible in the national systems of accounting because so much of it takes place outside the market, for example, in the form of child care or domestic work such as gathering water and fuel. When a man marries his housekeeper or nanny, the gross domestic product falls. Using this standard, judging the success or failure of globalization remains a patriarchal science, one that systematically denies the value of women's work (Waring 1988). As globalization moves more women into market work, they reduce the time spent doing work that is not officially counted and increase the time spent doing work that *is* counted, making economic growth appear to be more rapid than the reality (Folbre 2001).

Early attempts to address this bias, such as the measures of economic welfare originally proposed by

James Tobin (1978), have been mostly relegated to the footnotes of economics textbooks. However, the United Nations Development Program's Human Development Index, as well as the accompanying Gender-Related Development Index and Gender Empowerment Measure, represents important steps in bringing gender analyses into the evaluation of globalization (United Nations Development Programme 1995). Also, civil society organizations have increasingly promoted the adoption of gender-sensitive budgets as a tool for raising awareness of the impacts of budgetary expenditures on the lives of women and men (Çağatay and Ertürk 2004).

PART II: MONITORING THE IMPACT OF GLOBALIZATION ON HEALTH

As is already evident from the preceding sections, progress toward systematic assessments of the impact of globalization on health has been hampered by the lack of data and analytical tools with which to build the evidence base. Forecasting the impacts of globalization on population health begs the question of what processes and outcomes we should be measuring.

Part II describes the tools by which researchers and policy makers can monitor and evaluate the impacts of globalization on health. Daniel Reidpath in chapter 11 describes and offers a critique of summary measures of population health status (e.g., disability-adjusted life years and health-adjusted life expectancies) that have been promoted by the WHO (among other bodies) as tools for priority setting in health policy. As Reidpath reveals, this is not a value-free exercise.

In chapter 12, Eileen O'Keefe and Alex Scott-Samuel provide a guide to the burgeoning technique of health impact assessments (HIAs), which are increasingly recommended (and being adopted) for prospective evaluations of the impacts of policies on health outcomes. The potential utility of HIAs in the area of globalization is clear. For example, Deaton (2004) noted that when economists talk about globalization, they seldom pay attention to its health impacts, focusing instead on outcomes such as growth, poverty, and inequality. The introduction of HIAs offers the promise of changing that policy discourse and transforming the nature of the globalization debate. It is not fanciful to imagine that eventually it will become impossible for policy makers to introduce proposals such as trade liberalization without considering the health impacts in addition to macroeconomic outcomes.

PART III: THE INTERNATIONAL RESPONSES TO GLOBALIZATION

Global health threats, such as poverty, communicable diseases, and climate change, demand global solutions. Part III describes the roles and responses of the major international institutions in meeting these challenges. The main institutions of globalization include the international financial institutions (the World Bank and IMF), the WTO, the WHO, and national governments (particularly the G8).[4]

The International Financial Institutions

Of the various discontents expressed against globalization, none have been more charged, perhaps, than the reactions to the international institutions that were established with the mission of governing the world economy. The World Bank and the IMF both originated in World War II as a result of the Bretton Woods Conference in 1944. The World Bank's overarching mission is the eradication of poverty, as reflected by its motto, "Our dream is a world without poverty" (Stiglitz 2002).[5] By contrast, the IMF's mission is to maintain global macroeconomic stability through attention to matters such as government budget deficits, monetary policies, inflation rates, and terms of trade.

Both institutions have been castigated by street protestors (and even the occasional insider; see Stiglitz 2002) for imposing policy prescriptions on crisis-ridden poor countries that even affluent countries have not followed. The numerous "conditionalities" dictated by these lending institutions, as well as the imperious manner in which they have been perceived to conduct their business, have been singled out for criticism. To quote Joseph Stiglitz, the former chief economist of the World Bank:

For peasants in developing countries who toil to pay off their countries' IMF debts or the businessmen who suffer from higher value-added taxes upon the insistence of the IMF, the current system run by the IMF is one of taxation without representation. Disillusion with the international system of globalization under the aegis of the IMF grows as the poor in Indonesia, Morocco, or Papua New Guinea have fuel and food subsidies cut, as those in Thailand see AIDS increase as a result of IMF-forced cutbacks in health expenditures, and as families in many developing countries, having to pay for their children's education under so-called cost recovery programs, make the painful choice not to send their daughters to school. (Stiglitz 2002, p. 20)

That, in a nutshell, summarizes some of the chief complaints made by antiglobalizers against the so-called structural adjustment loans made by the IMF and World Bank throughout the 1980s and 1990s. Chapter 13 by Anna Breman and Carolyn Shelton provides a systematic overview of the controversial structural adjustment programs (SAPs). In an exercise resembling retrospective HIAs, the authors trace out the potential health impacts of SAPs on the citizens of recipient countries. They conclude based on their overview that the historical legacy of SAPs, viewed through the lens of public health, has been decidedly mixed. While SAPs did not universally result in detrimental health impacts (and in some instances yielded positive results), the majority of case studies in sub-Saharan Africa suggest that the prescribed policies (e.g., reduction in government expenditures, cost recovery, liberalization of markets, exchange rate devaluation) did in fact lead to health deterioration.

Since 1999, SAPs have been superseded by poverty reduction strategy papers (PRSPs), which developing countries must now submit in advance of receiving World Bank/IMF loans, as well as debt relief under the Heavily Indebted Poor Countries initiative. Unlike SAPs, which were unpopular as a result of being thrust upon indebted countries with minimal consultation,[6] PRSPs are supposedly "owned" by the recipient governments and developed through a broad-based participatory process involving civil society and development partners. As Sarah Wamala, Ichiro Kawachi, and Besinati Phiri Mpepo describe in chapter 14, PRSPs may signal an improvement on SAPs but still have some distance to go in recognizing and addressing issues such as equity and gender disparities. Although it is too soon to appraise the outcomes of PRSPs, already some skepticism has been voiced in some quarters that they are SAPs by another name. Critics outside of government suspect that the PRSP is more of a tool for government to mobilize international resources rather than a genuine plan for poverty reduction (see, e.g., the case study of PRSPs in Zambia in chapter 14).

The World Trade Organization

The WTO came into existence out of the General Agreement on Tariffs and Trade (GATT) on January 1, 1995, as a provision of the eighth (Uruguay) round of multilateral trade negotiations. Despite its relatively short period of existence, few other institutions of globalization have been subjected to such vocal criticisms, and for that reason, the WTO deserves a chapter by itself. Among other charges, the WTO has been accused of setting rules (e.g., TRIPS) that favor powerful multinational interests (e.g., pharmaceutical companies) so that they can block access to life-saving drugs. Antiglobalization protestors have also complained that the WTO is secretive, undemocratic, and unfair, frequently forcing poor countries to open their markets to products from the developed world while dragging its feet on opening up markets in the latter to agricultural products from less developed countries (Bourguignon et al. 2002).

The reality, like many other debates about globalization, is considerably more complex. Most public health experts concur that the provisions under TRIPS, while originally intended to encourage the creation of new knowledge (e.g., the development of medicines), have actually made patented drugs less accessible to people in poor countries. The recent controversy over poor countries' access to antiretroviral drugs illustrates this dilemma. While citizens of affluent countries might view the annual cost of US$10,000 for AIDS drugs an acceptable price to pay for continuing research and development, "it strikes almost everyone as immoral that people in the developing world cannot get access to these drugs whose manufacturing cost is only several hundred dollars for a year's supply" (Dollar 2001).

Where do we stand on other accusations leveled at the WTO? Contrary to the perception that the WTO is undemocratic, the organization is unusual among international institutions for operating on the basis of one vote per member state.[7] The WTO's trade negotiations do take place behind closed doors. On the other hand, the organization does put out a great quantity of background material pertaining to its deliberations, which are subject to intense public scrutiny (Bourguignon et al. 2002).

As related by M. Gregg Bloche and Elizabeth R. Jungman in chapter 15, an examination of the WTO's recent history reveals that it often rules in favor of public health protections. For example, Article XX(b) under the General Exceptions section of the General Agreement on Tariffs and Trade (GATT) (1994) allows countries to restrict trade on the basis of national health standards, provided those restrictions do not present discriminatory or unjustifiable barriers to trade. This provision was used, for example, by a WTO dispute settlement panel regarding a French ban on asbestos, which was upheld under a challenge from Canada.

The World Health Organization

Of the eight Millennium Development Goals adopted by the world community in 2000 (United Nations 2000), three are explicitly about health: goal 4, reduce mortality by two-thirds among children younger than five years of age by 2015; goal 5, reduce maternal mortality by three-quarters by 2015; and goal 6, halt and reverse the spread of HIV/AIDS, malaria, and other diseases. The remaining goals are also inextricably tied to health. For example, goal 1 (eradicate extreme poverty) could not be achieved without meeting the health goals (Sachs 2004), while goal 3 (promote gender equality by eliminating gender inequalities in primary and secondary education) is one of the surest routes to reducing infant mortality in developing countries (Caldwell 1986). According to Jeffrey Sachs (2004), these goals amount to nothing less than a "revolution" in public health thinking and practice. As Ruth Bonita, Alec Irwin, and Robert Beaglehole describe in chapter 16, the WHO seized the center stage in this campaign, chiefly through the Commission on Macroeconomics and Health (WHO 2001) appointed by the then director general, Gro Harlam Brundlandt (1998–2001).

The Commission on Macroeconomics and Health has not escaped subsequent criticism (see, e.g., Waitzkin 2003; Navarro 2004). By treating health as an instrument for economic growth, critics argued that the WHO had finally fallen into the clutches of neoliberal ideology that characterize the international financial institutions, the IMF, World Bank, and WTO. However, democratic and inclusive institutions such as the WHO are capable of responding to experience and criticism by adapting their policies. As Bonita and colleagues relate, the WHO has already begun to respond by announcing the establishment of a new Commission on the Social Determinants of Health and reaffirming the organization's commitment to the core values of social justice and health equity.

National Governments

Our book concludes with two chapters on the response of national governments to globalization. In chapter 17, Ted Schrecker and Ronald Labonte critically scrutinize the pledges made by developed countries, particularly the rich club of G8 nations, to make globalization work better for the world's poor. Contrary to the ringing rhetoric, they find that levels of foreign aid remain pitifully inadequate. None of the G8 nations currently comes close to meeting the target of spending 0.7% of annual national incomes on overseas development aid. The wealthiest country in the world, the United States, currently spends about 0.14% of national income on foreign aid, which ranks it dead last among the G8, and even the countries in the Organization for Economic Cooperation and Development. As Schrecker and Labonte remark, for Americans to meet the 0.7% spending target would require an additional daily sacrifice of only about 57 cents per person—less than a quarter of the cost of a hamburger.

Of course, foreign aid is not a panacea, as Schrecker and Labonte caution. Yet even a modest flow of aid could do untold good. For example, a typical poor country in sub-Saharan Africa with a gross national product (GNP) of US$300 per person per year currently expends about $3 per person per year (or 1% of GNP) on basic health services. According to the WHO Commission on Macroeconomics and Health, the cost of expanding access to a universal system of basic health services is around $36 per person per year (or 12% of GNP) (WHO 2001). That gap between needs and reality could easily be met with donor assistance. Indeed, "donors would hardly notice it—a few billion dollars a year is a rounding error in the U.S. budget" (Sachs 2004), where Americans currently spend about $5,000 per person per year on health care.

In the final chapter, Raymond R. Hyatt, Jr., turns his attention to the dark side of national spending priorities, namely, military expenditure. Chapter 18 updates and corroborates a classic empirical analysis (Woolhandler and Himmelstein 1985) on the relationships between national military spending and higher infant mortality and lower life expectancy. As nations divert a larger proportion of their state budgets toward arms, fewer resources remain available for other sectors, including health. Life expectancy at birth is reduced by between 3 and 6 months for each 1% of GNP spent on military programs. Moreover, this association is three times stronger in the poorest countries compared with middle-income and more affluent nations.

As pointed out by Sen (2002), the world powers are complicit in this process through the global arms trade. The permanent members of the United Nations Security Council together account for 80% of the world arms exports, much of it flowing to developing countries.[8]

MAKING SENSE OF GLOBALIZATION AND HEALTH

Globalization presents many challenges for the future health of the world's citizens, yet the same forces that present threats to health (e.g., the declining cost of distance and its impact on the spread of communicable disease) simultaneously represent opportunities for advancing health. The globally coordinated efforts to contain the SARS outbreak could not have been possible without the conquest of distance, whether in the form of WHO consultants traveling to afflicted regions to lend their expertise, or the possibility of electronic surveillance of outbreaks and the rapid transport of biological specimens for diagnosis.

Health does not need to be the inevitable hostage or the Cinderella of globalization. Global public goods—such as the Framework Convention on Tobacco Control or the Kyoto Accord on reducing greenhouse gas emissions—point to the way forward for containing global health threats.

The technological impetus behind the current wave of globalization is an unstoppable force, even though many of its attendant health threats could be controlled on the basis of current knowledge. No sane person would advocate halting or reversing the tide of globalization and condemning millions to truncated living standards. Indeed, that is not what antiglobalization street protestors are agitating for. Nobody—not even the "antiglobalizers"—are really against globalization per se (Sen 2002). Rather, people are protesting about real issues such as the absence of "voice" in international decision making, about inadequate levels of debt relief and foreign aid, and about the slow pace of leveling the playing field in agricultural trade—problems that have left millions of poor people behind, unable to benefit from the "gifts of globalization." These charges cannot be dismissed, even if the protestors occasionally get the diagnosis wrong by blaming globalization for a surfeit of the world's ailments. Globalization, like Darwinian evolution, is fundamentally amoral. It is up to the world's citizens, through globally coordinated actions, to meet its health threats or to harness its health dividends.

Notes

1. For example, the systematic looting and decimation of mahogany forests in South America, which seems to have been caused by a combination of opportunities to trade (i.e., the lucrative and illicit markets in North America) plus local poverty and corruption (Forero 2003).

2. Mangrove swamps are some of the world's most important ecosystems. They help to protect offshore coral reefs, because their roots filter out the silt flowing seaward from the land and thus act as a buffer for large waves. They perform all the Gaian functions of a tropical rainforest and they absorb more carbon dioxide per unit area than does ocean phytoplankton, a critical factor in global climate stability.

3. Though we hasten to add that a job lost in a rich country is a job gained by a worker in a poorer country. Nobody disputes that globalizations produces winners and losers.

4. One could also add to this list the International Labor Organization (ILO), civil society/nongovernmental organizations, and global public—private partnerships (GPPPs). For discussions of the roles of these other institutions, see, e.g., Elliott and Freeman (2003) on the ILO and Buse and Walt (2002) on GPPPs.

5. Some critics have turned this motto around to accuse the World Bank of creating poverty, not eradicating it.

6. See, e.g., Robert Klitgaard's (1990) characterization of IMF–World Bank structural adjustment teams "parachuting in" to countries on three-week "missions" to impose their various conditions.

7. In contrast to the decisions of the World Bank and IMF, where voting strength is weighted by the size of national financial contributions—see chapter 17.

8. "Indeed, the world leaders who express deep frustration at the 'irresponsibility' of anti-globalization protestors lead the countries that make the most money in this terrible trade" (Sen 2002, p. 8).

References

Alleyne, G. (2003). Globalization and Challenges for Caribbean Health. Michael Manley Memorial Lecture, The Michael Manley Foundation, Kingston, Jamaica.

Bettcher, D. & Lee, K. (2002). Globalization and public health. Glossary. J Epidemiol Comm Health 56:8–17.

Bourguignon, F., Coyle, D., Fernandez, F., et al. (2002). Making Sense of Globalization: A Guide to the Economic Issues. Centre for Economic Policy Research (CEPR) Policy Paper No. 8. London: European Commission Group of Policy Advisors.

Buse, K. & Walt, G. (2002). Globalisation and multilateral public-private health partnerships: issues for health policy. In: Lee, K., Buse, K. & Fustukian, S. (eds.), Health Policy in a Globalising World. Cambridge: Cambridge University Press, pp. 41–62.

Çağatay, N. & Ertürk, K. (2004). Gender and Globalization: A Macroeconomic Perspective. World Commission on the Social Dimension of Globalization Working Paper No. 19. Geneva: International Labour Office.

Caldwell, J. C. (1986). Routes to low mortality in poor countries. Pop Dev Rev 12(2):171–220.

Deaton, A. (2004). Health in an Age of Globalization [mimeo]. Princeton University.

Diamond, J. (1997). Guns, Germs, and Steel. New York: W.W. Norton & Co.

Diamond, J. (1998). Disasters waiting to happen. Guardian, U.K., January 6. Available at: http://healthandenergy.com/disasters_waiting_to_happen.htm.

Dollar, D. (2001). Is globalization good for your health? Bull World Health Org 79:827–833.

Dollar, D. (2004). Globalization, Poverty, and Inequality since 1980. World Bank Policy Research Working Paper 3333. World Bank: Washington, DC.

Dollar, D. & Kraay, A. (2001). Trade, growth, and poverty. Finance Dev 38(3):1–6.

Dugger, C. W. (2004). Roads lead to a new way of life fur rural Ethiopia. New York Times, November 8, p. A3.

Easton, B. (2004). The political economy of the diminishing tyranny of distance. J Econ Soc Policy (in press).

Ehrenreich, B. & Russell Hochschild, A. (eds.). (2002). Global Woman. Nannies, Maids, and Sex Workers in the New Economy. New York: Metropolitan Books.

Elliott, K. A. & Freeman, R. B. (2003). The role global labor standards could play in addressing basic needs. In: Heymann, J. (ed.), Global Inequalities at Work. New York: Oxford University Press, pp. 299–327.

Fischer, S. (2003). Globalization and its challenges. Richard T. Ely lecture. Am Econ Rev 93(2):1–30.

Folbre, N. (2001). The Invisible Heart. Economics and Family Values. New York: New Press.

Forero, J. (2003). A swirl of foreboding in mahogany's grain. New York Times, September 28, p. 14.

Friedman. T. L. (1999). The Lexus and the Olive Tree. Understanding Globalization. New York: Farrar, Straus, Giroux.

General Agreement on Tariffs and Trade (GATT). (1994). Available at: http://www.wto.org/English/docs_e/legal_e/legal_e.htm.

Goldsmith, E. (1996). Global trade and the environment. In: Mander, J. & Goldsmith, E. (eds.), The Case against the Global Economy. San Francisco: Sierra Club Books, pp. 78–91.

Honjo, K. & Kawachi, I. (2000). Effects of market liberalization on smoking in Japan. Tobacco Control 9(2):193–200.

Hutton, W. & Giddens, A. (eds.). (2000). Global Capitalism. New York: New Press.

International Labour Office. 2003. World Commission on the Social Dimension of Globalisation, International Labour Office, Geneva, Switzerland. Available at: http://www.ilo.org/public/English/wcsdg/index.htm.

Jaggar, A. M. (2002). Vulnerable women and neo-liberal globalization: debt burdens undermine women's health in the global south. Theor Med 23:425–440.

Jha, P. & Chaloupka, F. J. (eds.). (2000). Tobacco Control in Developing Countries. Oxford: Oxford University Press.

Klitgaard, R. (1990). Tropical Gangsters. New York: Basic Books.

Milanovic, B. (2003). The two faces of globalization: against globalization as we know it. World Dev 31(4):667–683.

Moorehead, A. (1966). The Fatal Impact. New York: Harper & Row.

Navarro, V. (2004). The world situation and WHO. Lancet 363:1321–1323.

Omran, A. R. (1971). The epidemiologic transition: a theory of the epidemiology of population change. Milbank Mem Fund Q 49(1):509–538.

Peto, R., Lopez, A. D., Boreham, J., Thun, M. & Health, C., Jr. (1994). Mortality from Smoking in Developed Countries 1950–2000. New York: Oxford University Press.

Sachs, J. D. (2004). Health in the developing world: achieving the Millennium Development Goals. Bull World Health Org 82:947–952.

Sachs, J. D. (2005). The End of Poverty. Economic Possibilities for Our Time. New York: Penguin Press.

Sen, A. (2002). How to judge globalism. Am Prospect 13(1):1–8.

Stiglitz, J. E. (2002). Globalization and Its Discontents. New York: W.W. Norton & Co.

Tobin, J. (1978). A proposal for international monetary reform. Eastern Economic Journal 4:153–159.

United Nations Development Programme. (1995). Human Development Report 1995. New York: Oxford University Press.

United Nations Development Programme. (1999). Human Development Report 1999. New York: Oxford University Press.

Waitzkin, H. (2003). Report of the WHO Commission on Macroeconomics and Health: summary and critique. Lancet 361:523–526.

Waring, M. (1988). If Women Counted. A New Feminist Economics. San Francisco: Harper & Row.

Woolhandler, S. & Himmelstein, D. U. (1985). Militarism and mortality. An international analysis of arms spending and infant death rates. Lancet 1:1375–1378.

WHO. (2001). Report of the Commission on Macroeconomics and Health. Geneva: World Health Organization.

Part I

The Health Consequences of Globalization

Chapter 2

Infectious Disease in the Age of Globalization

Lance Saker, Kelley Lee, and Barbara Cannito

There is currently much interest in the impact of globalization on the epidemiology of infectious diseases and on the capacity to effectively prevent, control, and treat these illnesses. The chief issues that raise concern are globalization's influence on the risk factors for specific infections, along with technological and other developments that may provide opportunities for improving the surveillance, monitoring, and reporting capacity of serious infectious diseases. In this chapter, we broadly explore the links between globalization and infectious diseases in relation to changes in four major spheres— economic, environmental, political and demographic, and technological. We highlight areas where the evidence suggests that processes of globalization have led to changes in the distribution, transmission rate, and, in some cases, management of infectious diseases.

GLOBALIZATION AND THE CHANGING NATURE OF INFECTIOUS DISEASE

In simple terms, an infection occurs when a *pathogenic* microorganism survives and multiplies within another, usually larger, organism or *host*. To do so, it must first reach the host using any of a number of *transmission systems* (box 2.1). The pathogen must then find a way to survive and multiply within the host (the *amplification process*). The transmission system used determines which factors are capable of enhancing or inhibiting the spread of a particular infectious disease, while the success of the amplification process is dependent on the presence or absence of many variables, including natural and acquired immunity, numbers of pathogens present, and favorable physiological circumstances or triggers. Crucially, these factors are themselves heavily influenced by ecological factors, such as the natural and built environment, social and cultural practices, and population size, age distribution, and density (May, 1994). Therefore, the rate at which new human infections are produced depends on a mixture of biological, environmental, and social factors. Also, the appropriate preventive and treatment strategy for a specific infectious disease will usually depend on the control of these factors.

Box 2.1 – Mechanisms of Transmission of Pathogens Causing Infectious Disease

1. Direct spread—e.g., from soil in tetanus
2. Blood-borne spread—e.g., through contaminated transfusions in hepatitis C
3. Sexual/intimate contact—e.g., in AIDS or syphilis
4. Airborne or droplet spread—e.g., influenza, tuberculosis
5. Fecal–oral spread—e.g., by consuming infected food or water in dysentery and cholera
6. Vector-borne (between humans)—e.g., via a mosquito in malaria and dengue fever
7. Vector-borne (from animals to humans)—e.g., from a deer via a tick in Lyme disease
8. Directly from an intermediate host—e.g., from snails in schistosomiasis

An infection that is directly transmitted between humans (or animals) is *contagious*.

A *vector* is an intermediary agent (usually a biting insect or arthropod) that spreads pathogens to humans. Infections transmitted in this way are called *vector-borne diseases*.

An infection that is transmissible from animals to humans is known as a *zoonotic infection*. Sometimes these may be transmitted by vectors.

Endemic infections are present at a constant level in a community or area; *epidemic* infections represent a sudden increase in numbers of infected and ill people.

Despite disagreements about what globalization is, it is clear that it is driven and constrained by several forces: economic processes, technological developments, political influences, cultural and value systems, and social and natural environmental factors. These varied forces have the potential to affect many of those biological, environmental, and social factors that determine whether a specific pathogen can survive and spread in the environment, infect particular individuals, and cause disease. Globalization may also affect measures to treat and prevent infectious diseases by influencing, for example, household incomes, the availability of health workers and other resources in health care systems, and the adoption and spread of health standards and principles through international and global agreements. At different levels, therefore, global change can either increase or decrease infections, depending on who you are and where you live. For poorer populations, there is substantial evidence to suggest that, so far, globalization has posed more negative than positive impacts on the risks from infectious disease.

ECONOMIC GLOBALIZATION AND INFECTIOUS DISEASE

Economic globalization describes the restructuring of the world economy from one centered on production and exchange relations between different countries to one operating on a global scale that cuts across national boundaries (Dicken, 1998). This process has accelerated since the end of the Second World War, particularly since the early 1970s with major events such as the collapse of the gold standard, oil crises, and increased debt burden.[1]

Fundamental changes to economies worldwide are believed to be having a range of impacts on the spread and control of infectious diseases.

World Trade Organization and Multilateral Trade Agreements

The emergence of the global economy has been facilitated, since 1944, by regional and international organizations that govern trade relations. Most notably, successive rounds of the General Agreement on Tariffs and Trade, and measures introduced by its more powerful replacement, the World Trade Organization, have sought to reduce barriers to trade. These international trade agreements have overseen an enormous increase in gross world production and world trade (Lang, 2001). In addition, populations living within market economies, or in countries engaged in market-oriented reforms, rose from 1 billion to roughly 5.5 billion during the 1990s (Lehmann, 2001).

There remains substantial debate about the overall benefits of trade on health. At a macroeconomic level, changes can influence the overall level of resources available to governments for health expenditure. Rapid economic transition in Central and Eastern Europe during the 1990s, for example, was found to have undermined government capacity to provide for health care, and marked increases in the rates of several infections were reported (Maclehose et al., 2002). The Asian financial crisis in the late 1990s had a similar impact on public health spending. Evidence suggests that this, in turn, had detrimental effects on the rates of certain infections such as tuberculosis (TB), HIV/AIDS, and other sexually transmitted diseases (STDs) (Wibulpolprasert, 1998). Reduced spending on vector-borne disease control programs in Africa during periods of structural adjustment has led to failures to control diseases such as malaria, as well as the resurgence of some parasitic infections such as African trypanosomiasis (sleeping sickness) (Sanders, Chopra, 2002). Furthermore, outbreaks of infectious diseases are themselves associated with significant costs in terms of lost trade and tourism revenue, and there is some evidence that fear of economic penalties has led authorities to underreport epidemics, risking serious public health consequences. More comparative empirical analysis of the effects of trade liberalization on the epidemiology of infectious diseases is much needed.

There are more specific consequences for infectious diseases from intensified trade in particular goods and services. The most obvious examples are trade in food products and pharmaceuticals.

The Global Trade in Food

Over recent decades, huge increases in international trade have transformed the availability of food products, particularly for inhabitants of high-income countries. The growing demand for year-round availability of fresh fruit and vegetables, for so-called ethnic foods, and for generic rather than local produce has led to a dramatic increase in the quantity of food transported across the world. Cheaper transport systems of global reach now allow companies to manufacture many food products in less expensive labor markets, using ingredients from different parts of the world, and then to transport them worldwide. Control over this extremely lucrative market is increasingly concentrated in the hands of a few very large transnational corporations (TNCs).

Mass production, handling procedures, environmental factors, new and emerging pathogens, and poor regulation are believed to be contributing to a marked increase in worldwide incidence of food-borne infections (Lang, 2001). Several factors may be responsible. First, the increasing reliance on producers abroad means that food may be contaminated during harvesting, storage, processing, and transport, long before it reaches overseas markets; for example, outbreaks of *Salmonella poona* infection in the United States associated with eating imported melons from Mexico have been linked to unhygienic irrigation and packaging practices at source farms. Low-income countries may also cultivate nonindigenous crops to meet the needs of the export market, and these may be more susceptible to indigenous pathogens. This happened when Guatemalan raspberries became contaminated with the protozoan *Cyclospora*, causing outbreaks of gastroenteritis in the United States and Canada (Swerdlow, Altekruse, 1998).

Second, centralized processing and mass distribution may lead to widespread dissemination of contaminated foods. This risk has been augmented by changes in methods of food production such as the rearing of huge poultry flocks in communal housing, a practice that generates large numbers of birds with common risk profiles. Similarly, outbreaks of *E. coli* 0157:H7 have been traced to hamburgers from multiple outlets of a fast-food chain in the United States, and clusters of gastroenteritis have been traced to flocks of poultry infected with *Salmonella typhimurium* throughout Europe (Altekruse et al., 1997). Contaminated animal feeds may also be widely disseminated throughout the world, as exemplified by the crisis caused by bovine spongiform encephalopathy (mad cow disease) in the United Kingdom.

"New" pathogens not previously associated with human illness, such as *Cyclospora* and *E. coli* 0157:H7, were first identified through epidemics of food-borne disease. Emerging zoonotic pathogens are ever more resistant to antimicrobial agents, largely because of widespread use of antibiotics in the animal reservoir; *Campylobacter* isolated from human patients in Europe has become increasingly resistant to fluoroquinolones drugs since these antibiotics were introduced for use in animals (Endtz et al., 1991). Overall, there is a need to understand better how the global trade in food has spread hitherto local risks more widely and has created new risks from increased economies of scale and changing methods of production.

The Global Trade in Pharmaceuticals

The potential health benefits and risks posed by trade liberalization to access to pharmaceuticals are varied. In theory, countries will benefit from enhancing the range of drugs available, particularly where there is little or no domestic capacity to produce such products, and foreign competition should exert pressure on prices overall. In practice, however, the effects on production and consumption are more complex given the changing structure of the pharmaceutical industry. Like the food industry, pharmaceuticals are increasingly dominated by a small number of large TNCs (Baris, McLeod, 2000).

The increasing availability of scientifically educated but cheap labor and local manufacturing facilities has led to the creation of a thriving generics industry in many developing world countries. However, increased access by large TNCs to markets in the developing world could undermine these local producers. Under the Agreement on Trade-Related Aspects of Intellectual Property Rights, domestic subsidies on drugs could be deemed an unfair trade advantage, and there may be a tightening of regulations around the production and trade of generic drugs.

An emerging global market for pharmaceuticals raises concerns about a greater focus on health conditions deemed most profitable, regardless of their global burden. How drugs will be developed for infectious diseases afflicting the poorest population groups within such a context remains unclear. Only 13 of the 1,223 new chemical entities commercialized between 1975 and 1997 were for tropical diseases (Pecoul et al., 1999), and no new drugs for TB have been developed for more than 30 years despite its enormous toll, perhaps because only 5% of the 16 million infected can afford medication (Global Alliance for TB Drug Development, 2005). These inequities contribute to the "10/90 gap," in which 90% of research funds address the health needs of 10% of the world's population (Global Forum for Health Research, 1999).

Unregulated access to, and inappropriate consumption of, pharmaceuticals in a global marketplace may worsen antimicrobial drug resistance. These factors are believed to have contributed to the spread of multidrug-resistant TB (MDR-TB) worldwide and may lead to further spread of resistance to antiretrovirals for HIV, particularly given the important role that the unregulated private sector plays in providing care for stigmatizing conditions (Brugha, 2003). Control of these diseases could therefore be jeopardized, and the misuse of pharmaceutical products facilitated, if sufficient regulatory mechanisms are not implemented alongside globalization of the pharmaceutical industry.

GLOBAL ENVIRONMENTAL CHANGE AND INFECTIOUS DISEASE

The environment consists of not only the natural world but also the built and social environments. It plays an important role in shaping human health. Local and global environmental change may be either natural or anthropogenic (i.e., human induced). Anthropogenic changes are increasingly linked to processes of globalization (McMichael, Haines, 1997). Over the past 50 years, huge increases in economic and industrial activity have led to unprecedented effects on air, land, and water environments, and the resulting changes have important and wide-ranging implications for infectious diseases.

Global Climate Change

Current concerns about global climate change can be divided into two main subjects: rising global average land and sea surface temperatures (global warming), and increasing frequency of extreme weather conditions in many parts of the world (see also chapter 5). These are etiologically linked, but since each is associated with different patterns of infectious disease, we discuss them separately here. In general, climate constrains the range of infectious diseases, while weather affects the timing and intensity of outbreaks (Dobson, Carper, 1993).

Global Warming

There is now substantial evidence that global average land and sea surface temperatures have been increasing since the mid-nineteenth century (see chapter 5). Most of this change has taken place since 1976, and 14 of the warmest years on record have occurred since 1980. Although the causes are controversial, the Intergovernmental Panel on Climate Change has concluded that much of the warming observed in the last 50 years can be attributed to human activity (Albritton et al., 2001).

Global warming may alter the range and prevalence of many infections, particularly insect vector-borne infections. Diseases carried by mosquito vectors are highly sensitive to meteorological conditions since these insects have fastidious temperature thresholds for survival and are especially susceptible to changes in average ambient temperature (Epstein, 2001a). *Anopheles* species mosquitoes can transmit *Plasmodium falciparum* malaria parasites only if the temperature remains above 16°C, and the eggs, larvae, and adults of *Aedes aegypti* mosquitoes that spread dengue fever and yellow fever are killed by temperatures below 10°C. Furthermore, within their survival range, warmth accelerates the biting rate of mosquitoes and the maturation of parasites and viruses within them (McArthur, 1972). Since insects have short life spans, this increases the chances of their having the two blood meals crucial to transmission—one from an infected person and the second for transmission of the pathogen to another person.

In some cases, global warming may be beneficial. For example, the incidence of schistosomiasis may drop if the temperature is too warm to sustain the snail host, and malaria transmission may diminish in an established endemic zone if this becomes too hot and dry. In temperate zones, shorter and milder winters may curtail the seasonal excess of deaths due to respiratory infections. Nevertheless, most of the anticipated effects of global warming will be adverse, since shifts in the climate mean and climate variability are likely to perturb the physical and biological systems to which human health is biologically and culturally adjusted (McMichael, Haines, 1997). Overall, global warming is expected to widen the geographical range within which climate is capable of sustaining transmission of several vector-borne infections and to increase the proportion of the world's population living in areas capable of sustaining malaria transmission (Martens et al., 1997).

The scientific difficulties of obtaining empirical proof that global warming is altering the transmission of infectious diseases are considerable (box 2.2). However, available evidence suggests that changes consistent with climate-change effects are occurring. Anopheline mosquitoes are found in parts of the

United States, and small outbreaks of locally transmitted malaria have occurred during unseasonably hot weather spells (Zucker, 1996). Increases in malaria incidence have coincided with record high temperatures and rainfall in Rwanda (Loevinsohn, 1994), while higher median temperature during the rainy season was also a strong predictor of dengue fever prevalence in Mexico (Koopman et al., 1991).

Box 2.2 – The Scientific Evidence for Global Environmental Change

Detecting the influence of the observed (and much larger predicted) changes in climate and weather on infectious diseases transmission is not obvious and straightforward. First, climate change is a gradual process, and its effects are hard to distinguish from the much larger natural variations that occur from season to season or year to year. Second, many nonclimatic factors may moderate the effects of climate change on the impact of infectious diseases. For example, changes in human behavior or levels of immunity, better socioeconomic conditions, and improved treatment and control programs may all reduce the extent to which a climate-driven increase in pathogen transmission is translated into clinical disease. A cast-iron case for climate change producing a direct increase in infectious disease prevalence would require standardized monitoring of the exposure (climate), the outcome (incidence of a particular infectious disease), and other determinants of disease (e.g., immunity, treatment, socioeconomic factors) over many years.

Such data sets are very rare, particularly for populations in developing countries with poor health and socioeconomic infrastructure, who are the most likely to experience the effects of climate change. There is the added ethical problem of not imposing control measures to prevent disease after such analysis is undertaken. It is therefore not surprising that a recent review of the evidence for climate effects on vector-borne diseases concluded that there was only relatively weak direct evidence for such effects so far, but this was due to "absence of evidence" rather than "evidence of absence" (Kovats et al., 2001). Direct evidence of climate change on infectious diseases may become more obvious with improved disease surveillance and as changes in climate accelerate. However, because climate change may be irreversible, at least within given time frames, it seems unacceptable to wait for these to occur before trying to assess the risk. In the meantime, the best estimation of the likely current and future impacts of climate change comes from theoretical consideration of the known effects of climate on disease transmission and from indirect assessment based on reported effects of climate on infectious diseases in the present or recent past.

___

Further substantiation comes from ecological changes occurring at high altitudes. Since temperature varies inversely with elevation above sea level, global warming should change ecologies at high altitudes to those more characteristic of lower altitudes before climate change occurred. This appears to be happening. In many mountainous regions, glaciers are in retreat and plants preferring lower temperatures have been displaced to higher altitudes (Patz et al., 1996). More directly, malaria is now prevalent in elevated regions where it did not previously exist, such as rural highland areas in Papua New Guinea, while in Mexico, the first reported cases of dengue at an altitude of 1,700 meters occurred during an unseasonably warm summer in 1988 (Githeko et al., 2000; Herrera-Basto et al., 1992).

In addition to vectors, many pathogens themselves multiply quicker and are more infectious in warmer temperatures. In Lima, Peru, researchers who analyzed the relationship between day-to-day variations in temperature and the incidence of infective diarrhea found that, over and above the seasonal pattern, incidence increased by 12% per 1°C temperature rise in the cool season and by 4% per 1°C in the hotter season, averaging an 8% increase per 1°C throughout the study. Checkley et al. (2000) estimated that an 0.3°C increase in average temperature over the past 30 years would be associated with a 2.4% increase in diarrhea over what would have been expected without climate change.

Oceanic warming is one of several factors that may be contributing to a worldwide proliferation of algae blooms in coastal waters. These been associated with outbreaks of gastroenteritis after shellfish meals and massive loss of marine life, with nutritional and other consequences. Local variations in oceanic climate may also support the proliferation of planktonic populations that harbor human pathogens, such as *Vibrio cholerae*. Coastal blooms of algae coincided with this pathogen's introduction into offshore waters in Peru in 1991 (Tamplin, Carrillo Parodi, 1991), while outbreaks of cholera in Bangladesh have been associated with variations in sea temperature (Huq et al., 1995).

Global Weather Change

In the last three decades, periods of drought, heat waves, thunderstorms, and hurricanes have devastated many countries, often with severe public health consequences. The increasing frequency of these extreme weather events (EWEs) has been linked to the buildup of heat in the earth's atmosphere and oceans.

EWEs increase infectious diseases in two ways. First, by creating disaster situations where basic public health measures break down and people are forced to live in cramped, unhygienic conditions, EWEs encourage epidemics of *crowd* infections such as gastroenteritis, respiratory ailments, and typhus (Epstein, 2001b). Intense rains and flooding may also overwhelm sanitation systems, and this has led to outbreaks of waterborne infectious diseases (MacKenzie et al., 1994).

Second, EWEs can alter ecosystems such that they advance the appearance and spread of specific infectious diseases. Since 1950, all known Rift Valley Fever outbreaks in east Africa, as well as many clusters of malaria, have followed periods of abnormally high rainfall. These provided plentiful breeding sites for the mosquito vectors of Rift Valley Fever and malaria (Linthicum et al., 1999). EWEs can provoke outbreaks of infectious disease by altering predator–prey relationships. Prolonged drought in the late 1980s is believed to have favored mice in the Southwest United States by killing off their predators. When intense rains arrived, mouse populations rose quickly; soon after, a previously unrecognized disease, hantavirus pulmonary syndrome, appeared. The causative hantavirus was isolated in mice living near patients' homes. When predators returned after a few months, the outbreak abated (Schmaljohn, Hjelle, 1997).

Vulnerability to Global Climate Changes

The health impacts of global climate change will depend not only on the biological consequences of this change but also on the overall vulnerability of societies and populations. In high-income countries, which are more likely to be located at the temperature-sensitive edge of disease transmission, public health measures are sufficiently effective to prevent diseases such as malaria from reemerging even when rising temperatures support the survival of vectors. In contrast, in many low-income countries in tropical climates, already in the midst of transmission zones, public health infrastructures are much weaker, and the increasing vogue for cutting back government expenditure means this is unlikely to change soon. Therefore, how these countries cope with the consequences of climate change may be more dependent on longstanding challenges for the public health system than on climate change per se. There continues to be debate on the relative vulnerability of populations, with the United Nations (2001) reporting that lower income countries would be worst hit by the predicted rises in global temperatures during the next century. Others argue that population responses to ecological changes are usually nonlinear, leading to a sudden deterioration or improvement in infection control once a threshold is crossed (Sutherst, 2001). Overall, it is necessary to take into account a range of factors when estimating vulnerabilities to health from climate change.

Water Supply

The last half century has seen an explosion in water development projects around the world (World Commission on Dams, 2001). While population growth and socioeconomic development have clearly contributed to these trends, it is likely that economic globalization has played an important role in recent decades. Greater economic activity, accompanied by technological advances, will raise the demand for water-related services, while changes in the pattern of goods and services that a society produces and demands will themselves increase the demand for water. Thus, natural water sources must increasingly be harnessed for storage and distribution. Trade liberalization has increasingly allowed private industry to play a role in water resources developments; these have been subjected to mixed amounts of regulation. Yet of all natural habitat changes, water projects have perhaps the greatest potential for increasing human susceptibility to infectious diseases.

Ecological Changes

Modification of the aquatic environment may alter the local ecology such that the spread of infections,

particularly those transmitted by vectors, is influenced. For example, a dam creates a water surface that is sometimes extensively exposed to sunlight, possibly helping malaria mosquitoes to proliferate, or an aquifer in which the snail hosts of schistosomiasis may survive and multiply. Alternatively, land cleared to make way for a dam may destroy the habitat of blackflies, which spread onchocerciasis (river blindness).

Overall, most research suggests that the construction of dams in tropical areas is associated with increases in prevalence of endemic vector-borne infections, principally malaria and schistosomiasis, but also filariasis and onchocerciasis (see box 2.3 for description of infections following Nile water projects). In some cases, however, reduced rates of vector-borne infection have been reported (Hunter et al., 1993). Ecological changes may also increase the incidence of non-vector-transmitted infections, such as diphyllobothriasis (caused by the fish tapeworm) in the Siberian and Volga regions of the former USSR and, in tropical and subtropical regions, toxic cyanobacteria, which have been linked to outbreaks of gastroenteritis and liver cancer in China (Carmichael et al., 2001; 2002; Ding et al., 1999).

Box 2.3 – Infection and Water Projects along the Nile River

The Low Dam at Aswan was constructed in the 1930s to allow perennial irrigation of the Nile Valley. Within twenty years, local prevalence of schistosomiasis rose from about 10% to 75% (Khalil Bey, 1949). In 1942–1943, a malaria epidemic in the region followed an invasion by Anopheles gambiae mosquitoes from the Sudan and caused 130,000 deaths (Farid, 1977). Further increases in schistosomiasis prevalence were reported after the creation of the Aswan High Dam at Lake Nasser in the 1960s. Throughout the 1970s and part of the 1980s, local inhabitants continued to show high prevalence of schistosomiasis (Strickland, 1982). This led to fears that endemic schistosomiasis would spread south to the Sudan via infected fishermen. Large-scale application of snail control since the 1970s, however, and other major control efforts have led to important improvements. Lymphatic filariasis has increased twentyfold in the southern Nile delta since the 1960s. This may have been primarily due to an increase in breeding sites for Aedes mosquitoes, which followed a rise in the water table as a result of extension of irrigation. The spread of Rift Valley fever has been associated with dams and irrigation systems in Egypt and Sudan (Centers for Disease Control and Prevention, 1994a).

While large water projects may produce dramatic changes in rates of infectious diseases, the overall consequences of small-scale water developments are potentially much larger. These cover a far greater total area and are more closely associated with human settlements, less well served by health facilities, and less subject to planning, construction, and operation regulations than large dams.[2] In addition, breeding sites for mosquitoes tend to be in shallow backwaters (Hunter et al., 1993). In several African countries, small dams have been closely associated with increases in malaria, schistosomiasis, dracunculiasis, onchocerciasis, and lymphatic filariasis. Irrigation schemes created to support rice or sugar cane cultivation have been particularly associated with vector-borne infections (DukhaNiña et al., 1975; Hunter et al., 1993).

Displacements, Disruptions, Distant Effects, and Migrations

Water resource developments are often associated with physical and social disruption of communities. Frequently, communities are forced to live in unpleasant conditions that favor epidemics of crowd infections. People may also move to live in previously unsettled forests or deserts where they are exposed to new vector-borne diseases. Dams are often situated in remote areas where poverty and illiteracy are rife and where, consequently, people are especially at risk if they do not receive education to modify their behavior (e.g., to not drink or bathe directly in a reservoir contaminated with human waste or effluent). If decontamination processes are inadequate, a dam may increase the potential for infections in distant communities that are reliant on its output. Sometimes the risk of infection decreases in one community at the expense of another. For instance, a rural reservoir may help decrease the prevalence of epidemics in a distant urban population by providing better downstream sanitary facilities, but may increase the local infection rate by progressively degrading the water environment and impoverishing the resident community.

Although ecological changes per se may be responsible, decreased rates of infection with water developments usually follow deliberate efforts to control particular infections, such as malaria in the Panama Canal project. Vector-borne infections decrease when local communities make greater use of pesticides, bed nets, and antimalarials or when living standards and prosperity rise (Service, 1989). Simple developments, such as the provision of a water pump that provides communities with access to clean water for bathing, have caused dramatic reductions in rates of infections such as schistosomiasis (Tchuente et al., 2001). Such examples can be informative for mediating the health impacts of global changes. New water storage, irrigation, and hydropower projects may increase economic prosperity, ensuring a more plentiful supply of food, which can reduce the prevalence of many infectious diseases. Development projects can also facilitate greater investment in local health care facilities. These are often set up primarily for the benefit of migratory workers but nevertheless may contribute favorably to the health of indigent communities (World Commission on Dams, 2001). Thus, the challenge is not to oppose the often necessary development of a region's water resources, but to ensure that these are constructed in a way that brings positive, sustainable, and equitable health benefits to both local and geographically distant communities. In too many cases, past experience and other health information have been ignored, with negative and avoidable consequences.

Land Clearance and Deforestation

Land clearance, particularly of tropical rainforests, has increased dramatically in the last half century. Much of this has been driven by the need to provide settlements, fuel, and land for growing populations. However, the global expansion and liberalization of trade has also played an important role in making deforestation more financially attractive to countries mired in debt. Increasing demand for forest hardwood in wealthy countries has made logging a lucrative trade, and there is rising foreign investment in clearing forests for plantations (FAO, 2001). Pulp milling, mining, hydropower, and livestock rearing are also highly profitable. To develop their national economies, many countries have cleared land for agriculture or to build roads to improve access to economically important regions, often in remote areas (McMichael, 1993). These developments have influenced the intensity and pattern of infectious diseases because land clearance creates new local habitats that inhibit or encourage pathogens, or it facilitates or impedes contact between humans and pathogens (Walsh et al., 1993). In addition, loss of biodiversity affects the chances of discovering new drugs for the treatment of infections. Once again, it is difficult to conclusively prove that an episode of land clearance has altered the prevalence of a particular infection. Nevertheless, there is growing evidence of a changing burden of viral, bacterial, and parasitic illnesses in many parts of the world.

"New" or "Emergent" Infections

Worldwide, since 1975, more than thirty "new" or "emergent" human infections have appeared (World Health Organization, 1996). The appearance of a completely new agent is a rare occurrence, and most of these seem to be caused by existing pathogens that have been brought out of obscurity, or given selective advantage, by changing ecological or social conditions. Land clearance facilitates these changes. Certain animals, typically rodents, proliferate in land cleared of forest and become infected with a "new" pathogen. People who move to live and work at the edge of a previously unexplored forest come into contact with these animals, and the "new" pathogen then has a chance of being transferred to humans. Alternatively, land clearance may lead to the recognition of an existing but previously unknown human infection by increasing the numbers of people living in a formerly sparsely populated area and making better diagnostic facilities available (Wilson, 1995a). Several new infections, such as Venezuelan hemorrhagic fever and Oropouche fever in tropical South America, have been described in association with episodes of deforestation (Tesh, 1994). In both these examples, studies strongly suggested that changes following land clearance, such as the increasing availability of food and habitats that encouraged proliferation of virus-carrying rats and growing contact between humans and rodents, were responsible. Recently, deforestation in parts of Africa has led to increased incidence and distribution of yellow fever, originally a disease of monkeys (Walsh et al., 1993).

Vector-Borne Infections

The destruction of forest ecosystems often produces local environments that are highly conducive to mosquito breeding, leading to epidemics of malaria (Walsh et al., 1993). Land clearance may also destroy local mosquito habitats, but other disease-transmitting mosquito species often adapt and become more prominent, setting up new malaria cycles (Sharma, 1991). In contrast, replanting forests may facilitate the reemergence of malaria caused by formerly inhibited species (Singh, Tham, 1990).

The process of deforestation has created vast new swathes of open land, which may act as "motorways," allowing mosquitoes and other vectors to migrate to regions they would hitherto have been unable to reach. In this way, infections such as malaria and Chagas disease have spread across Africa and South America, respectively. Deforestation and economic adversity have also spawned much poor-quality housing in South America, which has provided excellent breeding conditions for the triatomine bugs that spread Chagas disease. In combination, these factors have probably helped to spread this infection widely across the continent and to establish itself in urban settings (Schofield, 1988).

The increasing numbers of people living close to remaining forest areas often compensates for the destruction of local vector habitats. For example, an epidemic of cutaneous leishmaniasis occurred when people moving to the Brazilian city of Amazonias were encouraged to settle in housing estates in newly cleared forest, where they encountered vectors for this infection (Walsh et al., 1993). Lyme disease, an ancient but previously rare bacterial infection, has returned to prominence in North America, Europe, and temperate Asia. This is thought to be partly due better transportation, which has increased human access to forests (Steere, 1994).

Pharmacological Implications of Loss of Biodiversity

Plants are an extremely important source of medicinal compounds. In technologically advanced countries, around 50% of prescription drugs derive from natural compounds; this proportion is far greater in more traditional societies (McMichael, 1993). Many antibiotics, such as streptomycin, neomycin, and amphotericin, originate from tropical soil fungi. Other plants produce toxins, which have been used to control agricultural pests and disease-carrying vectors (McMichael, 1998). Deforestation is leading to massive destruction of plant life, eliminating many possible future therapeutic agents, and threatening our prospects for developing new drugs, insecticides, and herbicides. This is particularly worrying in light of the enormous challenges posed by the global rise in antimicrobial resistance and the emergence of new infectious diseases.

GLOBAL DEMOGRAPHIC CHANGE AND INFECTIOUS DISEASE

Globalization and Population Mobility

Trends in Population Mobility

Population mobility is not a new phenomenon, but since the middle of the twentieth century it has been characterized by unprecedented volume, speed, and geographical range (Collin, Lee, 2003). Extensive research[3] suggests that people move in search of a better life and employment prospects or to escape an insecure situation. Globalization is contributing to these trends in several ways. Macroeconomic policies adopted to integrate countries into the global economy can lead to economic instability and insecurity, especially for the low skilled and poor. Increased trade in cash crops can threaten the livelihoods of rural communities through the loss of arable land, encouraging populations to relocate to urban areas. Differences in wage levels can lead to movement of workers within and across countries. Increasing uniformity of expertise worldwide means that demand for skilled workers, including health workers, in high-income countries can be satisfied by recruiting educated migrants from other high-income countries or, increasingly, from poorer countries. At the same time migration has become easier, less permanent, and less daunting.

Population Mobility and Infectious Disease

Human migration has been a source of epidemics throughout history, several of which have changed whole societies (Wilson, 1995b). Indeed, efforts in international health cooperation during the nineteenth century were focused on preventing infections spreading from one country to another (Gushulak, MacPherson, 2000). For several reasons, population mobility and the incidence and spread of infections are closely linked. First, the conditions that lead people to migrate are akin to those that favor the emergence of new infections and the breakdown of structures and systems to control well-understood infections. Second, the process of migration, in particular, mass migration, can present significant psychological, socioeconomic, and even physical challenges that themselves increases the risk of infection. On arrival, migrants may be more susceptible to a range of infectious diseases, such as respiratory infections that are associated with poor housing. Third, migration brings people into contact with new microbes and vectors, as well as new gene pools, immunological makeups, cultural preferences, behavioral patterns, and technologies, all of which influence the risk of infection.

The link between infectious diseases and population mobility must thus be understood in relation to the different forms, conditions, and patterns of migration, which have very different influences on the distribution and spread of infectious diseases.

Refugees and Displaced Persons

The last fifty years has seen huge increases in the number of refugees and internally displaced persons (see chapter 9). Although it is difficult to demonstrate a direct link with the processes of globalization, worldwide economic, political, and environmental change can contribute indirectly to the conditions leading to conflict and how they are resolved. Most of the world's refugees reside in camps or temporary shelters in low-income countries, where conditions favor epidemic infections, often of a devastating intensity. For example, within one month in 1994, around 50,000 Rwandans died in epidemics of cholera and dysentery that broke out refugee camps (Wilson, 1995a). Outbreaks of malaria and other vector-borne diseases are common when refugees who live in nonendemic regions and are not immune travel to endemic areas (Molyneux, 1997). Crowded conditions may facilitate rapid mixing of different strains of bacterial or viral DNA, which may encourage the emergence of new infections or multidrug-resistant pathogens.

Long-Term Migration

More permanent migration can lead to contact between populations from geographically or environmentally remote regions. Since human populations often show different degrees of susceptibility to specific infectious agents, this form of migration can accelerate and amplify the spread of infections to new communities and areas. Populations are more susceptible if they come from regions with low regional prevalence of particular infections, or if they have a less heterogeneous genetic mix. These factors were probably responsible for the devastating epidemics of influenza and smallpox that killed up to half the indigenous population of the Americas within a few decades of contact with Europeans in 1492. In modern times, the reemergence of TB in urban areas of many high-income countries has been attributed to migrant populations from South Asia who, upon arrival, face living conditions that enable the infection to spread (Gushulak, MacPherson, 2000). The long-term impact of migration of parasite genes, notably drug resistance, is also very important.

Migration to Developed Countries

In high-income countries infectious epidemics are uncommon because public health infrastructures are usually able to prevent, detect, and treat imported diseases. In these settings, migration is more important in facilitating the spread of "nonclassical" infectious diseases, of which there are two main categories (Gushulak, MacPherson, 2000). First are certain chronic infections that are more prevalent in immigrant communities and that may present after an immigrant has settled into the host country. The danger is that the individual may unknowingly spread the infection to others; this is particularly worrying if the index case is resistant to conventional antibiotic treatment, as in MDR-TB. Immigrants presenting with "exotic" infections may pose diagnostic difficulties to a health service with little experience of these diseases.

A second type of problem occurs when an infection, formerly eradicated or rendered unimportant in the host country following vaccination or other health prevention program, is reintroduced by immigrants from regions where it remains endemic or highly prevalent. Levels of immunity in the host community are often low or absent, leaving its members susceptible to new and virulent diseases. Again, lack of awareness and expertise in diagnosing and treating such infections among local health practitioners may exacerbate the problem. It may also be difficult to persuade people to accept vaccination programs for diseases thought to be extinct or rare.

Migration to or within Low-Income Countries

Considerable evidence now suggests that in low-income countries the consequences of migration are at least as severe, and probably worse, compared to high-income countries. This is probably due to weaker public health infrastructures and greater population susceptibility. The risk of serious epidemics caused by isolated cases of imported disease is much greater, and migrating populations may fall victim to epidemics if traveling brings them into contact with new infections. Temporary migration of people from nonendemic to endemic regions has also allowed migrants to import diseases to a nonimmune population on their return home. In southern Sudan, this led to a severe outbreak of anthroponotic visceral leishmaniasis, with around 100,000 deaths in a population of fewer than one million (Seaman et al., 1996).

Economic migration has played a crucial in the evolution of the HIV/AIDS epidemic in low-income countries. The basic living and working conditions of migrant workers have been accompanied by changes in sexual behavior that heighten their risk of contracting STDs. This is then often compounded by poor access to health care and preventative services. The migrant labor system in apartheid South Africa, for example, permitted miners to travel and work in urban areas but denied this right to their families. A flourishing market for commercial sex workers emerged, facilitating the spread of HIV/AIDS and other STDs to rural areas. Other research has highlighted the association between mobile armed forces, including peacekeeping forces, and the spread of HIV/AIDS (Minas, 2001).

In low-income countries, migration often accompanies economic development projects. In the early phases, this is usually temporary and involves single males, who are especially at risk for STDs. Developments may also provide new migratory routes, which have sometimes allowed infections to spread from endemic to previously unaffected areas (Hunter et al., 1993). The economically driven movement of domestic animals can also spread disease-carrying vectors, for instance, ticks in Australia (Petney, 2001).

Urbanization

Since 1800, the proportion of the world's population living in large towns or cities has grown from around 5% to 50%. If current trends continue, urban areas will be home to two-thirds of the world's people (around 7 billion) by 2030. Urban population growth is a function of both rural emigration and the expansion of existing city populations, although the relative importance of these varies by region (McMichael, 2000). Globalization has influenced the pace and nature of urbanization by substantially impacting on both of these forces. Political and economic pressures have displaced many subsistence farmers and farm workers in developing countries. At the same time urban employment opportunities have emerged, for instance, in the growing tourism industry or in the production of manufactured goods that rely on cheap labor. Although these processes of change are not dissimilar to the trends in urbanization experienced in Europe during the Industrial Revolution, the more rapid pace and scale of transition being experienced today are exceeding the capacity of many governments to effectively plan and manage it.

The Urban Physical Environment

Rapid and unplanned population growth places huge strains on a city's infrastructure. This is most dramatically evidenced in the emergence of growing number of "megacities" (more than 10 million inhabitants) in the developing world. In these, overcrowding, poor housing, inadequate sanitation and solid waste removal, and unsafe drinking water are extremely common. Socioeconomic inequalities are rife. Urban health care services are typically grossly overstretched, and their provision may be distorted to cater for the needs of the rich urban elite. These conditions are ideally suited to the transmission of pathogens through the air, human waste, or insect vectors. The high density of nonimmune people allows many crowd infections to establish sustained outbreaks of disease (McMichael, 1993), and cities are often great concentrators of infections. Overcrowding, high levels of air pollution and malnutrition increase susceptibility to chronic respiratory infections. While the expansion of urban areas can actually reduce the prevalence of parasitic infections by destroying the breeding grounds of some vectors, it can also increase disease by creating new opportunities for vectors and hosts to flourish. Nonbiodegradable plastic containers in which rainwater collects have provided urban breeding sites for *Aedes aegypti* mosquitoes, which in turn spread dengue fever (Barrera et al.,

1995). These developments have contributed to a major expansion in urban dengue over the last forty years (see box 2.4) (Gibbons, Vaughn, 2002). Urban areas may also encroach on rural environments where insect or arthropod vectors thrive, facilitating exposure to vector-borne infections. Other, less obviously hazardous features of the urban environment may also contribute to the spread of infections. Distribution of sewage-contaminated vegetables from urban gardens led to the dissemination of cystercercosis in Mexico City (Vasquez Tsuji et al., 1996).

Box 2.4 – Dengue

Dengue fever is caused by several flaviviruses and is responsible for an estimated 50–100 million episodes of illness annually, including 24,000 deaths from dengue hemorrhagic fever. In the past 60 years, the incidence, distribution, and clinical severity of dengue have increased dramatically. In Southeast Asia, for instance, cases have increased almost twentyfold since the 1950s. Currently, more than two-fifths of the world's population lives in areas potentially at risk from dengue. As well as population growth, other, more subtle, forces have played a role in this increase. Uncontrolled urbanization has led to inadequate management of water and waste, providing a range of large water stores and disposable, nonbiodegradable containers that become habitats for the larvae of the mosquito vectors. Similarly, trade in car tires has facilitated the spread of mosquito vectors to new regions. Air travel has allowed humans to import new serotypes of the virus; the exposure of humans to multiple serotypes is thought to cause the more severe immune reactions that characterize dengue hemorrhagic fever. Tourism places residents of nonendemic countries at risk; in some studies, up to 8% of travelers returning with febrile illnesses were found to have dengue. Man-made environmental changes, such as the construction of new dams, may cause increases in incidence, and global warming is also a potential threat. Despite advances in biotechnology, there is still no dengue animal model, and a vaccine may yet be many years away.

Cities are major contributors to global environmental change at a macro level, due to the annexation of nonurban habitats, production of industrial waste, and individual activities of their vast numbers of inhabitants. These transformations have implications for the impact of infectious diseases, as previously described. Global warming, for instance, may be contributing to the recent appearance of certain infectious diseases in urban areas where they did not previously exist. In addition, since most urban settlements are located within 75 miles of the sea, city dwellers are especially vulnerable to the effects of EWEs, such as hurricanes and floods (Wilson, 1995a).

The Urban Social Environment

Rapid and large-scale urbanization increases susceptibility to infection through changes in the social environment. Traditional, often rural based, cultural restraints are often challenged, leading to greater risk-taking behaviors. This is exacerbated by the greater human contact urban settings afford. In many cities, the growing intensity and diversity of sexual activity and use of illicit drugs has escalated the incidence of STDs. Increasing human travel to and from urban settings also facilitates the spread of disease. In combination, these factors may have played an important role in the rapid and extensive spread of HIV/AIDS during the 1980s and 1990s (Minas, 2001).

Rural–Urban Migration

Migration of rural people can add to the urban burden of infectious disease. Rural migrant communities who have traveled from nonendemic areas have suffered outbreaks of infections such as schistosomiasis and cutaneous leishmaniasis, which were endemic in their respective destination cities (Mott et al., 1990). Urban inhabitants may also be at risk from new infections brought in by rural immigrants. This may be either through the introduction of new vectors (e.g., mosquitoes) or animal hosts (e.g., snails in fisherman's buckets that spread schistosomiasis) or through direct transmission of pathogen through the air (respiratory infections) or in infected blood (in South America more than 50% of blood transfusion products are serologically positive for Chagas disease) (Schumunis, 1985). These factors are believed to have created peri-urban endemic foci of previously rural infections in African and South American cities.

GLOBAL TECHNOLOGICAL CHANGE AND INFECTIONS

During the past 100 years, enormous advances in technology have revolutionized most aspects of human activity. This section considers the impact on infectious diseases of three technologies crucial to process of globalization: information and communication, transportation, and medical technologies.

Information and Communication Technologies

Unprecedented advances in information and communication technologies (ICTs) have fundamentally altered the speed and nature of communications in personal and professional settings. Optimists claim that their arrival heralds widespread benefits for poorer countries. They have the potential to reduce the threat of infections in several ways.

First, with the improvements in satellite and media technology, news about natural disasters and other catastrophic events now travels quicker and with greater immediacy across the globe than before. This means that international and domestic responses to these may be organized more rapidly and appropriately than in the past, perhaps preventing or controlling major epidemics of infectious disease.

Second, the Internet is an invaluable means of providing access to continuing medical education and lifelong learning far from well-funded centers of excellence. Expert guidance on how to treat complex infections, for instance, a case of MDR-TB, will help the patient and the professional responsible and will have a wider beneficial impact on public health.

Third, advances in communications along with medical technologies have raised hopes that they may be used to deliver a variety of previously unavailable services to poor and remote locations. This is exemplified by the growth of "telemedicine," whereby emergency clinical advice and specialized consultations are provided from a geographically remote site (Fraser, McGrath, 2000). Although a number of encouraging pilot projects are up and running, there are real challenges in sustaining these services in regions where resources are limited (Wright, 1999).

Fourth, the growing sophistication and availability of geographical information systems (GIS) may be used to link relevant information about individual cases of infectious disease and can provide a tool to investigate and control outbreaks (Aron, Patz, 2001). They are already contributing to the control of many vector-borne diseases where local capacity is appropriately developed, such as schistosomiasis in China (Xiaonong et al., 2002) and malaria and sleeping sickness in Africa (Molyneux, 2001). GIS programs are an essential tool for forecasting epidemics that follow El Niño/Southern Oscillation (ENSO) events (Kovats, 2000). In some countries, ICTs are being used to coordinate and improve responses to epidemics in emergency situations (Chandrasekhar, Ghosh, 2001).

The use of ICTs in developing countries is limited by affordability, access, and education. The relative merit of investing heavily in these should be carefully scrutinized, because there is a danger that an overemphasis on ICT projects could divert resources from basic public health activities such as the provision of clean water, sanitation, primary education, and basic health care.

TRANSPORTATION TECHNOLOGIES

The Growth in Short-Term Travel

During the last 50 years, advances in transportation technology have facilitated dramatic increases in short-term travel for tourism, work, and transportation of traded goods. Instead of single, longer excursions, there is a growing tendency for people to make several, shorter trips to multiple destinations. Increasingly, these journeys extend to tropical regions or relatively unexplored destinations (Clift, Page, 1996). Business travel has increased in similar fashion as the globalization of financial services, trade, and industry has made international mobility of personnel vital. The speed and volume of cargo moved across the world each day have also increased hugely (Pedersen, 2000). All of these have implications for the spread of infectious diseases.

Short-Term Travel and Infectious Diseases

Most travel-related illness consists of injuries and accidents. However, infections pose perhaps the greatest threat to global health since they can be rapidly spread to large numbers of people living in widely dispersed areas and communities across the world. Human and cargo traffic facilitates the movement of pathogens (Aron, Patz, 2001). Since most infectious diseases have an incubation period exceeding thirty-six hours, and any part of the world can now be reached within this time frame, the potential for rapid geographical spread is apparent.

Travelers may be exposed to a variety of pathogens that they have not previously encountered and therefore are not immune to. Classic examples are gastroenteritis due to *Giardia* or cholera, hepatitis A and B, malaria, and yellow fever. Migrants who travel on holiday to their country of birth are especially at risk of endemic vector-borne diseases, particularly malaria, since they may erroneously believe that their previous residence in the country confers them with immunity despite many years of absence (Habib et al., 2000). Travelers are more likely to indulge in risky sexual behavior, and they have a higher than average chance of contracting STDs; the growth of sex tourism has major implications for both resident and visiting populations (Clift, Carter, 2000). Means of transport can themselves facilitate the spread of contagious infections: epidemics of TB, influenza, and cholera have been disseminated on commercial airplane flights, and cruise ships have been associated with outbreaks of *Legionella* pneumonia (Centers for Disease Control and Prevention, 1994b, 1995a; Wilson, 1995b). Some infections are associated with specific types of travel, for instance, outbreaks of meningitis during the annual Haj.

As overseas trips become shorter, infections are increasingly declaring themselves after the traveler has returned home. In 1996, 10,000 cases of malaria were reported in the European Union, all of which were imported from abroad (Heymann, Rodier, 1998). Fatal cases of yellow fever have been reported in returning Swiss and American tourists who had traveled to endemic countries without receiving vaccination (Gubler, 1998). Travel-related illness may give rise to public health concerns that precipitate a disastrous fall in tourist revenue. Efforts to prevent travel associated diseases may thus produce significant economic benefits to host countries (Behrens, Grabowski, 1995).

The greatest concern is that travelers may return to spread new infections to residents of their home country. Although cases of rare and exotic diseases, such as viral hemorrhagic fevers (e.g., Ebola, yellow, and Lassa fevers), are the subject of enormous media interest, outbreaks of gastrointestinal or respiratory diseases, such as hepatitis A, *Cryptosporidium*, and TB are far more common (Gubler, 1998). People may also return carrying pathogens that are particularly virulent or unusually resistant to antibiotics (Cookson et al., 1995). There is a risk that resistant strains may be spread to developing countries by travelers from wealthy regions, perhaps even before the relevant antibiotic has been introduced in the destination country. This may lead to epidemics of difficult and expensive to treat infections, such as MDR-TB or methicillin-resistant *Staphylococcus aureus*, which could be devastating if health care facilities are inadequate (Ayliffe, 1997).

Transport of Goods and Infectious Diseases

Transport of certain nonhuman goods risks spreading human infections directly or indirectly. Direct risks arise when people are exposed to materials that may themselves contain pathogens. For example, animal tissues transported for scientific purposes may contain dangerous organisms that can spread to human handlers. In Marburg, Germany, seven people died from viral hemorrhagic fever after handling blood and tissues sent from African green monkeys in Uganda (Wilson, 1995b). These dangers seem especially relevant as researchers consider using animals as the source of tissues and organs for transplantation.

Vehicles of transportation have themselves spread pathogens to new areas. The international trade in used car tires has helped disseminate mosquito vectors for dengue fever (Gubler, 1998). Sea freight may have introduced an epidemic of cholera to South America (Anderson, 1991): *Vibrio cholerae* was isolated in ballast, bilge, and sewage from cargo ships off the continent. Mosquitoes can survive on international flights and have probably been responsible for cases of malaria in destination countries.

Indirect risks occur when transported materials alter ecosystems in ways that facilitate breeding of pathogens or vectors that spread infections. For instance, alien plant species may provide new protective habitats for mosquito vectors, causing outbreaks of malaria. Plant pathogens spread by transport can decimate crops leading to famine; malnourished populations are left more susceptible to infectious diseases (Wilson, 1995b).

Medical Technologies

New medical technologies and techniques are disseminated across the world with increasing speed, and more people than ever can potentially benefit from scientific advances. This is a consequence not only of advances in ICTs but also of greater scientific collaboration and interchange of ideas, which are themselves features of globalization. For instance, there is much interest and considerable international collaboration in the development of new vaccines. Although vaccines already prevent more than 3.2 million deaths per year, the benefits of existing products have not been fully realized, particularly in developing regions (World Health Organization, 1996). There are also currently no vaccines for many of the most important infections in tropical regions. Although developments in biotechnology, for example, advances in DNA sequencing technology, have raised hopes for prevention of many of these infections (Jordan Report, 1998), many obstacles prevent the full application of modern technologies to these problems. Most important, there is currently little financial incentive for pharmaceutical companies, who are responsible for most new developments, to invest in such projects (Lang, Wood, 1999). A variety of nonprofit initiatives have attempted to rectify this lack of investment, including grants provided by the Gates Foundation and the Special Program for Research an Training in Tropical Diseases (Schwartz, Rabinovich, 1999).

Advances in technology are often offset by new vulnerabilities (Wilson, 1995a). Modern medical techniques applied with inadequate training and resources have had disastrous consequences. For example, hospital outbreaks of Ebola disease in the Congo and of Lassa fever in Nigeria both followed the use of insufficiently sterilized needles and surgical implements (Centers for Disease Control and Prevention, 1995b; Fisher-Hoch et al., 1995). Trade in blood products has spread viral and other infections between countries. Widespread and inappropriate use of antibiotics has led to dramatic increases in antimicrobial resistance. Use of vaccines derived from animal sources may transfer unknown infections from animals to humans. The intentional distribution of anthrax spores in the United States in the autumn of 2001 highlighted the threat posed by the use of infectious agents for terrorist purposes (Polyak et al., 2002). Alarmingly, in some cases terrorist groups have recruited scientists, physicians, and engineers and have even built laboratories for the development of toxins (Olson, 1999). Since 2001, the regulatory framework surrounding the exchange of pathogens for scientific purposes has tightened significantly. What is less known is the extent to which trade, legal or illicit, notably following the end of the Cold War, has spread potentially dangerous samples more widely. Economic and political instability in the former Soviet Union, for example, has led to fears that such materials are no longer stored in a secure environment and some even cannot be wholly accounted for. Appropriate regulation of such substances by all countries is clearly needed.

CONCLUSION

Globalization has, potentially, both positive and negative consequences for the infectious disease burden. The existing literature remains limited, although it is expanding and illustrative of the wide-ranging issues for research and policy. From this literature, a number of conclusions may be drawn.

First, globalization appears to be causing profound and sometimes unpredictable changes in the ecological, biological, and social conditions that shape the burden of infectious diseases in certain populations. There is accumulating evidence that these changes have led to alterations in the prevalence, spread, geographical range, and control of many infections. There is also a weight of theoretical, experimental, and empirical research suggesting the potential for much greater change in the future. Changes have been both positive and negative, in different cases increasing or decreasing the infectious disease burden. Furthermore, different facets of globalization overlap and interlock, such that the same process is often responsible for a range of impacts on infectious diseases, and the prevalence of a specific infection may be influenced by several aspects of globalization concurrently. There is a need for greater understanding of these complex linkages through case studies, computer modeling, and improved surveillance systems.

Second, individuals and population groups show varying degrees of gains and losses from economic globalization, and thus differential vulnerability to infectious diseases. Thus, crude assessments of globalization as "good" or "bad" are neither accurate nor useful. Nevertheless, there is increasing evidence that infectious diseases affect the poor disproportionately because of inequities in basic living conditions (e.g., clean water, housing, sanitation), in the availability of and access to health care, in standards of diet and nutrition, and in migration patterns. An assessment of the degree of vulnerability faced by different people can then form the basis of appropriate policy response.

Third, epidemiology in general and surveillance in particular offer useful analytical tools and methods for identifying and measuring transborder patterns of infectious disease arising as a consequence of globalization. An approach that defines population across a wide spectrum of variables, which are not delineated by territorial space, is needed in studying how globalization may be changing the distribution of infections both within and across countries and regions of the world (e.g., the spread of SARS in 2002–2003).

Fourth, attention to the linkages between globalization and infectious diseases so far shows a disproportionate focus on selected acute and epidemic infections. There is a need to recognize and respond to a broader range of infectious disease impacts than currently.

Fifth, inadequate surveillance and monitoring systems means that we may currently be underestimating the infectious disease burden faced by poorer countries. There is a particular need to develop surveillance systems that can be used effectively in low-tech, developing world contexts. It is also imperative to ensure that, when changes in disease patterns are detected, the information is transmitted to those able to implement appropriate actions.

Sixth, the impact of globalization on infectious diseases supports the need for appropriate forms of global governance on key issues to improve systems for prevention, control, and treatment. National level efforts and international health cooperation, notably through international health regulations, are reliant on voluntary cooperation by governments. This is not always forthcoming. In addition, these regulations do not incorporate key nonstate actors such as nongovernmental organizations and the private sector. There is a need to put greater responsibility on global players, notably TNCs, for their actions, which may contribute to the infectious disease burden both directly and indirectly. There is a clear collective need for international standards of practice and for regulatory mechanisms to enforce such practice.

In this context, there is a need for greater attention to be paid to the impacts on the infectious disease burden of policy decisions taken in other sectors such as trade and investment, large infrastructure projects (e.g., dam building), migration, agriculture, transportation, and communications. There is a need to integrate health impact assessment as part of decision-making processes in these sectors and to establish long-term monitoring after policy decisions or infrastructure changes are implemented.

Seventh, there is need for enhanced training on the global dimensions of infectious diseases. Medical practitioners would benefit from greater understanding of the potentially changing profile of infectious diseases as a result of increased population mobility, intensified trade in goods and services, climate change, and other factors linked to globalization. In many cases, international training exchange programs are required to enable the sharing of experiences and ideas across national contexts.

Finally, it is clear that improving action on the impact of globalization on infectious disease on an a priori basis is a highly cost-effective policy intervention. Resources committed to infectious diseases prevention, treatment, and control, in a globalizing world, is a worthwhile investment. As well as the costs of prevention, treatment, and control of the disease, countries risk losing substantial revenues from reduced trade, investment, and tourism. These economic costs can be imposed indiscriminately. In addition, given the integrated nature of the global economy, including capital flows, population mobility, and trade in goods and services, there is shared interest in investing greater resources in strengthening global capacity surrounding infectious diseases.

Notes

1. For a detailed discussion, see Held et al. (1999).
2. Large dams are defined as those greater than fifteen meters in height or with a reservoir capacity of more than 3 million cubic meters.
3. E.g., see Boyle et al. (1998), Castles and Miller (1998), and Skeldon (1997).

References

Albritton DI et al. *IPPC Working group I for policy makers, third assessment report, climate change 2001: The scientific basis.* Cambridge, UK, Cambridge University Press, 2001.

Altekruse SF et al. Emerging foodborne diseases. *Emerging Infectious Diseases*, 1997, 3:285–293.

Anderson C. Cholera epidemic traced to risk miscalculation. *Nature*, 1991, 354(6351):255.

Aron JL, Patz JA. *Ecosystems change and public health: A global perspective.* Baltimore, MD, John Hopkins University Press, 2001.

Ayliffe GA. The progressive intercontinental spread of methicillin-resistant *Staphylococcus aureus*. *Clinical Infectious Diseases*, 1997, 24:S74–S79.

Baris E, McLeod K. Globalization and international trade in the twenty-first century: opportunity for and threats to the health sector in the south. *International Journal of Health Services*, 2000, 30:187–210.

Barrera R et al. Public service deficiencies and *Aedes aegypti* breeding sites in Venezuela. *Bulletin of the Pan American Health Organization*, 1995, 29: 193–205.

Behrens RH, Grabowski P. Travellers' health and the economy of developing nations. *Lancet*, 1995, 346:1562.

Boyle P et al. *Exploring contemporary migration.* Harlow, UK, Longman, 1998.

Brugha R. Antiretroviral treatment in developing countries: the peril of neglecting private providers. *British Medical Journal*, 2003, 326:1382–1384.

Carmichael WW et al. Human fatalities from cyanobacteria: chemical and biological evidence for cyanotoxins. *Environmental Health Perspectives*, 2001, 109:663–668.

Castles S and Miller MJ. *The age of migration: International population movements in the modern world.* London, MacMillan, 1998.

Centers for Disease Control and Prevention. Rift Valley Fever—Egypt, 1993. *Morbidity & Mortality Weekly Report*, 1994(a), 43:693, 699–700.

Centers for Disease Control and Prevention. Update: outbreak of Legionnaires' disease associated with a cruise ship. *Morbidity & Mortality Weekly Report*, 1994(b), 43:574–575.

Centers for Disease Control and Prevention. Exposure of passengers and flight crew to *Mycobacterium tuberculosis* on commercial aircraft, 1992–1995. *Morbidity & Mortality Weekly Report*, 1995(a), 44:137–140.

Centers for Disease Control and Prevention. Update: outbreak of Ebola viral hemorrhagic fever—Zaire. *Morbidity & Mortality Weekly Report*, 1995(b), 44:468–469.

Chandrasekhar CP, Ghosh J. Information and communication technologies and health in low income countries: the potential and the constraints. *Bulletin of the World Health Organization*, 2001, 79:850–855.

Checkley W et al. Effects of El Niño and ambient temperature on hospital admissions for diarrhoeal diseases in Peruvian children. *Lancet*, 2000, 355: 442–450.

Clift S, Carter S. *Tourism and sex.* London, Pinter, 2000.

Clift S, Page S. *Health and the international tourist.* London, Routledge, 1996.

Collin J, Lee K. *Globalization and transborder health risk in the UK.* London, Nuffield Trust, 2003.

Cookson B et al. International inter- and intrahospital patient spread of a multiple antibiotic-resistant strain of *Klebsiella pneumoniae. Journal of Infectious Diseases,* 1995, 171:511–513.

Dicken P. *Global Shift: Transforming the world economy.* 3rd ed. London, Sage, 1998.

Ding WX et al. Genotoxicity of microcystic cyanobacteria extract of a water source in China. *Mutation Research,* 1999, 442:69–77.

Dobson A, Carper R. Biodiversity. *Lancet,* 1993, 342:1096–1099.

DukhaNiña NN et al. The malaria problem and malaria control measures in northern Afghanistan. First Report. Malaria in Afghanistan. *Meditsinskaia Parazitologiia i Parazitarnye Bolezni,* 1975, 44:338–344.

Endtz HP et al. Quinolone resistance in campylobacter isolated from man and poultry following the introduction of fluoroquinolones in veterinary medicine. *Journal of Antimicrobial Chemotherapy,* 1991, 27:199–208.

Epstein PR. Climate change and emerging infectious diseases. *Microbes & Infection,* 2001(a), 3:747–754.

Epstein PR. Infectious diseases. In: Munn T, ed., *Encyclopaedia of global environmental change,* Chichester, Wiley, 2001(b):357–363.

FAO. *The state of the world's forests.* Rome, Food and Agriculture Organization, 2001.

Farid MA. Irrigation and malaria in arid lands. In: Worthington EB, ed., *Arid land irrigation in developing countries. Environmental problems and effects.* Oxford, Pergamon, 1977:413–429.

Fisher-Hoch SP et al. Review of cases of nosocomial Lassa fever in Nigeria: the high price of poor medical practice. *British Medial Journal,* 1995, 311:857–859.

Fraser HS, McGrath SJ. Information technology and telemedicine in sub-saharan Africa. *British Medical Journal,* 2000, 321:465–466.

Gibbons RV, Vaughn DW. Dengue: an escalating problem. *British Medical Journal,* 2002, 324:1563–1566.

Githeko AK et al. Climate change and vector-borne diseases: a regional analysis. *Bulletin of the World Health Organization,* 2000, 78:1136–1147.

Global Alliance for TB Drug Development. No R&D in 30 years. New York, 2005. http://www.tballiance.org/ 2_3_C_NoRandDin30years.asp (accessed March 1, 2006).

Global Forum for Health Research. *The 10/90 report on health research.* Geneva, World Health Organization, 1999.

Gubler DJ. Population growth, urbanization, automobiles and aeroplanes: the dengue connection. In: Greenwood B, De Cock K, eds., *New and resurgent infections: Prediction, detection and management of tomorrow's epidemics,* Chichester, John Wiley and Sons, 1998:118–129.

Gushulak B, MacPherson DW. Population mobility and infectious diseases: the diminishing impact of classical infectious diseases and new approaches for the 21st century. *Clinical Infectious Diseases,* 2000, 31:776–780.

Habib NA et al. Travel health and infectious disease. In: Parsons L, Lister G, eds. *Global health: A local issue,* London, Nuffield Trust, 2000:124–133.

Held D et al. *Global transformations, politics, economics and culture.* Stanford, Stanford University Press, 1999.

Herrera-Basto E et al. First reported outbreak of classical dengue fever at 1,700 meters above sea level in Guerrero State, Mexico, June 1988. *American Journal of Tropical Medicine & Hygiene,* 1992, 46:649–653.

Heymann DL, Rodier GR. Global surveillance of communicable diseases. *Emerging Infectious Diseases,* 1998, 4:362–365.

Hunter JM et al. *Parasitic diseases in water resources development.* Geneva, World Health Organization, 1993.

Huq A et al. Coexistence of Vibrio cholerae 01 and 0139 Bengal in plankton in Bangladesh. *Lancet,* 1995, 345:1249.

Jordan Report. *Accelerated development of vaccines 1998.* Washington, DC, National Institute of Allergy and Infectious Diseases, 1998.

Khalil Bey M. The national campaign for the treatment and control of bilharziasis from the scientific and economic aspects. *Journal of the Royal Egyptian Medical Association,* 1949, 32:820.

Koopman JS et al. Determinants and predictors of dengue infection in Mexico. *American Journal of Epidemiology,* 1991, 133:1168–1178.

Kovats RS. El Niño and human health. *Bulletin of the World Health Organization,* 2000, 78:1127–1135.

Kovats RS et al. Early effects of climate change: do they include changes in vector-borne diseases? *Philosophical Transactions of the Royal Society of London Series B Biological Sciences,* 2001, 356: 1057–1068.

Lang J, Wood SC. Development of orphan vaccines: an industry perspective. *Emerging Infectious Diseases,* 1999, 5:749–756.

Lang T. Trade, public health and food. In: McKee MG, Stott R, eds., *International cooperation in health,* London, Oxford University Press, 2001:81–108.

Lehmann JP. Developing economies and the demographic and democratic imperatives of globalization. *International Affairs,* 2001, 77:69–82.

Linthicum KJ et al. Climate and satellite indicators to forecast Rift Valley fever epidemics in Kenya. *Science,* 1999, 285:397–400 [comment].

Loevinsohn ME. Climatic warming and increased malaria incidence in Rwanda. *Lancet,* 1994, 343:714–718.

MacKenzie WR et al. A massive outbreak in Milwaukee of cryptosporidium infection transmitted through the public water supply. *New England Journal of Medicine,* 1994, 331:161–167.

Maclehose L et al. Responding to the challenge of communicable disease in Europe. *Science*, 2002, 295:2047–2050.

Martens WJM et al. Sensitivity of malaria, schistosomiasis and dengue to global warming. *Climatic Change*, 1997, 35:145–156.

May R. Changing diseases in changing environments. In: Cartledge B, ed., *Health and the Environment*. Oxford, Oxford University Press, 1994:150–171.

McArthur RH. *Geographical ecology*. New York, Harper and Row, 1972.

McMichael AJ. *Planetary overload: Global environmental change and the health of the human species*. Cambridge, Cambridge University Press, 1993.

——. The influence of historical and global changes upon the patterns of infectious diseases. In: Greenwood B, De Cock K, eds., *New and resurgent infections: prediction, detection and management of tomorrow's epidemics*. Chichester, New York, John Wiley and Sons, 1998:17–31.

——. The urban environment and health in a world of increasing globalization: issues for developing countries. *Bulletin of the World Health Organization*, 2000, 78:1117–1126.

McMichael AJ, Haines A. Global climate change: the potential effects on health. *British Medical Journal*, 1997, 315:805–809.

Minas IH. Migration, equity and health. In: McKee M, Garner P, Stott R, eds., *International co-operation and health*. Oxford, Oxford University Press, 2001:151–174.

Molyneux DH. Patterns of change in vector-borne diseases. *Annals of Tropical Medicine & Parasitology*, 1997, 91:827–839.

——. Vector-borne infections in the tropics and health policy issues in the twenty-first century. *Transactions of the Royal Society of Tropical Medicine & Hygiene*, 2001, 95:233–238.

Mott KE et al. Parasitic diseases and urban development. *Bulletin of the World Health Organization*, 1990, 68:691–698.

Olson KB. Aum Shinrikyo: once and future threat? *Emerging Infectious Diseases*, 1999, 5:513–516.

Patz JA et al. Global climate change and emerging infectious diseases. *Journal of the American Medical Association*, 1996, 275:217–223.

Pecoul B et al. Access to essential drugs in poor countries, a lost battle? *Journal of the American Medical Association*, 1999, 281:361–367.

Pedersen PO. *The changing structure of transport under trade liberalisation and globalization and its impact on African development*. Working paper 00.1. Copenhagen, Centre for Development Research, 2000.

Petney TN. Environmental, cultural and social changes and their influence on parasite infections. *International Journal for Parasitology*, 2001, 31:919–932.

Polyak CS et al. Bio terrorism-related anthrax: international response by the Centers for Disease Control and Prevention. *Emerging Infectious Diseases*, 2002, 8:1056–1059.

Sanders D, Chopra M. Globalization and the challenge of health for all: a view from sub-Saharan Africa. In: Lee K, ed., *Health impacts of globalization: Towards global governance*. London, Palgrave Macmillan, 2002:105–116.

Schmaljohn C, Hjelle B. Hantaviruses: a global disease problem. *Emerging Infectious Diseases*, 1997, 3(2):95–104.

Schofield CJ. Biosystematics of the Triatominae. *Biosystematics of haematophagous insects*. Oxford, Oxford University Press, 1988:285–312.

Schumunis G. Chagas disease and blood transfusion. In: Dodd RY, Barker LF, eds., *Infection, immunity and blood transfusion*. New York, Liss, 1985: 127–145.

Schwartz B, Rabinovich NR. Stimulating the development of orphan (and other) vaccines. *Emerging Infectious Diseases*, 1999, 5:832.

Seaman J et al. The epidemic of visceral leishmaniasis in western Upper Nile, southern Sudan: course and impact from 1984 to 1994. *International Journal of Epidemiology*, 1996, 25:862–871.

Service MW. *Irrigation: Boon or bane?* Baco Raton, FL, CRC Press, 1989.

Sharma VP, Kondrachine AV. *Forest malaria in Southeast Asia: Proceedings of an informal consultative meeting*. New Delhi, World Health Organization/Medical Research Council, 1991.

Singh YP, Tham A. *Case history of malaria control through the application of environmental management in Malaysia*. World Health Organization, Geneva, 1990.

Skeldon R. *Migration and development: A global perspective*. Harlow, UK, Longman, 1997.

Steere AC. Lyme disease: a growing threat to urban populations. *Proceedings of the National Academy of Sciences of the United States of America*, 1994, 91:2378–2383.

Strickland GT. Providing health services on the Aswan High Dam. *World Health Forum*, 1982, 3:297–300.

Sutherst RW. The vulnerability of animal and human health to parasites under global change. *International Journal for Parasitology*, 2001, 31:933–948.

Swerdlow DL, Altekruse SF. Food-borne diseases in the global village: what's on the plate for the 21st century. In: Schield MW et al., eds., *Emerging infections 2*. Washington, DC, American Society for Microbiology, 1998: 273–293.

Tamplin ML, Carrillo Parodi C. Environmental spread of *Vibrio cholerae* in Peru. *Lancet*, 1991, 338:1216–1217.

Tchuente LA et al. Impact of installation of a water pump on schistosomiasis transmission in a focus in Cameroon. *Transactions of the Royal Society of Tropical Medicine & Hygiene*, 2001, 95:255–256.

Tesh RB. The emerging epidemiology of Venezuelan hemorrhagic fever and Oropouche fever in tropical

South America. *Annals of the New York Academy of Sciences*, 1994;740:129–137.

United Nations. *Climate change 2001: Impacts, adaptation and vulnerability*. New York, United Nations, 2001.

Vasquez Tsuji O et al. Soil contamination with *Toxocara* sp. eggs in public parks and home gardens from Mexico City. *Boletin Chileno de Parasitologia*, 1996, 51:54–58.

Walsh JF et al. Deforestation: Effects on vector-borne disease. *Parasitology*, 1993, 106:S55–S75.

Wilson ME. Infectious diseases: an ecological perspective. *British Medical Journal*, 1995(a), 311:1681–1684.

Wilson ME. Travel and the emergence of infectious diseases. *Emerging Infectious Diseases*, 1995(b), 1:39–46.

World Commission on Dams. *Dams and development: A new framework for decision-making*. United Nations Environment Program, 2001.

World Health Organization. *The world health report 1996: Fighting disease, fostering development*. Geneva, World Health Organization, 1996.

Wibulpolprasert S et al. *The economic crisis and responses by health sector in Thailand in 1997–1998*. Paper presented at Regional Consultation on Health Implications of the Economic Crisis in the South-East Asia Region, March 23–25, 1998, Thailand.

Wright D. The sustainability of telemedicine projects. *Journal of Telemedicine & Telecare*, 1999, 5:S107–S111.

Xiaonong Z et al. Schistosomiasis control in the 21st century. Proceedings of the International Symposium on Schistosomiasis, Shanghai, 4–6 July 2001. *Acta Tropica*, 2002, 82:95–114.

Zucker JR. Changing patterns of autochthonous malaria transmission in the United States: a review of recent outbreaks. *Emerging Infectious Diseases*, 1996, 2:37–43.

Chapter 3

Globalization and Tobacco

Derek Yach, Heather Wipfli, Ross Hammond, and Stanton Glantz

Tobacco has followed the trends of globalization since Columbus first encountered it upon his arrival in the New World (Hobhouse 1989, Kiernann 1991). On the wave of exploration, discovery, and cultural interaction, tobacco spread at an incredible speed. Within 100 years, tobacco could be found growing and traded in all major regions of the world. Tobacco production and use rapidly increased in the late nineteenth century throughout North America and Europe with the onset of the industrial revolution, laissez-faire economic policies, and increasing international exchange of capital, goods, persons, concepts, and values (Kiernann 1991). The rapid pace of globalization during the late twentieth century further extended mass consumption of tobacco products, especially in low- and middle-income countries. At the turn of the twenty-first century, transnational tobacco companies (TTCs) operate in more than 180 countries, more than 1.1 billion people smoke, and the Marlboro Man is one of the most widely recognized advertising symbols in the world (Madeley 1999, Jha et al. 2002, Ourusoff 1992).

The current global presence and seemingly deep cultural foundations of tobacco use often blur the realities behind tobacco's origins and traditional significance. Tobacco industry representatives often point out that tobacco use has been an established practice for centuries in the countries in which they operate, including new markets in Asia, Africa, and the newly independent states of Europe (Holmes 1997, Rupert and Frankel 1996). While tobacco was first introduced to these regions around 400 years ago, the way tobacco is used and by whom is changing rapidly as a result of industry production, penetration, and marketing. Seventy-five percent of the world's cigarette market is controlled by just four companies: Philip Morris (PM), British American Tobacco (BAT), Japan Tobacco (JT), and the China National Tobacco Corporation (Crescenti 1998). The latter's share is attributed almost entirely to its near monopoly over the enormous Chinese market, but the others have been tireless in their pursuit of worldwide sales. In line with other global industries, the tobacco industry has used numerous elements of globalization to sell their products, including trade liberalization, foreign direct investment, and marketing.

In 2002, PM, BAT, and JT had combined tobacco sales of more than $121 billion (World Bank 2003b). The transnational tobacco industry's worth and its effective use of global trade, communication, and financial liberalization are fueling a global public health tragedy.

Tobacco-related diseases are responsible for nearly 5 million premature deaths in 2003 (figure 3.1) and are forecasted to kill more than 10 million people per year by 2030, with 70% of these deaths occurring in low- and middle-income countries (WHO 2002). However, the global public health response to tobacco uses modern information technologies and interactive virtual networks to spread information, coordinate activities, and elicit responses from local, national, and international authorities (Wipfli et al. 2001).

Tobacco demonstrates the effects of globalization on efforts to regulate consumer products, on traditional understandings of industry/government/nonprofit relationships, and on efforts to provide for the "global public good" (Taylor and Bettcher 2000). The development of minimum global regulatory standards in the form of the World Health Organization (WHO) Framework Convention on Tobacco Control (FCTC) is reworking domestic and international tobacco policies. By providing an ongoing and institutionalized platform for multilateral cooperation on tobacco control, the FCTC promotes the adoption

and implementation of effective tobacco control strategies worldwide (Taylor and Bettcher 2000). The FCTC is in essence an attempt to develop a form of health governance capable of effectively regulating transnational corporations (Collin 2004). Its negotiation entailed wrestling with fundamental questions about the social impacts of globalization, particularly the relationship between trade and health, state sovereignty, and resolution of how to distribute benefits and costs resulting from international treaties. The negotiations also illuminated the important and evolving role of low- and middle-income countries and nongovernmental organizations (NGOs) in determining the future direction of global public health policy.

In this chapter we review the evolving economic and social system sustaining the growing tobacco epidemic in order to identify how globalization is affecting the industry, governments, and tobacco control advocates. It is divided into four main sections. In the first section we recall the key historical events that led to the worldwide prominence of tobacco use and the global rise of tobacco-related death and disease. In the second section we examine the scientific evidence base regarding the health effects of active and passive smoking and review the globalization of the public health response to the tobacco epidemic. In the third section we describe the FCTC negotiating process and final treaty text. In the fourth section we analyze some of the remaining major challenges resulting from working within a global system, in particular, those challenges associated with developing coherent domestic and international policies and the permanent need to anticipate the unintended consequences of national and global regulations. Finally, we conclude by identifying new directions and resources for global tobacco control and predicting some of the main challenges that lie ahead.

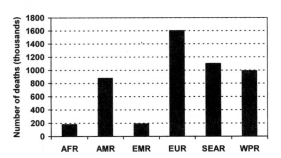

FIGURE 3.1. Tobacco Deaths by Region 2002. AFRs, African region; AMRs, American region; EMRs, eastern Mediterranean region; EURs, European region; SEARs, Southeast Asian region; WPRs, western Pacific region. *Source:* WHO (2002).

GLOBALIZATION OF THE TOBACCO EPIDEMIC

Little more than 400 years ago, tobacco was only used by Native Americans for medicinal and ceremonial purposes (Kiernann 1991). Europeans first encountered tobacco when Columbus brought back a few leaves and seeds from his first voyage to America in 1492 (table 3.1). Over the following century, tobacco was established as a commodity in Europe, and

TABLE 3.1. Tobacco Timeline

Global Spread and Initial Control Effort

1492	Tobacco encountered by Columbus
1556–1559	Tobacco introduced in France, Spain, Portugal, Japan
1560	Tobacco introduced to East Africa
1564	Tobacco introduced to England
1600	Tobacco introduced to India
1604	King James I writes *A Counterblaste to Tobacco*
1620–1640	Tobacco prohibited in Japan, New Amsterdam (New York), and China, where use or distribution of tobacco is punishable by decapitation

Birth of the Modern Industry and Rise of the Cigarette

1832	Invention of rolled cigarette in Turkey
1839	Discovery of flue-cured yellow tobacco
1852	Invention of safety matches
1880	Invention of Bonsack machine
1905	Tobacco removed from U.S. Pharmacopoeia
1907	Breakup of American Tobacco Company

Scientific Discovery

1950	Three key case–control studies linking smoking to lung caner
1962	U.K. Royal College report
1964	U.S. Surgeon General's report on active smoking
1986	U.S. Surgeon General's report on secondhand smoke
1994	International Agency for Research on Cancer monograph on secondhand smoke

Recent Tobacco-Control Developments

1998	Master Settlement Agreement, public release of industry documents
1999	BAT purchases Rothmans, JT purchases RJR international
2003	FCTC is adopted by the member states of WHO

global travel and trade spread the weed throughout Africa and Asia (Hobhouse 1989).

As tobacco spread, it was often seen as an "evil plant" associated with savages from the New World, and use of tobacco was viewed as a sin. It was also not long before the addictive qualities began to be recognized and initial health concerns arose. In 1604, King James I issued his *Counterblaste to Tobacco*, where he wrote: "Smoking is a custom loathsome to the eye, hateful to the nose, harmful to the brain, dangerous to the lungs" (James 1604). In addition, he increased the import tax on tobacco by 4,000% (from 2 pence/pound to 6 shilling 10 pence/pound) with the *initial* aim of stamping out the tobacco trade (Arents 1938). By 1640, tobacco was banned in New Amsterdam (New York), Japan, Turkey, and China—where use or distribution of the plant was punishable by decapitation (Borio 1997).

Despite these early attempts at control, the habit-forming nature of tobacco resulted in its permanent establishment wherever it was introduced. This boundless market has become a revolutionary fact of economic history (Kiernann 1991). By 1604 the British had established tobacco as the key cash crop of the self-sufficient Virginia colony (Hobhouse 1989). Over the following two centuries, the rapid expansion of tobacco production in the American colonies helped finance American independence and helped fuel the transatlantic slave trade. While historically the United States was the main supplier of tobacco to the world, since the 1960s the bulk of tobacco production has moved to low- and middle-income countries, where production grew by 128% between 1975 and 1998, while falling by 31% in developed countries (Jacobs et al. 2000). (See figure 3.2.) U.S. land devoted to tobacco growing was halved in the last decades of the 1900s, while it almost doubled in China, Malawi, and the Republic of Tanzania (Mackay and Eriksen 2002).

As the international tobacco trade grew, national

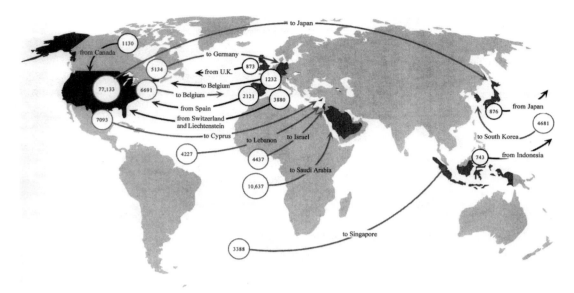

FIGURE 3.2. Modern Trade Flow of Tobacco Leaf (in metric tons of cigarettes). *Source:* Mackay and Eriksen (2002). Permission provided by WHO.

treasuries quickly recognized that significant revenues could be generated from the sale and taxation of tobacco, and it was not long before initial tobacco control laws were repealed (Jha and Chaloupka 2000). Even James I backed down from his attempts at tobacco prohibition after enjoying the revenues that could be gained from tobacco taxes (Arents 1938). In 1776, economic theorist Adam Smith suggested that tobacco represented one of the few commodities governments should tax, because the tax revenue generated would allow poor people to "live better, work cheaper, and to send their goods cheaper to market" (Smith 1776). Two centuries later, nearly every government in the world taxes tobacco. Their motives have mainly been to generate revenue, but in recent years taxation has also been used, by at least some governments, as a way of reducing the health damage caused by tobacco and for covering the economic and social costs of tobacco use (World Bank 1999).

EVOLUTION OF THE TRANSNATIONAL TOBACCO INDUSTRY

Like modern globalization, contemporary tobacco use has its roots in the industrial revolution and the laissez-faire economic policies of the late nineteenth century. Until the latter half of the 1800s, tobacco consumption was nearly entirely confined to chewing, snuff, and pipe smoking. By contrast, in 2003, mass-manufactured cigarettes, together with hand-rolled bidis consumed in South Asia, accounted for 85% of all tobacco consumed worldwide (table 3.2) (FAO 2003). Three major inventions led to the popular use of cigarettes. First was the discovery of a standard method for producing flue-cured tobacco leaves in Virginia in 1839. Flue-cured "yellow" tobacco resulted in a mild-flavored smoke more appealing to the general public than the harsh dark tobacco previously available. In 2003, Virginia flue-cured tobacco was the predominant type of tobacco produced, with increasing share in total tobacco production worldwide (FAO 2003). Second was the invention in 1852 of safety matches, making smoking much more convenient. Third was the invention in 1880 of the first practical cigarette-making machine by James Bonsack. One Bonsack machine could perform the work of forty-eight workers and significantly cut the cost of manufacturing (Duke Homestead Historical Site 2004). In 1884, James Duke formed a partnership with James Bonsack in which he gained an advantageous leasing arrangement over two cigarette-making machines. By the end of the year, Duke had produced 744 million cigarettes, more than the national total in 1883 (Borio 1997). Over the next century, cigarette

TABLE 3.2. Total Cigarette Consumption 1970–2000 (million sticks)

	1970	1975	1980	1985	1990	1995	2000
Levels of Development							
Developed	1,462,484	1,671,140	1,755,758	1,705,064	1,604,389	1,588,411	1,496,606
Developing	1,093,936	1,381,203	1,917,390	2,503,841	2,982,487	3,126,193	3,344,068
Transition	580,797	656,639	687,635	715,036	647,541	659,302	703,195
World	3,261,565	3,853,906	4,452,619	5,060,363	5,328,264	5,308,016	5,710,889

Source: Guindon and Boisclar (2003).

manufacturing became more and more mechanized, making many workers redundant. In 2002, more than 5.5 trillion cigarettes were produced a year—nearly 1,000 for every man, woman, and child on the planet (Mackay and Eriksen 2002).

The cost savings associated with his arrangement with Bonsack allowed Duke to sell his cigarettes cheaper than his competitors. In 1890, following a series of price wars, Duke merged with several competitors to form the American Tobacco Company (Duke Homestead Historical Site 2004). Over the next two decades, the American Tobacco Company virtually controlled tobacco production and trade worldwide. However, in 1907 the U.S. Justice Department filed an antitrust suit against the company. In 1911 the company was broken into several major companies that together dominated the global tobacco business in the twentieth century, including the American Tobacco Company, R.J. Reynolds, Liggett & Meyers Tobacco Company, Lorillard, and BAT.

Prior to the 1980s, the large tobacco companies largely exported cigarettes from facilities in the United States and Western Europe. The past 25 years has witnessed a complete transformation and globalization of the tobacco industry. The major TTCs have established a presence in almost every country on the planet. The three largest TTCs now own or lease manufacturing facilities in more than 50 countries each (Hammond 1998). Three main factors have fuelled this expansion: the opening up of formerly closed economies in the former Soviet Union, Eastern Europe, and China, pressure on countries by the World Bank and International Monetary Fund to liberalize foreign investment laws and privatize state-owned tobacco companies, and the expansion of free trade areas in Asia and Latin America (Hammond 1998).

The multinational tobacco companies were some of the first foreign companies to establish operations in the Soviet Union and Eastern Europe following the collapse of communist governments there in the late 1980s. Taking advantage of pressure from the international financial institutions on these countries to quickly liberalize their economies and privatize state-owned industries, the companies spent billions purchasing and modernizing state tobacco monopolies across the region. These purchases were quickly followed by advertising and promotion campaigns on a scale never seen in these countries, campaigns that sought to link smoking with freedom, affluence, and other "Western" values. In China, the political leadership's decision to pursue a path of economic liberalization and membership in the World Trade Organization has presented unprecedented opportunities for the multinational tobacco companies to establish a foothold in the world's largest cigarette market (Frankel and Muson 1996). Since the late 1990s, these companies have signed numerous cooperation agreements with Chinese tobacco companies to modernize manufacturing facilities, improve crop yields, and build tobacco processing plants.

Thinking about the Chinese smoking statistics is like trying to think about the limits of space.
—Fletcher (1992)

Since the early 1980s, pressure on developing countries from the International Monetary Fund and World Bank to privatize state-owned industries and liberalize foreign investment laws, as well as countries' desperate need for foreign exchange earnings, has led to the selling off of most of the world's state-owned tobacco companies. Between 1991 and 2001 alone, there were more than 140 mergers and acquisitions involving international tobacco companies in countries as diverse as Spain, Hungary, Indonesia, Vietnam, and Mexico (Callard et al. 2001). In most cases, subsidiaries of sophisticated multinational tobacco companies replaced sleepy, inefficient state-owned industries. When the TTC took over these new markets, they replaced high-priced, poor-quality products that helped to limit smoking mostly to older men who had the money and taste for harsh, tar-heavy local brands, with jazzier international brands and marketing campaigns that targeted the untapped markets of women and young people. Also driving these purchases has been the emergence of regional free trade areas in the Americas and Asia, which has encouraged these companies to locate manufacturing facilities within these areas in order to take advantage of lower tariffs.

The other major change in the global tobacco industry over the past decade has been a series of huge mergers and acquisitions among the major international players. Beginning in April 1999 with the purchase by BAT of Carolinian-based Rothmans, the fourth largest tobacco company at the time, followed a few weeks later by JT's purchase of the overseas operations of U.S.-based R.J. Reynolds, the size and global reach of the largest tobacco companies have been transformed. In 2002, the combined tobacco revenues of PM, BAT, and JT was greater than the combined gross national product of Albania, Bahrain, Belize, Bolivia, Botswana, Cambodia, Cameroon, Estonia, Georgia, Ghana, Honduras, Jamaica, Jordan, Macedonia, Malawi, Malta, Moldova, Mongolia, Namibia, Nepal, Paraguay, Senegal, Tajikistan, Togo, Uganda, Zambia, and Zimbabwe (Jacobs et al. 2000). In many ways, the tobacco industry at the start of the twenty-first century appears to be returning to the monopolistic structure broken apart nearly 100 years before. (See figure 3.3.)

Increasingly open international borders and the expansion of global tobacco trade have also resulted in increased opportunities for smuggling. In 2002, it was estimated that around one-quarter of internationally traded cigarettes entered the black market, making cigarettes the world's most widely smuggled legal consumer product (WHO 2002). From a world export total of 846 billion cigarettes in 2000, some 227 billion did not reappear as imports (Framework Convention Alliance 2002). Smuggling is commonly misunderstood as arising from tax differentials between countries or states, but this is a relatively small part of the smuggling problem (Framework Convention Alliance). Most cigarette smuggling results from organized large-scale tobacco smuggling, which involves the diversion of large consignments of cigarettes into the black market while in transit (Merriman et al. 2000). By diverting cigarettes while they are in the wholesale distribution chain, large-scale smugglers avoid all tobacco taxes.

Total loss of tax revenues by governments due to cigarette smuggling around the world is estimated at US$25–30 billion annually (Jha and Chaloupka 2000). Tobacco manufacturers and wholesalers, on the contrary, are not harmed by tobacco smuggling since they make their profit when the product is first sold, before it enters the transit trade. Moreover, they gain from smuggling in many ways. Smuggling gives the companies access to closed markets and increases the supply of cheap cigarettes by reducing the average cigarette price, thus stimulating demand. Moreover, the existence or even the threat of large-scale smuggling allows tobacco company lobbyist to argue against increased tobacco taxes. The commercial benefits of smuggling have led some companies to support and, in some cases, participate in the illicit tobacco trade, viewing it as just another distribution channel to be monitored and managed alongside legal, duty-paid sales. Evidence that BAT and other tobacco companies have encouraged and participated in tobacco smuggling has resulted in some governments suing tobacco companies to recover lost taxes (Beelman 2004).

INDUSTRY INFLUENCE OVER TOBACCO REGULATION

The global tobacco industry manufactures and aggressively markets the only legal product that kills when used as intended. Often containing more than 600 additives and numerous carcinogens, the modern

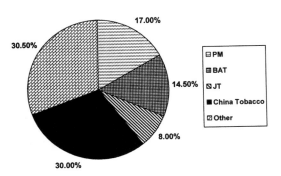

17.00%

30.50%

14.50%

8.00%

30.00%

PM
BAT
JT
China Tobacco
Other

FIGURE 3.3. Global Cigarette Market Share 2002.
Source: Fletcher (2004).

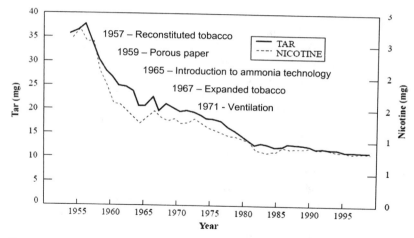

FIGURE 3.4. The Changing Cigarette. Values before 1968 are estimated from available data. *Source:* NCI (2002).

cigarette is a highly engineered product (Bollinger and Fagerstrom 1997). Numerous changes have been made to the cigarette over the decades to make it appear less harmful and taste better and to increase its addictiveness (figure 3.4). These alterations include the introduction of filter tips, addition of flavorings such as honey and vanilla, use of ammonia technology to increase the effects of nicotine on the brain, and utilization of ventilation and dilution techniques to obtain misleading measurements of tar and nicotine (Bollinger and Fagerstrom 1997). Industry whistleblower Jeffrey Wigand described the continual evolution of the cigarette when he said: "What the [tobacco] industry wants people to believe is that a cigarette is nothing but a natural product grown in the ground, ripped out, stuffed in a piece of paper and served up. It's not. It's a meticulously engineered product. The purpose behind a cigarette . . . is to deliver nicotine—an addictive drug" (Dawson 1999).

The effects of nicotine in tobacco on the body have long been recognized. In 1890, tobacco appeared in the U.S. Pharmacopoeia, an official U.S. government listing of drugs (Fritschler 1969). It was dropped in 1905 after tobacco companies threatened that as long as tobacco was included, the tobacco-growing states would not support the passage of the 1906 Food and Drug Act, the legislation that created the Food and Drug Administration (FDA) (Fritschler 1969). Despite irrefutable evidence regarding how nicotine affects the body, the FDA still cannot regulate nicotine in tobacco. In 1996, with the support of

U.S. President Bill Clinton, the FDA declared it had authority over tobacco products and announced a series of new regulations (Federal Register 1996). These regulations brought fierce opposition from tobacco companies, who sought to challenge the FDA in court. In 2000, after multiple decisions by lower courts, the U.S. Supreme Court ruled in a 5–4 decision that Congress did not intend to delegate jurisdiction over tobacco products to the FDA (FDA v. Brown & Williamson Tobacco Corp. 2000). In the decision, the Court cited the Pure Food and Drug Act of 1906 and repeated congressional rejections of FDA authority over tobacco despite evidence that "tobacco use, particularly among children and adolescents, poses perhaps the most significant threat to public health in the United States" (FDA v. Brown & Williamson Tobacco Corp. 2000).

Early political lobbying by tobacco companies, and the subsequent U.S. decisions not to establish standards over tobacco products, has had global implications. The lack of regulatory mechanisms in the United States has certainly influenced the fact that tobacco has also existed in a regulatory "no-man's land" internationally. For example, until the adoption of the FCTC, in only a few countries were tobacco companies required to disclose the contents of their cigarettes or provide customers basic information regarding the products they are consuming. Tobacco companies benefited from the unregulated international environment, especially in low- and middle-income countries that lacked the domestic capacity to challenge industry activities and educate the public regarding the health risks associated with tobacco consumption.

Political lobbying remains a strategic activity of the TTCs. Its well-funded and sophisticated corporate lobbying machine aims to resist restrictive legislation that would reduce their sales and to realign national and international laws so as to enlarge its corporate rights and reduce its corporate responsibilities (Saloojee and Dagli 2000). This lobbying effort is undertaken by the companies themselves, as well as through third parties, and targets governments, international institutions, and the media.

In Central and South America, for example, PM and BAT, working through the U.S. law firm Covington & Burling, developed the "Latin Project" to counter regulations aimed at creating smoke-free workplaces and public places (Pan American Health Organization 2002, Barnoya and Glantz 2002). Argentina provides the clearest case of successful lobbying conducted under this project. On September 30, 1991, the Argentine Senate approved the "Neri Bill," which sought to end all tobacco advertising, promotion, and sampling and severely limit smoking in public places. A strong tobacco industry lobbying campaign ensued, relying heavily on media debates and industry consultant Carlos Alvarez, who was Argentine President Menem's chief scientific advisor. Alvarez met numerous times with the president and other senators and developed a briefing packet arguing that the proposed smoking restrictions lacked a solid scientific basis (Barnoya and Glantz 2002). On October 13, 1991, President Menem vetoed the law.

In the Middle East, the major TTCs operating in the region formed the Middle East Working Group, which later became the Middle East Tobacco Association, to promote and defend the interests of the companies in the region (Hammond and White 2002). Companies enlisted prominent political figures to provide information and lobby for them, including an Egyptian member of Parliament, a former assistant secretary general of the Arab League and even, at one point, the secretary general of the Gulf Cooperation Council Health Ministers who was also the Kuwaiti undersecretary for health (Hammond and White 2002). In Africa, the industry developed the International Tobacco Growers' Association (ITGA) to lobby on their behalf. The ITGA, along with other international consortiums such as the International Council

on Smoking Issues, later known as the International Tobacco Information Centre, targeted the United Nations, the Food and Agriculture Organization (FAO), and WHO in particular (WHO 2000a).

The U.S. Congress has also remained a vital lobbying target. During the first half of 1998, for example, the industry reportedly spent more than US$43 million on lobbying against federal tobacco legislation sponsored by Senator John McCain. The industry's advertising campaign against the bill was, according to the dean of communications at the University of Pennsylvania, Kathleen Hall Jamieson, the highest amount ever spent in a sustained issue advocacy campaign in the United States (Saloojee and Dagli 2000).

INDUSTRY ADVERTISING
AND PROMOTION

The tobacco industry has been at the forefront of advertising and promotion since the late 1800s. Duke, an aggressive advertiser, devised new and startling methods that dismayed his competitors and was always willing to spend in advertising a proportion of his profits that seemed appalling to more conservative manufacturers (Duke Homestead Historical Site 2004). Tobacco provided one of the first demonstrations that advertising could create demand for a product when no previous demand existed and has significantly contributed to the notion that consumption is an act of the imagination—that is, that one buys not just the product but also the attributes for which the product is merely a vehicle (USDHHS 2000). Through the years, tobacco industry advertising has used images of rebellion, health, fitness, stress relief, wealth, weight loss, and sex appeal to construct and perpetuate social attributes linked to cigarette smoking. The most infamous of all cigarette ad campaigns, Phillip Morris's Marlboro Man, associated cigarettes with the American West and a masculine approach to life that rejected concerns surrounding the potential health risks associated with daily pleasures. Launched in the early 1960s, the campaign transformed a stagnant American brand into a transnational business phenomenon and "one of the quintessential global brands" (Klein 2000). It was declared the number one advertising icon of the twentieth century by *Advertising Age* magazine (Yach and Bettcher 2000).

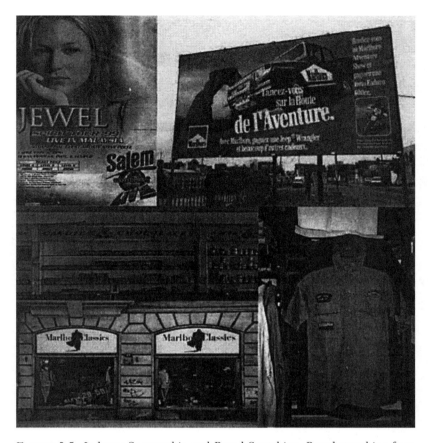

FIGURE 3.5. Industry Sponsorship and Brand Stretching. Brand stretching from top left (*clockwise*): music concert in Malaysia, Mary Assunta; adventure concert in Senegal, Anna White; Camel active wear, Thailand, Ross Hammond; Marlboro men's store, Czech Republic, Ross Hammond; convenience store, Malaysia, Ehsan Latif. Reproduced with permission.

Industry marketing increasingly taps into globalization trends to develop a "global mental framework" in association with their cigarettes to overcome markets that have thus far resisted the industry's onslaught—a strategy employed to associate cigarettes with modernity, prosperity, and internationalism (Yach and Bettcher 1999, Collin 2003). In India, for example, where traditional use of bidis and chewing tobacco remains the preferred form of tobacco use, the industry uses global brands to encourage young smokers to switch to manufactured cigarettes (Crescenti 1998). The industry uses every conceivable medium to promote cigarettes, including television, newspapers and magazines, billboards, and the Internet. The companies also use a whole host of "indirect advertising" methods, including sponsoring sporting events and teams; promoting music concerts and parties; placing their brand logos on T-shirts, backpacks, and other merchandise popular among children; sponsoring adventure contests; and giving away free cigarettes and brand merchandise in places where youth gather, such as rock concerts and shopping malls (CTFK 2001). (See figure 3.5.)

Marketing and promotional strategies in low- and middle-income countries are particularly targeted at women, capitalizing on Western images of independence, equality with men, glamour, and sophistication to break down the traditional taboos against female smoking (figure 3.6). Images of beauty and weight loss/management are used to falsely associate them with cigarette smoking in female-targeted tobacco advertising (CTFK 2001).

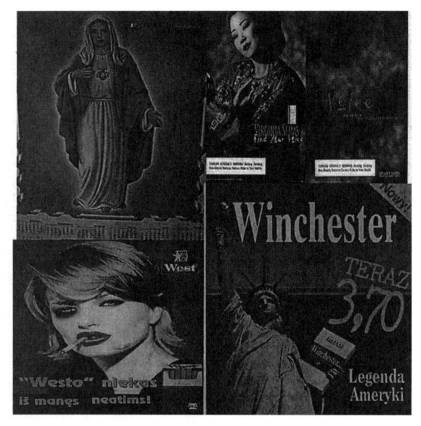

FIGURE 3.6. Examples of Tobacco Advertising Targeted at Women. International tobacco ads from top left (*clockwise*): Virgin Mary calendar, Philippines, Bobby del Rosario; Find Your Voice, Asia, Campaign for Tobacco Free Kids; American legend, Poland; "I'd rather be beaten than do without my cigarettes," Poland, Katarzyna Stanclik.

RISE OF THE CIGARETTE

The rise of popular cigarette use over the past century has been astounding (table 3.2). In the 1960s, 50% of the U.S. adult male population and more than 80% of adult men in Japan smoked; by 1970 nearly 75% of men smoked in Poland (Mackay and Eriksen 2002, Zatonski and Przewozniak 1992). In 2003, thanks to aggressive tobacco control programs, smoking prevalence had decreased to 25% and roughly 40% among U.S. and Polish men, respectively (Shafey et al. 2003). In Japan, where tobacco control policies have been extremely difficult to institute, approximately 50% of men continue to smoke (Shafey et al. 2003). While prevalence rates in most high-income countries have begun to decline, prevalence in low- and

middle-income countries continues to grow. Between 1970 and 2000, cigarette consumption in low- and middle-income countries rose more than threefold, from 1.1 billion to 3.3 billion cigarettes, while cigarette consumption in developed countries rose only slightly (Guindon and Boisclair 2003).

In many low- and middle-income countries, prevalence rates among men approach and exceed the 60% mark (Shafey et al. 2003). While the global prevalence of tobacco use remains significantly higher among men (47%) than among women (12%), this is changing quickly (WHO 2002). In some countries, such as Sweden and Norway, female smoking rates have overtaken male smoking rates (Shafey et al. 2003). In many countries where female prevalence has been traditionally low, industry penetration and marketing are

TABLE 3.3. GYTS Results: Percentage of Boys and Girls Smoking

	Boys currently smoking cigarettes	Girls currently smoking cigarettes	Boy:Girl ratio
Overall / Median	15.0	6.6	1.9:1.0
Africa	10.4	4.6	2.2:1.0
Burkina Faso	28.6	9.6	3.0:1.0
South Africa	21.0	10.6	2.0:1.0
Americas	16.6	12.2	1.2:1.0
Columbia	31.0	33.4	0.9:1.0
United States	17.7	17.8	1.0:1.0
Eastern Mediterranean	22.8	5.3	4.3:1.0
Jordan	22.0	9.9	2.2:1.0
Europe	33.9	29.0	1.2:1.0
Bulgaria	26.0	39.4	0.7:1.0
Czech Republic	34.0	35.1	1.0:1.0
Southeast Asia	13.5	3.2	4.2:1.0
Indonesia	38.9	4.7	8.3:1.0
Myanmar	19.0	3.2	5.9:1.0
Western Pacific	11.0	6.4	1.7:1.0
Palau	20.0	23.3	0.9:1.0

Source: CDC (2004).

resulting in increasing prevalence among females, especially among young women. Evidence from the Global Youth Tobacco Survey (GYTS) shows that girls thirteen to fourteen years of age were more likely to smoke than are boys of the same age in Bulgaria, Denmark, Ireland, Italy, Malta, Norway, Slovenia, and the United Kingdom (table 3.3) (CDC 2004). Moreover, in Asian countries that traditionally had very low female smoking rates (< 10%), GYTS data show much lower male:female smoking ratios among the youth (GYTS Collaborating Group 2003).

Tobacco consumption also has a very strong and complex social class gradient. In most countries, individuals with the highest educational standards are less likely to smoke. In China, individuals with no schooling are nearly seven times more likely to smoke than are individuals with a college degree, while uneducated adults in Brazil are five times more likely to smoke than are adults who received at least a college degree (WHO 2004a). In Poland in 1996, the risk of dying during middle age due to tobacco-related disease was 5% among people with higher education and nearly double (9%) among persons with only primary and secondary education levels (Bobak et al. 2000). However, it does not follow simply that moderate increases in education lead immediately to less

tobacco consumption (figure 3.7). In many low- and middle-income countries, increasing urbanization, increases in educational levels and the associated marginal increases in income often result in higher consumption patterns (Yach 1990).

Countries, development agencies, donors, and multilateral agencies are recognizing the broad social implications of tobacco use (World Bank 2003a, Efroymson et al. 2001b). Studies show that poor smokers can spend a significant portion of their household income on tobacco. In Bulgaria, low-income households with at least one smoker spent up to 10% of their total income on tobacco products (Sayginsoy

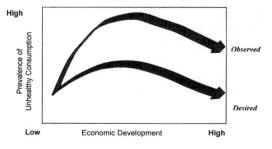

FIGURE 3.7. Rise in Income Leads to Rise in Unhealthy Consumption. *Source:* WHO (2004b).

et al. 2002). In the Minhang District of China, smokers surveyed reported spending 17% of their household income on cigarettes (WHO 2004b). The money that poor households spend on tobacco products has very high opportunity costs. In Bangladesh, for example, it is estimated that if the money spent on cigarettes were spent on food instead, it could save more than 10 million people from malnutrition (Efroymson et al. 2001a). In Morocco, the average amount spent by poor households on tobacco was virtually the same as the amount spent on education and more than half the amount spent on health care (Nassar 2003). In addition, most tobacco farmers are barely making a living producing a crop that is labor and input intensive and brings with it a host of health and environmental dangers, from pesticide exposure to nicotine poisoning (WHO 2004a).

GLOBAL RESPONSE TO TOBACCO

In the early 1900s, the negative health effects of tobacco were still not known. Growing rates of lung cancer were most often ascribed to atmospheric pollution from coal smoke. Cigarettes were commonly advertised with the endorsement of physicians carrying slogans such as "more doctors smoke Camels," "soothe the throat," or "aid digestion" (Brown & Williamson Tobacco Company 1964). However, with the growth of cigarette smoking, studies addressing the health effects of smoking began to appear. In the 1930s, scientists in Germany were making statistical correlations between cancer and smoking (Lickint 1929, Müller 1939). In 1938, Dr. Raymond Pearl of Johns Hopkins University reported that smokers do not live as long as nonsmokers (Pearl 1938). The year 1950 marked a watershed event with the publication of three key case–control studies all linking smoking to higher risk of lung cancer (Doll and Hill 1950, Levin et al. 1950, Wynder and Graham 1950). In 1953, Ernst Wynder demonstrated that cigarette tar caused tumors on the backs of mice, and Richard Doll and Bradford Hill followed up their 1950 article with a nationwide prospective survey of British doctors (Wynder et al. 1953, Doll and Hill 1954).

Broad public acceptance of the link between smoking and cancer, as well as the principal birth of modern tobacco control efforts, can be largely accredited to the release of the Royal College of Physicians report in 1962 in the United Kingdom and first U.S.

Surgeon General's report in 1964, both entitled "Smoking and Health." The reports concluded that cigarette smoking is causally related to lung cancer and recommended legislative action to control its use (Royal College of Physicians 1962, U.S. Public Health Service 1964). Elsewhere in the world, early calls for tobacco control measures were also heard. In 1963, the *South African Medical Journal* urgently called on the South African government to ban smoking in public places and on public transport, eliminate tobacco advertising, require health warnings, and increase taxation of cigarettes (South African Medical Journal 1963). It took, however, more than twelve years for the South African government to enact even one of the recommendations, and another twenty years after that to develop an effective multipronged tobacco control program.

Since the 1950s, tens of thousands of scientific articles originating from researchers throughout the world have implicated active and passive smoking in causing a wide variety of diseases and other adverse health effects. This global evidence base constitutes the largest and best-documented body of literature linking any behavior and environmental agent to disease in humans (USDHHS 1994). Key scientific findings continue to be made by researchers. Research continues to reaffirm that tobacco kills wherever it is consumed, and patterns of smoking-related diseases differ somewhat from country to country. In India and China, for example, studies show that while the relative risks of cardiovascular disease appear lower than in Western countries, smoking seems very important in increasing the risk of tuberculosis, a major disease in both countries (Gajalakahmi et al. 2003, Liu et al. 1998). Economic research increasingly plays a key role in building the evidence base for effective tobacco control policies. Researchers in India, Poland, and South Africa have made important contribution regarding tobacco economics and the effects of economic globalization, as has the World Bank.

INDUSTRY EFFORTS TO
UNDERMINE THE SCIENTIFIC
EVIDENCE BASE

Despite overwhelming evidence, the tobacco industry has fought hard to discredit the conclusions of the international scientific community that their products kill. In 1954 the industry created the Tobacco Industry

Research Committee to conduct its own scientific studies and on January 4, 1954, it released the "Frank Statement to Cigarette Smokers" in 448 newspapers throughout the United States. In the Frank Statement, the industry stated: "We accept an interest in people's health as a basic responsibility, paramount to every other consideration in our business.... We believe the products we make are not injurious to health.... We always have and always will cooperate closely with those whose task it is to safeguard the public health" (American Tobacco Companies 1954). This statement is often cited as the official start of the industry's decades-long campaign of public deceit regarding the health effects of active and passive smoking.

At the same time, the industry also began to mass-market filtered cigarettes and later low-tar formulations that promised a "healthier" smoke. The strategy was effective, and cigarette sales boomed. It took nearly fifty years for the scientific community to conclude that allegedly "reduced risk" products, including "light" and "low tar" cigarettes, do not offer any protection to smokers (NCI 2002, McNeill 2004). Conversely, false perceptions regarding the harmful nature of these products and the way smokers use them have actually resulted in higher tobacco-related morbidity and morality. These findings have intensified concerns regarding new "reduced risk" products being developed and marketed by the industry.

In 1998, as a condition of settling ongoing litigation with the Attorney General of Minnesota, the tobacco industry made available to the public millions of confidential documents dating back to the early 1930s (Ciresi et al. 1999). A further settlement required that the industry make the Minnesota documents available to all on the Internet and to add additional documents that were produced in other smoking and health litigation for a period of ten years (Master Settlement Agreement 1998). These documents offer a unique insight into the industry's role in influencing public policy and in shaping the conduct and public perception of science (Ciresi et al. 1999). The documents proved that the companies were themselves aware of the harmful effects of smoking since the mid-1950s and implemented a strategy to hide this information and undermine the growing evidence base. In particular, the industry used its own research institutes to produce contradictory results, paid scientists to challenge established scientific methods such as epidemiology, and publicly rejected

claims that their products were dangerous or addictive (Hurt and Robertson 1998, Drope and Chapman 2001, Ong and Glantz 2001). Moreover, industry documents prove that the industry targeted vulnerable population groups such as women, ethnic minorities, young people, and the poor and penetrated major national and international public health bodies (Perry 1999, Hastings and McFadyen 2000, Bialous and Yach 2001, Ong and Glantz 2001).

Starting in 1999, international tobacco control activists began gathering evidence from the documents that suggested that WHO tobacco control policies may have been affected by tobacco company practices aimed at influencing funding, policy, and research priorities (Ong and Glantz 2000). These findings led the WHO director general to appoint a committee of independent experts to assess whether those fears were justified and what, if any, was the long-term effect within WHO. The committee found that tobacco companies fought WHO's tobacco control agenda by, among other things, staging events to divert attention from the public health issues raised by tobacco use, attempting to reduce budgets for scientific and policy activities carried out by WHO, pitting other United Nations agencies against WHO, seeking to convince developing countries that WHO's tobacco control program was a "first-world" agenda carried out at the expense of the developing world, distorting the results of important scientific studies on tobacco, and discrediting WHO as an institution (Zeltner et al. 2000). The committee concluded that the tobacco companies' activities slowed and undermined effective tobacco control programs around the world and that the tobacco companies' subversion of WHO's activities had resulted in "significant harm" to global public health.

The release of the inquiry conclusions received global media coverage and helped encourage numerous other countries and regions to undertake their own independent document inquiries into industry influence on their public institutions and policy-making processes. The United Kingdom parliamentary inquiry provided hard evidence that BAT played an important role in conspiracy that allowed cigarette smuggling to happen (House of Commons 2000). The Pan American Health Organization's inquiry report, *Profits over People* (2002), revealed a well-planned industrywide strategy to undermine tobacco control initiatives throughout Central and South America. The broad implications of industry influence on high-level policy makers revealed in the WHO Eastern Mediterranean Regional Office's inquiry report, *Voices of Truth*, helped to convince Her Majesty Queen Rania Al-Abdullah of Jordan to host an international conference on tobacco litigation and public inquiries (White and Hammond 2002).

GLOBAL IMPACT OF TOBACCO CONSUMPTION

Industry efforts to deny the science and deceive the public could not change the public health impact of active and passive smoking. In fifty years of observations of doctors in the United Kingdom, Doll found that prolonged cigarette smoking from early adult life tripled age-specific mortality rates (Doll et al. 2004). Between 1930 and 1990. Lung cancer rates among U.S. males went from 5 to more than 75 in 100,000, a 1,4 00% increase in fifty years (Peto et al. 1994). (See figure 3.8.) Once an extremely rare disease, lung cancer became a leading form of cancer for both men and women in high-income countries.

Cardiovascular disease and chronic obstructive lung diseases also increased rapidly in high-income countries as a result of increased tobacco use (Peto et al. 1994).

The changing disease burden in these countries reflected an "epidemiological transition" from the infectious disease epidemics of the past to high rates of chronic diseases. Public health campaigns in high-income countries were initially slow to reflect this disease transition; however, aggressive tobacco control campaigns appear to be having some impact on reduced death rates from heart disease and lung cancer incidence (Fichtenberg and Glantz 2002). Between 1985 and 2000, lung cancer deaths in men dropped in many European countries, including the United Kingdom (38% decrease), Finland (36%), Netherlands (29%), Luxembourg (24%), Austria (23%), and Ireland (22%) (Boyle et al. 2003).

However, the same cannot be said for low- and middle-income countries, where the full scale of the tobacco epidemic lies ahead. In the twentieth century, three out of four tobacco-related deaths occurred in high-income countries. Current projections indicate that by 2030, of the 10 million annual worldwide deaths from tobacco, 70% will occur in low- and middle-income countries (WHO 2002). In China alone, annual smoking deaths are expected rise from 1 million to 3 million by 2050 (Liu et al. 1998). Due to a delay of approximately twenty years between smoking and death, this disease burden is based on

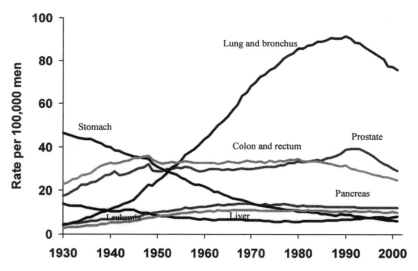

FIGURE 3.8. The Spectacular Rise of Lung Cancer Death Rates among U.S. Men. Data are cancer death rates per 100,000 U.S. men, age adjusted to the 2000 U.S. standard population. *Note*: due to changes in International Classification of Disease coding, numerator information has changed over time. Rates for cancers of the liver, lung and bronchus, and colon and rectum are affected by these coding changes. *Source*: Jemal et al. (2004).

tobacco consumption trends measured in the late 1990s, which is largely limited to the adult male population in low- and middle-income countries. Large increases in female prevalence could send this estimate even higher. Unlike high-income countries, increasing rates of chronic disease are occurring simultaneously with the infectious diseases of the past as well as the devastating impact of HIV/AIDS. Low- and middle-income countries experience what Yach et al. (1992) have coined the "epidemiological trap," saddling their health care systems with considerable new health costs while having to continue to treat infectious disease.

DOMESTIC TOBACCO CONTROL MOBILIZES

As the tobacco epidemic grew, so too did public health demands for urgent action to control tobacco consumption. Domestic forerunners in tobacco control included Canada, Finland, Norway, Singapore, and the United States. Their early efforts eventually framed the basis of current global tobacco control efforts.

The exact mix of early tobacco control policy responses adopted differed from country to country, reflecting their underlying political, social, and economic realities. Singapore and Finland were able to institute comprehensive national tobacco control legislation in the 1970s that included advertising bans, health warnings on all cigarette packages, indoor-smoking prohibitions, and tobacco taxes. Norway passed a comprehensive national advertising ban in 1975 but did not consistently increase tobacco taxes.

In the United States, longstanding linkages between the federal government and the tobacco industry, combined with early preemption at the federal level, led advocates to focus on the state and the local level. Tobacco control advocates in the United States quickly learned that the local level provided many advantages when combating the industry. First, the costs of running election and public health campaigns are much lower than at the state or national level, and political leaders are much more accessible and sensitive to the interests of their constituents. Moreover, tobacco industry efforts to lobby at the local level are much easier to uncover for the public and can easily backfire. Most important, the substantial controversy generated by tobacco companies in opposition to local

regulation often leads to substantial public debate. For example, the tobacco industry recognized as early as the 1970s that enactment of policies restricting or ending smoking in public places would severely undermine the social acceptability of smoking and create an environment that would make it much easier for smokers to stop smoking and that would discourage young people from starting (Drope and Chapman 2001). Subsequent scientific research has confirmed this concern; smoke-free workplaces are associated with a 29% reduction in cigarette consumption (Fichtenberg and Glantz 2002). The industry therefore aggressively fought local clean indoor air measures (often working through surrogates with undisclosed links to the tobacco industry, e.g., "hospitality associations") (Muggli et al. 2001, Hirschorn and Bialous 2001). Protracted public debates led to considerable discussion and raised public awareness of the dangers of second-hand smoke. This public awareness then facilitated the implementation and enforcement of local indoor smoking restrictions, once they were passed.

The local experience with clean indoor air in the United States demonstrates that the process of developing and implementing policy is an integral part of making the policy itself work. In Norway, there was a notable fall in smoking rates during and immediately after the widespread discussion that led up to the 1975 legislation (Crofton and Simpson 2002). However, after the laws had been passed, discussion died away and taxation rates were not continuously raised. Smoking rates fell more slowly, evened out, and then tended to rise (Crofton and Simpson 2002). In Sweden, a strong tobacco control alliance has continuously generated public discussion, and smoking rates have continued to decline. In 2003, Sweden had the lowest smoking rates in Europe (Shafey et al. 2003). In other countries, health advocates quietly passed many admirable tobacco control laws with little public debate or education about the need for these laws. As a result, public support for the laws was never articulated, and there is no political pressure to fully implement and enforce them. In France, for example, excellent tobacco control laws have been passed without building public support first, and courts have imposed large fines on tobacco companies for breaking the law against tobacco promotion. However, smoke-free public places are rarely carried out in practice because the public does not insist on its enforcement (Crofton and Simpson 2002). In Canada,

Australia, and Singapore, tobacco control activities have successfully roused public opinion, and in each case excellent legislation has been passed and is effectively implemented, including restrictions on indoor smoking.

INTERNATIONAL COLLABORATION AND NETWORKING

The increasing international activities of the major tobacco companies throughout the 1980s and 1990s led to increasing collaboration and coordination between domestic tobacco control activists. International interaction was encouraged through large tobacco control conferences, such as the World Conference on Tobacco or Health first held in 1967, and the emergence of the Internet. Thailand provided one of the first opportunities for tobacco control advocates to collaborate internationally. Throughout the 1980s the U.S. government used the notoriously aggressive office of the U.S. Trade Representative to open up Asian markets to U.S. tobacco companies (Frankel 1996b). The U.S. government successfully pressured Japan, South Korea, and Taiwan to allow American companies to sell cigarettes and demanded that the companies be allowed to advertise, hold giveaway promotions, and sponsor concerts and sports events. In each of these countries, the state-run monopoly was overtaken by the jazzier American brands in free competition. The result was the creation of new demand, especially among women and young people. After South Korea opened its market to U.S. companies in 1988, for example, the smoking rate among male Korean teens rose from 18.4% to 29.8% in a single year. The rate among female teens more than quintupled from 1.6% to 8.7% (Taylor et al. 2000).

After previous successes, the tobacco companies were anticipating another relatively easy victory in Thailand (Frankel 1996a). However, this did not happen. Shortly after the U.S. Trade Representative filed its complaint against Thailand requiring that they allow U.S. cigarette makers free market access in the country, Prakit Vateesatokit, a staunch Thai tobacco control advocate, attended the Asia-Pacific Association for Control of Tobacco (Vateesatokit 2003). There he met Greg Connolly, a veteran tobacco control advocate from Massachusetts. With his assistance, Vateesatokit and his public health colleagues

were able to enlist the support of the Thai government and the state-run monopoly, got themselves appointed to the official delegation that fought the U.S. trade demands, and pleaded Thailand's case before the multilateral forum of the General Agreement on Tariffs and Trade, the predecessor to the World Trade Organization. Connolly and other international experts also assisted in drafting and implementing one of the world's strictest tobacco control policies. The Thai experience quickly became a regional example, as other countries turned to Vateesatokit and his international colleagues for information and advice on how to best confront the tobacco industry in Asia.

The emergence of the Internet as a low-cost, rapid communications medium transformed tobacco control. Before the Internet, the tobacco industry could send its "experts"—often without disclosing their relationship to the tobacco industry—into a country, state, or locality, accomplish its political or public relations mission (e.g., arguing that second-hand smoke is not dangerous or that ventilation was a reasonable and feasible solution to the problems created by second-hand smoke), and then be gone before any of the local public health advocates realized who they were. With the Internet, it is possible for public health activists to rapidly learn who these people are and what are their connections to the industry. South Africa provided one of the first illustrations of this. Following the dramatic political changes brought about by the end of the apartheid regime in the early 1990s, new political support for the development of tobacco control legislation emerged. In response, the tobacco industry significantly increased their lobbying activities in the country by sponsoring media workshops, lobbying the hospitality sector, creating front groups to oppose proposed tobacco control measures, and reaching out to law makers. South African public health officials turned to international tobacco control experts for information and advice in preparation for the legislative process that lay ahead. Reflecting on one of the first preparatory meetings to discuss proposed legislation adjourned by the minister of health, a South African public health official recalled, "I'm pretty sure they [the tobacco industry representatives] thought they were coming into a developing country where the knowledge base about the tobacco industry's behavior was poor. But we [public health officials] had been fully briefed—through our links with international colleagues—on everybody who was going to be before us. We knew all their arguments and that they could be countered easily" (Malan and Leaver 2003:130).

The international relationships established in South Africa led to the All Africa Tobacco Control Conference in Harare, Zimbabwe, in 1993. The conference brought experienced tobacco control advocates from high-income countries together with emerging tobacco control advocates in African countries to discuss industry tactics, provide evidence-based counterarguments, and increase media attention on the issue. The impact of this conference and the collaboration that followed was apparent during the Framework Convention on Tobacco Control (FCTC) negotiations. The African "block" was among the most prepared to negotiate for the strongest and most effective tobacco control interventions to be part of the FCTC final text.

Initial and haphazard tobacco control networking over the Internet received a major boost in 1992 when the American Cancer Society turned over control of GLOBALink (then mainly a domestic U.S. online tobacco control network) to the International Cancer Union. The world of cyberspace soon proved to be an inexpensive way to distribute information anywhere in the world and link advocates. The network's homepage contains news bulletins, electronic conferences, live interactive chat, and full-text databases (including news, legislation, and directories). In 1997, GLOBALink received the Tobacco or Health Award from WHO for its unique ability to bring together advocates for tobacco control policy (WHO 2003b).

GLOBALIZATION OF TOBACCO LITIGATION

International tobacco control networking has been effective in linking experts from a range of sectors and has broadened the scope of international tobacco control collaboration. International collaboration regarding litigation, for example, is improving efforts to hold the tobacco industry liable for the harm caused by their products. Following their successful battle against the industry, members of the Minnesota legal team met with representatives from the WHO. In follow-up, Roberta Walburn, one of the key lawyers involved in the Minnesota case, spent a year at WHO as a Global Health Leadership Senior Fellow advising them on international litigation and the development

of the FCTC. Building on the U.S. experience, lawyers in several countries have brought individual suits against the tobacco industry to obtain compensation for tobacco-related health care costs and to challenge illegal industry activities, such as smuggling. Such cases have been filed in Argentina, Ireland, Israel, Finland, France, Japan, Norway, Sri Lanka, Thailand, and Turkey (Daynard 2000). Governments other than the United States have also filed third-party suits in the United States, including Guatemala, Venezuela, Bolivia, Nicaragua, Canada, and the European Union, which sued the tobacco industry for its involvement in large-scale cigarette smuggling (Daynard 2000). Notably, the European Union dropped the smuggling case in April 2004 after accepting US$1 billion from the tobacco companies to "help strengthen border controls" (Financial Times 2004).

Globalization of tobacco litigation faces numerous hurdles because of differences in legal systems, including (i) contingency fee compensation (which allows lawyers to finance the cases with the expectation that, while they will lose many cases, the sums of money they can earn from major victories will permit them to take the risks associated with mounting major cases against well-financed and aggressive defendants such as the tobacco industry); (ii) punitive damages to punish manufacturers in most international markets; (iii) class actions removing potential economies of scale; and (iv) awarding of defense costs whereby if defendants prevail, they can be reimbursed for reasonable defense costs.

GLOBAL ADVOCACY AND PARTNERSHIPS

Increased networking among NGOs has also helped to intensify public debate and media coverage of tobacco issues. World No Tobacco Day (WNTD), for example, has become an increasingly large international event. On WNTD 2000, new legislation was announced in Brazil, South Africa, Lebanon, the European Union, Malaysia, and Switzerland. In Pakistan, cricket superstar Imran Khan called on international sport—both players and organizations—to stop accepting sponsorship from tobacco companies, while in Thailand, 10,000 people marched and sang songs. In India, the first tobacco control website in Hindi was launched, and in the Philippines, a mock parliament attended by more than 200 children passed a resolution asking the real congress to pass laws regulating the manufacture, sale, and marketing of cigarettes. In Mauritius, two NGOs announced their decision to request BAT for compensation relating to the cost of treating diseases caused by tobacco. These activities represent only a small handful of the initiatives that took place around the globe on May 31, 2000 (Wipfli et al. 2001).

WNTD 2002 happened to fall on the opening game of the Fédération Internationale de Football Association (FIFA) World Cup in Japan and Korea. WHO therefore launched a Smoke-Free Sports campaign in which it partnered with FIFA for a Smoke-free World Cup, got tobacco control messages incorporated into the World Cup opening ceremony, and placed tobacco control posters alongside other commercial advertisements around the opening game's pitch. This partnership alone distributed tobacco control messages to a global audience of approximately 356.2 million on WNTD 2002 (Soccerphile 2002). Other partnerships developed through the WNTD Smoke-Free Sports campaign included the International Olympic Committee for a Smoke-Free Winter Olympics in Salt Lake City and the Fédération Internationale de Volleyball, which also made its 2002 world championships in Germany smoke-free. By years end, few global sporting associations were still sponsored by tobacco.

As a result of domestic action and international collaboration, there are new leading tobacco control countries in the world, including Thailand, Poland, South Africa, and Brazil. Thailand and South Africa belong to a growing number of countries that have enacted total bans on tobacco advertising and marketing. Brazil recently joined Canada in requiring picture-based health warnings. Thailand, along with Canada, requires companies to disclose the ingredients in their cigarette brands, while Poland and South Africa also have strict labeling requirements. Brazil has been among the first countries to ban labels such as "light" or "low tar" that imply that one tobacco product is less harmful than another. Due to tobacco taxes, cigarettes in Brazil, Thailand, and Poland are much less affordable than in many other, high-income countries (Guindon et al. 2002). In addition, Thailand requires that 1% of tobacco tax revenues be used to fund public health initiatives through the Thai Health Promotion Foundation. The foundation not only supports domestic initiatives, but also supports tobacco control research in neighboring countries. The

domestic activities in these four countries have significantly lowered smoking rates: in South Africa, from well more than 50% in the early 1990s to 42% in 1998; in Thailand, from 49% in 1986 to 38% in 1999; and, in the most dramatic case, in Poland, from peak levels of 65–75% in the mid-1970s to 39% in 1998 (de Beyer and Bridgen 2003).

THE WHO FRAMEWORK CONVENTION ON TOBACCO CONTROL

By the mid-1990s, social, economic, and political globalization was having an ever-greater impact on national tobacco control efforts. In Singapore, for example, the effectiveness of the advertising ban in place since 1970 began to weaken as advertising from neighboring Malaysia increasingly crossed the border via the electronic media. In Europe, membership in the European Union often meant repealing certain elements of hard-fought comprehensive tobacco control legislation. In Sweden, for example, framed health warnings were initially reduced from 20% of the pack to just 4% and no longer appeared in a frame. In Canada, effective tobacco taxes were reduced due to increased cigarette smuggling. There was also a growing awareness regarding the public health tragedy on the rise as a result of the global assault by TTCs. It became increasingly clear to tobacco control advocates throughout the world that simply exporting the national experiences of high-income countries to low- and middle-income countries was not enough to counter an unregulated global tobacco industry. Despite many individual successes, domestic tobacco control groups recognized the need for multinational cooperation and effective international action to control transnational factors.

In 1994, at the ninth World Conference on Tobacco or Health in Paris, Ruth Romer, a tobacco control advocate from California, and her protégée Allyn Taylor, a doctorate student from Columbia University, drafted the following resolution:

National Governments, Ministries of Health, and the WHO should immediately initiate action to prepare and achieve an International Convention on Tobacco Control to be adopted by the United Nations as an aid to enforcement of the

International Strategy for Tobacco Control adopted at the Ninth World Conference on Tobacco or Health. (World Conference on Tobacco or Health 1994)

This resolution marked the first international forum in which the FCTC was formally discussed.

Although the World Health assembly endorsed the idea of the FCTC in 1996, institutional commitment to the treaty came in 1998 when Gro Harlem Brundtland took over as director general of WHO and created the Tobacco Free Initiative (TFI) as one of two cabinet projects. TFI's mission was to control the rise and spread of the tobacco epidemic through the promotion of national action and international cooperation. TFI established global leadership in four priority areas: (1) global information management, (2) development of nationally and locally grounded action, (3) the establishment of strong and effective partnerships, and (4) global regulation and legal instruments. The development of the FCTC was the prime vehicle through which the WHO planned to develop global regulation over the tobacco industry (Yach and Bettcher 2000).

The Framework Convention on Tobacco Control (FCTC) was developed as a scientific, evidence-based approach to global tobacco control. The term "framework convention" is used to describe a variety of legal agreements that, unlike more comprehensive forms of treaties, do not attempt to resolve all significant issues in a single document. Rather, states first adopt the framework convention, which creates an institutional forum in which states can cooperate and negotiate for the conclusion of separate protocols containing detailed substantive obligations or added institutional commitments (Taylor 1996).

The FCTC marked the first time that the member states of WHO enacted the organization's power under Article 19 of its constitution to negotiate and sign a binding treaty aimed at protecting and promoting public health. It also represents the first time that nation-states have cooperated worldwide to form a collective response to the cause of avoidable chronic disease.

PRENEGOTIATION PREPARATIONS

In preparation for the FCTC negotiations, WHO established numerous global partnerships and initiated global multisectoral cooperation for tobacco control. First, TFI initiated a Policy Strategy Advisory Committee (PSAC) to gain policy coherence on tobacco control, solidify support for WHO activities, and expand the base of advocacy and action. PSAC included representatives from the World Bank, United Nations Children's Fund, World Self Medication Industry, International Nongovernmental Coalition Against Tobacco, the Campaign for Tobacco Free Kids, and the U.S. Centers for Disease Control and Prevention. In addition, WHO advocated for and in 1999 was successful in being asked by the United Nations Secretary General to convene the Ad-Hoc Interagency Task Force on Tobacco Control (United Nations Conference on Trade and Development 2000). The task force replaced the former United Nations tobacco focal point that had been situated within the United Nations Conference on Trade and Development and, in doing so, shifted the tobacco debate within the United Nations from one of addressing supply first, to putting health first and supply second. Fifteen United Nations organizations as well as the World Bank, the International Monetary Fund, and the World Trade Organization participate in the task force's work.

In 1999, WHO also obtained funding from the United Nations Foundation to develop partnerships with civil society to raise awareness and counter global marketing practices of the tobacco industry. Based on the successful California counteradvertising campaign that had pioneered the strategy of exposing the tobacco industry's behavior, the "Don't Be Duped" campaign sought a new language, a new idiom, and a new sense of purpose and direction for tobacco control—replacing the traditional "No Smoking" sign with an image of two Marlboro cowboys riding into the sunset with one confiding in the other that he has cancer (Subramaniam 1998). The campaign engaged and supported nationally based tobacco control champions and became an important avenue to accessing nongovernmental partners to support and advocate for the FCTC.

WHO also sparked early civil society participation in the FCTC process when it held its first-ever public hearings in October 2000. All interested parties, including the tobacco industry, were invited to present their views on the FCTC. In two days of testimonies, more than 90 pubic heath groups took the floor, along with representatives from all four major tobacco companies (WHO 2000b). Public health representatives expressed extreme concern about the impact of tobacco use, especially in low- and middle-income countries, and made specific demands of the FCTC. Most tobacco industry representatives discounted the usefulness of global regulation. The one notable exception was PM, which supported reasonable international regulations (Phillip Morris 2000). The hearings were widely reported in the world's press and helped to intensify tobacco control debate. Although some tobacco industry representatives challenged the evidence base linking passive smoking to disease, the public hearings did provide the first truly global forum in which tobacco companies admitted the addictive and deadly effects of active smoking.

The World Bank's 1999 publication *Curbing the Epidemic* provided perhaps the single most important tool in preparing for the FCTC negotiations. The report identified a virtuous circle of cost-effective interventions that enhance revenues and promote health (World Bank 1999). In doing so, it provided a credible evidence base for global regulation and helped to reverse the longstanding perception that the tobacco industry was economically too beneficial to developing countries to allow for effective health regulation (Collin 2004). The FCTC working groups, created to consolidate the scientific evidence for the WHO convention and possible protocols, cited the World Bank report as the empirical evidence supporting the demand for reduction strategies in its proposed draft of the FCTC (WHO 2000c). The Intergovernmental Negotiating Body accepted this proposed draft as the base text from which to initiate negotiations. In doing so, the potentially divisive issue of demand–supply was resolved before the negotiations even began.

NEGOTIATIONS

Those who have done; those who want to do; those who want to but cannot do; and those who do not want to do.
—*Ambassador Felipe de Seixas Correa,*
Intergovernmental Negotiating Body Chair

Much of the formal FCTC negotiations can be summed up by the quote above from Ambassador Correa from Brazil, chair of the Intergovernmental Negotiating Body, the formal body charged with negotiating the treaty. Generally speaking, four types of states participated in the negotiations. First, there was

a dedicated group of high-income countries that had instituted strong tobacco control policies domestically and fought to institutionalize effective measures globally through a strong FCTC. These countries, including Canada, Australia, and New Zealand, often championed the public health proposals emanating from the NGOS and took a stand against the vested interests of the tobacco industry. A second group of mainly low- and middle-income countries that were in the process of developing new tobacco control programs believed a strong FCTC could help build domestic momentum and increase the long-term effectiveness of their policies. These countries, including South Africa, Thailand, and Poland, often took on leadership roles and formed important alliances with other countries in their region. A third group of low-income states, with little or no capacity to institute effective tobacco control programs, looked to the FCTC for assistance in fending off the onslaught of the TTCs. These states, including tobacco-producing states in Africa, such as Tanzania, and smaller Asian states, such as Cambodia, joined important regional negotiating blocks. By getting their priorities incorporated into the blocks' formal negotiating position, these small states were able to increase their political impact on the negotiations. Finally, there was a small group of high-income states, home to the TTCs, that largely fought against strong commitments in the FCTC and, at times, threatened to derail the entire process.

Persistent leadership by low- and middle-income countries throughout the FCTC negotiations does much to explain the strength of the final text (Collin 2003). In part, this leadership was due to the sheer number of countries participating in the negotiations. Delegates from 171 member states attended the final negotiating session in February 2003. The broad participation of developing countries in the negotiating process reflects the global nature of tobacco production, use, and control, as well as the increasing recognition of tobacco as a sustainable globalization and development issue. As Remi Parmentier of Greenpeace wrote following his invitation to the final session of the FCTC negotiations,

[The FCTC negotiations] epitomize all the same dynamics which I'd faced in the run up to the World Summit on Sustainable Development: developing countries being saddled with rising health costs to feed the profits of northern multinationals,

U.S. double standards designed to serve America first, and the same kind of cynical arm-twisting rich-country politics. . . . (Parmentier 2003:1)

Civil society participation in the formal FCTC negotiations, albeit heavily circumscribed, was enhanced when WHO increased the number of international tobacco control NGOs with which it had "official relations." This formal status allowed the designated NGOs to observe proceedings and "make a statement of an expository nature" at the discretion of the chair. The significance of a broader and diversified base of NGOs formally participating in the negotiation sessions lay not in the NGOs' official statements but in the lobbying opportunities afforded by this status and their ability to generate global media debates (Collin 2004).

The impact of civil society was greatly enhanced by the development of the Framework Convention Alliance (FCA). The FCA was a loose alliance of NGOs formed to support the development and ratification of an effective FCTC. The FCA served to increase communication between NGOs already engaged and sought to systematically reach out to and support new and small NGOs, particularly in developing countries. By the end of the negotiations, the FCA was composed of more than 200 NGOs from more than 90 countries and had established itself as an important lobbying alliance. Throughout all the negotiating sessions, the FCA held lunch seminars on various technical aspects of the convention and distributed a bulletin each day to all delegates that highlighted a different area of interest to the FCTC—as well as identified the best and worse negotiating positions the day before by awarding "orchid" and "dirty ashtray" awards to specific states. The technical seminars and the distribution of information over the years evolved into what former WHO executive director for noncommunicable disease and mental health Derek Yach called "the best university of global tobacco control" (Simpson 2003).

Most important, FCA members were powerful at localizing the global FCTC process by raising domestic political debates regarding the FCTC negotiations. In the lead-up to the FCTC's adoption and in the year after its adoption, FCA members were very effective in getting the local news media to cover the FCTC. The NGO activities undertaken around FCTC process, and the media coverage it received, had a major impact on global debate and changing social understandings in relation to tobacco and its consumption.

The Final Text and Implications

The WHO member states unanimously adopted the final text of the FCTC in May 2003. The treaty went into effect in February 2005 after forty countries had ratified it. By May 2006, more than 160 countries had signed the treaty and more than 126 countries had ratified it.

Many universal elements of national tobacco control policy are contained as core provisions of the FCTC final text (table 3.4). Some of the key provisions included are a comprehensive ban on tobacco advertising, promotion, and sponsorship (with an exception for countries, e.g., the United States, that deem such a ban unconstitutional); a ban on descriptors that misleadingly convince smokers that such products are safer than standard cigarettes (e.g., by use of the term "lights" in Marlboro Lights); and a mandate to place rotating warnings on tobacco packaging, covering at least 30% of display areas, with encouragement for even larger, graphic warnings. The FCTC also encourages countries to implement smoke-free workplace laws, take measures to address tobacco smuggling, and increase tobacco taxes (WHO 2003).

Notably, the word "trade" never appears in the FCTC. Throughout the negotiations, an alliance of the majority of developing countries and NGOs fought to secure specific language prioritizing public health and tobacco control over trade agreements. Although the final text does not include any specific reference to health over trade, the first line of the convention's preamble reads, "The parties to this convention, determined to give priority to their right to protect public health. . . ." In line with the content of the rest of the convention, this wording could be interpreted in the case of trade disputes involving tobacco that reach the international trade bodies, including the World Trade Organization, as having the intent to allow nondiscriminatory national control of tobacco even if they adversely affect trade. Only hours after the completion of the negotiations, World Trade Organization Director-General Supachai Panitchpakdi spoke out in support of the FCTC, stating, "I congratulate all of those who worked so hard to bring about this important agreement. . . . When dealing with the pressing problems of our age, whether they relate to improving health standards or eradicating poverty,

TABLE 3.4. Key Demand Reduction Provisions of the FCTC

Article 6: Price and tax measures to reduce the demand for tobacco

Recognizes that price and tax measures are an effective and important means of reducing tobacco consumption, especially among young people

Article 8: Protection from exposure to tobacco smoke

Requires parties to adopt and implement effective legislative, executive, administrative, and/or other measures "providing for protection from exposure to tobacco smoke in indoor workplaces, public transport, indoor public places and, as appropriate, other public places"

Article 9: Regulation of the contents of tobacco products

Obligates countries to require that manufacturers and importers of tobacco products disclose to governmental authorities information about product contents and emissions; measures for public disclosure must be adopted

Article 10: Regulation of tobacco product disclosures

Future Conference of the Parties is to develop guidelines that can be used by countries for the testing, measuring, and regulation of contents and emissions; parties must adopt pertinent measures at the national level

Article 11: Packaging and labeling of tobacco products

Requires parties to adopt and implement effective measures requiring large, clear health warnings, using rotating messages approved by a designated national authority; provides that these warnings should cover 50% or more of the principle display areas and must occupy at least 30%

Requires the parties adopt and implement effective measures to ensure that tobacco product packaging and labeling do not promote a tobacco product by any means that are false, misleading, deceptive, or likely to create an erroneous impression about its characteristics, health effects, hazards, or emissions

Article 12: Education, communication, training, and public awareness

Requires the adoption of legislative, executive, administrative, or other measures that promote public awareness and access to information on the addictiveness of tobacco, the health risks of tobacco use and exposure to smoke, the benefits of cessation, and the actions of the tobacco industry

Article 13: Tobacco advertising, promotion, and sponsorship

Requires, in accordance with constitutional limitations, a comprehensive ban on all tobacco advertising, promotion, and sponsorship; requires countries with constitutional limitations to apply a series of restrictions on all advertising, promotion, and sponsorship

Article 14: Demand reduction measures concerning tobacco dependence and cessation

Requires creation of cessation programs in a range of settings, including diagnosis and treatment of nicotine dependence in national health programs, establishment of programs for diagnosis, counseling and treatment in health care facilities and rehabilitation centers, and collaboration with other countries to increase the accessibility of cessation therapies

---

there can be no doubt that the nations of the world must work together" (Panitchpakdi 2003:1). This announcement was evidence that the highest levels of the trade regime had heard and acknowledged the public health goals behind the FCTC. In many ways, this reflects what George Soros has urged those committed to making globalization work to do—avoid trying to reframe the World Trade Organization and instead develop international norms and standards that would be the basis for deciding trade disputes (Soros 2002). FCTC, for tobacco, joins the Codex Alimentaries Commission (jointly led by WHO and FAO) for food safety, labeling, and advertising in an era of globalization as established international norms for health. Revision of the international health

regulations will be the next step in developing a set of global norms to promote health.

From the outset of the FCTC negotiations, there was a fear that tobacco-growing developing countries would argue that they would bear the consequences of reduced demand for tobacco in direct employment loss and gain few of the benefits because their populations had low smoking rates. Anticipating this, WHO supported the FAO and World Bank to produce empirical evidence to show that demand reduction would take many decades to influence supply, that subsidies in the United States and European Union were a bigger threat to farmers in countries such as Malawi and Zimbabwe, and that for sound economic reasons they should start reducing their national dependence on tobacco. The financial provisions are sensitive to the legitimate concerns of the countries and were negotiated after WHO and European Community Development Commissioners had stated that European Community development funds could be used, on request, for countries wanting to transition out of tobacco production. These provisions have also been included, in brief, in the Global Strategy for Diet, Physical Exercise, and Health in order to address similar concerns raised by sugar producers from developing countries (WHO 2004b).

At the outset of the formal FCTC negotiation process, there was the possibility of simultaneously negotiating the treaty's core text and initial protocols (World Health Assembly 1999). While the negotiations of specific protocols proved infeasible before the core text of the FCTC was agreed upon, a consensus arose around some topics for initial protocols, including cross-border advertising and smuggling. In 2002, the United States held an international conference on illicit trade in tobacco with the aim of identifying how an FCTC protocol and other international mechanisms could assist countries in combating smuggling. U.S. incentive to initiate international action arose from emerging evidence that terrorist organizations are involved in tobacco smuggling and use smuggling profits to finance terrorist activities. The European Union has united with the United States against smuggling because of its desire to reduce the significant economic costs resulting from lost taxes. Some tobacco companies have also indicated that they are supportive of efforts to reduce illicit tobacco trade and are willing to cooperate. The industry cites the explosion in the production of counterfeit cigarettes for their seemingly "irrational" support for more stringent controls (Burgess 2004).

While it is too early to meaningfully appraise the long-term impact of the FCTC on globalization trends, its broader implications on the politics of tobacco control are already evident (Collin 2003). A senior vice president for corporate affairs at PM advised an industry conference that, whether or not the FCTC is ratified, "the treaty has had a significant influence on us, simply because it has accelerated the pace of regulation in individual countries" (Davies 2003). Many governments around the world, signatories and nonsignatories alike, have responded by taking new measures for tobacco control to better align themselves with the treaty, and have prepared to sign and/or ratify the treaty in the future. New Zealand,

for example, needed only one further law regarding the size of warning labels on tobacco products to come into compliance with and ratify the FCTC. The Indian Parliament responded to the FCTC by passing the Cigarettes and Other Tobacco Products Act of 2003 and approved India's ratification of the treaty. Malta altered its Tobacco Control Act and implemented the 2003 Smoking in Public Places Act in April 2004, both in order to comply with its ratification of the FCTC in September 2003.

GLOBALIZATION AND TOBACCO: REMAINING CHALLENGES

Despite the FCTC, numerous elements of the global tobacco environment continue to threaten the public's health. Government inconsistencies toward the tobacco industry at home and abroad also continue. The U.S. Congress, for example, has made some attempts to reform its own activities toward the TTCs since its notorious trade promotion activities in the 1980s. In 1997 it passed the Doggett Amendment banning the use of government funds to promote the sale or export of tobacco products and barring U.S. agencies from seeking the removal of "nondiscriminatory" restrictions on tobacco marketing. However, both Democratic and Republican administrations have since sought to force countries to lower tariffs on tobacco products, despite evidence that lower tariffs lead to increased tobacco consumption. The Chinese government has also given some indications that they are interested in expanding the export business of the Chinese National Tobacco Company, despite warnings that this could result in increases in tobacco consumption.

The tobacco industry is also extremely effective at circumventing new tobacco control legislation. Analysis of the U.S. Federal Trade Commission reports since 1998, for example, shows that overall industry expenditures on marketing in the United States have gone up considerably despite the new limited marketing restrictions resulting from the Master Settlement Agreement in 1998. Expenditures have largely shifted away from billboards toward point-of-sale displays and behind-the-scenes tactics focused on delivering tobacco merchandise to local providers (Federal Trade Commission 2001). As a result, local providers have become increasingly important in the sale of tobacco products. Data from the United States indicate that 42% of convenience store profits come from tobacco products (Feldman 2004). As tobacco control policies refocus on the point of sale, there will undoubtedly be resistance from this important partner of the tobacco industry. In the end, the Master Settlement Agreement appears to have had little effect on cigarette advertising in magazines and on the exposure of young people to these advertisements (King and Siegel 2001). Similar results should be expected in countries whose government does not control all forms of marketing.

Already, there are some indications that tobacco companies are preparing markets for a post-FCTC environment (table 3.5). There has been an increase, for example, in the amount of nonbranded products, and companies besides the top TTCs are gaining market share (Feldman 2004). These products are often produced on the black market and bypass many national laws, as well as FCTC provisions, including antismuggling, warning labels, and taxes. The exact role of the TTCs in the production and marketing of these illegal products is not known, but they are increasingly calling for better regulations and border controls over these products. There is also a rise in industry investment in smokeless tobacco and production of other new "reduced-risk" products. The market share of smokeless tobacco has dramatically increased over the past few years in many countries, and the pubic health community is currently playing catch-up regarding the impact of these new products on health and tobacco control (Feldman 2004).

TABLE 3.5. Gearing Up to Circumvent the FCTC

FCTC Restriction	TTC Tactic to Circumvent
Tax	Smuggle, bootleg, use old machines, promote smokeless products, promote self-rolling
Ad bans	Public relations, celebrities, point-of-sale advertising
Smoke-free public areas	"Privatize" public space, "members only" restaurants and bars
Product regulation	Market products with lower carcinogens, lower carbon monoxide and nitrogen dioxide
Education/information	Industry-funded campaigns to control public messages

Another element of the new tobacco environment is that major effort underway by the top tobacco companies to remake their public image through new corporate social responsibly programs. In relation to tobacco, TTCs are increasingly recognizing the scientific literature on the health effects of active smoking, funding youth prevention programs, and even in some cases voicing support at the national level for ratification of the FCTC. They are also active in nontobacco activities, such as sponsoring the arts and supporting community programs. There is evidence that these programs are working. By 2004, the stock value of PM/Altria completely recovered from losses incurred as a result of litigation and stockholder distrust (Feldman 2004). In 2004, BAT was awarded the Stakeholder Communication Award in the new PricewaterhouseCoopers Building Public Trust Awards (Broughton 2004).

While corporate social responsibly programs appear to be an industrywide strategy, the rationale behind supporting increased regulation does not appear to be the same among the companies, nor are their approaches to the future global business alike. PM/Altria appears to be taking a much more proactive approach toward supporting domestic and global regulation than the other three major TTCs. An internal PM memo from 2001 states, "[W]e're convinced that regulation is good for our tobacco businesses" (Desel 2001). There are multiple reasons that this may be the case. First, as the only one of the four TTCs based in the United States, PM has been and remains the most vulnerable target for massive litigation. Second, the global breadth of the company, especially in the food sector, forces it to be more proactive in protecting its reputation as a responsible international player. Third, as the industry leader, PM has the most to gain from global tobacco control restrictions. Moody's Investors Service reports, for example, that more restrictions on advertising would make PM's merchandising strength an ever-greater competitive advantage. Marlboro is by far the most popular global brand and is rapidly growing in popularity in comparison to other global brands (Feldman 2004). The Marlboro brand represents 50% of Phillip Morris/Altria's tobacco revenues. Stronger regulations also provide PM a competitive advantage and huge return on their investment in the area of reduced-risk products. Formal governmental regulation, such as FDA control in the United States, could also provide a form of protection against legal punitive damages already mentioned above as a particularly present threat to PM's business.

The truth remains that tobacco company interest in regulations and public service is a reflection of how they feel it will benefit their business. When questioned about the ethics of targeting the world's poor, a manager at Rothmans Export Ltd. (part of BAT) replied: "It would be stupid to ignore a growing market. I can't answer the moral dilemma. We are in the business of pleasing our shareholders" (Sweeney 1988). It is largely this narrow corporate philosophy, involving an exclusive commitment to shareholders rather than accountability to all stakeholders, including customers, that results in an acceptable defense of corporate profits in the face of unimaginable global inequity and unsustainable globalization. Industry support for any restrictions must be understood within this context, and the unintended consequences of tobacco control regulations must be analyzed and anticipated. Allowing the tobacco industry to remake itself into a responsible corporate citizen and shed its current pariah status could jeopardize future efforts at regulation.

CONCLUSION: THE FUTURE

The FCTC process has galvanized global action for tobacco control. Throughout the negotiations, there has emerged a stronger sense of global solidarity concerning the need for joint action between countries in diverse regions and at different levels of development. But it has also led many in public health to believe they now have solved the problem and can move on to obesity and other global health issues. Complacency could be the biggest future challenge to global tobacco control. Major funders of international tobacco control have already announced they will reduce their support; few countries have used their tobacco excise taxes to create the type of dedicated and sustainable infrastructure needed to address tobacco control over decades; and all this time the tobacco industry makes progress in finding new ways of marketing their products in an environment in which they are no larger pariahs.

As countries adopt the provisions of the FCTC into national laws, and protocols are developed, there will be gradual progress on tobacco control. Many countries may well reach Canada's 2% per annum decline in prevalence—some may reach South Africa's

5–6% per annum decline. But this should not be regarded as acceptable. Accelerated approaches to tobacco control that extend beyond the FCTC provisions need to be developed so that future deaths from an entirely man-made globalized epidemic can be prevented.

References

American Tobacco Companies (1954). Frank Statement. http://www.library.ucsf.edu/tobacco/docs/html/190 1.01/ (accessed April 7, 2004).

Arents G (1938). Early Literature of Tobacco [booklet]. Privately printed for distribution at the Library of Congress. http://www.tobacco.org/resources/history/ Tobacco_Historynotes.html (accessed April 7, 2004).

Barnoya J, Glantz S (2002). Tobacco industry success in preventing regulation of secondhand smoke in Latin America: The "Latin Project" *Tobacco Control*, 11:305–314.

Beelman M (2004). Philip Morris Accused of Smuggling, Money-Laundering Conspiracy in Racketeering Lawsuit. Washington, DC: Center for Public Integrity. http://www.publicintegrity.org/dtaweb/report .asp?ReportID=84&L1=10&L2=10&L3=0&L4=0& L5=0) (accessed June 30, 2004).

Bialous SA, Yach D (2001). Whose standard anyway? How the tobacco industry determines the International Organization for Standardization (ISO) standards for tobacco and tobacco products. *Tobacco Control*, 10(2):96–104.

Bobak M, Jha P, Nguyen S, Jarvis M (2000). Poverty and smoking. In: Jha P, Chaloupka F, eds. *Tobacco Control in Developing Countries*. Oxford: Oxford University Press, 41–62.

Bollinger CT, Fagerstrom KO (1997). *The Tobacco Epidemic*. Basel: Karger Press.

Borio G (1997). The History of Tobacco. History Net. http://www.historian.org/bysubject/tobacco (accessed April 7, 2004).

Boyle P, Onofio A, Maisonneuve P, Severi G, Robertson C, Tubiana M, Veronesi U (2003). Measuring progress against cancer in Europe: has the 15% decline targeted for 2000 come about? *Annals of Oncology*, 14:1312–1325.

Broughton M (2004). Chairman's Speech to the British American Tobacco Annual General Meeting, London, April 21. http://www.bat.com/oneweb/ sites/uk_3mnfen.nsf (accessed April 26, 2004).

Brown & Williamson Tobacco Company (1964). A Review of Health References in Cigarette Advertising, 1927–1964. Bates #696000889. Brown & Williamson Tobacco Company.

Burgess P (2004). Philip Morris to back EU counterfeit fight. *Washington Post*, April 6.

Callard C, Collishaw N, Swenarchuk M (2001). *An Introduction to International Trade Agreements and*

*Their Impact on Public Measures to Reduce To-
bacco Use.* Ottawa: Physicians for a Smoke-Free
Canada.

CDC (2004). Global Youth Tobacco Survey. Centers for
Disease Control and Prevention. http://www.cdc
.gov/tobacco/global/GYTS (accessed April 7, 2004).

Ciresi MV, Walburn RB, Sutton TD (1999). Decades of
deceit: document discovery in the Minnesota tobacco litigation. *William Mitchell Law Review,*
25(2):477–566.

Collin J (2003). Transnational tobacco companies and
cognitive globalization. In: Lee K, ed., *Health Impact of Globalization: Towards Global Governance.*
Hampshire, UK: Palgrave, 61–85.

Collin J (2004). Tobacco politics. In: *Development,*
47(June 1):91–96

Crescenti MG (1998). The new tobacco world. *Tobacco
Journal International,* 3:51.

Crofton J, Simpson D (2002). *Tobacco: A Global Threat.*
Oxford: Macmillian Education.

CTFK (2001). How Do You Sell Death? Washington,
DC: Campaign for Tobacco Free Kids. http://tobac-
cofreekids.org/campaign/global (accessed April 14,
2004).

Davies D (2003). External Forces: Facing the Future.
Barcelona: Tabexpo, November 26. http://www
.philipmorrisinternational.com/pages/eng/press/spe
eches/DDavies_20031126.asp (accessed April 26,
2004).

Dawson A (1999). The insider scoop. *C-Health News,*
December 7. http://www.canoe.ca/Health9912/07
_smoking (accessed on April 7, 2004).

Daynard R (2000). Tobacco litigation worldwide. *British
Medical Journal,* 320(7227):111–113.

De Beyer J, Brigden WL (2003). *Tobacco Control Policy:
Strategies, Successes, and Setbacks.* Washington,
DC: World Bank.

Doll R, Hill AB (1950). Smoking and carcinoma of the
lung: preliminary report. *British Medical Journal,*
2:739–748.

Doll R, Hill AB (1954). The mortality of doctors in relation to their smoking habit: a preliminary report.
British Medical Journal, 4877, 1451–1455.

Doll R, Peto R, Boreham J, Sutherland I (2004). Mortality in relation to smoking: 50 years' observations on
male British doctors. *British Medical Journal,*
328:1519.

Drope J, Chapman S (2001). Tobacco industry efforts at
discrediting scientific knowledge of environmental
tobacco smoke: a review of internaitoal industry
documents. *Journal of Epidemiology and Community Health,* 55 (8):588–594.

Duke Homestead Historical Site (2004). A Brief History of the Duke Family and Its Tobacco Empire.
Duke Historical Society. http://www.ibiblio.org/duke-
home/family (accessed April 7, 2004).

Efroymson D, Ahmed S, Townsend J, et al. (2001a).
Hungary for tobacco: an analysis of the economic
impact of tobacco consumption on the poor in
Bangladesh. *Tobacco Control,* 9:78–89.

Efroymson D, Must E, Tanudyaya F (2001b) *A Burning
Issue: Tobacco Control and Development.* Dhaka,
Bangladesh: PATH Canada.

FAO (2003). *Projections of Tobacco Production, Consumption and Trade to the Year 2010.* Rome: Food
and Agriculture Organization.

FDA v. Brown & Williamson Tobacco Corp. (2000). 529
U.S. 120.

Federal Register (1996). Part 897: Cigarettes and Smokeless Tobacco, 61(168):44395–44618. http://www.fda
.gov/cdrh/registration/fr/44615.pdf (accessed March
22, 2006).

Federal Trade Commission (2001). *Cigarette Report for
2001.* Washington, DC: Federal Trade Commission.

Feldman M (2004) *Tobacco Research,* March 9. New
York: Merrill Lynch.

Fichtenberg C, Glantz S (2002). Effect of smoke-free
workplaces on smoking behaviour: systematic review. *British Medical Journal,* 325:188.

Framework Convention Alliance (2002). The FCTC
and tobacco smuggling NGO. Briefing for the International Conference on Illicit Trade in Tobacco
New York, July 30–August 1. http://www.ash.org
.uk/html/international/html/icittbrief.html (accessed
June 30, 2004).

Frankel G (1996a). Thailand resists US brand assaults.
Washington Post, November 18, p. A01.

Frankel G (1996b). US aided cigarette firms in conquests
across Asia. *Washington Post,* November 17, p. A01.

Frankel G, Muson S (1996). Vast China market key to
smoking disputes. *Washington Post,* November 20,
p. A01.

Fritschler, AL (1969). *Smoking and Politics: Policymak-
ing and the Federal Bureaucracy.* Englewood Cliffs,
NJ: Prentice Hall.

Gajalakahmi V, Peto R, Kanaka TS, Jha P (2003). Smoking and mortality from tuberculosis and other diseases in India. *Lancet,* 363:507–515.

Guindon E, Boisclar D (2003). Past, Current and Future
Trends in Tobacco Use. HNP Discussion Paper,
Economics of Tobacco Control Paper 6. Washing-
ton, DC: World Bank.

Guindon E, Tobin S, Yach D (2002). Trends and affordability of cigarette prices: ample room for tax increases and related health gains. *Tobacco Control,*
11:35–43.

GYTS Collaborating Group (2003). Differences in
worldwide tobacco use by gender: findings from the
Global Youth Tobacco Survey. *Journal of School
Health,* 73(6):207–215.

Hammond R (1998). Consolidation in the tobacco industry. *Tobacco Control,* 7:426–428.

Hammond R, White C (2002). Multinational Tobacco
Industry Activity in the Middle East: A Review of
Internal Industry Documents. Cairo: World Health
Organization, Regional Office for the Eastern
Mediterranean.

Hastings G, McFadyen L (2000). A day in the life of
an advertising man: review of internal documents

from the UK tobacco industry's principle advertising agencies. *British Medical Journal*, 321(7257): 366–371.

Hirschorn N, Bialous S (2001). Secondhand smoke and risk assessment: what was in it for the tobacco industry? *Tobacco Control*, 10:365–382.

Hobhouse H (1989). *Forces of Change: An Unorthodox View of History*. New York: Arcade.

Holmes C (1997). Big tobacco exhales—in Russia. Cox News Service, September 14. As cited in: Hammond R (1998). Addicted to Profit: Big Tobacco's Expanding Global Reach. Washington DC: Essential Action. http://www.essentialaction.org/addicted/country.html (accessed March 22, 2006).

House of Commons (2000). *The Tobacco Industry and Health Risks of Smoking*. London: House of Commons Select Health Committee.

Hurt RD, Robertson CR (1998). Prying open the door to the tobacco industry's secrets about nicotine. *Journal of the American Medical Association*, 280(13)1173–1181.

International Union Against Cancer (1997). WHO Award goes to GLOBALink. *UICC Newsletter*, 3(2):1.

Jacobs R, Gale HF, Capehart TC, Zhang P, Jha P (2000). The supply-side effects of tobacco control policies. In: Jha P, Chaloupka F, eds. *Tobacco Control in Developing Countries*. Oxford: Oxford University Press, 311–342.

James I (1604). A Counterblaste to Tobacco. http://darkwing.uoregon.edu/~rbear/james1.html (accessed April 7, 2004).

Jemal A, Tiwari R, Murray T, Samuels A, Ward E, Feuer EJ, Thun M (2004). Cancer statistics, 2004. *CA Cancer J Clin*, 54:8–29.

Jha P, Chaloupka F, eds. (2000). *Tobacco Control in Developing Countries*. Oxford: Oxford University Press.

Jha P, Ranson MK, Nguyen SN, Yach D (2002). Estimates of global and regional smoking prevalence in 1995, by age and sex. *American Journal of Public Health*, 92(6):1002–1006.

Kiernann VG (1991). *Tobacco a History*. London: Hutchinson Radius.

King C, Siegel M (2001). The master settlement agreement with the tobacco industry and cigarette advertising in magazines. *New England Journal of Medicine*, 345:504–511.

Klein N (2000). *No Logo*. London: Flamingo.

Levin ML, Goldstein H, Gerhardt PR (1950). Cancer and tobacco smoking. *Journal of the American Medical Association*, 143:336–338.

Lickint F (1929). Tabak und Tabakrauch als ätiologischer Factor des Carcinoms. *Zeitschrift für Krebsforschung*, 30:349–365.

Liu BQ, Peto R, Chen ZM, Boreham J, Wu P, Li JY, Campbell YC, Chen JS (1998). Emerging tobacco hazards in China: 1. Retrospective proportional mortality study of one million deaths. *British Medical Journal*, 317(7170):1411–1422.

Mackay J, Eriksen M (2002). *The Tobacco Atlas*. Geneva: World Health Organization.

Madeley J (1999). British American Tobacco: the smokescreen. In: Madeley J, ed., *Hungry for Power*. London: UK Food Group, 80–89.

Malan M, Leaver R (2003). Political change in South Africa: new tobacco control and public health policies. In: de Beyer J, Weaverly Brigden L, eds. *Tobacco Control Policy: Strategies, Successes, and Setbacks*. Washington, DC: World Bank, 121–153.

Merriman D, Yurekli A, Chaloupka F (2000). How big is the worldwide cigarette smuggling problem? In: Jha P, Chaloupka F, eds., *Tobacco Control in Developing Countries*. Washington, DC: World Bank, 365–392.

McNeill A (2004). Harm reduction. *British Medical Journal*, 328:885–887.

Muggli M, Forster J, Hurt R, Repace J (2001). The smoke you don't see: uncovering tobacco industry scientific strategies aims against environmental tobacco smoke policies. *American Journal of Public Health*, 91(9):1419–1423.

Müller FH (1939). Tabakmissbrauch und Lungencarcinom. *Zeitschrift für Krebsforschung*, 49:57–85.

Nassar H (2003). The economics of tobacco in Egypt. A New Analysis of Demand. HNP Economics of Tobacco Control Discussion Paper No. 8. Washington, DC: World Bank.

NCI (2002). *Monograph 13: Risks Associated with Smoking Cigarettes with Low Tar Machine-Measured Yields of Tar and Nicotine*. Bethesda, MD: National Cancer Institute, U.S. Department of Health and Human Services.

Ong EK, Glantz SA (2000). Tobacco industry efforts subverting the International Agency for Research on Cancer's second-hand smoke study. *Lancet*, 355:1253–1259.

Ong E, Glantz G (2001). Constructing "sound science" and "good epidemiology": tobacco lawyers, and public relations firms. *American Journal of Public Health*, 91(11):1749–1757.

Ong E, Glantz SA (2001). Tobacco industry efforts subverting International Agency for Research on Cancer's second-hand smoke study. *Lancet*, 355(9211):1253–1259.

Ourusoff A (1992). What's in a name? What the world's top brands are worth. *Financial World*, September 1, pp. 32–49.

Pan American Health Organization (2002). *Profits over People*. Washington, DC: Pan American Health Organization.

Panitchpakdi S (2003). Director General Supachai Welcomes WHO Tobacco Agreement. WTO News, March 3. http://www.wto.org/english/news_e/news03_e.htm (accessed February 17, 2006).

Parmentier R (2003). Tobacco Control: Don't Trade Away Public Health. International Center for Trade and Sustainable Development, Paris, April 1.

Pearl R (1938). Tobacco smoking and longevity. *Science*, 87(2253):216–217.

Perry CL (1999). The tobacco industry and underage youth smoking: tobacco industry documents from the Minnesota litigation. *Archives of Pediatric and Adolescent Medicine*, 153(9):935–941.

Peto R, Lopez AD, Boreham J, Thun M, Heath C Jr (1994). *Mortality from Smoking in Developed Countries 1950–2000*. Oxford: Oxford University Press.

Phillip Morris (2000). Submission to the WHO Public Hearings on a Proposed Framework Convention on Tobacco Control. http://www3.who.int/whosis/fctc/fctc.cfm (accessed April 25, 2004).

Royal College of Physicians (1962). *Smoking and Health*. London: Royal College of Physicians.

Rupert J, Frankel G (1996). In ex-Soviet markets, US brands took on role of capitalist liberator. *Washington Post*, November 19, p. A01.

Saloojee Y, Dagli E (2000). Tobacco Industry tactics for resisting pubic policy on health. *Bulletin of the World Health Organization*. 78(7):902–910.

Sayginsoy O et al. (2002). Cigarette Demand, Taxation, and the Poor. A Case Study of Bulgaria. HNP Discussion Paper No. 4, Economics of Tobacco Control. Washington, DC: World Bank.

Shafey O, Dolwick S, Guindon E (2003). *Tobacco Country Profiles 2003*. Geneva: American Cancer Society.

Simpson B (2003). Smoke out! *Johns Hopkins Public Health* (spring):34.

Smith, Adam (1776). *The Wealth of Nations*. Canaan E, ed. Chicago: University of Chicago Press, 1976.

Soccerphile (2002). 2002 Most Watched Ever. http://www.soccerphile.com/soccerphile/archives/wc2002/ne/nov24 (accessed April 26, 2004).

Soros G (2002). *George Soros on Globalization*. Cambridge, MA: Perseus Book Group.

South African Medical Journal (1963). Cigarettes and smoking [editorial]. 37(39):944–975.

Subramanian C (1998). Advocacy for Policy Change. NGO and Media Workshop. Geneva: World Health Organization.

Sweeney J (1988). Selling cigarettes to the Africans. *The Independent Magazine*, October 29, p. xxviii.

Taylor A (1996). An international regulatory strategy of global tobacco control. *Yale Journal of International Law*, 21(2):257.

Taylor A, Bettcher D (2000). WHO Framework Convention on Tobacco Control: a global "good" for public health. *Bulletin of the World Health Organization*, 78(7):920–929.

Taylor A, Chaloupka F, Guindon E, Corbett M (2000). The impact of trade liberalization on tobacco consumption. In: Jha P, Chaloupka F, eds., *Tobacco Control in Developing Countries*. Oxford: Oxford University Press, 353–364.

United Nations Conference on Trade and Development (2000). Ad Hoc Inter-Agency Task Force on Tobacco Control—Report of the Secretary General, UNCTAD, Substantive Session of 2000. ECOSOC Document E/2000/21. New York: UNCTAD.

USDHHS (1994). Preventing Tobacco Use among Young People: A Report of the Surgeon General. Rep. No. 23. Atlanta, GA: U.S. Department of Health and Human Services.

USDHHS (2000). Reducing Tobacco Use: A Report of the Surgeon General. Rep. No. 29. Atlanta, GA: U.S. Department of Health and Human Services.

U.S. Public Health Service (1964). Smoking and Health: Report of the Advisory Committee to the Surgeon General of the Public Health Service. PHS Publ. No. 1103. Washington, DC: U.S. Department of Health, Education, and Welfare, Public Health Service, Centers for Disease Control and Prevention.

Vateesatokit P (2003). Tailoring tobacco control efforts to the country: the example of Thailand. In: de Beyer J, Weaverly Brigden L, eds. *Tobacco Control Policy: Strategies, Successes, and Setbacks*. Washington, DC: World Bank, 154–178.

White C, Hammond R (2001). *Voices of Truth*. Vol. 1. Cairo: WHO Eastern Mediterranean Regional Office.

WHO (2002). World Health Report. Geneva: World Health Organization.

WHO (2000a). *Tobacco Company Strategies to Undermine Tobacco Control Activities at the World Health Organization—Report of the Committee of Experts on Tobacco Industry Documents*. Geneva: World Health Organization.

WHO (2000b). Public Hearings on the Framework Convention on Tobacco Control. Geneva: World Health Organization. http://www.who.int/geneva-hearings/ (accessed April 25, 2004).

WHO (2000c). *Proposed Draft Elements for a WHO Framework Convention on Tobacco Control: Provisional Texts with Comments of the Working Group*. Geneva: World Health Organization.

WHO (2003a). *WHO Framework Convention on Tobacco Control*. World Health Assembly Resolution 56.1, May 21. Geneva: World Health Organization.

WHO (2003b). *World No Tobacco Day Awards: 1988–2000*. Geneva: World Health Organization. http://www.euro.who.int/tobaccofree/projects/20030910_2 (accessed April 25, 2004).

WHO (2004a). *Tobacco and Poverty: A Vicious Cycle. World No Tobacco Day 2004*. Geneva: World Health Organization.

WHO (2004b). *WHO Global Strategy on Diet, Physical Activity and Health*. A57/9, April 17. Geneva: World Health Organization.

Wipfli H, Bettcher D, Subramaniam C, Taylor A (2001). Confronting the tobacco epidemic: emerging mechanisms of global governance. In: McKee M, Sott R, eds., *International Co-operation and Health*. London: Oxford University Press, 189–231.

World Bank (1999). *Curbing the Epidemic: Governments and the Economics of Tobacco Control*. Washington, DC: World Bank.

World Bank (2003a). The Economics of Tobacco Use and Tobacco Control in the Developing World—A Background Paper for the High Level Round Table on Tobacco Control and Development Policy. Washington, DC: World Bank.

World Bank (2003b). Phillip Morris/Altria, British American Tobacco, Japan Tobacco 2002 Annual Reports in World Development Indicators. Washington, DC: World Bank.

World Conference on Tobacco or Health (1994). Appendix 5: Resolutions from the Ninth World Conference on Tobacco or Heath. Paris. http://web.idrc.ca/en/ev-28852-201-1-DO_TOPIC (accessed April 26, 2004).

World Health Assembly (1999). *Towards a Framework Convention on Tobacco Control.* Resolution WHA 52.18. Geneva: World Health Organization.

Wynder EL, Graham EA (1950). Tobacco smoking as a possible etiologic factor in bronchogenic carcinoma. *Journal of the American Medical Association,* 143:329–336.

Wynder EL, Graham EA, Croninger AR (1953). Experimental production of carcinoma with cigarette tar. *Cancer Research,* 13:855–864.

Yach D (1990). Tobacco-induced disease in South Africa. *International Journal of Epidemiology,* 19(4): 1122–1123.

Yach D, Bettcher D (1999). Globalization of tobacco marketing, research, and industry influence: perspectives, trends and impacts on human welfare. *Development,* 42(4):25–30.

Yach D, Bettcher D (2000). Globalization of tobacco industry influence and new global responses. *Tobacco Control,* 9:206–216.

Yach D, McIntyre D, Saloojee Y (1992). Smoking in South Africa: the health and economic impact. *Tobacco Control,* 1:272–280.

Zatonski W, Przewozniak K (1992). Tobacco smoking in Poland. In: Zatonski W, Przewozniak K, eds. *Health Consequences of Tobacco Smoking in Poland.* Warsaw: Arial, 24–44.

Zeltner T, Kessler D, Martiny A, Randera F (2000). *Tobacco Industry Strategies to Undermine Tobacco Control Activities at the World Health Organization.* Geneva: World Health Organization.

Chapter 4

The Rapid Shifts in Stages of the Nutrition Transition: The Global Obesity Epidemic

Barry M. Popkin and Michelle Mendez

Over the past fifteen years, there have been increasingly rapid changes in the structure of dietary intakes, levels of physical activity, and the prevalence of obesity throughout the developing world (Popkin, 2002b). Modern societies seem to be converging on a diet high in saturated fats, sugar, and refined foods and low in fiber—often termed the "Western diet"—and on lifestyles characterized by lower levels of physical activity. These developments, which are reflected in nutritional outcomes such as changes in average stature, body composition, and morbidity patterns, have been described as part of the "nutrition transition" (Popkin, 2002a).

In this chapter, we examine the types of shifts in food availability, dietary intake patterns, and obesity that have taken place in developing countries during a period of rapid globalization and urbanization. The accelerated pace of globalization—defined broadly as the greater flow of information, capital, goods, and services—and urbanization experienced by developing countries in recent decades is believed to play a major role in these shifts. For example, globalization may promote shifts in occupational structures as industries develop in response to world markets; enhanced access to nontraditional foods as a result of changing prices, production practices, and trade; and greater access to modern mass media programming. Similarly, urbanization has been accompanied by a rise in modern technologies that influence activity levels in work, leisure, and transportation; increased access to modern media; and enhanced access to a variety of foods across all seasons of the year. Because of the multiple shared paths through which urbanization and globalization may influence diet, activity, and health in developing countries, it is difficult to unravel effects of these forces.

In addition to structural changes, developing countries undergoing rapid urbanization and globalization are experiencing widespread sociocultural changes such as the rise of mass media and other modern marketing tools—factors that play an important role in influencing tastes and preferences (Lang, 1999; Evans et al., 2001; Chopra et al., 2002). Growing foreign investment has contributed to the rise of fast food restaurants and Western-style supermarkets, which may influence consumer food choices by offering greater variety, quality, convenience, and competitive prices in high-value-added foods, in addition to perceived higher social desirability (Regmi and Gehlar, 2001; Reardon and Berdegué, 2003). Over time, these changes in the food environment are expanding beyond large urban centers and into smaller cities and towns, mirroring the pattern that occurred over time in industrialized countries. For example, in China, Western-style supermarkets are now found in smaller cities and towns along the eastern coast and in the interior (Reardon and Berdegué, 2003).

WHAT IS THE NUTRITION TRANSITION?

The nutrition transition is described in detail in figure 4.1. In stage 1, famine begins to recede as income rises. In stage 2, changes in diet and activity pattern lead to the emergence of new disease problems and increased disability. In stage 3, behavioral change begins to reverse the negative tendencies and make possible a process of "successful aging" (see Manton and Soldo, 1985; Crimmins et al, 1989). The changes are all driven by a range of factors, including urbanization, economic growth, technical change, and culture. For convenience, the patterns can be thought of as historical developments; however, "earlier" patterns are not restricted to the periods in which they first arose, but continue to characterize certain geographic and socioeconomic subpopulations. In addition to differences in timing, there is substantial variation in the pace with which each of these stages takes place around the globe. In some parts of the developing world, the pace of dietary change in stage 2—in which the consumption of energy-dense foods increases—has been extremely rapid.

Two historic processes of change are closely linked to the nutrition transition. One is the demographic transition—the shift from a pattern of high fertility and mortality to one of low fertility and mortality (typical of modern industrialized countries). The second is the epidemiological transition, first described by Omran (1971): the shift from a pattern of high prevalence of infectious disease, associated with malnutrition, periodic famine, and poor environmental sanitation, to one of high prevalence of chronic and degenerative disease, associated with urban-industrial lifestyles (see also Olshansky and Ault, 1986). The diet and activity shifts that characterize the nutrition transition are likely accompanied by reduced susceptibility to (and mortality from) early infections and increased risk of overnutrition and related chronic diseases in later life.

DYNAMICS OF THE FOOD SYSTEM

There is substantial evidence that diets of the developing world are shifting rapidly, particularly with respect to dietary fats, caloric sweeteners, and animal-source foods (ASFs; Popkin, 2002b; Popkin and Du, 2003). Broad-based evidence of these shifts comes from data on global availability (production) of food for human consumption, which provide an estimate of intakes (FAOSTAT, 2004). In addition, we provide evidence from country case studies that directly estimate intakes.

Edible Oil

In the popular mind, the Westernization of the global diet continues to be associated with increased consumption of animal fats. Yet the nutrition transition in developing countries typically begins with major increases in production and imports of oilseeds and vegetable oils, rather than meat and milk. Principal vegetable oils include soybean, sunflower, rapeseed, palm, and peanut (groundnut) oil. With the exception of peanut oil, global availability of each has approximately tripled between 1961 and 1990. In the past two decades, a period of rapid globalization and urbanization, intakes of edible oils in developing countries increased steadily, rising from 133 to 181 kcal per capita between 1980 and 1990 and further increasing to 216 kcal per capita by 2000. In contrast, the consumption of visible animal fats remained fairly steady from 1980 to 1990 (27–30 kcal per capita) but increased to 39 kcal per capita by 2000.

Fat intake increases with rising national incomes. Over time, though, there have been dramatic changes in the relationship between aggregate income and fat consumption. The changing relationship is displayed in figure 4.2. Most significantly, by 1990, even poor nations had access to a relatively high-fat diet, when a diet deriving 20% of energy

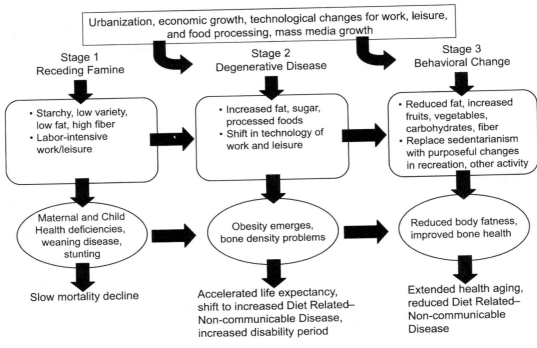

FIGURE 4.1. Stages of the Nutrition Transition. *Source:* Popkin (2002a).

(kcal) from fat was associated with having a mean gross national product (GNP) of only $750 per capita. In 1962, the same dietary fat level (20% of energy) was associated with having a GNP of $1,475 (both GNP values are in 1993 US$).

This dramatic change arose principally from a major increase in the consumption of vegetable fats in low-income countries. In 1990, edible oils accounted for a greater proportion of dietary energy than did animal fats for countries in the lowest 75% of the per capita income distribution (all of which have incomes below $5,800 per capita). The change in edible vegetable fat prices, supply, and consumption is unique because it affected rich and poor countries equally, but the net impact is relatively much greater on low-income countries.

Caloric Sweeteners

Sugar (sucrose) is the world's predominant sweetener. For this chapter, however, we describe more broadly shifts in intakes of caloric sweeteners instead of added sugar, because there is such a range of noncalorie sweeteners used today. High-fructose corn syrup is a prime example, because it is the sweetener used in all U.S. soft drinks (Popkin and Nielsen, 2003; Bray et al., 2004). The overall trends show a large increase in the availability of caloric sweeteners (see table 4.1). In 2000, about 306 kcal of sweeteners was consumed per person per day, about a third more than in 1962; caloric sweeteners also accounted for a larger share of both total energy and total carbohydrates consumed.

Not surprisingly, table 4.1 shows that all measures of caloric sweetener intakes increase significantly as a country's GNP per capita and urbanization increase. However, the interaction between income growth and urbanization is important. Figure 4.3 shows the relationship between the proportion of energy from different food sources and GNP, for two different levels of urbanization (see Drewnowski and Popkin, 1997, for a description of the analysis). In the less urbanized case (figure 4.3A), the share of sweeteners increases sharply with GNP, from about 5% to about 15%. In the more urbanized case, the share is much higher at lower national income levels (more than 15%) and hardly increases with rising income. The analysis confirms previous observations that people living in urban areas consume diets distinct from those of their rural counterparts (Popkin and Bisgrove, 1988; Solomons and Gross, 1995).

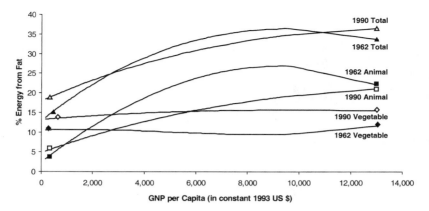

FIGURE 4.2. Relationship between the Percentage of Energy from Fat and GNP per Capita, 1962 and 1990. Nonparametric regressions run with food balance data from Food and Agricultural Organization of the United Nations and GNP data from the World Bank for 134 countries. *Source:* Guo et al. (2000, 4). Reprinted with permission from the University of Chicago Press.

Animal-Source Foods

The revolution in ASFs refers to the increase in demand and production of meat, fish, and milk in low-income developing countries. International Food Policy Research Institute's Christopher Delgado has studied this issue extensively in a number of seminal reports and papers (summarized in Delgado et al., 1999; Delgado, 2003). Most of the world's recent growth in production and consumption of these foods has taken place in developing countries. Developing countries will produce 63% of meat and 50% of milk in 2020. This global food pattern shift is transforming the grain markets for animal feed. It also leads to resource degradation, rapid increases in feed grain imports, rapid concentration of production and consumption, and social change.

A critical reason for this increase in intake of ASFs is the continued decline in the real prices of ASFs over the past several decades. Delgado (2003) has shown that these price shifts, fueled by cheap feed grain costs in the West, represent a key component of this shift in consumption.

A case study on food pattern changes from China based on data from the China Health and Nutrition Survey (CHNS) is useful for summarizing food pattern changes for a typical fast growing economy (table 4.2). The shifts in the Chinese diet follows a classic Westernization pattern (for more detail on these Chinese changes, see Popkin et al., 1993; Du et al., 2002). Case study data from China also indicate that consumption patterns closely reflect changes in food availability.

First, intake of cereals decreased considerably during the past two decades in both urban and rural areas and among all income groups (table 4.2). During the eight-year period from 1989 to 1997, the total intake of cereals decreased by 127 g per capita per day (67 g for urban residents and 161 g for rural residents). The decrease in the low-income group was the largest, at 196 g per capita, compared with their counterparts in mid- and high-income groups (86 g and 85 g, respectively). However, there remains an inverse relationship between income and cereal intake. For example, in 1997, the intake in low-, mid-, and high-income groups was 615 g, 556 g, and 510 g per capita, respectively.

The shift away from coarse grain consumption such as millet, sorghum, and corn is a key component of this change. CHNS data showed a 38 g decrease in refined cereals between 1989 and 1997 but an even larger decrease in coarse cereal consumption of 89 g.

Second, consumption of animal products increased, more so for the rich than for the poor and more for urban than rural residents. As shown in table 4.2, urban residents' intake of animal foods per capita per day in 1997 was higher than for rural residents (178.2 g for urban vs. 116.7 g for rural) and also showed a larger increase (46.7 g vs. 36.8 g) from 1989 to 1997. The amount and growth of intake of animal foods were positively associated with income levels. The intake level and the increase in the high-income group from 1989 to 1997 were almost three times those in the low-income group.

TABLE 4.1. World Trends in Caloric Sweetener Intake for GNP and Urbanization Quintiles (1962 Values)

	Quintile 1	Quintile 2	Quintile 3	Quintile 4	Quintile 5	Total
Quintiles of GNP (using 1962 GNP levels for each country)						
Caloric Sweetener (kcal/capita/day)						
1962	90	131	257	287	402	232
2000	155	203	362	397	418	306
Total Carbohydrates (kcal/capita/day)						
1962	1,464	1,552	1,542	1,627	1,677	1,572
2000	1,690	1,670	1,752	1,779	1,693	1,717
Total Energy (kcal/capita/day)						
1962	2,008	2,090	2,157	2,411	2,960	2,322
2000	2,346	2,357	2,716	2,950	3,281	2,725
% Total Energy: Caloric Sweetener						
1962	4.5	6.2	11.9	12	13.5	9.5
2000	6.4	8.3	13.4	13.7	12.7	10.9
% Total Carbohydrates: Caloric Sweetener						
1962	6.2	8.5	16.8	17.7	24.4	14.6
2000	9	12.1	20.6	22.4	24.6	17.7
GNP						
1962	216	478	983	2,817	12,234	3282
2000	435	839	2,836	5,915	28,142	7198
% Urban						
1962	10	21.6	37.3	46.7	66.2	36.1
2000	27.7	41.3	58.7	70	78	54.9
Quintiles of % Urban (using the 1962 values for % urban for each country)						
Caloric Sweetener (kcal/capita/day)						
1962	79	131	236	335	389	232
2000	151	201	339	403	441	306
% Total Energy: Caloric Sweetener						
1962	3.8	6.3	11	13.2	13.8	9.5
2000	6.5	8.1	12.3	13.7	13.9	10.9
% Total Carbohydrates: Caloric Sweetener						
1962	5.4	8.5	15.4	20.3	24.1	14.6
2000	6	12.1	19.2	22.7	25.7	17.7
GNP						
1962	287	734	1294	4696	9606	3282
2000	653	1796	2898	11739	20568	7198
% Urban						
1962	7.1	20.4	33.9	47.6	73	36.1
2000	27	42.3	57.6	64.9	84	54.9

Source: Popkin and Nielsen (2003); FAO (2004).

Third, and partly as a result of this change, data from the CHNS also show a shift in the diet away from carbohydrates to fat (table 4.3). Energy from carbohydrates fell for all residents, and by more than 20% for urban residents. Energy from fat increased sharply, from 19.3% in 1989 to 27.3% in 1997. Other data show that more than 60% of urban residents consumed more than 30% of energy from fat in 1997.

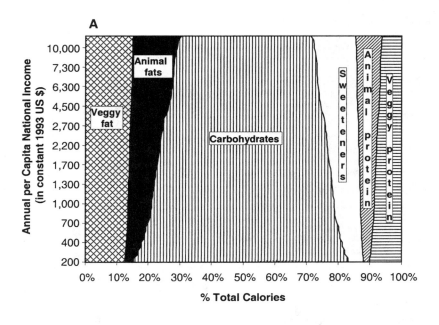

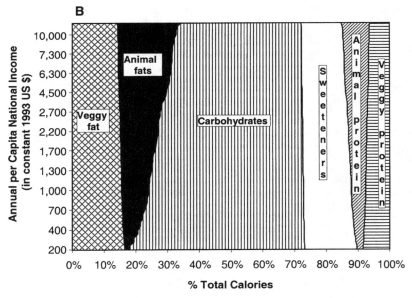

FIGURE 4.3. Relationship between the Proportion of Energy from Each Food Source and GNP per Capita and Urbanization. A: Proportion of the population residing in urban areas placed at 25%, 1990. B: Proportion of the population residing in urban areas placed at 75%, 1990. *Source:* Drewnowski and Popkin (1997) Nutrition Reviews 55:31. Reprinted with Permission from ILSI Press. Food balance data from the FAOUN; GNP data from the World Bank; regression work by UNC-CH.

TABLE 4.2. Shift in Consumption in the Chinese Diet (CHNS, 1989–1997) for Adults 20–45 Years of Age (mean intake in grams/capita/day)

Food	Urban		Rural		Low Income		Mid Income		High Income		Total	
	1989	1997	1989	1997	1989	1997	1989	1997	1989	1997	1989	1997
Total grains	556	489	742	581	811	615	642	556	595	510	684	557
Coarse	46	25	175	54	226	68	98	43	78	30	135	46
Refined	510	465	567	527	585	546	544	513	517	479	549	511
Fresh vegetables	309	311	409	357	436	356	360	357	335	325	377	345
Fresh fruit	14.5	36	15	17	5.5	8	13	18	26	38	15	21.7
Meat and meat products	73.9	97	44	58	36	40	58	64	67	96	53	67.8
Poultry and game	10.6	16	4.1	12	4.1	7	6.6	10	7.7	20	6.1	12.7
Eggs and egg products	15.8	32	8.5	20	6	14	11	22	16	32	11	22.7
Fish and seafood	27.5	31	23	27	12	16	29	26	33	40	25	27.9
Milk and milk products	3.7	4	0.2	0.9	0.8	0.1	0.2	1.4	3.5	3.6	1.3	1.7
Plant oil	17.2	40	14	36	13	32	16	37	16	42	15	37.1

Finally, specific examination of the combined effect of these various shifts in the structure of rural and urban Chinese diets shows an upward shift in the energy density of the foods consumed (Popkin and Du, 2003). Energy intake from foods and alcohol per 100 g of food in both urban and rural Chinese adult diets increased by 13% between 1989 and 1997. These are very rapid shifts.

CRITICAL RELATED REDUCTIONS IN PHYSICAL ACTIVITY

There are several changes in physical activity occurring jointly. One is a shift away from high-energy-expenditure activities such as farming, mining, and forestry toward the service sector, which includes such sedentary jobs as travel agent, clerk, or typist (for details, see Popkin, 1999). Reduced energy expenditures within the same occupation are a second change. Other major changes relate to mode of transportation and activity patterns during leisure hours.

China again provides interesting illustrations. Table 4.4 shows the decreased proportion of urban adults (male and female) working in occupations where they participate in vigorous activity patterns. In rural areas, however, there has been a shift for some toward increased physical activity linked to holding multiple jobs and more intensive effort. For rural women, there is a shift toward a larger proportion engaged in more energy-intensive work, but there are also sections where light effort is increasing. In con-

TABLE 4.3. Shifts in Energy Sources in the Chinese Diet for Adults 20–45 Years of Age (CHNS, 1989–1997) (%)

	% Energy from Fat				% Energy from Carbohydrates			
	89	91	93	97	89	91	93	97
Urban	21.4	30	32	32.8	65.8	58	55	53.3
Rural	18.2	23	23	25.4	70	65.6	65.2	62.1
Low income	16	19	20	23	72.9	69.2	68.6	64.5
Middle income	20.3	25	26	27.1	67.5	62.6	62.2	60.3
High income	21.5	30	32	31.6	65.4	57.5	55.4	54.8
Total	19.3	25	26	27.3	68.7	63.2	62.1	59.8

TABLE 4.4. Distribution of Work-Related Energy Expenditure among Adults 20–45 Years of Age (CHNS 1989, 1997)

		Light (%)		Vigorous (%)	
		1989	1997	1989	1997
Urban	Male	32.7	38.2	27.1	22.4
	Female	36.3	54.1	24.8	20.8
Rural	Male	19	18.7	52.5	59.9
	Female	19.3	25.5	47.4	60

trast, for rural men there is a small decrease in the proportion engaged in light work effort.

China also provides evidence of dramatic shifts in activity levels during transportation and leisure. In China, 14% of households acquired a motorized vehicle between 1989 and 1997. One study showed that the odds of being obese were 80% higher ($p < 0.05$) for men and women in households that owned a motorized vehicle compared to those that did not own a vehicle (Bell et al., 2002). Television ownership has skyrocketed in China, leading to greater inactivity during leisure time (see Du et al., 2002).

Obesity changes are very rapid, and these dietary and activity shifts have important consequences for nutritional status, and thus for health. In a series of papers published in a recent issue of *Public Health Nutrition*, the current levels of overweight in countries as diverse as Mexico, Egypt, and South Africa are shown to be equal to or greater than those in the United States. Moreover, the current rate of change in obesity in lower and middle-income countries is much greater than that in higher income countries (see Popkin, 2002a, for an overview).

Figure 4.4A presents the level of obesity and overweight in several illustrative countries from different regions (the United States, Brazil, Mexico, Egypt, Morocco, South Africa, Thailand, and China). Most interesting is that, despite having substantially lower incomes, many of these countries have levels of overweight and obesity comparable to or only slightly lower than those in the United States. Figure 4.4B shows how quickly overweight and obesity status has emerged as a major public health problem in some of these countries. Compared with the United States, where the annual increase in the prevalence of overweight and obesity is about 0.25, the rates of change are very high in countries in Asia, North Africa, and

Latin America—two to five times greater than in the United States.

The burden of obesity is shifting toward the poor: a large number of low- and moderate-income countries already have a greater likelihood that adults residing in lower income or lower educated households are overweight and obese relative to adults in higher income or higher education households (Monteiro et al., 2004). This study, based on multilevel analysis of thirty-seven nationally representative data sets, shows that countries with a GNP per capita greater than about $1,700 are likely to have a greater burden of obesity among the poor than among the wealthy. It also provides some idea of the set of risk factors causing obesity and other noncommunicable diseases that are changing rapidly, including poor diets, inactivity, smoking, and drinking. Not only in urban areas but also most rural areas in the developing world, there are more more overweight than underweight adult women (Mendez et al., 2005).

DISCUSSION

Overall, the global trends in obesity can be attributed to a number of factors, including urbanization, income and food price changes, and other aspects of globalization such as the introduction of modern technology related to work, transportation, and leisure. Clearly, many of the forces noted under globalization were initiated earlier and fit under longer term economic development, and the same holds for cultural changes. But for simplicity, we address here four major forces: urbanization, and two aspects of globalization—income and food price changes, as separate from the mass media and cultural shifts, and techological changes. The relative contributions of each of these factors to the observed global trends in obesity seem to be fairly evenly split: about 25% of the change is related to cultural factors, modern advertising, and other elements affecting food choice and dietary patterning; 30%, to the economic forces of food and price changes; 30%, to technological shifts linked with reduced energy expenditures at work, travel, home production, and leisure; and the remainder, to urbanization. In this chapter we have summarized attempts to parcel out these dynamic shifts and the relative importance of each.

Throughout the developing world, there have been dramatic changes in patterns of diet and activity,

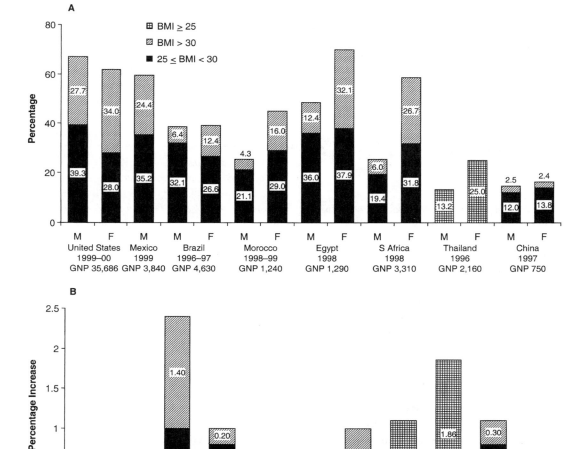

FIGURE 4.4. Obesity Patterns and Trends A: Patterns in the United States and across the developing world. B: Trends among adults in the United States and in selected developing countries: annual percentage increase in prevalence. GNP in 2002 US$. BMI, body mass index; F, female; M, male. *Source:* Popkin (2002a).

as well as in levels of overweight and obesity, during this period of accelerated globalization and urbanization. The effects of globalization and urbanization on dietary and activity patterns and nutritional status in developing countries are complex. These forces are associated with potentially beneficial dietary shifts such as increases in energy sufficiency and reduced micronutrient deficiency, but also appear to promote potentially obesogenic shifts such as increased intakes of edible oils, animal foods, and caloric sweeteners. While there have been substantial reductions in undernutrition in this period of rapid development and social change, overweight has become an increasing problem. Among adult women, overweight now exceeds underweight in almost all developing countries, particularly in the most urbanized countries.

Food availability and intake data suggest that potentially adverse shifts in dietary composition are taking place at a much higher speed than more beneficial changes: there has been relatively little change in consumption levels of fruits and vegetables but very large increases in edible oils, ASFs, and added sugar and caloric sweeteners over short periods of time. Case study data confirm that China experienced large increases in consumption of dietary fats, oils, and ASFs in the 1990s. As a result of these changes, mean intakes of ASFs in China have reached levels similar to maximum amounts recommended in U.S. guidelines (USDA, 2000). Numerous studies have shown that consumption of energy-dense (high-fat, added sugar) foods tends to promote excessive energy intakes (Rolls, 2000). These adverse dietary shifts have undoubtedly contributed to the rise in overweight and obesity observed throughout the developing world.

With globalization, many developing countries are experiencing large shifts in food imports. Between 1990 and 1998, there were large increases in trade in processed grain products, while trade in unprocessed bulk grains has declined (Regmi and Gehlar, 2001). Similarly, there have been large increases in trade in oils (Williams, 1984). At the same time, foreign direct investment in the food industry, notably supermarkets and fast food restaurants, has expanded several-fold in many countries (Bolling and Somwaru, 2001; Reardon and Berdegué, 2003). For example, between 1989 and 1998, sales by U.S.-owned food processing affiliates in South America grew from US$5 billion to US$15 billion, and sales in Asia increased from US$5 billion to US$20 billion (Bolling and Somwaru, 2001). Furthermore, globalization is associated with occupations that involve spending more time away from home. Thus, in many countries, intakes of processed foods, ready-to-eat meals and snacks, and street vendor, restaurant, and fast food meals have increased (Regmi and Gehlar, 2001). These eating patterns are associated with the higher intakes of fat, sugars, and energy. These shifts in imports and eating patterns have been accompanied by marketing of brands and shifts in cultural norms that have influenced tastes (Chopra et al., 2002). These changes in food availability, occupational structures, and marketing strategies promote consumption of processed, energy-dense foods.

There are several underlying reasons for the large shifts in edible oil consumption in developing countries (Drewnowski and Popkin, 1997). Technological breakthroughs in the development of high-yield oilseeds and in the refining of high-quality vegetable oils greatly reduced the cost of baking and frying fats, margarine, butterlike spreads, and salad and cooking oils in relation to animal-based products (Williams, 1984). Worldwide demand for vegetable fats was fueled by health concerns regarding the consumption of animal fats and cholesterol. Furthermore, a number of major economic and political initiatives led to the development of oil crops not only in Europe and the United States but also in South East Asia (palm oils) and in Brazil and Argentina (soybean oils) (USDA 1966).

Delgado has written perceptively about the ASF revolution in low-income developing countries, documenting the increase in demand for and production of meat, fish, and milk (Delgado et al., 1999, 2001; Delgado, 2003). As relative commodity prices decrease and incomes increase, people usually increase the diversity of their diet and shift into higher priced commodities and processed convenience foods. While average income growth explains overall growth, urbanization and population growth also help to explain the greater increase in ASF demand in developing countries relative to developed countries. From 1975 to 1999, animal products drove the expansion of production in developing countries, which now account for more than half the world's meat production (Delgado, 2003). In contrast, growth in ASF production in the developed world is now flat—the market is saturated. Since 81% of the world's people live in developing countries, small shifts in their diets result in huge changes in the world market. Since 1970, relative prices of food have dropped considerably, most dramatically for beef (Delgado, 2003). Due to market saturation and technological changes that increase productivity, the ASF revolution is projected to level off by 2020.

Many countries have experienced large increases in consumption of caloric sweeteners. Sugar is the world's predominant sweetener, but there are marked increases also in consumption of high-fructose corn syrup (Bray et al., 2004). Increasing sugar and sweetener use has been linked with industrialization and with the proliferation of processed foods and beverages that have caloric sweeteners added to them (e.g., tea, coffee, cocoa, soft drinks). For a detailed review of the way the world's diet has changed with respect to added caloric sweeteners, see Popkin and Nielsen (2003).

As shown using data from China, these emerging, potentially adverse dietary patterns are especially marked in urban areas. Compared to rural dwellers, urban residents continue to consume higher levels of fats and animal foods, along with lower intakes of vegetables. However, the dietary effects of globalization appear to be expanding into areas designated as rural. With marked increases in oils and ASF consumption in rural areas, the disparity between urban and rural intakes has become smaller over time. Rural consumption of these foods is particularly high in areas that are highly urbanized in terms of infrastructure and resources. Only areas with very low levels of urbanicity have maintained traditional diets, low in fat and ASFs. "Urban" dietary patterns are likely to become more common throughout developing countries as the process of rural development—or increased urbanicity in rural areas—continues.

Disturbingly, there is evidence that the adverse changes in dietary intakes associated with globalization are taking place at all levels of socioeconomic status and likely contribute the rising levels of low-income obesity observed in some developing countries. In China, although low-income adults consumed lower levels of animal foods and oils than do higher income adults, the rate of increase ASF and edible oil consumption is, overall, faster in low-income groups (Du et al., 2004). Relatively high levels of overweight were observed in women of low socioeconomic status in numerous developing countries, resulting in relatively small disparities in overweight between groups with high and low socioeconomic status.

These dietary shifts have occurred along with increased sedentarism in occupational activity and commuting and in the nature of leisure time activity (e.g., from increased television watching) (Bell et al., 2001, 2002; Hu et al., 2002). Because of their tendency to promote overconsumption, the dietary changes currently taking place in developing countries may help to explain energy imbalance and obesity, as individuals fail to adapt their energy intakes to match reduced energy expenditure levels. Together, these shifts in diet and activity have contributed to the rising obesity observed throughout the developing world, at all income levels and increasingly in rural areas (Mendez et al., 2004). The high speed of change is also a concern, as individuals exposed to undernutrition earlier in life are also making these dietary shifts. Individuals with very poor nutrition in early life may be at greater risk of adverse consequences from

overnutrition later, including diabetes, cardiovascular disease, and weight gain from these dietary shifts (Schroeder et al., 1999; Barker, 2001; Reddy, 2002; Sawaya et al., 2003).

The dietary changes associated with globalization are of great concern not only regarding obesity but also because of the implications for risk of obesity-related chronic disease. Large increases in the prevalence of numerous obesity-related chronic diseases have been documented around the developing world, including diabetes and cardiovascular diseases (Yusuf et al., 2001; Kumanyika et al., 2002). A large body of evidence, including data from clinical trials, shows that diets lower in meats and fats and richer in fruits and vegetables reduce blood pressure and risk of diabetes incidence as much or more than costly pharmacological treatments (Vollmer et al., 2001; Knowler et al., 2002).

Developing countries may benefit from preventive measures that minimize further adverse shifts in diet, rather than attempting to reverse shifts after new dietary patterns are even more established as cultural norms. Given that adverse dietary and activity patterns appear to be widespread geographically and socioeconomically, strategies with broad reach are appropriate, such as the use of mass media. The experience in Brazil suggests that mass media nutrition education efforts may be effective for reaching some population groups. Another important component of obesity prevention may involve working with the food industry. In the United States, increases in portion sizes in commercial food products may have contributed to higher intakes of energy-dense foods and exceed standard serving sizes (Nielsen and Popkin, 2003; Young and Nestle, 2003). Working with or regulating the restaurant and supermarket industries to maintain appropriate portion sizes may help to minimize excess intakes. Pricing has also been shown to play a key role in food choices in both developed and developing countries (Guo et al., 1999; French, 2003). The use of subsidies or other incentives to ensure that fresh fruits and vegetables are affordable may help to promote healthier food choices. Since high intakes of meats are associated with increased risk of hypertension and cardiovascular disease, developing countries should continue to explore agricultural and educational policies that promote the production and consumption of pulses as protein substitutes. Tastes and preferences begin to be established in early life (Hill, 2002). Therefore, schools may provide an important opportunistic venue through which preferences for more healthy options can be encouraged. Workplaces also provide an opportunity to encourage or provide opportunities for exercise and healthier diets, and efforts in some countries have targeted work sites (Doak, 2002). Dietary policies should be accompanied by programs to address country-specific barriers to maintaining high levels of physical activity, such as efforts to facilitate safe active commuting and the promotion of physical activity during leisure time.

References

Barker D, ed. (2001). Fetal Origins of Cardiovascular and Lung Disease. New York City: Marcel Dekker, Inc.

Bell AC, Ge K, and Popkin BM (2002). The road to obesity or the path to prevention? Motorized transportation and obesity in China. Obes Res 10: 277–283.

Bell C, Ge K, and Popkin BM (2001). Weight gain and its predictors in Chinese Adults. Int J Obes 25: 1079–1086.

Bolling C, and Somwaru A (2001). U.S. food companies access foreign markets through investment. ERS Food Rev 24(3): 23–28.

Bray GA, Nielsen SJ, and Popkin BM (2004). Consumption of high-fructose corn syrup in beverages may play a role in the epidemic of obesity. Am J Clin Nutr 79: 537–543.

China Health and Nutrition Survey (1989–1997). Data Sets. http://www.cpc.unc.edu/projects/china/data/datasets.html.

Chopra M, Galbraith S, and Darnton-Hill I (2002). A global response to a global problem: the epidemic of overnutrition. Bull World Health Org 80: 952–958.

Crimmins EM, Saito Y, and Ingegneri D (1989). Changes in life expectancy and disability-free life expectancy in the United States. Pop Dev Rev 15: 235–267.

Delgado C, Rosegrant M, and Meijer S (2001). Livestock to 2020: The Revolution Continues. Paper presented at the annual meetings of the International Agricultural Trade Research Consortium (IATRC), Auckland, New Zealand, January 18–19, 2001. http://www.iatrcweb.org/publications/proceedings.

Delgado CL (2003). Rising consumption of meat and milk in developing countries has created a new food revolution. J Nutr 133: 3907S–3910S.

Delgado CL, Rosegrant MW, Steinfeld H, Ehui SK, and Courbois C (1999). Livestock to 2020: The Next Food Revolution. Washington, DC: International Food Policy Research Institute, Food and Agriculture Organization of the United Nations, International Livestock Research Institute.

Doak C (2002). Large-scale interventions and programmes addressing nutrition-related chronic diseases and obesity: examples from 14 countries. Public Health Nutr 5(1A): 275–277.

Drewnowski A, and Popkin BM (1997). The nutrition transition: new trends in the global diet. Nutr Rev 55: 31–43.

Du S, Lu B, Zhai F, and Popkin BM (2002). The nutrition transition in China: a new stage of the Chinese diet. In: Caballero B, Popkin BM, eds. The Nutrition Transition: Diet and Disease in the Developing World. London: Academic Press, pp. 205–222.

Du S, Mroz TA, Zhai F, and Popkin BM (2004). Rapid income growth adversely affects diet quality in China—particularly for the poor! Soc Sci Med 59: 1505–1515.

Evans M, Sinclair RC, Fusimalohi C, and Liava'a V (2001). Globalization, diet, and health: an example from Tonga. Bull World Health Org 79(9): 856–862.

FAOSTAT (2004). Food Balance Sheets. Food and Agricultural Organization of the United Nations. http://faostat.fao.org/faostat/.

French SA (2003). Pricing effects on food choices. J Nutr 133(3): 841S–843S.

Guo X, Popkin BM, Mroz TA, and Zhai F (1999). Food price policy can favorably alter macronutrient intake in China. J Nutr 129: 994–1001.

Guo X, Mroz TA, Popkin BM (2000). Structural changes in the impact of income on food consumption in China, 1989–1993. Econ Dev Cult Change 48: 737–760.

Hill AJ (2002). Developmental issues in attitudes to food and diet. Proc Nutr Soc 61(2): 259–266.

Hu G, Pekkarinen H, Hanninen O, Yu Z, Huiguang T, Zeyu G, and Nissinen A (2002). Physical activity during leisure and commuting in Tianjin, China. Bull World Health Org 80(12): 933–938.

Knowler WC, Barrett-Connor E, Fowler SE, Hamman RF, Lachin JM, Walker EA, Nathan DM, and Diabetes Prevention Program Research Group (2002). Reduction in the incidence of type 2 diabetes with lifestyle intervention or metformin. N Engl J Med 346(6): 393–403.

Kumanyika S, Jeffery RW, Morabia A, Ritenbaugh C, Antipatis VJ, and Public Health Approaches to the Prevention of Obesity Working Group of the International Obesity Task Force (2002). Obesity prevention: the case for action. Int J Obes Relat Metab Disord 26(3): 425–436.

Lang T (1999). Diet, health and globalization: five key questions. Proc Nutr Soc 58(2): 335–343.

Manton KG, and Soldo BJ (1985). Dynamics of health changes in the oldest old: new perspective and evidence. Milbank Mem Fund Q Health Soc 63: 206–285.

Mendez MA , Monteiro CA, and Popkin BM (2005). Overweight now exceeds underweight among women in most developing countries! Am J Clin Nutr 81: 714–721.

Monteiro CA, Conde WL, Lu B, Popkin BM (2004). The burden of disease due to under- and over-nutrition in countries undergoing rapid nutrition transition: a view of Brazil. Am J Public Health 94: 433–444.

Nielsen SJ, and Popkin BM (2003). Patterns and trends in portion sizes, 1977–1998. JAMA 289(4): 450–453.

Olshansky SJ, and Ault AB (1986). The fourth stage of the epidemiologic transition: the age of delayed degenerative diseases. Milbank Q 64: 355–391.

Omran AR (1971). The epidemiologic transition: a theory of the epidemiology of population change. Milbank Mem Fund Q 49(4 pt 1): 509–538.

Popkin BM (1999). Urbanization, lifestyle changes and the nutrition transition. World Dev 27: 1905–1916.

Popkin BM (2002a). An overview on the nutrition transition and its health implications: the Bellagio meeting. Public Health Nutr 5(1A): 93–103.

Popkin BM (2002b). The shift in stages of the nutrition transition in the developing world differs from past experiences. Public Health Nutr 5(1A): 205–214.

Popkin BM, and Bisgrove E (1988). Urbanization and nutrition in low-income countries. Food Nutr Bull 10(1): 3–23.

Popkin BM, and Du S (2003). Dynamics of the nutrition transition toward the animal foods sector in China and its implications: a worried perspective. J Nutr 133: 3898S–3906S.

Popkin BM, Ge K, Zhai F, Guo X, Ma H, and Zohoori N (1993). The nutrition transition in China: a cross-sectional analysis. Eur J Clin Nutr 47: 333–346.

Popkin BM, and Nielsen SJ (2003). The sweetening of the world's diet. Obes Res 11: 1325–1332.

Reardon T, and Berdegué JA (2003). The rapid rise of supermarkets in Latin America: challenges and opportunities for development. Dev Policy Rev 20: 371–388.

Reddy KS (2002). Cardiovascular diseases in the developing countries: dimensions, determinants, dynamics, and directions for public health action. Public Health Nutr 5(1A): 231–237.

Regmi A, and Gehlar M (2001). Consumer preferences and concerns shape global food trade. Food Rev 24(3): 2–8.

Rolls BJ (2000). The role of energy density in the overconsumption of fat. J Nutr 130(2 suppl): 268S–271S.

Sawaya AL, Martins P, Hoffman D, and Roberts SB (2003). The link between childhood undernutrition and risk of chronic diseases in adulthood: a case study of Brazil. Nutr Rev 61(5 pt 1): 168–175.

Schroeder DG, Martorell R, and Flores R (1999). Infant and child growth and fatness and fat distribution in Guatemalan adults. Am J Epidemiol 149(2): 177–185.

Solomons NW, and Gross R (1995). Urban nutrition in developing countries. Nutr Rev 53: 90–95.

USDA (1966). U.S. Fats and Oils Statistics, 1909–65. Statistical Bulletin No. 376, Economic Research Service. Washington, DC: U.S. Department of Agriculture.

USDA (2000). Dietary Guidelines for Americans. Washington, DC: Department of Agriculture, Center for Nutrition Policy and Promotion. http://www.health.gov/dietaryguidelines/dga2000/document/contents.htm.

Vollmer WM, Sacks FM, and Svetkey LP (2001). New insights into the effects on blood pressure of diets low in salt and high in fruits and vegetables and low-fat dairy products. Curr Control Trials Cardiovasc Med 2(2): 71–74.

Williams GW (1984). Development and future direction of the world soybean market. Q J Intl Agr 23: 319–37.

Young LR, and Nestle M (2003). Expanding portion sizes in the US marketplace: implications for nutrition counseling. J Am Diet Assoc 103(2): 231–234.

Yusuf S, Reddy S, Ounpuu S, and Anand S (2001). Global burden of cardiovascular diseases. Part I: general considerations, the epidemiologic transition, risk factors, and impact of urbanization. Circulation 104(22): 2746–2753.

Chapter 5

Global Climate Change and Human Health

A. J. McMichael and G. Ranmuthugala

Humans, like all other species, depend upon the biosphere's complex biophysical and ecological systems for their health and survival. This natural environment not only provides the basics—air, food, and water—but also provides a range of life-supporting environmental "goods" (e.g., clothing materials, shelter, and energy) and "services" (e.g., constancy of prevailing climate, maintenance of the hydrological cycle, pollination of food plants, and the uptake of carbon dioxide and production of oxygen via plant photosynthesis).

Over many millennia, human societies have increased the "carrying capacity" of their local environment by modifying it, exploiting the local resources, and supplementing local supplies of food and other materials via trade. The major stages of cultural evolution have seen human societies move from hunter-gatherer existence to agrarianism (coupled increasingly with urban living), to industrialization, and now to an "information age." These cultural and technological changes have required a tradeoff between increases in human population density via immediate gains in environmental carrying capacity, and the potential longer term weakening of the life-supporting capacity of local environments.

During the nineteenth and twentieth centuries, the scale of human impact on the environment increased rapidly as human numbers expanded almost tenfold and as the material intensity and energy intensity of economic activity increased. Global economic activity increased approximately twentyfold in the twentieth century alone. The aggregate world population, 6.6 billion in 2006, is anticipated to reach around 8.5–9 billion by 2050. The total human carrying capacity of the earth is uncertain—and depends, of course, on future patterns of consumption and waste generation.

Along with human numbers, the average levels of consumption of materials and energy are rising globally, as are humankind's waste products. Hence, we face today various unfamiliar problems posed by global environmental changes. The best known of these is global climate change. This modern phenomenon is occurring in response to the excessive emission of greenhouse gases by human societies, especially the release of carbon dioxide from fossil fuel combustion.

Climate change and the other global environmental changes have a particular contemporary significance. Environmental health hazards have, until recently, been largely confined to local issues, such as microbial and chemical water pollution and urban air pollution. In the last two decades, however, various historically unprecedented global environmental changes have emerged as human domination of the earth's surface has rapidly increased (Vitousek et al., 1997). These changes include human-induced changes in the gaseous composition of the lower atmosphere (climate change) and middle atmosphere (stratospheric ozone depletion); loss of soil fertility in all continents; depletion of freshwater supplies, including many major underground aquifers; depletion of fisheries; disruption of global elemental cycles (especially nitrogen, carbon, and phosphorus); and a high rate of loss of species and local populations. These global environmental changes are likely to have important consequences for the health of human populations.

Recognition, during the past decade, of these large-scale risks to human health has influenced several major international scientific assessments to pay increasing attention to the relationship between these global changes and human health. Indeed, there is nascent realization that understanding the impacts of global environmental changes on human well-being and health is central to the public debate on the achievement of "sustainability"—since, from an anthropocentric perspective, the ultimate goal of "sustainability" is to optimize human experience (well-being, comfort, security, health, survival) into the indefinite future. Accordingly, the third assessment by the United Nation's Intergovernmental Panel on Climate Change (IPCC, 2001b) and the recent assessment by the Millennium Ecosystem Assessment project have given substantial emphasis to estimating current and future risks to human health.

Over the past two decades, there has been substantial work done to estimate the health risks due to stratospheric ozone depletion. Of all the global environmental changes, that one, in process terms, is the simplest. Various human-produced industrial gases, especially halogenated compounds (e.g., the chlorofluorocarbons), destroy the ozone molecules in the stratosphere, and this allows a greater penetration to the earth's surface of incoming solar ultraviolet radiation—although this has so far been largely confined to the higher latitudes. This increase in exposure to solar ultraviolet radiation, particularly UV-B, necessarily increases the risk of melanoma and non-melanocytic skin cancers in some parts of the world, including southern Australia, southern South America, northern Europe, and Canada. Other probable risks to health include increases in incidence of ocular cataracts, several other eye disorders such as pterygium, squamous cell carcinoma of the cornea, and conjunctiva, and the several health consequences of immune system suppression (Lucas and Ponsonby, 2002; McMichael et al., 2003a).

Estimating the population health risks due to ecosystem disruption, biodiversity losses, disruption of global elemental cycles (especially nitrogen and phosphorus), the degradation of fertile soils, and the depletion of freshwater supplies is much less straightforward. Much of this work is only now getting under way, typically in response to international and national multidisciplinary reviews of these particular topics. A major contemporary example, mentioned above, is the series of reports now appearing from the wide-ranging international work, conducted during 2001–2004, of the Millennium Ecosystem Assessment. The conceptual framework, including specific concepts and methods pertaining to well-being and health, are discussed in the initial major publication of this project (Millennium Ecosystem Assessment, 2003).

To date, however, the most intensive and best-developed health risk assessments have been done in relation to global climate change, current and future. In the remainder of this chapter we therefore concentrate primarily on that example of global environmental change and its attendant health impacts.

First, though, there is need for brief consideration of the relationship between globalization and global environmental change.

RELATIONSHIP OF GLOBAL ENVIRONMENTAL CHANGE TO "GLOBALIZATION"

"Globalization" reflects the scale, intensification, and connectedness of human economic, technological, and cultural activities. At first sight, it seems likely that there is a close, intrinsic connection between globalization and large-scale environmental change. After all, as industrialization spreads, so does the emission of greenhouse gases. As tropical countries strive to increase export income, so forests—undervalued by prevailing short-term market economics—are cleared. This results in both the sale of timber and the conversion of land into farming, while also releasing additional carbon dioxide into the atmosphere. More generally, as trade internationalizes and liberalizes, countries that exploit their particular points of comparative economic-production advantage to produce export commodities often do so to the detriment of local ecosystems and of the natural resource base. Many other such points of current connection between globalization and global environmental changes could be identified.

Historically, one of the most cited historical examples of the impact of "globalizing" interconnectedness on human health is the entry of plague into fourteenth-century Europe from the Orient, and its subsequent devastating spread. This resulted from plague-infected, flea-infested rats being transported on ships from East–West trading ports in the Black Sea to Italian seaports. In later centuries, the introduction of quarantine and other control strategies helped control the spread of this and other infectious diseases across transnational borders. Today's globalization process, however, is characterized by a market-driven intensification of productivity and trade and increased human mobility, all underwritten by rapid advances in science and technology. This poses a much greater challenge to infectious disease control, environmental stewardship, and social management, requiring strategies that transcend national borders.

Meanwhile, increasingly, we strive to attain a "sustainable" future world—and this will presumably be a globalized world. Achieving such a future world will necessarily entail uncoupling the environmentally and socially damaging aspects of today's globalization activities from the ongoing connection process in our increasingly "global village." This is possible, in principle, because the seemingly close linkage between globalization and global environmental changes is neither intrinsic nor inevitable. The challenge will be to achieve this uncoupling and to transform the (potentially beneficial) globalizing process with a newly forged set of sustainability-oriented values, policies, and practices.

CLIMATE VARIABILITY AND CHANGE

Several climate-related terms warrant early clarification. "Weather" refers to transient climatic conditions, from day to day, as opposed to the longer term conditions that define the prevailing "climate." Within the short term, climate is what you expect, while weather is what you get. "Climate change" generally refers to long-term change—over decades, centuries, or even millennia—in the average state of one or more meteorological parameters (e.g., temperature and/or rainfall). "Climate variability" refers to shifts in patterns of the natural climate system that are relatively short term—over years or decades—but that go beyond individual weather events.

Scientific understanding of the "modes" of climate variability between years has increased considerably in recent years. There has been particular interest in the El Niño Southern Oscillation (ENSO) cycle, which displays an approximately half-decadal variation. ENSO arises from the complex interplay, across the Pacific Ocean, between anomalies and surface winds blowing along the equator and ocean currents and temperatures (National Research Council, 2001), resulting in warm (El Niño) and cold (La Niña) phases. ENSO effects are experienced around the low- to mid-latitude globe, causing variations in rainfall and temperature over much of the tropics, subtropics, and some temperate areas (IPCC, 2001a). Over the past quarter century, ENSO warm events (El Niño) have been more frequent, persistent, and intense than in the previous 100 years.

Beyond natural and human-induced climate variability, long-term human-induced climate change is of increasing concern. The *Third Assessment Report* of the United Nations' IPCC, a large and authoritative international body of scientific review, concluded that the global average temperature increased by about 0.6°C plus or minus 0.2°C during the twentieth century (IPCC, 2001a). The IPCC concluded that the 1990s was almost certainly the warmest decade since record keeping began in mid-nineteenth century and that 1998 was the single warmest year. This general increase in temperature has been accompanied by a reduction in the frequency of extreme low temperatures since 1950 and a small increase in the frequency of extreme high temperatures. An important conclusion of the IPCC (2001a, p. 3) was this: "There is new and stronger evidence that most of the warming observed over the last 50 years is attributable to human activities." (Note that the oft-heard popular debate about whether global warming is natural or due to human actions is simplistic. The processes can, and apparently do, occur concurrently.)

During the twentieth century, rainfall and other precipitation appears to have increased by 0.5–1.0% per decade over most of the middle- and high-latitude land areas of the northern hemisphere, while decreasing by about 0.3% per decade over most of the northern hemisphere's subtropical land areas (10° N to 30° N). Over the same period, precipitation appears to have increased by 0.2–0.3% per decade over tropical land areas (10° S to 10° N). No consistent changes in precipitation have been detected in the southern hemisphere, and there are insufficient data to establish trends in precipitation over the oceans (IPCC, 2001a). During that same century, there were small increases in global land areas experiencing severe drought and severe wetness—including an increase in the frequency and intensity of droughts in parts of Africa and Asia in recent decades. There have been no significant trends in the frequency or intensity of storms, however, either in the tropics or in the temperate regions.

Global ocean heat content has increased since the late 1950s, the period for which data are available. However, parts of the southern hemisphere oceans and Antarctica have not warmed. The global sea level rose approximately 0.15 meters during the twentieth century. The IPCC concluded that warming has contributed significantly to last century's sea-level rise, due both to the expansion of water at higher temperatures and to the melting of alpine glacier ice.

Global climate change, occurring in response to human action, reflects the modern configuration of population size and economic activities. This has caused an increase in the atmospheric concentration of greenhouse gases—the energy-trapping gases that amplify the natural "greenhouse effect" that keeps most of the earth comfortably above freezing point. The greenhouse gases comprise, principally, carbon dioxide (mostly from fossil fuel combustion and forest burning), plus various other heat-trapping gases such as methane (from irrigated agriculture, animal husbandry, and oil extraction), nitrous oxide, and various human-made halocarbons.

The concentration of carbon dioxide in the lower atmosphere (troposphere) has increased by approximately one-third since 1750, from 275 ppm to 370 ppm (IPCC, 2001a). Over the past twenty years, about three-fourths of carbon dioxide emissions from human activity have been linked to the burning of fossil fuels. The remaining emissions are predominately due to land-use change, especially deforestation. At the current atmospheric concentrations, the land and ocean together take up about half of these carbon dioxide emissions—the rest remain in the atmosphere. There have also been significant increases in methane and nitrous oxide in the atmosphere. The atmospheric concentration of some other greenhouse gases is increasing more slowly or decreasing as a result of emission controls in response to international agreements.

Over the coming century, as shown in figure 5.1, world average temperature is predicted to increase within the range 1.4–5.8°C (IPCC, 2001a). This anticipated increase will be greater at higher latitudes and will be greater in winter than in summer. Meanwhile, overall, rainfall will increase. However, many parts of the terrestrial globe will become drier, and in other areas precipitation events are expected to become more severe (thus increasing the risk of flooding).

IMPACTS OF CLIMATE CHANGE

In recent decades, many nonhuman physical and biological systems have undergone changes that are reasonably attributable to the recent global warming. This includes the retreat of glaciers, the diminution of sea ice, and the earlier occurrence of bird nesting, flowering, and insect migrations (IPCC, 2001b; Root et al., 2003). The IPCC has assessed that this overall pattern indicates the incipient impact of warming around the world. So, given these changes in nonhuman systems, what impacts might we expect on human settlements, food production, environmental security, and, more generally, well-being and health?

The human impacts of climate change and consequent environmental changes will differ between locations and geographical settings. Further, the vulnerability of each human population depends on locality, level of material resources, information base, technological assets, and type of governance. Overall, the human species, via its social organization and cultural practices, is better buffered against environmental stressors than are all other plant and animal species. Hence, *Homo sapiens* is likely to be affected less soon and less sensitively by climate change than are most other species.

Nevertheless, the IPCC's *Third Assessment Report* stated:

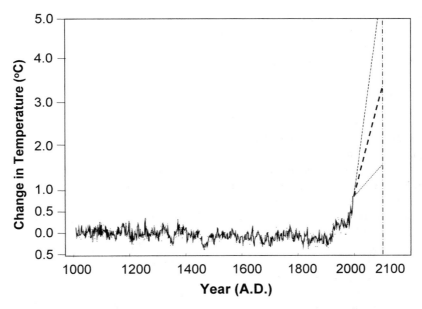

FIGURE 5.1. Reported Variations in Earth's Average Global Surface Temperature since 1000 A.D. Data are supplemented by estimated range of increases over the coming century in response to recent and ongoing buildup of atmospheric greenhouse gas concentration. Note also the rapid rise in temperature of around 0.4°C since 1975. Dotted lines show approximate range of temperature increases estimated to the year 2100. The central estimate (dashed line) is 2–3°C. *Source:* Based on data from IPCC (2001a).

There is emerging evidence that some social and economic systems have been affected by the recent increasing frequency of floods and droughts in some areas. However, such systems are also affected by changes in socioeconomic factors such as demographic shifts and land-use changes. The relative impacts of climatic and socioeconomic factors are generally difficult to quantify.... Human systems that are sensitive to climate change include mainly water resources; agriculture (especially food security) and forestry; coastal zones and marine systems (fisheries); human settlements, energy and industry; insurance and other financial services; and human health. The vulnerability of these systems varies with geographic location, time and social, economic and environmental conditions. (IPCC, 2001b, pp. 4–5)

Climate Change and Food Production

Climatic influences on world food production are of particular interest. There has been particular research interest in cereal grains, which account for approxi-

mately two-thirds of the world's total world energy for human populations. Most of the grain is consumed directly, while some is consumed via its conversion into beef, pork, and chicken. Annual global cereal yields became a little less stable during the 1990s, and there has been a steady decline in annual per-person production during the period 1996–2002 (Lang and Heasman, 2004). Could this be partly due to changing climatic conditions? There are, of course, many influences upon food production—ecological, commercial, consumer driven, and political. However, temperature, rainfall, and soil moisture are fundamentally important to agriculture and horticulture. These act not only via the central process of photosynthesis, and thus grain growth, but also via weather disasters, influences on crop pests and diseases, and loss and spoilage.

The impact of standard scenarios of climate change, over three time slices during this coming century, has been modeled by several groups of scientists, working particularly with climate change scenarios from the Hadley Research Centre, U.K. Meteorology Office, and the European Community Hamburg Centre (Parry et al., 1999; Shah and Strong, 2000). These studies incorporate estimates of future trends in population growth, economic development, governmental policies on pricing, world food trading, and agricultural technological developments. Overall, these modeling studies have found that the imposition of climate change would cause a net decline in total global yield of grain.

The models forecast marked differences in the impact of climate change on local cereal production in regions around the world. In short, they indicate that it will become a world of "winners and losers"—the former generally being in temperate zones (including the developed countries of Europe and North America, along with China and much of South America), while the latter tend to be in low-latitude countries where food insecurity is already widespread (including South Asia, parts of the Middle East, North Africa, much of sub-Saharan Africa, and Central America).

A research task yet to be properly undertaken is the conversion of such estimates of changes in food yields to estimates of risks to human nutrition, especially child stunting and development; adult malnutrition, dysfunction, and disease risk; and premature mortality.

Climate Change and Human Health: Overview

The health impacts of climate change do not entail novel processes and unfamiliar disease outcomes (in contrast to the recent surprise appearances of HIV/AIDS and human mad cow disease). Rather, they entail climate-induced changes in the frequency or severity of familiar health risks—such as floods, storms, and fires; the mortality toll of heat-waves; the range and seasonality of infectious diseases; the health consequences of altered freshwater supplies; and the many repercussions of economic dislocation and population displacement.

Overall, most of the health impacts of climate change are likely to be adverse (IPCC, 1996, 2001b). However, some impacts would be beneficial. For example, milder winters would reduce the normal seasonal wintertime peak mortality in temperate countries, and in currently hot regions, a further increase in temperatures might reduce the viability of disease-transmitting mosquito populations.

Several recent reports have suggested that we may now be seeing some early impacts of climate change on infectious diseases. For example, tick-borne (viral) encephalitis in Sweden appears to have increased in response to a succession of warmer winters over the past two decades (Lindgren and Gustafson, 2001), and there is some, though still inconclusive, evidence of malaria ascending in the eastern African highlands in association with local warming (Patz et al., 2002). Meanwhile, the intensification of the ENSO over the past quarter century, a presumed consequence of global climate change, has been accompanied by a strengthening interannual association with diarrheal disease in Bangladesh (Rodo et al., 2002). Climatologists anticipate that, under conditions of global warming, the ENSO will become more energetic, thereby acquiring greater amplitude (IPCC, 2001a). Indeed, the great severity of the recent national drought in Australia in 2002–2003 has been attributed in part to climate change as a source of the extremity of this unusually hot, dry episode (Nicholls, 2004).

In the past, epidemiologists have had little interest in studying the relationship of climatic variations to human health. This may have reflected a general assumption that there are few opportunities for direct intervention to reduce adverse health impacts from climatic influences. However, the position has changed markedly following the recognition of "anthropogenic" global climate change. Further, in addition to the forecast gradual rise in the earth's mean surface temperature, an increase in climatic variability is likely (IPCC, 2001a). Indeed, many scientists now consider human health and safety to be more endangered by an impending increase in extreme and anomalous weather events than by changed average climate conditions (National Research Council, 2001).

MAJOR CATEGORIES OF HEALTH IMPACTS

There are several generic categories of health impacts due to climate change: (i) those that arise from relatively direct impacts of alterations in temperature, precipitation, and extreme weather events; (ii) those that occur in response to climate-induced changes in ecological processes and systems; and (iii) those that result from the economic and demographic dislocation of human communities. These various pathways are illustrated in figure 5.2.

Direct Effects

The more direct and immediate impacts include those due to changes in exposure to very cold and

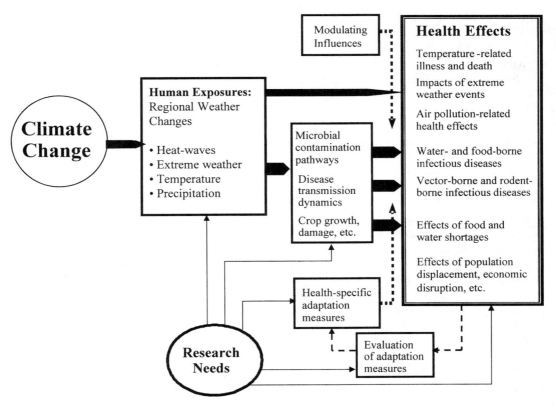

FIGURE 5.2. Climate Change and Health: Pathways of Influence, Adaptation, Research, and Evaluation. Modulating influences are diverse nonclimatic factors that affect climate-related health outcomes, such as material standard of living, population growth and demographic change, public health infrastructure, access to health care, and quality of health care. Adaptation (discussed further below) includes actions, planned or unplanned, that reduce the risk of adverse health outcomes, such as public education, the use of protective technologies, vaccination programs, disease surveillance, monitoring, use of climate forecasts and health-impact forecasts, and development of emergency-management and disaster-preparedness programs. *Source:* Based on Patz et al. (2000).

very hot weather extremes, and those due to increases in extreme weather events (floods, tropical cyclones, storm surges, and droughts). Climate change would also directly increase the production of certain air pollutants, such as tropospheric ozone (the formation of which is affected by both temperature and level of sunlight), and may affect the concentration and geographic range of various aeroallergens (spores and molds) that contribute to asthma, hay fever, and other allergic disorders.

Thermal Stress

Under normal physiological conditions, the human body endeavors to maintain a core temperature of around 37°C. Thermal stress results from exposure to extreme cold or hot weather when the physiological mechanisms for maintaining core body temperature are challenged. The association between weather (mainly temperature) and mortality has been well established in studies albeit predominantly from developed countries experiencing temperate climates. Each population displays a characteristic pattern of level of daily deaths (and hospitalizations) in relation to concurrent and immediately preceding daily temperature (Wilkinson et al., 2002). Presence of preexisting disease (particularly of the cardiovascular and respiratory systems), socioeconomic status, and housing type determine vulnerability to the effects of thermal stress (Hales et al., 2003). Being elderly and living alone also increases the risk, posing an important challenge to the developed nations in particular, with aging populations (Koppe et al., 2004).

Typically, daily death rates increase with extremes of both heat and cold, hence described as displaying a U-shaped relationship. Therefore, in temperate countries, usually experiencing higher mortality during winter, climate change would result in a decrease in the winter mortality peak, offset by the increases in summer heat-related mortality. The net balance of future changes in hot and cold effects remains both contentious and, anyway, is highly variable among different geographic regions and states of economic development and between urban and rural populations (McMichael et al., 2006). Developing nations undergoing rapid industrialization are likely to experience an overall increase in heat-related mortality due to increasing heat island effect. This is a phenomenon characterized by higher daytime and nighttime temperatures in built up areas, compared to surrounding areas, resulting from loss of vegetation and the use of heat-absorbing and heat-retaining man-made substances for building and road construction.

Human populations have the capacity to adapt to a great extent physiologically and technologically, and by behavioral change, to gradual changes in climate. However, sudden changes in weather can have a significant impact on human physiology and therefore health. Global warming is likely to cause an overall increase in the number of extreme heat events and a reduction in extreme cold weather (Houghton et al., 2001; Koppe et al., 2004). In Europe, for example, the annual increase of warm extremes during the period 1976–1999 was twice as much as the corresponding decrease in extreme cold events (Koppe et al., 2004). This does not, however, eliminate the importance of extreme cold weather events.

The impact of extreme events is estimated using episode analysis, which cannot then be used to estimate future risks from predicted increased climate variability. Examining the impact of these events will, however, help in adaptation assessment (Kovats et al., 2003). Vulnerability of individuals with preexisting disease to the effects of heat can mask, to some extent, the impact of an extreme heat event on human health due to the effect being attributed to the underlying disease. For a death to be classified as directly heat related, the core body temperature has to be recorded before or immediately after death. Presentation with a cardiovascular or respiratory problem would overshadow the significance of body temperature. Alternatively, the discovery of a body after death, by definition, excludes the possibility of classifying the death as directly heat related, unless by exclusion of other causes. In spite of these limitations, deaths from direct heat-related illness have been shown to increase during heat waves (Centers for Disease Control and Prevention, 1995). Another approach is to report "excess deaths," whereby the number of deaths that occurred during the extreme event is compared with the number of deaths for the same period in previous years (Institut De Veille Sanitaire, 2003).

The increase in deaths observed with extreme temperature events is partly attributed to forward displacement of deaths that may have otherwise occurred in the immediate future. This phenomenon, known as mortality displacement, has been reported with extreme heat and cold and is demonstrated by a compensatory decrease in deaths that follows (Huynen et al., 2001; Rooney et al., 1998; Sartor et al., 1995). Similarly, the impact of extreme temperatures may not be visible immediately, and lag periods are often used to examine the impact (Ebi and Patz, 2002). The lag period for extreme events may differ depending on suddenness of onset, intensity, and duration of extreme event. Generally, heat events demonstrate shorter lag periods compared to cold events.

The association between temperature and nonfatal outcomes is less well researched. Traditionally, heat-related illness referred to dehydration, heat stroke, and heat exhaustion; hypothermia described cold-related illness. However, as with temperature-related mortality, it is becoming evident that extreme weather, both hot and cold, also increases hospital admissions from respiratory and cardiovascular disease (Afza and Bridgman, 2001; Jones et al., 1982; McGregor et al., 1999; Rusticucci et al., 2002; Semenza et al., 1999; Stewart et al., 2002). Illness leading to presentation to the primary care provider and hospital admissions are significant nonfatal outcomes that need to be assessed in relation to climate change, as these impose a burden on health care services. Knowing the impact on such outcomes in relation to current and predicted climate change can assist in the management and allocation of health service resources.

There is still uncertainty surrounding the climate variable or variables that most affect health. Weather variables do not act independently to influence health. Maximum temperature is often used as the exposure variable against which health outcome is assessed. However, heat waves occur during synoptic conditions that also result in higher than average overnight (minimum) temperatures and increased humidity. Photochemical ground-level ozone, an air pollutant, is also known to occur in high levels during heat waves. The extent to which these variables influence health, and interact with each other to affect human health, may vary according to local conditions and needs further assessment. These are important considerations in light of rapid industrialization, urbanization, and population pressures faced by many nations.

INTERACTION BETWEEN
WEATHER AND AIR POLLUTION

Air pollutants, by themselves, are harmful to human health. The production of ground-level photochemical ozone, an air pollutant that is the main component of urban smog, is favored by high atmospheric temperature due to acceleration of the photochemical reaction (Patz and Balbus, 2001). The relationship between ambient temperature and ozone levels is not linear, with a stronger correlation reported when temperatures exceed 32°C (Patz and Balbus, 2001). Apart from high temperatures, high-pressure systems, increased water vapor concentration, and increased emission of precursor pollutants such as volatile organic carbons and nitrogen oxides also increase ozone production. These conditions are more likely to occur with climate change. So is increased cloud cover, which may help reduce ozone production (Patz and Balbus, 2001).

It is estimated that, globally, air pollution causes 5% of tracheal, bronchial, and lung cancers; 2% of cardiorespiratory mortality; and 1% of respiratory infection mortality, amounting to about 0.8 million deaths and 7.9 million disability-adjusted life years (DALYs; one DALY equals the loss of one healthy life year) (World Health Organization, 2002). The proportion of these outcomes attributable to climate change is not known.

Extreme Weather Events

Some uncertainty remains as to changes in the regional frequency of extreme weather events because of climate change. However, climatologists are increasingly able to downscale their climate forecasting models, focusing with higher resolution on regional and local environments. In the meantime, despite the potentially great impact of extreme climatic conditions and weather events on deaths, injuries, and consequent diseases (infections, malnutrition, and mental health disorders), the estimation of the future profile of health should be treated as no more than an indicative exercise.

There are diverse health impacts of changes in the frequency and intensity of extreme weather events such as storms and floods. These events can directly affect health through injuries and deaths from trauma and drowning. Loss of housing, sanitary facilities, social structure, and access to clean water (through contamination of existing water supplies) can lead to increased transmission of communicable disease (Balbus and Wilson, 2000; Greenough et al., 2001; Hales et al., 2003). Transmission of vector-borne disease typically increases because the disrupted conditions favor vector breeding and human contact. In the long term, mental strain and physical illness may result from economic losses due to damage to agriculture and livestock. Coastal and low-lying areas are more susceptible to cyclones and storms, as are environmentally degraded areas (Hales et al., 2003). Impoverished and dense populations, poor housing structures, and poor access to medical services, water, and sanitation increase vulnerability of populations (Balbus and Wilson, 2000; Hales et al., 2003). At the same time, urbanization also increases the risk of flash flooding because the land is made incapable of absorbing precipitation (Greenough et al., 2001).

Hurricane Mitch, centered in the Honduras in 1998, resulted in tens of thousands of cases of malaria, dengue fever, acute respiratory illness, and diarrhea (Forum, 1999; Guill and Shandera, 2001). An estimated 9,600 people were killed and 1 million people were left homeless as a result of this tropical cyclone turned category 5 hurricane. The impact on an economy reliant on farming was severe, with extensive loss of banana, coffee, corn, and sugar crops (Forum, 1999; Hales et al., 2003). It is likely that the severity of the impact was amplified by the extensive deforestation for farming on hillsides and lower mountain slopes.

The impact of drought is predominantly through lost food production, presenting as malnutrition and famine in developing countries (Greenough et al., 2001; Hales et al., 2003). Crop production may improve in some regions such as northern Europe, but this impact is likely to be overshadowed by the reduced yield in developing countries, where an estimated 790 million people are already undernourished (Houghton et al., 2001). The dry conditions that accompany droughts also increase the risk of wildfires, which in turn can cause or exacerbate respiratory illness, burns, and traumatic injuries (Greenough et al., 2001).

There is other evidence suggesting that floods and hurricanes adversely affect mental health (Hales et al., 2003; Krug et al., 1998). Several levels of posttraumatic stress and depression were reported in a group of adolescents six months after experiencing Hurricane Mitch (Goenjian et al., 2001). There has been little research yet on the impact of drought on mental health.

Indirect Effects (Especially Infectious Diseases)

The indirect category of health impact refers, in particular, to climate-related changes in the transmission patterns of infectious diseases and changes in regional food-producing ecosystems. These changes in health risks reflect disturbances of complex ecological processes. In the longer term, these indirect impacts on health are likely to have greater magnitude than the more direct impacts (IPCC, 2001b).

For vector-borne infectious diseases, the geographic range, seasonal activity, and abundance of vector organisms (and, in some cases, their intermediate hosts) are affected by various meteorological factors (temperature, precipitation, humidity, surface water, and wind) and biotic factors (vegetation, host species, predators, competitors, parasites, and human interventions). Further, the rate of maturation of pathogens within the vector organism is typically sensitive to temperature, in a curvilinear fashion, such that a particular absolute increment of warming, at different parts of the temperature range, yields very different increases in transmissibility.

Mathematical modeling studies have, in general, forecasted that an increase in worldwide average temperature and associated changes in rainfall patterns would cause a net increase in the geographic range of potential malaria transmissibility (IPCC, 2001b; Martens et al., 1999). However, some localized decreases may also occur in regions that become too hot or dry, such as in the Sahel region of sub-Saharan Africa. Downscaled modeling studies of future malaria transmissibility under climate change conditions have also been carried out, at higher geographic resolution, for various countries such as Zimbabwe, Australia, and Canada.

Temperature-related changes in the life-cycle dynamics of both the vector species and the pathogens (protozoa, bacteria, and viruses) would increase the potential transmission of many other vector-borne infectious diseases such as dengue fever (one the world's great vector-borne viral infectious diseases, transmitted by mosquito) and leishmaniasis (transmitted by the sand fly) (see also chapter 2). Several different types of models, either biologically based or statistically based, have been used to forecast the future patterns of potential transmission of dengue fever. For example, a study using a statistically based model of the observed recent correlation of climatic variables with the geographic range of *Aedes aegypti*, the principal mosquito vector for dengue fever, indicates that under future climate change conditions dengue fever would extend its range and seasonality in various parts of the world (Hales et al., 2002). Figure 5.3 presents a map, based on that modeling technique, of the potential transmission probabilities for dengue, globally, later in the twenty-first century under a standard scenario of climate change. This study demonstrates some of the uncertainties when estimating the future impact of climate change. Transmission probabilities were generated based on projected population change, with and without considering climate change. It was estimated that, if humidity (which influences vector breeding and survival) did not change, the population at risk of dengue would increase from a baseline of about 30% of the world's population in 1990 (1.5 billion people) to 35% (3.5 billion people) in 2085. Altering the humidity scenario increased the population at risk to 52% of the world's population (5.2 million people) by 2085 (Hales et al., 2002). As recognized by Hales et al. (2002), these estimates did not take into account other important influences on actual risk of dengue transmission, such as changes in social and economic conditions.

Figure 5.4 illustrates the application of the same modeling technique to a particular geographic region, in this case Australia (McMichael et al., 2003b). It is evident from the two maps for 2050 that the potential transmission zone for dengue fever, as a function of the climatically receptive zone for the

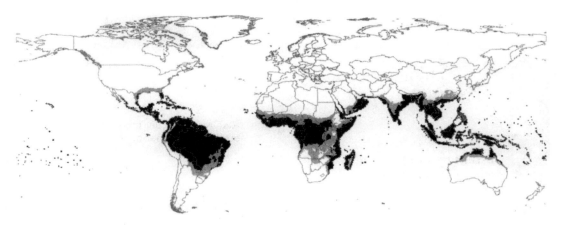

FIGURE 5.3. Estimated Baseline World Population at Risk of Dengue Fever in 1990 (Black) and Increase in Population at Risk by 2085 (Gray). Map was modeled using global circulation models to forecast future climatic conditions, linked with a statistical model of the current relationship between climatic variables and the geographic range of the principal mosquito vector for dengue fever. *Source:* Figure provided by S. Hales, based on Hales et al. (2002).

mosquito vector, will increase as warming ensues and as rainfall extends farther south, especially in the northwestern coastal region.

In Australia, Ross River virus disease (transmitted by mosquitoes) has increased in geographic range since 1990 (Tong et al., 2001). Using data from the past two decades in Australia, a combination of heavy rainfall and high temperatures has moderate capacity to "predict" recent epidemics of Ross River virus disease (Woodruff et al., 2002). This also suggests that climate change will result in an increase in future transmission in some regions of Australia, while in other regions drying may lessen transmission risk. Note, however, that some of these vector-borne diseases are inherently complex to model, since important nonhuman host (reservoir) species are also involved in the transmission cycles. In the case of Ross River virus disease, this entails various vertebrate species, including kangaroos in particular, other mammals, and perhaps some bird species.

Geographic information systems (GIS) enable the linking of climatic, geographic, and epidemiological information. Recent developments in GIS are facilitating the construction of predictive models. GIS can incorporate remotely sensed satellite data, assessing factors such as vegetation change that may be influence vector distribution and transmission potential for endemic disease. In Africa, for example, the MARA/ARMA (Mapping Malaria Risk in Africa) collaboration has used GIS with a robust database to assess how climate change affects disease risk down to the district level. From this analysis, a model has been developed that describes the climatic limitations on the distribution of the *Anopheles* mosquito vectors and the *Plasmodium* parasites.

Climate change would also affect the transmission of water-borne infectious diseases via several mechanisms, including intensification of rainfall episodes, leading to flooding that causes contamination of drinking water supplies. Bacterial water-borne illnesses such as gastroenteritis due to coliform bacteria, giardiasis, and cholera may thus be affected; so, too, would various protozoal water-borne infectious diseases such as cryptosporidiosis. Similarly, warmer temperatures would tend to increase the summer seasonal peaks of food-borne bacterial enteric infections, such as those due to salmonella and campylobacter (Hall et al., 2002).

In low-income countries, with poor hygiene and resources, rates of serious child diarrheal disease would rise. High temperatures may accelerate the multiplication of pathogens that cause food to spoil, resulting in gastrointestinal infections. The sensitivity of child diarrhea to variations in climatic conditions has been well demonstrated in time-series studies in Lima, Peru, and in Fiji (Checkley et al., 2000; Singh et al., 2001). For example, Singh et al. (2001) found a positive association between annual average temperature and the incidence of diarrhea in adults in eighteen Pacific Island nations. In a second study in Fiji,

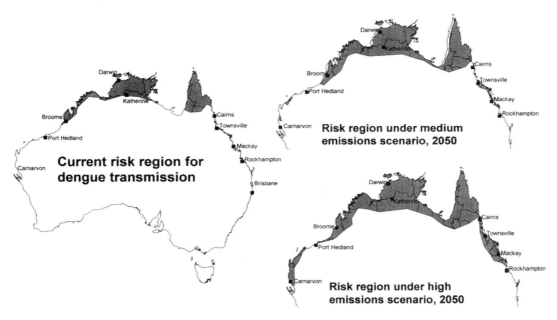

FIGURE 5.4. Dengue Fever in Australia, Current and Future. Map presents model-based estimates of the geographic region suitable for maintenance of *Aedes aegypti*, the principal mosquito vector for dengue fever. The current risk region, on the left, is compared with those for two alternative climate change scenarios in 2050 (as modeled by the Australian Commonwealth Scientific and Industrial Research Organization). *Source:* Figure based on McMichael et al. (2003b).

they found positive associations between diarrhea and temperature and between diarrhea and extremes in rainfall.

EFFECTS OF ECONOMIC, SOCIAL, AND DEMOGRAPHIC DISRUPTION

This third main category of health impact from climate change is difficult to model quantitatively—but, given the usual experience of displaced or economically disrupted populations elsewhere, a range of adverse health consequences is near certain. Refugee populations experience various risks to health, including mental health problems, malnutrition, infectious diseases, and the physical hazards of new and improvised living environments (see chapter 9). Several small island states are already registering growing concern about sea-level rise, and this concern itself may jeopardize well-being and mental health. Economic downturns and unemployment induce a similar range of risks to health. Further, such disturbances can create conflict situations, both internally within the affected community and in its external relations with other communities.

These anticipated climate change-related health consequences of economic disruptions, of rising sea level, and of population displacement for reasons of physical hazard, land loss, unemployment, and civil strife may not become evident for several decades. Further, it will often not be easy to attribute such outcomes to climate change in situations where there are many, often interrelated, causal influences involved.

PREVENTIVE STRATEGIES: MITIGATION AND ADAPTATION

The reduction of population health risks from climate change requires two complementary strategies. First, the fundamentally important option is mitigation—that is, the reduction of greenhouse gas emissions. Second, we can implement adaptation measures to reduce the health impacts of current and already-committed climate change.

Mitigation strategies to halt and reverse global

climate change require participation by all nations. Although industrialized countries have, historically, largely driven global environmental change, mitigation cannot be effective unless all countries are prepared to contribute to the requisite global decrease in emission of greenhouse gases. This may be on a negotiated "differentiated" basis, with agreement to converge at a common per capita level of emissions later this century. Carbon cycle models indicate that, in order to stabilize the atmospheric carbon dioxide concentration at 450 ppm, anthropogenic carbon dioxide emissions would need to drop well below 1990 levels within a few decades. (In recognition of this, the British government has committed itself to achieving a national 60% reduction in greenhouse gas emissions by 2050.) Clearly, the much-debated Kyoto Protocol is merely a first, small attempt to decrease global greenhouse gas emissions. However, in mid-2004, even this modest first-step level of international commitment had not been ratified and implemented.

Adaptive capacity is formally defined by the IPCC (2001b, p. 982) as "the ability of a system to adjust to climate change (including climate variability and extremes) to moderate potential damages, to take advantage of opportunities, or to cope with the consequences." In human societies, adaptive capacity varies with wealth, access to technology, education and information, skills levels, societal infrastructure, access to resources and management capabilities, and developmental status. It also depends on various structural and politically determined characteristics, including social-cultural rigidity, international connectedness, and political flexibility (Woodward et al., 2000). Since adaptation is, in general, wealth dependent, poorer countries are less able to act to lessen the impacts of climate change (McMichael et al., 2003a).

In 2003, Europe was affected by an intense prolonged heat wave and by severe floods. During the two-week heat wave, there were more than 30,000 excess deaths across Europe—of which over 15,000 were in France alone (Kovats et al., 2004). Such nations, however, have a good capacity to recover and to take subsequent adaptive action, thereby minimizing the long-term impact on the community. In contrast, the long-term impacts on disadvantaged populations such as a rural community or a developing nation may be greater and need to be assessed separately. To date, there has been relatively little research on how climate change affects the health of such populations.

Similarly, the impact of climate change on regions that normally experience less climate variability is not well established.

We are already committed to experiencing some degree of global climate change over coming decades, despite any mitigation actions we might take now. This is ensured by the generally persistent nature of greenhouse gases within the atmosphere. Hence, it is important to begin assessing, for each particular population, its vulnerability to climate change and its adaptation options. Adaptive actions range from strengthening flood defenses to improved building design, improved public health infrastructure, enhanced vaccination programs and disease-vector control programs, more robust and ecologically sustainable local food production, strengthened disaster-medicine preparedness, and weather watch-warning systems for early alerts for extreme weather events.

THE CHALLENGE TO EPIDEMIOLOGISTS AND OTHER POPULATION HEALTH RESEARCHERS

Over the past decade, the advent of global climate change and other global environmental changes has begun to influence the environmental health research agenda (Martens and McMichael, 2002; Kovats et al., 2003). In particular, the growing interest in elucidating the relationship between climatic conditions and population health has prompted three main types of epidemiological research:

1. Empirical studies, based on recent data, of the causal relationship between climatic variations or trends and health outcomes
2. Studies seeking evidence of recent or current health impacts attributable to (now predominantly human-induced) climate change
3. Estimations of the likely range of health impacts of plausible climatic-environmental scenarios over coming decades, increasingly using formal modeling techniques

The examples that follow illustrate each of these three categories of research tasks. The examples given are skewed toward studies of relatively straightforward causal relationships. In contrast, causal relationships that are complex, systems based, and high in uncertainties and those that are seemingly frankly nonestimable are much less tractable to formal research—at least within our current methodological repertoire. Of course, for all such climate-health relationships, the usual considerations of epidemiological research apply, including the role of confounding variable and interactive processes (Balbus, 1998).

To illustrate the above point about inherently complex relationships, consider first the impacts on agricultural yields of climate change (along with the oft-concurrent influences of other large-scale environmental changes, e.g., land degradation, water supply depletion, shifts in plant pests and diseases, and acidification due to globally amplified nitrogen fixation). Changes in food yields have consequences for local/regional food availability, nutritional status, child development, and survival—and for conflict situations. However, estimating the actual population-level burden of malnutrition and childhood stunting attributable to climate change is problematic given the confounding due to regional differences in economic and trading circumstances and to the overlay of infectious disease and other factors that interact with nutritional status. Currently, therefore, we must address such relationships in largely qualitative terms.

Empirical research into causal relationships has included studies of how thermal stress affects mortality in diverse populations, how high temperatures and air pollution jointly affect cardiorespiratory morbidity and mortality, how climatic variability (especially that associated with the approximately half-decadal ENSO cycle) affects outbreaks of mosquito-borne infectious diseases, and how climatic variations affect rates of food poisoning and diarrheal disease. In all these studies, estimates of additional rates of disease incidence or death are made, and relative risks can be derived.

The second research category—the search for early evidence of health impacts—has been stimulated by the persuasive documentation of changes in many nonhuman physical and biotic systems over the past two decades in association with, and now attributed to, regional warming (IPCC, 2001a). Birds, bugs, and buds are responding to earlier springtime weather; ice caps, glaciers, and sea ice are diminishing. However, detecting and attributing changes in human health outcomes are much more difficult: our culture (behavior, technology, etc.) buffers us against direct exposure to environmental change, and there are many concurrent influences (confounders) on any particular health outcome. Nevertheless, as mentioned earlier in this chapter, several recent studies

have reported plausible climate-related changes in certain infectious diseases. These include tick-borne encephalitis in Sweden (Lindgren and Gustafson, 2001), cholera in Bangladesh (Rodo et al., 2002), and malaria in certain highland regions of eastern Africa (Patz et al., 2002). It is also emerging that the tempo of extreme weather events has been increasing in many regions, with resultant increases in human death and injury, as well as associated increases in infectious disease and mental trauma.

The World Health Organization has, for the first time, reported an estimation of the current level of health impact of climate change. In its *World Health Report 2002*, the World Health Organization estimated that climate change, by the year 2000, was responsible for 2.4% of diarrheal disease worldwide up to 6–7% of malaria and dengue in specified groups of countries. This estimation, as part of the larger *Global Burden of Disease 2000* (Ezzati et al., 2004), was necessarily based on an interpolation between the reference level of health impact for the period 1961–1990 (currently viewed as the baseline period for the modeling of future climate change scenarios) and the estimated scenario-based health impacts for 2030.

The third category of research is less familiar to conventional epidemiological researchers and therefore warrants exploration in a little more detail.

SCENARIO-BASED HEALTH RISK ASSESSMENTS

Epidemiologists are familiar with the task of estimating future trends in disease incidence. Where there is a high level of information and certainty about the recent and current levels of the underlying causal exposure, as with occupational asbestos exposure, and where the causal relationship (e.g., asbestos as the cause of mesothelioma) is well characterized, then formal *prediction* of future disease incidence can be made. Where there is certainty about recent trends in disease incidence but incomplete understanding about the underlying causal determinants, then *projection* of trends can reasonably be made, for at least the near term. However, where there is considerable uncertainty about the future exposure conditions, several decades hence—as with global climate change—while there is good understanding and certainty about how climatic conditions affect health risks, then *scenario-based health risk assessment* becomes appropriate.

The techniques for conducting scenario-based health risk assessments have been the focus of much effort, and some controversy, over the past decade. Most of the published research has been in relation to vector-borne infectious diseases, particularly malaria and dengue fever. The "exposure" variable comprises the geographically gridded estimates of future climate scenarios, particularly location-specific average annual temperature and average monthly precipitation.

The main points of contention have been these:

1. A choice must be made between biological, or process-based, models versus statistical-empirical models. The former assume that the basic relationships between meteorological variables and the biology of vector organism and parasite are sufficiently well known and parameterized. The latter eschew such assumptions and work from the current observable relationship between regional meteorological conditions and regional transmission of the disease of interest.

2. Models necessarily simplify a more complex real world. A balance must be struck between clarity and computability, on the one hand, and sufficiently detailed inclusion of meteorological-biological information, on the other. However, argument persists as to the extent to which we should, and can, "horizontally integrate" into the model any foreseeable future changes in population characteristics (e.g., wealth levels, technology, and public education) that affect vulnerability to disease transmission. Further, the estimation of model errors is at present intractable and can only be assessed by sensitivity testing to see which parameters, when varied, cause large differences in estimates.

3. Related to the above two points, validation of predictive integrated models is, by definition, difficult. Analogues can be sought in recent past experience, where climate variability or change appears to approximate future climatic changes. Validation, thus, asks, how well does the model predict the observed past trends in the outcome variable? However, such opportunities are limited.

Overall, then, there is a range of research tasks and methods applicable to understanding and forecasting the impacts of climate change on human health (Martens and McMichael, 2002). For this topic area, and for research into the health impacts of global environmental changes generally, there is a particular need for epidemiologists to work in an interdisciplinary context. The ways in which environmental, ecological, and associated social changes translate into risks to health are often complex and may require a more systems-based approach to elucidation and modeling.

CONCLUSIONS

The topic of "global environmental change" is coming onto the population health research agenda, rapidly. There is increasing interest on the part of general public and policy makers in understanding the full range of likely consequences of these large-scale, often complex changes. During the past two decades there has been, in particular, a growing awareness of the risks to health posed by global climate change.

Assessing the impact of climate change on health is, however, a complex task. There are often difficulties in obtaining data; there is frequent interaction of climatic-environmental influences on health with factors such as level of economic development, the state of public health systems, and individual and population behavior, and much of the focus of the work lies in estimating the future health impacts of plausible scenarios of climate change and other environmental changes.

As the earth's atmosphere continues to change in response to human actions, we anticipate increasing temperatures around the world, altered precipitation patterns, and some increases in the intensity and frequency of natural climatic variability. There is some early evidence of adverse effects of climate change on human health, but more systematic research and assessment is needed. Given the uncertainty of future climatic trends, and the complex interactions (of climate with economy, population profile, social structure, etc.), it is not possible to use traditional predictive methods to estimate future health impacts. Rather, scenario-based health risk assessment must be used. This, in turn, requires an interdisciplinary approach, bringing and understanding of complex causal processes, and a capacity to incorporate multiple variables into complex causal models.

The health impact of climate change will be very uneven around the world. It is therefore important to estimate the likely attributable burdens of health risk within specific groups or populations. Identifying vulnerable groups or populations is, of course, a priority task in policy terms, enabling targeted intervention to lessen risks.

As a final word, the better the job done by health researchers in this important, emerging topic area, the better we will understand the implications for human well-being and health of the great human-induced changes occurring today in the earth's environment. This must become an important criterion in the evolving discourse on how to achieve an ecologically and socially sustainable future world.

References

Afza M, Bridgman S (2001). Winter emergency pressures for the NHS: contribution of respiratory disease, experience in North Staffordshire district. *J Public Health Med* 23: 312–313.

Balbus JM (1998). Human health. In Feenstra JF, Burton I, Smith JB, Tol RSJ, eds. *Handbook on Methods for Climate Change Impact Assessment and Adaptation Strategies.* Nairobi: United Nations Environment Program and Institute of Environmental Studies, chapter 10.

Balbus JM, Wilson ML (2000). *Human Health and Global Climate Change: A Review of Potential Impacts in the United States.* Arlington, VA: Pew Centre for Global Climate Change.

Centers for Disease Control and Prevention (1995). Heat-related mortality—Chicago, July 1995. *MMWR* 44: 577–579.

Checkley W, Epstein LD, Gilman RH, Figueroa D, Cama RI, Patz JA, Black RE (2000). Effect of El Nino and ambient temperature on hospital admissions for diarrhoeal diseases in Peruvian children. *Lancet* 355: 442–450.

Ebi KL, Patz JA (2002). Epidemiological and impacts assessment methods. In: Marten P, McMichael AJ, eds. *Environmental Change, Climate and Health.* Cambridge: Cambridge University Press, pp. 120–143.

Ezzati M, Lopez AD, Rodgers AA, Murray CJL (2004). *Comparative Quantification of Health Risks: Global and Regional Burden of Disease Attributable to Selected Major Risk Factors.* Geneva: World Health Organization.

Forum (1999). Environmental impact of Hurricane Mitch. *Environ Health Perspect* 107: A139–140.

Goenjian AK, Molina L, Steinberg AM, Fairbanks LA, Alvarez ML, Goenjian HA, Pynoos RS (2001). Posttraumatic stress and depressive reactions among Nicaraguan adolescents after Hurricane Mitch. *Am J Psychiatry* 158: 788–794.

Greenough G, McGeehin M, Bernard SM, Trtanj J, Riad J, Engelberg D (2001). The potential impacts of climate variability and change on health impacts of extreme weather events in the United States. *Environ Health Perspect* 109: 191–198.

Guill CK, Shandera WX (2001). The effects of Hurricane Mitch on a community in Northern Honduras. *Prehosp Disast Med* 16: 166–171.

Hales S, de Wet N, Maindonald J, Woodward A (2002). Potential effect of population and climate changes on global distribution of dengue fever: an empirical model. *Lancet* 360: 830–834.

Hales S, Edwards SJ, Kovats S (2003). Impacts on health of climate extremes. In: McMichael AJ, Campbell-Lendrum DH, Corvalan CF, Ebi KL, Githeko A, Scheraga JD, Woodward A, eds. *Climate Change and Human Health: Risks and Responses.* Geneva: World Health Organization, pp. 79–102.

Hall GV, D'Souza RM, Kirk MD (2002). Food borne disease in the new millennium: out of the frying pan into the fire? *Med J Aust* 177: 614–618.

Houghton JT, Ding Y, Griggs DJ, Noguer M, van der Linden PJ, Xiaosu D (2001). *Climate Change 2001: The Scientific Basis.* Cambridge: Cambridge University Press.

Huynen MM, Martens P, Schram D, Weijenberg MP, Kunst AE (2001). The impact of heat waves and cold spells on mortality rates in the Dutch population. *Environ Health Perspect* 109: 463–470.

Institut De Veille Sanitaire (2003). *Impact Sanitaire de la Vague de Chaleur en France Survenue en août 2003 Rapport d'Étape—29 Août 2003* (Progress report on the heat wave 2003 in France). Saint Maurice: Institut De Veille Sanitaire (National Institute of Public Health Surveillance).

IPCC (2001a). *Climate Change 2001: The Scientific Basis.* Contribution of Working Group I to the Third Assessment Report of the Intergovernmental Panel on Climate Change. Cambridge: Cambridge University Press.

IPCC (2001b). *Climate Change 2001: Impacts, Adaptation and Vulnerability.* Contribution of Working Group II to the Third Assessment Report of the Intergovernmental Panel on Climate Change. Cambridge: Cambridge University Press.

Jones TS, Liang AP, Kilbourne EM, Griffin MR, Patriarca PA, Wassilak SG, Mullan RJ, Herrick RF, Donnell HDJ, Choi K, Thacker SB (1982). Morbidity and mortality associated with the July 1980 heat wave in St. Louis and Kansas City, Mo. *JAMA* 247: 3327–3331.

Koppe C, Kovats S, Jendritzky G, Menne B (2004). *Heat-Waves: Risks and Responses.* Denmark: World Health Organization.

Kovats S, Ebi KL, Menne B (2003). *Methods of Assessing Human Health Vulnerability and Public Health Adaptation.* (Health and Global Environmental Change Series No. 1.) Copenhagen: World Health Organization.

Kovats S, Wolf T, Menne B (2004). Heatwave of August 2003 in Europe: provisional estimates of the impact on mortality. *Eurosurveill Wkly Arch* 8: 11. http://www.eurosurveillance.org/ew/2004/040311 .asp#7.

Krug EG, Kresnow M, Peddicord JP, Dahlberg LL, Powell KE, Crosby AE, Annest JL (1998). Suicide after natural disasters. *N Engl J Med* 338: 373–378.

Lang T, Heasman M (2004). *Food Wars*. London: Earth-scan.

Lindgren E, Gustafson R (2001). Tick-borne encephalitis in Sweden and climate change. *Lancet* 358: 16–18.

Lucas RM, Ponsonby AL (2002). Ultraviolet radiation and health: friend and foe. *Med J Aust* 177: 594–598.

Martens WJM, Kovats RS, Nijhof S, de Vries P, Livermore MTJ, Bradley D, Cox J, McMichael AJ. (1999) Climate change and future populations at risk of malaria. *Global Environ Change* 9(suppl): S89–S107.

Martens WJM, McMichael AJ, eds. (2002). *Environmental Change, Climate and Health: Issues and Research Methods*. Cambridge: Cambridge University Press.

McGregor GR, Walters S, Wordley J (1999). Daily hospital respiratory admissions and winter air mass types, Birmingham, UK. *Int J Biometeorol* 43: 21–30.

McMichael AJ, Campbell-Lendrum D, Ebi K, Githeko A, Scheraga J, Woodward A, eds. (2003a). *Climate Change and Human Health: Risks and Responses*. Geneva: World Health Organization.

McMichael AJ, Woodruff R, Hales S (2006). Climate change and human health: present and future risks. *Lancet* 367: 859–869.

McMichael AJ, Woodruff R, Whetton P, Hennessy K, Nicholls N, Hales S, Woodward A, Kjellstrom T (2003b) *Human Health and Climate Change in Oceania: A Risk Assessment 2002*. Canberra: Commonwealth of Australia.

Millennium Ecosystem Assessment (2003). Ecosystems and human well-being: a framework for assessment. In: Alcamo J, Ash NJ, Butler CD et al., eds. *Ecosystems and Human Well-being*. Washington, DC: Island Press, pp. 71–84.

National Research Council (2001). *Abrupt Climate Change*. Washington, DC: National Academy Press.

Nicholls N (2004). The changing nature of Australian droughts. *Climate Change* 63: 323–336.

Parry M, Rosenzweig C, Iglesias A, Fischer G, Livermore M (1999). Climate change and world food security: a new assessment. *Global Environ Change* 9: S51–S67.

Patz J, Balbus J (2001). Global climate change and air pollution: interactions and their effects on human health. In: Aaron J and Patz J, eds. *Ecosystem Change and Public Health*. Baltimore, MD: John Hopkins University Press, chapter 13.

Patz JA, Hulme M, Rosenzweig C, Mitchell TD, Goldberg RA, Githeko AK, Lele S, McMichael AJ, Le Sueur D (2002). Climate change: regional warming and malaria resurgence. *Nature* 420: 627–628.

Patz JA, McGeehin MA, Bernard SM, Ebi KL, Epstein PR, Grambsch A, Gubler DJ, Reither P, Romieu I, Rose JB, Samet JM, Trtanj J (2000). The potential health impacts of climate variability and change for the United States: executive summary of the Report of the Health Sector of the US National Assessment. *Environ Health Perspect* 108: 367–376.

Rodo X, Pascual M, Fuchs G, Faruque ASG (2002). ENSO and cholera: a nonstationary link related to climate change? *Proc Natl Acad Sci USA* 99: 12901–12906.

Rooney C, McMichael AJ, Kovats RS, Coleman MP (1998). Excess mortality in England and Wales, and in Greater London, during the 1995 heatwave. *J Epidemiol Community Health* 52: 482–486.

Root TL, Price JT, Hall KR, Schneider SH, Rosenzweig C, Pounds JA (3002). Fingerprints of global warming on wild animals and plants. *Nature* 421: 57–60.

Rusticucci M, Bettolli ML, de los Angeles HM (2002). Association between weather conditions and the number of patients at the emergency room in an Argentine hospital. *Int J Biometeorol* 46: 42–51.

Sartor F, Snacken R, Demuth C, Walkiers D (1995). Temperature, ambient ozone levels, and mortality during summer 1994, in Belgium. *Environ Res* 70: 105–113.

Semenza JC, McCullough JE, Flanders WD, McGeehin MA, Lumpkin JR (1999). Excess hospital admissions during the July 1995 heat wave in Chicago. *Am J Prev Med* 16: 269–277.

Shah MM, Strong MF (2000) *Food in the 21st Century: From Science to Sustainable Agriculture*. Washington, DC: World Bank.

Singh RB, Hales S, de Wet N, Raj R, Hearnden M, Weinstein P (2001). The influence of climate variation and change on diarrheal disease in the Pacific Islands. *Environ Health Perspect* 109: 155–159.

Stewart S, McIntyre K, Capewell S, McMurray JJ (2002). Heart failure in a cold climate. Seasonal variation in heart failure-related morbidity and mortality. *J Am Coll Cardiol* 39: 760–766.

Tong SL, Bi P, Hayes J, Donald K, MacKenzie J (2001). Geographic variation of notified Ross River virus infections in Queensland, Australia, 1985–1996. *Am J Trop Med Hygiene* 65: 171–176.

Vitousek PM, Mooney HA, Lubchenco J, Melillo JM (1997). Human domination of earth's ecosystems. *Science* 277: 494–499.

WHO (2002). *World Health Report 2002: Reducing Risks, Promoting Healthy Life*. Geneva: World Health Organization.

Wilkinson P, McMichael T, Kovats S, Pattenden S, Hajat S, Armstrong B (2002). International study of temperature and heatwaves on urban mortality in low and middle income countries (ISOTHURM). *Epidemiology* 13: S81–S81.

Woodruff RE, Guest CS, Garner MG, Becker N, Lindesay J, Carvan T, Ebi K (2002). Predicting Ross River virus epidemics from regional weather data. *Epidemiology* 13: 384–393.

Woodward A, Hales S, Litidamu N, Phillips D, Martin J (2000). Protecting human health in a changing world: the role of social and economic development. *Bull World Health Organ* 78: 1148–1155.

Chapter 6

Car Culture, Transport Policy, and Public Health

Tord Kjellstrom and Sarah Hinde

Globalization is an economic force, the logical outcome of the elimination of "old-fashioned" barriers to trade, capital movement, investment, and enterprise (Stiglitz, 2002). There are strong lobbying forces for making the globe into one market, whose power has arisen from strong economic growth in developed countries and the expansion of the domain of multinational enterprises. The principles of globalization are described in box 6.1. The International Monetary Fund has underpinned pressures toward globalization with demands—placed primarily on developing countries—to "open up" national economies and markets, providing opportunities for the entry of global businesses (Stiglitz, 2002). In some cases, this liberalization has led to positive economic and social development for the country concerned, but negative experiences have also been common (Stiglitz, 2002). A number of public health problems described in this book are associated with the economic and social changes driven by globalization, and car reliance is no exception.

Today's reliance on the automobile in most developed countries (and, increasingly, in developing countries) has arisen from what may be described as a "perfect fit" between the principles and processes of globalization, the nature of automobile transport, and the actions of the car industry. There are many aspects to this close intertwining of car reliance and globalization:

- The automotive and related sectors include some of the most powerful global economic actors.
- Motor vehicles facilitate trade, employment, and enterprise around the world.
- The automotive industry was a leader in relation to mass consumption and multinational expansion.
- A car-based transport system is believed to conform to the values underpinning globalization (e.g., commodification, individualized consumption, minimal government intervention, and privatization of profits).

- The automobile is a commodity that supports an immensely profitable global industry.

Box 6.1 – The "Washington Consensus": A Foundation for Economic Globalization

During the 1980s conservative economists in the U.S. Treasury, the World Bank, and the International Monetary Fund developed an agreement on what constituted "good development policies" (Stiglitz, 2002):

- Liberalized financial transactions across borders
- Less government intervention, relying on market wisdom
- Privatization
- Free trade
- Low inflation
- Less government borrowing
- Low proportion of gross domestic product from aid or loans

These principles have become the foundation for globalization to date and the focus of much of the criticism of globalization.

The integral role of car reliance in globalization sets it up as a far-reaching and potent influence on global population health. Evidence is accumulating on the sheer breadth and extent of impact of the motor vehicle on health, with many common problems emerging in developed and developing countries. The global impacts of car reliance are described in this chapter. The automobile is entrenched within broader processes of globalization, and the resulting global health impacts call for public health interventions at this international level, as well as in national and local environments.

A feature of globalization is that multinational enterprises have grown in recent years to the extent that their overall market capital value is larger than the gross domestic product (GDP) of some countries. The largest corporations, such as General Electric, Cisco Systems, Exxon-Mobil, General Motors, Toyota, and Mitsubishi, have a value similar to the GDP of medium-sized developed countries such as the Netherlands or Australia (Bradshaw and Wallace, 1996). The car is responsible for 10% of employment in developed countries, and in each of the G7 countries, car and oil manufacturers generate the most revenue (Urmetzer et al., 1999). Car and oil manufacturers team with players from the construction, engineering, and other industries to form the "road lobby," who together are a powerful force in the global economy (Paterson, 2000). Urmetzer et al. (1999) declare that "the most powerful corporations in the world either manufacture cars or are involved in the exploration and refinement of oil" (p. 355).

Globalization depends on mobility—the movement of dollars, people, ideas, and goods. The motor vehicle is the predominant instrument for mobilizing people and goods in most countries. It brings people face to face, transports goods between factories and retail outlets, and moves people between homes, workplaces, and shops. The car also supports mobility in the global sense by supplying connections with airplanes and ships. The globalized economy rests on the web of journeys and transactions that take place via the automobile.

As well as being instrumental in supplying mobility, the car industry itself was also a leader in innovation and expansion, both essential to globalization. Indeed, the car industry itself was the home of "Fordism"—namely, the advances in management and manufacturing techniques that enabled mass production of commodities. Mass production, and in turn mass consumption, was the basis for a "regime of accumulation" that underpinned economic growth in developed countries throughout the twentieth century. The automotive industry was also at the cutting edge in terms of expanding into the global sphere, as one of the first industries with multinational operations, including the generation of global commodity chains (Paterson, 2000).

Reliance on the private motor vehicle as the preeminent means of transport fits well with the principles and values of globalization (box 6.1), but the result is a disproportionate division of the social and economic costs and benefits. Freund and Martin (1996) point out that mobility has been successfully commodified by the car industry—a public need that has been converted into a "socially subsidized system of private consumption" (Freund and Martin, 1996, p. 27). Thus, mobility has become a commodity to be purchased in the economy, and the economic costs are borne by the individual car owner, and society more widely, while the profits are accrued by industry.

It is perceived that car transport requires a low

level of government intervention, but this belief is strongly disputed. Laird et al. (2001) suggest that Australia's "road deficit" is around A$19 billion a year. The externalities of a car-based transport system, including the health impacts, lie outside the domain of private industry and are borne by society. Often the most disadvantaged groups bear the brunt of these externalities, not to mention the environmental, social, and health impacts to be incurred by future generations.

The automobile industry has been instrumental in the process of globalization, placing it as an important force in the global economy as we progress into the twenty-first century. While global car reliance has contributed in many ways to positive social and economic outcomes, it also brings with it a host of global population health consequences.

TRANSPORT—ITS PURPOSES AND FEATURES

Globalization and Transport in Developing Countries

Globalization and its focus on enhanced trade increase the need for efficient transport systems in developing countries (Galbraith, 2001). Many countries undergoing rapid economic development are making major investments in transport, particularly road transport as a reflection of an advancement of the global car culture. The rapid developments in the most important current "economic boom" country, China, are an indication of current global trends. According to media reports, new car sales have increased by 30% in China in 2004, to a great extent facilitated by easily available bank loans. The Chinese government has put brakes on this development, but a pattern has been established. One sign of the establishment of a Chinese car culture is the reduction of bicycle production (Worldwatch Institute, 2003) and the restrictions of the size of bicycle lanes in Shanghai, Beijing, and other cities.

Another sign of the spread of global car culture is the ambitious plans for highway construction in developing countries. For instance, an Asian Highway Network over more than 140,000 km is planned (ESCAP, 2004) to facilitate the increasing trade and travel links within Asia and beyond. A Trans-Asian Railway system is also projected (ESCAP, 2004), but

it will not reach as many parts of Asia as the highway network.

Urbanization is a major factor in these developments. The number of cities with more than one million people in developing countries is rapidly increasing, and meeting the transport needs within and between cities has become a major challenge for authorities. Cities can be planned for "walkability" and "livability" with the daily transport needs met primarily by "active transport" (walking or bicycling) or public transport (Kirdar, 1997), but the transport planners are often too wedded to private motor vehicle mobility to fully consider the alternatives (Vuchic, 1999).

At the local level, mobility and transport can promote public health, because it

- Enables people to participate in a distributed job market
- Allows family members to live in one part of town and work in another
- Brings attractive and/or necessary products, from faraway places (including food, therefore creating opportunities to maintain a balanced diet during all seasons)
- Broadens access to leisure and sports activities, as well as to social contacts with family and friends
- Improves access to health care

The Health Hazard Panorama

The different types of transport are also associated with their own combinations of health hazards. Transport-related health impacts can be analyzed from the viewpoint of the hierarchy of exposure factors that contribute to environmental health effects described with the DPSEEA (driving forces, pressure, state, exposure, effect, and action) framework (Kjellstrom and Corvalan, 1995; Corvalan et al., 1996) (figure 6.1). The driving forces are as follows:

- Demographic, including population growth and aging
- Economic, as in increased demand for transport from a growing economy, shifts in demand from changing industry, changing work travel patterns
- Social, such as changing patterns of social, shopping, leisure, and sports activities, changing attitudes to transport "norms"

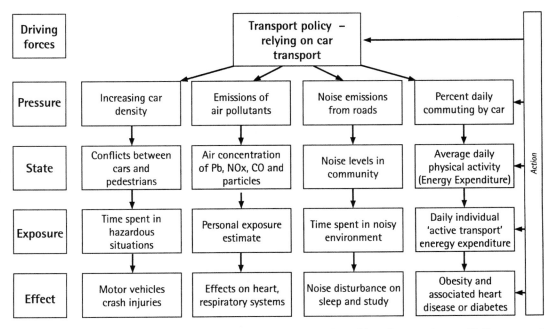

FIGURE 6.1. The DPSEEA Framework to Define Environmental Health Indicators. *Source:* Kjellstrom et al. (2003).

- Technological, through telecommunications reducing transport need, more energy-efficient car engines, more convenient and pleasant public transport modes

Out of these driving forces, different pressures on the transport environment emerge: more need for transport, more cars, more trucks, more air pollutant emissions, more noise emissions, and so forth. The increased pressures lead to a deterioration of the state of the environment, leading to higher exposures to hazards among people that spend time in the affected environment. Eventually, the exposures lead to health effects. Preventive actions can be taken at each level of the hierarchy of this "cause–effect" framework.

In this chapter we analyze primarily the transport and health issues related to motor vehicle transport of people, which has emerged in the last fifty years as the dominating area of health concern in relation to transport. It is important to note, though, that both personal and freight transport creates health hazards.

Table 6.1 summarizes the public health aspects that are considered in this chapter (Kjellstrom et al., 2003). The degree of health risk in a typical developed country (New Zealand used as a model) is indicated with the number of asterisks, combining assessments of the prevalence of exposure to hazard and the relative risk of injury or disease.

When interpreting health impact data, it should be remembered that the injury or disease "victim" may be riding in the vehicle causing the hazard (crash, air pollution, noise, etc.) but may also be in or on another vehicle (e.g., bicycle hit by car), may be walking or standing at the roadside, or may happen to live in the vicinity of a heavily traveled road. Even people living far away from such roads may be affected by motor vehicle air pollution covering large geographic areas, or by the environmental impacts of greenhouse gas emissions from motor vehicles.

Traffic crash injuries may occur with any mode of transport on its own, but many of these injuries are due to crashes involving vehicles or people using the same road space, for example, pedestrians hit by cars, bicyclists hit by buses, and motorcyclists hit by trucks. Health risks due to crashes for different modes of transport therefore appear quite different based on the numbers of injured people or the numbers of vehicles involved in a crash. Cars are the most common vehicles on the roads, and their drivers and passengers contribute the greatest proportion of injured people, but the few motorcyclists have a much higher risk of being injured per vehicle-kilometer traveled.

TABLE 6.1. Types of Health Hazards Related to Transport and Their Relative Importance at the National Level

Transport Mode	Crashes/ "Accidents"	Air Pollution	Noise	Physical Exercise Reduction	Community Disruption	Other Environmental Factors
Walking	*					
Bicycle	*					
Motorcycle	**	*	**	***	*	*
Car	***	***	***	**	***	***
Bus	*	**	**	*	*	*
Truck	***	**	**		***	***
Train	*	*	*	*	*	*
Ferry		*		*		*
Airplane	**	*	***		**	**

The numbers of asterisks indicate the degree of health risk in a typical developed country, in this case New Zealand as a model.

Source: Based Kjellstrom et al. (2003).

Air pollution from transport is due to the by-products of using energy to move the vehicles, usually provided by a liquid fossil fuel combustion engine (petrol or diesel). Fossil fuel engines emit air pollution where the vehicle is driven, while electric- or fuel-cell-driven vehicles transfer the air pollution problem to the power plant or fuel production plant where the energy is converted to fuel. Only walking and bicycling generate no health-damaging air pollution.

Traffic noise, physical exercise reduction, community disruption, and other environmental health hazards are also outcomes of motor vehicle transport. The extent to which the different health hazards materialize for each mode of transport in a specific location is determined by local geographical, meteorological, social, and physical planning conditions.

The global cost of traffic crash injuries has been estimated at US$518 billion (Jacobs et al., 2000). The total cost of *all* health impacts is likely to be several times higher. Apart from health hazards, different modes of transport affect society via physical damage and economic loss due to collisions, energy consumption, the ecological effects of air pollution, greenhouse gas emissions, and so forth.

Some may argue that the transport-related health hazards are a "necessary evil" of a modern economy. Perhaps this is so, but like so many modern health hazards, the level of hazard exposure in a population can be reduced by applying appropriate preventive policies and actions (Kjellstrom et al., 2003). The situation in developed countries is in many ways different from the situation in developing countries; however, lessons can be gained from the evidence collected around the world. Moreover, international comparisons and dialogue on this issue are a valuable opportunity to ameliorate and prevent further hazards and damage arising from the increasingly car reliant nature of many countries.

Mobility of People, Travel Profiles, and Exposure to Hazards

One should not confuse the need for mobility in daily life with the demand for motor vehicle transport. Mobility involves people being able to interact with other people as a part of social life and to transport goods and people to different locations for economic or social activities. In traditional local economies, most of this mobility is achieved on foot or on human-propelled vehicles, whereas urbanization and the broadening of the geographic scale of economic and social activities create challenges for these types of transport. Appropriate planning of urban areas can reduce the need for longer distance travel (Kirdar, 1997; Vuchic, 1999). However, exposure to transport hazards cannot be totally avoided.

In order to estimate health risks of transport the amount of *exposure* to hazards needs to be quantified. Fundamental variables in transport exposure assessment are the mode of transport used as well as

TABLE 6.2. Typical Weekly Travel Profile in New Zealand, by Age and Mode of Travel, 1997–1998

Age (years)	Walking	%	Passenger	%	Driver	%	Bus	%	Bicycle	%
0–14	1 hr	15	4 hrs	70	0	0	30 min	10	15 min	<5
15–24	1 hr 45 min	20	3 hrs 45 min	40	3 hrs 30 min	35	45 min	10	15 min	<5
25–64	1 hr	10	1 hr 30 min	70	6 hrs	70	15 min	<5	<5	<5
65+	1 hr	20	1 hr 15 min	55	2 hrs 30 min	55	<15 min	<5	<5	<5

Travel times are rounded to the nearest fifteen minutes. Percentage travel times are rounded to the nearest 5%.

Source: Based on data in LTSA (1999).

the duration of exposure to each transport mode (walking, bicycling, driving in a car, etc.). More specific risk variables that can be defined for the individual include, for example, which position in a car the person is in, the use of seatbelts, and the speed of the vehicle.

People use a variety of transport modes to carry out their everyday mobility. The predominant means of transport for most people in industrial countries is by private car, either as a driver or a passenger, as in the example of New Zealand (table 6.2). People in all age groups use cars and motorcycles for more than three-quarters of their travel; the next most common means of transport is walking (10–20%), followed by bus (5–10%), and cycling (<5%). Children spend four hours per week as car passengers, while young adults spend approximately seven hours per week in cars (table 6.2). This type of data based on travel surveys is of great importance to assess hazard exposures and public health risks from transport and the degree of car reliance in a specific population.

Similar surveys in other developed countries show that the total distance driven in cars (or on motor cycles) each year increases and that public transport use is decreasing, with a few exceptions in cities engaged in major efforts to improve public transport. Motorcycle riding has a particularly high risk of injury compared to cars (WHO, 2004). In many developing countries, the relatively low price of motorcycles, the small space they take on the road, and the hot climate make the motorcycle an attractive choice at the early stages of motorization. Over time, the motorcar becomes the vehicle of choice, and motorcycle use decreases.

Bicycling and walking are directly related to people's daily physical activity. In New Zealand, bicycling has declined by almost 20% since the 1989–1990 Travel Survey (NZMFE, 2002). The greatest decrease in cycling has occurred in school-age children, and it is thought to be due to concerns about child safety, in keeping with patterns observed in other countries (e.g., the United Kingdom). Cycling has also declined as a means of transport to work in New Zealand, from 5.7% of commuters in 1986 to 4.0% in 1996 (Statistics New Zealand, 1996). This type of travel profile data is becoming increasingly available for cities around the world (Kenworthy, 1997; Tiwari, 1997). This will facilitate health impact assessments and transport planning that takes public health issues into account.

Private Motor Vehicle Ownership and Use

The United States has the highest rate of motor vehicle ownership in the world (76 cars per 100 people), followed by Canada, Australia, New Zealand, and Italy. Generally, the richer a country is, the higher the rate of motor vehicle ownership (figure 6.2). A high rate of car ownership is an important "driving force" behind the public health impacts associated with automobiles.

Vehicular travel is undertaken for commuting to work or school, carrying out work, shopping, visiting people, or other recreational purposes. Most motor vehicle trips are short, particularly in urban areas. In rural areas, longer trips are more common. Over a typical year the kilometers add up: the average car travels 9,700 km/year in Japan, 10,900 km/year in Sweden, and 12,700 km/year in New Zealand (International Road Federation, 2005). In the twelve months ending October 2001, Australian automobiles together drove the distance to the planet Pluto and

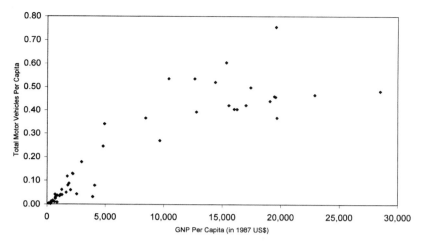

FIGURE 6.2. The Relationship between Affluence and Motor Vehicle Ownership in Selected Countries. *Source:* Ingram and Liu (1998).

back, twenty-three times, and passenger vehicles contributed three-quarters of this distance traveled (Australian Bureau of Statistics, 2003).

Public transport provides the main alternative to the private car for travel to work (Laird et al., 2001). According to the World Bank (2000) the cities of the world with the lowest use of public transport for work commuting are found in the countries where vehicle ownership is high. For instance, in Auckland, New Zealand, only 6% of commuting is done by public transport. In Melbourne, the figure is 16%, and in Stockholm, 37% (World Bank, 2000). One can assume that the vast majority of commuters use private cars or cars provided by the employer ("company cars"). Comparable figures for cities in Asian countries are given in table 6.3. In some Asian cities, as much as 60–90% of work-related trips are taken by public transport. For example, in Tokyo the figure is 62%, and this city is served by a very efficient public transport system.

Walking and Bicycling

Walking is an essential means of transport for children, young people, and older adults, and it provides daily exercise; for these groups, around 25% of all journeys in New Zealand are made on foot (LTSA, 2000). The extent to which walking is a feasible option for travel to work or for other regular travel depends on the geographic layout of a city and the availability of other transport. City planning that creates "walkability"

TABLE 6.3. Proportion of Daily Trips on Public Transport (Work Trips) or Nonmotorized Transport in Cities in Different Areas

City or Area	% Work Trips on Public Transport	% Daily Trips by Nonmotorized Transport
American cities	12	
Australian cities	20	
Seoul		12
Surabaya	29	53
Kuala Lumpur	31	28
Bangkok	31	14
European cities	44	
Asian cities	55	32
Manila	73	30
Jakarta	40	
Tokyo	62	45
Singapore	72	
Hong Kong	89	

Source: Assembled from data in Kenworthy (1997).

(Vuchic, 1999), and convenient links to public transport for longer journeys can have a great impact on people's travel habits.

Bicycling is another form of minimally polluting, health-promoting active transport, at least for the common short trips (<2 km). To ensure bicycling is an attractive, safe, and secure option for these trips, cities have to make special arrangements, such as

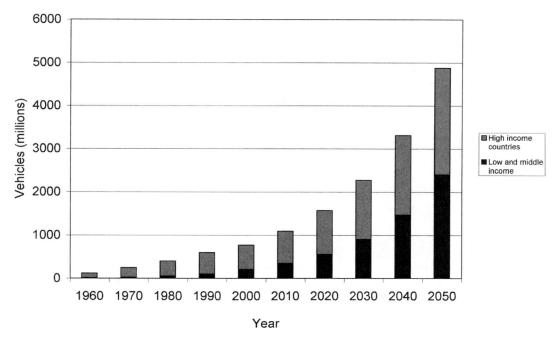

FIGURE 6.3. Growth of World Motor Vehicle Fleet, 1960–2050, in Selected High-, Middle-, and Low-Income Countries. *Source:* WHO (1997); Ingram and Liu (1999).

provision of bicycle paths and secure bicycle parking (Hathway, 2000). These arrangements are much less costly than building roads and car parks, and they take much less space.

An issue of importance for public health is the extent to which children walk or bicycle for their daily mobility needs. The current debate in many countries about the increasing obesity rate has made special reference to children's physical activity. Increasingly in affluent countries, parents are chauffeuring their children to and from school, often with just one parent driving and one child passenger (LTSA, 1999). In both rural and urban areas of New Zealand, the number of children making school trips as a car passenger has doubled during the 1990s. The reasons for these changes are partly explained by longer distances to school in rural areas (due to school closings), reduction in provision of school buses, and combining of child and parent travel needs. Safety concerns are also behind this chauffeuring trend, in terms of both pedestrian accidents involving the child and "stranger danger" from people that could harm the walking child (Kearns, 2001).

GLOBAL MOTOR VEHICLE TRANSPORT TRENDS

In 2003, some 41 million new passenger vehicles rolled off the world's assembly lines, five times as many as in 1950 (Worldwatch Institute, 2003). The global passenger car fleet now exceeds 750 million vehicles and may approach 5 billion by 2050 (Ingram and Liu, 1999). The development over time appears exponential (figure 6.3).

The trend in rising motor vehicle ownership in Asia is the fastest in the world (WHO, 2004). In such countries as the Philippines, Thailand, India, and China, the number of vehicles has more than doubled in 10 years. In most developing countries, the growth in motor vehicles has not been matched by sufficient growth in the road infrastructure or public transport provision, leading to major congestion and environmental deterioration in many places. Manila in the Philippines and Mumbai in India offer two vivid examples of such urban planning crises and consequent air pollution problems (Larssen et al., 1996a, 1996b).

Globalization has created the consolidation of national car manufacturing companies in a number of key countries (e.g., United States, United Kingdom, Germany, Italy, France, Japan, Sweden, South Korea) into larger global companies or consortia of companies. For instance, the Swedish car company Saab is now part of General Motors, and Volvo is part of Ford. In a manner similar to the development of the tobacco business, the important new markets for car companies are developing countries, and any significant expansion of their business has to be created in those countries. For example, every day in 2003, some 11,000 more cars merged onto China's roads alone, which added 4 million new private cars during the year (Worldwatch Institute, 2003). A recent analysis of the future trends of the global car market forecasted that, by 2020 (Pemberton, 2004), 100 million new cars would be produced each year, with most of the growth in developing countries. In a few decades, the world may need to cope with one billion motor vehicles (Tunali, 1996).

The type of motor vehicle produced and used is also a major feature of the global trend in motorization. The two-wheeled motorcycle is the vehicle of choice at early stages of motorization. The proportion of two-wheelers among all motor vehicles is in the range 50–95% in Asian countries (WHO, 2004). In Vietnam, the growth in motorcycle numbers during one year (2001) was as high as 29%, and during the same year road deaths increased by 37% (WHO, 2004).

Another type of vehicle that has featured strongly in the recent trends of global motorization is the sports utility vehicle (SUV), which is a mixture of a car and a light truck, often with four-wheel drive, a high wheel base, heavy chassis, and an extra strong engine. The SUVs are therefore emitting greater amounts of air pollutants than do typical cars, they consume more fuel per kilometer driven, and their design makes them inherently more accident prone than cars (Worldwatch Institute, 2003). The global growth of the number of SUVs has been very rapid, partly stimulated by special tax concessions for these vehicles in the United States. Based on current trends, by 2030 as many as half of the world's passenger vehicles may be SUVs or light trucks (Worldwatch Institute, 2003).

The rates and trends presented in this section have demonstrated how the motor vehicle has become entrenched in the economies and societies of developed and developing countries around the world. The trend toward ever-greater reliance on the car arose from the particular social, cultural, and economic characteristics of the automobile and its related industries, which are described next.

CAR RELIANCE AS A SOCIOCULTURAL PHENOMENON

What Is Car Reliance?

There is a small but growing literature dedicated to explaining the current state of car reliance in developed countries around the world. Car reliance may be defined as "a set of institutional policies and practices wherein the use of the car is embedded in the ways in which we organize our lives" (Urmetzer et al., 1999, p. 355). Put more simply, car reliance is the way society systematically preferences the automobile over other modes of transport.

Sociological approaches have variously analyzed the car in terms of its broad role in modernity and globalization, how it has permeated the cultures and economies of nations, and through to its role in the daily life of individuals. Together, this field of research reveals how the motor vehicle has become so entrenched in the lives and minds of people in most developed countries and more recently some developing countries. While theoretical positions and specific arguments might vary, the descriptions and explanations in the sociological research on car reliance tend to be unanimous on three matters:

1. The motor vehicle is highly esteemed.
2. Car use is socially reproduced, hence "car reliance."
3. Car reliance shapes the way people go about their everyday activities.

The Motor Vehicle Is Highly Esteemed

Starting out as a curious invention of the nineteenth century, the motor vehicle has become so widespread and ordinary that in many countries "a way of life without the motor vehicle is nearly unimaginable" (Hinde and Dixon, 2005, p. 50). The motor vehicle has come to be esteemed in a multiplicity of ways: it is regarded as a source of freedom and liberation, a thing of beauty, and an icon of prosperity, while also being regarded as a convenient, necessary, and almost invisible instrument in daily life. However, many researchers argue that this high esteem is most often based on prevalent myths about the automobile and is therefore unfounded.

The car was first promoted as a source of freedom and liberation. In the early twentieth century, Henry Ford declared, "I will build a motor car for the great multitude" (quoted in Brinkley, 2003), and ultimately, he was correct. The motor vehicle became esteemed as a sign of getting ahead in the world, and the "masses" came to aspire to car ownership: "Hoover's slogan in the 1924 election was 'a chicken in every pot; two cars in every garage'" (Paterson, 2000, p. 266). Later, baby boomer teenagers were aided in their quest for "sex, drugs and rock and roll" by the motor vehicle, which allowed them "an easy escape route from restrictive home environments" (Widmer, 2002, p. 68). Further, Davison (2004) argues that the motor vehicle became an instrument and symbol of liberation for women, whose routines were facilitated and enhanced by the use of a motor vehicle. Even today, the motor vehicle is regarded by most as a symbol of independence, even those who choose not to travel by automobile (Jensen, 1999).

Although the car is esteemed in many ways, this fondness is not necessarily well founded. Jensen (1999) points out that despite the perception that automobile signifies freedom and independence, there are significant numbers of people in car-reliant nations who get by well without a motor car every day. There is also a convincing argument that society's obsession with transport has actually reduced freedom for some, particularly for women, children, and the elderly (Ker and Tranter, 2003). Most significantly, as described below, the growing dominance of the motor vehicle has, in turn, led to reliance on the automobile and limited people's scope *not* to use the automobile.

Beyond the utility of the motor vehicle in providing freedom and escape, society's esteem for the motor vehicle is also aesthetic. Wollen and Kerr's (2002) collection of photographs and essays highlights the ways the car has been artistically portrayed in cinema, literature, poetry, and so on. They argue that cars can also be "artworks in their own right" (Wollen, 2002). This aesthetic admiration might even be regarded as emotional. Davison's (2004) account of the history of the automobile in Melbourne, Australia, described

how "like a human love affair, our love affair with the car unfolded, step by step, from its first moment of distant admiration through casual acquaintance, infatuation and deep bonding to taken-for-granted familiarity"(p. xii).

Paterson (2000) asserts that the motorcar has become "perhaps *the* symbol of progress for most of the twentieth century" (p. 263). Paterson argues that the motorcar gained the dominant economic status it enjoys today not only due to the particular features of the motor vehicle (e.g., it facilitates the movement of goods and people in the economy) but also because of the role of the car and associated industries in advancing industrialization and globalization and, most important, because of the ongoing financial, and rhetorical, support the automotive industry and its products have received from governments (Paterson, 2000).

The favor conferred upon the automobile by governments could have multiple bases. Private motor vehicles are a very visible sign of affluence and a household item that people are willing to spend a sizable proportion of their income to buy. The motor vehicle industry creates a lot of jobs, not only in the manufacturing of the vehicles and their parts, but also in the support industries dealing with repair, maintenance, petrol supply, road building, advertising, and other economic activities. All of these appear to contribute positively to the GDP of the country and boost economic growth. Multinational corporations in the motor vehicle industry are in a position to make multimillion-dollar investments in developing countries; the new "car society" offers training and employment in the support industries across the country. The globalization of a transport system focused on private motor vehicles may seem as a great enhancement of economic progress and human well-being.

However, the negative side effects (and economic externalities) of this rapid growth of motor vehicle manufacture and use are often overlooked. They are not always easy to identify and quantify, and many of the health impacts will not appear until after years of delay (Kjellstrom et al., 2003). Market forces alone cannot lead countries to the most efficient transport system when considerable external costs are ignored or difficult to predict. Transport is just one essential part of the infrastructure for a well-functioning society. The important driving forces of population and economic growth create rapidly increasing needs also for housing, various human services, and industrial facilities. An integrated approach to planning of the location of housing, industry, and services, as well as development of the transport system with due consideration given to public transport, walking, and bicycling (Vuchic, 1999), are needed to moderate the dramatic and problematic growth of private motor vehicle transport as an element of globalization.

The Social Reproduction of Car Use

An intriguing aspect of the place of the motor vehicle in modern societies is the self-replicating nature of a car-based transport system. Dupuy (1999) notes that "thirty years ago, American oil industry and road engineers discovered the 'magic circle' of automobile development" (p. 1). He describes how this manifests in many ways, the most obvious of which is the effect on the physical surroundings—roads, freeways, car yards, petrol stations, and parking lots—that further encourages the use of the car. However, the automobile is also rooted in the social environment in more subtle ways: the cultural norms and values that surround the motor vehicle, making it acceptable and desirable, and the economic processes that facilitate increasing ownership and use of the car. Even the very nature of social interaction has come to be shaped by, and therefore reliant on, the automobile. These processes together may be described as the "social reproduction" of the automobile and underpin the notion of "car reliance" as opposed to car use.

The motor vehicle has affected the nature of space, and time, in developed societies. The automobile allowed for changes to the landscape such as suburbanization; splitting business, retail, and residential land uses; fragmenting communities across space; and the emergence of car-only environments (e.g., roads and car parking spaces) (Sheller and Urry, 2000). This new kind of landscape not only was shaped by automobile transport, but in turn rendered automobile transport the only realistic option for citizens. The sheer distances that must be covered, as well as the nature of urban design and transport planning that favors the car, often prohibit other forms of mobility, especially walking (Mees, 2000). Thus, as Freund and Martin (1996) suggest, "the auto was transformed from a choice into a requirement" (p. 14).

Hinde and Dixon (2005) provide an account of the economic and social processes that led to the motor vehicle becoming entrenched in the way of life of Australians. These processes include pricing, distribution, and ownership rates in providing incentives to citizens to own and use a motor vehicle. The important role of actors—in government, industry, and civil society—who create these economic incentives is also highlighted. Moreover, a historical perspective illustrates how the cultural processes of esteem (briefly described above) and the normalization of the motor vehicle meant that, while the physical landscape was increasingly accommodating the motor vehicle, the car was also taking root in people's hearts and minds (Hinde and Dixon, 2005).

Finally, the very nature of social interaction has changed due to the motor car (see, e.g., Beckmann, 2001; Urry, 2000; Sheller and Urry, 2000). Our lives now take place over relatively long distances. In addition, the speed and flexibility of car transport have led to a change in our experience of time. Time horizons become shortened as destinations become more accessible, and products and information may be delivered more swiftly. People's expectations, relationships, and routines are adjusted accordingly.

Car Reliance and Everyday Life

As Wollen (2002) describes eloquently, the car has transformed "the food we eat, the music we listen to, the risks we take, the places we visit, the errands we run, the emotions we feel, the movies we watch, the money we spend, the stress we endure and the air we breathe" (p. 11).

Miller (2001) points out that using an automobile is like "second-nature" because cars require "no conscious mediation in their daily employment" (p. 3). This was illustrated by a qualitative study of women in suburban Sydney and a nearby rural area in Australia (Dowling, 2000). While most of the women interviewed acknowledged that they might prefer not to drive, the car had become vital to achieving their aspirations and performing their routines. The women, especially the mothers, had complex schedules involving crossing long distances within short periods of time. For example, the study included a single mother who in the morning drops off her six children at primary school, high school, and paid work, visits people and shops during the day, and then picks the children up and takes them to friends' places in the evening (Dowling, 2000).

HEALTH BENEFITS OF MOTOR VEHICLE TRANSPORT

Does the Car Confer Any Health Benefits to Individuals?

The population-level health effects of car reliance are relatively well documented, but little attention has been paid to the relationship between car reliance and health at the level of the *individual*. In the research that has been done, in contrast to the range of detrimental *population* effects, it appears that car ownership is positively correlated with health for individuals. Specifically, there are studies that show car ownership is associated with better health outcomes and that lack of car ownership is associated with poorer outcomes. These associations have only begun to be identified and explained, but the relationship must be at least partly due to the context: a society that is structured according to the automobile will create numerous advantages for car owners and users.

Macintyre et al. (1998) explain that car ownership has been generally ignored as affecting health in its own right, generally being treated as a proxy for class or income. These authors remind us that, previously, public health researchers never thought that the automobile could be important for health. Macintyre et al. (1998) dispute this assumption by listing some of the ways access to a motor vehicle could be health promoting

> by increasing access to employment, shops selling healthy food at affordable prices, leisure facilities, social support networks, health services and open space; and by reducing exposure to dangers such as mugging, rape or assault . . . [and] may provide ontological security, and thereby health, through its capacity to protect passengers from external threats, to express the owner's personality, and confer prestige. (p. 659)

Macintyre et al. (1998) went on to demonstrate that car ownership is positively associated with health, independent of its correlation with socioeconomic status. The study also showed that the car is related to health beyond its relationship with psychological

markers such as self-esteem. A later study (Macintyre et al., 2001) similarly demonstrated that income, class, housing, and car ownership are each related to health independently; that is, these variables are not all proxies for a common underlying construct (e.g., class).

Using the concept of "ontological security," Hiscock et al. (2002) used qualitative interviews to explore how car and public transport use are related to well-being. Specifically, ontological security consists of three dimensions: a sense of (1) protection, (2) autonomy, and (3) prestige. The researchers found that people's descriptions of their motor vehicle use reflected all three dimensions of ontological security. However, their interviews with public transport users also revealed that ontological security can be obtained using alternative transport modes. For example, the car is felt to provide "protection" in the form of shielding from the weather, avoidance of contact with others, and therefore lower risk of mugging. Alternately, public transport provides protection in the form of perceived reduced risk of being involved in a traffic accident or being stranded due to car breakdown. There are large numbers of people who own and gain ontological security from their motor vehicle, but the authors challenge the view that the car is the only transport mode that provides these psychosocial benefits.

There is also research that shows that lack of car ownership can be associated with ill-health outcomes. Bostock (2001) shows people in poverty often cannot get access to a car or afford to use public transport; they therefore mainly have to walk. She described how walking through their home neighborhood provides a constant reminder of their disadvantaged situation. In addition, walking with tired children is often stressful, especially in bad weather, carrying shopping bags. More broadly, the limited transport options of disadvantaged people mean that they have difficulty in accessing "hospitals, holidays and human resources" (Bostock, 2001). Disadvantage and its associated poor health outcomes are compounded among those individuals of low socioeconomic status who cannot access a motor vehicle.

Consistent with these findings, Bromley and Thomas (1993) point out that the retail revolution of providing cheap, large-scale shopping centers in suburban locations has led to an ever-increasing dependency on cars to access cheap and diverse products, including food. This change in the retail market has led to the emergence of a disadvantaged "carless" shopper who can only access shops in central locations and therefore must pay more for fewer choices.

Health Aspects of the Individual versus the Population

A car-reliant society creates social conditions that render the motor vehicle so essential to daily life that its absence is felt in the form of compounded disadvantage, and even health. Despite a general awareness among the public of the negative environmental consequences of the automobile, and their belief in the importance of reducing car use, this does not translate into behavioral change by individuals. People describe a range of activities and opportunities that the car confers, such as the opportunity to select educational opportunities for their children (Dowling, 2000) and access to holidays or other activities not accessible by other transport modes (Jensen, 1999). The car has become so entwined with people's aspirations that they "simply will not do without" the opportunities that they believe only the car can facilitate (Jensen, 1999). While there is a very clear-cut rationale for reducing car reliance as a major *population* health problem, there is some evidence to suggest that a transition away from car reliance might also negatively affect the health of certain groups or *individuals*.

PUBLIC HEALTH CHALLENGES

Road Traffic Injuries

The most obvious health impact of land transport is in road traffic injuries. This is well established in health statistics from all countries with significant motorization. During the 1960s and 1970s, in most industrialized countries, the mortality and morbidity rates (in relation to population) were increasing, and since then safety measures have made the rates decrease in spite of continued increase of motorization (WHO, 2004).

Sweden and the United Kingdom have some of the lowest recorded traffic mortality rates in the world (table 6.4). The ranking of rates will depend on how it is estimated, as seen by comparing the two variables presented in the table: deaths per 100,000 population and deaths per 10,000 vehicles. The rates by popula-

tion should ideally be age-adjusted, but these rates are crude—on average, the age-adjusted traffic crash mortality rates per 100,000 people in 2000 were 11.8 in high-income countries, with an expectation of a reduction to 7.8 by 2020 (WHO, 2004). All regions of developing countries had higher rates, which are also expected to increase by 2020. For example, the table highlights the extraordinarily high rate in a developing country such as Botswana in 1998 (32.1 deaths per 100,000 people). Elsewhere, very high rates have been reported in and predicted for Latin America: 26.1 and 31.0 deaths per 100,000 people for 2000 and 2020, respectively (WHO, 2004).

While road fatalities are likely to be accurately represented in the official statistics, less severe road injuries are significantly underreported. Studies comparing police report figures with hospital admissions and community survey data in New Zealand show that only a portion (50–70%) of serious crash injuries are reported (Morrison and Kjellstrom, 1987; Begg et al., 1990; Alsop and Langley, 2001). Similar gaps in official accident statistics are observed in other countries, including the United Kingdom, United States, Sweden, and Germany (Bruhning, 1997). For several categories of road user, fewer than 60% of traffic crash injuries were reported to police/transport authorities. In developing countries, the underreporting in official statistics may be an even greater problem. If the underreporting was constant over time and similar for all road users, one could make an adjustment of the official statistics, but this may still seriously underestimate injuries among bicyclists and child pedestrians.

The highest risks for motor vehicle crash mortality and morbidity occur in the fifteen to twenty-nine age group (figure 6.4). The rates go down after twenty-nine years of age and then increase again after age sixty. The rates among men are generally about twice the rates for women.

The situation in a developing country, Thailand, is shown in figure 6.5, with Swedish and Australian data included for comparison. The increase of the mortality rates from 1998 through 2001 is striking, and by 2001 the higher rates among the elderly have started to appear.

Another way of expressing the health impact of traffic crashes on different age, sex, and ethnic groups is to calculate the disability-adjusted life years (DALYs) (Murray and Lopez, 1996). The DALYs express the "preventable" extent of lost "healthy life" for a particular population group or disease/injury

TABLE 6.4. International Comparison of Crude Road Death Rates, 1998

Country	Vehicles per Capita	Road Deaths	Deaths per 100,000 Population	Deaths per 10,000 Vehicles
United States	0.77	41,471	15.3	2.0
Australia	0.64	1,763	9.4	1.5
Japan	0.61	10,805	8.5	1.4
New Zealand	0.61	502	13.3	2.2
Germany	0.60	7,792	9.5	1.6
Canada	0.59	2,934	9.7	1.6
Norway	0.56	352	8.0	1.4
Sweden	0.51	531	6.0	1.2
United Kingdom	0.48	3,581	6.1	1.3
Ireland	0.41	458	12.4	3.0
South Korea	0.28	10,416	22.7	8.0
Botswana	0.07	495	32.1	48.0

Source: Based on data from LTSA (2002) and the WHO website, http://www.who.int/research/en

category. Injuries contribute 12% of the total global burden of disease, and a quarter of these injuries are due to motor vehicle crashes (WHO, 2004). This means that 3% of the global burden is due to traffic crash injuries, which is similar to the contribution from other major risk factors: tobacco (4.1%), alcohol (4.0%), unsafe drinking water, and sanitation (3.7%) and indoor air pollution from solid fuels (2.6%) (WHO, 2002). The ranking of road traffic injuries among different causes of death and disability was ninth in 1990 and is expected to rise to third in 2020 (Murray and Lopez, 1996). As highlighted above, the increasing prominence of this health risk is likely to occur primarily in developing countries.

Motorcyclists face the highest risk of injury per hour of traveling, with an injury mortality rate of 440 per hundred million hours traveled (about seventeen times the injury rate of car occupants) (table 6.5). The risks to pedestrians and bicyclists per kilometer or hour traveled are high compared with car travel, but it should be remembered that cars and other motor vehicles are the primary causes of these risks. The exceptionally low risk of death in a collision for bus or rail travel (table 6.5) is an important consideration in assessing the overall health impacts of different transport modes and systems.

In developing countries, the risk of dying in a collision for the various modes of transport is different from developed countries, because motorization is still at an early stage (Tiwari, 1997). For example, the annual road deaths in Delhi during its early motorization in 1985 was approximately 1,100, 42% of whom were pedestrians, 23% motorcyclists, 12% bicyclists, and 10% bus passengers. Private car passenger deaths were very few (<2%) (Mohan and Bawa, 1985). However, almost all of the pedestrians and bicyclists killed were hit by a car, bus, truck, or motorcycle.

The risk of injury (per hour traveled) to pedestrians in New Zealand is highest at either end of the age spectrum (LTSA, 1999). Primary-school-age children are vulnerable because they are less visible than are adults and have less experience and judgment in negotiating busy roads. Older adults are also at increased risk of injury, due to a combination of increased physical frailty and decreased agility and sensory perception.

Air Pollution (Vehicle Emissions)

Vehicles with internal combustion engines emit air pollutants, including particulate matter (dust), carbon monoxide, nitrogen oxides, and a variety of hydrocarbons. Lead emissions are remaining major environmental health problems in those countries where lead addition to petrol is still allowed.

Nitrogen oxides and hydrocarbons can oxidize

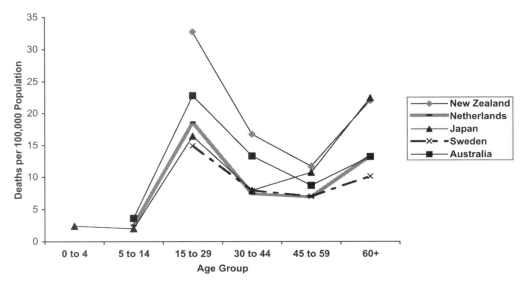

FIGURE 6.4. Age-Specific Motor Vehicle Crash Mortality Rates for Men in Five Countries. *Source:* WHO (2004).

oxygen in air to ozone if exposed to high levels of sunlight. This "secondary air pollutant" is becoming an increasing health problem in areas with high motor vehicle usage, due to the increasing amounts of air pollutants from vehicles, and possibly to increasing ultraviolet radiation at ground level caused by stratospheric ozone layer depletion. Very fine dust particles (particulate matter less than 2.5 μm in diameter [$PM_{2.5}$]) are also secondary pollutants.

The combustion of petrol or diesel in a typical vehicle engine produces emissions of particles containing combustion products as well as toxic gases. Some of the exhaust gases (particularly nitrogen oxides and sulfur dioxide) also form small particles when they condense in the cooler air. The particles are generally very small ($PM_{2.5}$), and these small particles can readily be inhaled into the alveoli in the lung. These fine particles are the most likely to be the pollutant of main concern for the mortality effect (WHO, 2000a), but the toxic gas emissions, carbon monoxides, nitrogen oxides, and volatile organic chemicals also cause health effects (U.S. EPA, 1998; WHO, 2000a; Kjellstrom et al., 2002).

The serious health effects of air pollution became evident in 1952 when the infamous "London Fog" incident killed at least 4,000 people during a winter week when PM air pollution was in the range of 1,000–2,000 μg/m³. The daily mortality increase above "normal" was approximately 100%. Since then, hundreds of studies of health effects of air pollution have documented the health risks in detail (Brunekreef and Holgate, 2002). All types of air pollution sources are health risks (coal smoke, wood smoke, and motor vehicle exhausts), and air pollution levels many times lower than those recorded during the London Fog incident can increase mortality rates (Kjellstrom et al., 2002). In fact, the World Health Organization air quality guidelines are based on an international agreement that there is no lower threshold for this health risk (WHO, 2000a).

The relative increase of daily mortality, above the background mortality, is about 0.1% per μg/m³ increase in PM_{10}, but the increase of longer term annual mortality in relation to the annual PM_{10} level is considered to be much greater (0.43% per μg/m³ PM_{10}) (Kunzli et al., 2000). Recent research indicates that the long-term (annual) dose–response relationship may be even higher (Pope et al., 2002; Scoggins et al., 2004).

A major health risk assessment conducted for three European countries (Kunzli et al., 2000), using the current evidence about the long-term mortality

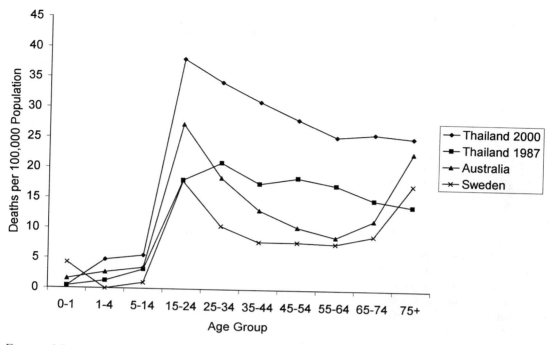

FIGURE 6.5. Age-Specific Motor Vehicle Crash Mortality for Men in Thailand, Sweden, and Australia. *Source:* Based on data WHO (2004).

effect of PM, found that the estimated number of deaths associated with PM exposure from motor vehicles was approximately twice as many as the deaths due to traffic crashes (table 6.6). These results were based on a very detailed analysis of exposures and health effects. The results made a major contribution to the recognition of the importance of motor vehicle air pollution in Europe, leading to the establishment of a Transport, Health and Environment Pan-European Program (THE PEP, 2004) by the World Health Organization and the United Nations Economic Council for Europe. In New Zealand, an assessment using the same methodology as the European study (Fisher et al., 2002) indicated that the mortality impact of motor vehicle air pollution for the whole country was similar to the crash road toll (table 6.6).

Traffic Noise

Noise is known to have an adverse impact on health, particularly for communities located close to major traffic routes, airports, or noisy industries. Annoyance, sleep disturbance, and interference with communication are the most commonly reported effects that

could contribute to stress-related health problems (Berglund and Lindvall, 1995). A review of seven community surveys (Hunt, 1989) identified these impacts and also vibration from passing traffic as commonly reported problems.

Survey respondents indicated that traffic noise

TABLE 6.5. Traffic Crash Deaths per Passenger-Kilometers (PK) and Passenger-Hours (PH) Traveled in European Union Countries in 2001–2002

Mode of Travel	Deaths per 100 Million PK	Deaths per 100 Million PH
Roads (total)	0.95	28
Motorcycle	13.8	440
Pedestrian	6.4	75
Bicycle	5.4	25
Car	0.7	25
Bus	0.07	2
Ferry	0.25	16
Aircraft	0.035	8
Rail	0.035	2

Source: WHO (2004).

TABLE 6.6. Air Pollution Mortality (for Adults
Thirty Years of Age) and the Road Toll, 1996

Country	Population (Million)	Traffic Accident Deaths (A)	Mortality Due to Traffic Air Pollution (B)	Ratio B:A
France	58.3	8,919	17,629	2.0
Austria	8.1	963	2,411	2.5
Switzerland	7.1	597	1,762	3.0
New Zealand	3.7	502	399	0.8

Source: Based on data from Kunzli et al. (2000) and Fisher et al. (2002).

caused most disturbance in the early morning and late night and that "stop/start" traffic conditions were more annoying than continuous traffic flow (Hunt, 1989). This is in accordance with the finding of studies of airport noise (Berglund and Lindvall, 1995). The disturbance of such noise is more related to the hourly frequency of loud aircraft movements than to the loudness of the noise. A recent study of airport noise effects comparing school children in Munich before and after a new airport was opened and the old airport closed (Hygge et al., 2002) showed that short-term and long-term memory, reading ability, and speech perception were all affected by the noise exposure. These are the kinds of effects that compound through the life course by reducing children's cumulative learning at school and in turn negatively affecting their future livelihood.

In recent years, considerable research has been carried out in Europe on the association between noise exposure, increased blood pressure, and morbidity and mortality in ischemic heart disease (van Kempen et al., 2002). The degree of association with traffic noise, in particular, is still uncertain, but at an individual level the risk is likely to be low. However, with significant exposure of large populations (an estimated 30% of the population in Europe is regularly exposed to road traffic noise above 55 dB[A]) and the common occurrence of high blood pressure and heart disease, even a small increase in individual risk can result in large disease burdens in a population. For the Netherlands, an estimated 1–2% of the total burden of disease could be attributed to traffic noise (this is a larger attributable risk than for most other specific risk factors). A similar analysis for Denmark (Ohm et al., 2003) concluded that between 200 and 500 premature deaths each year may be due to traffic noise.

Physical Inactivity

Active transport can be defined as modes of transport that confer more exercise than motor vehicle use. This includes walking, cycling, and using public transport (Mason, 2000). It has been shown that physical activity through active transport has a very important role to play in obesity and disease prevention (Koplan and Dietz, 1999). Inactivity leads to an elevated risk of chronic diseases such as cardiovascular disease and diabetes. Up to one-third of deaths caused by coronary heart disease, diabetes, and colon cancer are linked to a sedentary lifestyle (Roberts et al., 1996). Sedentary people have displayed a risk of fatal cardiovascular events up to 100% greater than that of active people (Berlin and Colditz, 1990). British data suggest that people who are physically inactive are twice as likely to develop coronary heart disease and three times as likely to suffer a stroke (Sustrans, 2001). Using data from the 1996–1997 New Zealand Health Survey, Tobias and Roberts (2001) estimated that physical inactivity accounts for the death of 2,600 New Zealanders each year—that is, 9% of all deaths.

Conversely, participation in physical activity reduces the risk of all-cause mortality, being linked to the prevention of colon, breast, and lung cancers and being associated with improvements in mental health and musculoskeletal health (Roberts et al., 1996). Being physically active is also related to the reduction of risk factors, including overweight/obesity, high blood pressure, and high blood cholesterol. One of the most effective means of managing mild to moderate hypertension is physical activity (Sustrans, 2001).

Obesity accounts for a significant share of the mortality burden from diseases such as diabetes (44–46%), coronary heart disease (22–25%), and hypertension (57–66%) (Galgali et al., 1998). Recent field experiments in Denmark have investigated cycling to test the effects of physical activity on health. The Copenhagen Heart Study, which involved 13,375 women and 17,265 men twenty to ninety-three years of age, found that cycling has a strong health protective function. Even after adjustment for other risk factors, such as leisure-time physical activity, those who did not cycle to work experienced a 39% higher mortality rate than those who did (Andersen et al., 2000; WHO, 2000b). A British study found that men who live in households with no cars and have to walk and cycle every day have a lower rate of death from ischemic heart disease than men who travel to work by car; those men who use public transport have a death rate between these two levels (Public Health Alliance, 1991).

By replacing one or two 3–5 km journeys per day with walking or cycling, the recommended daily exercise level of thirty minutes per day can be easily achieved without specific physical activity time being allocated (WHO, 2000b). There is a convergence of policy goals between the health and the transport sectors. Daily routine exercise, via active transport, provides a means to improve health while helping to lower negative externalities of motorized vehicle use, thus moving toward sustainable transport goals (Davis, 1999).

The term "obesogenic environment" has been coined for living environments that discourage physical activity or encourage consumption of high-fat or high-sugar foodstuffs (Egger and Swinburn, 1997). Research is emerging that makes it possible to quantify the relationship between obesity and transport habits. The first detailed study of this issue (Frank et al., 2004) found that riding in a car and walking have opposite associations with the prevalence of obesity in suburban areas in the United States. Each additional hour per day spent in a car increased the likelihood of obesity by 6%, and each additional kilometer walked per day decreased the likelihood of obesity by 4.8%. These are large effects, and the results need to be confirmed in longitudinal (incidence) studies. The town planning or land-use mix was also strongly associated with obesity (Frank et al., 2004). "Walkable"

neighborhoods had the lowest prevalence of obesity even after adjusting for socioeconomic variables. Urban sprawl and town planning that favors motor vehicle travel over "active transport" are increasingly acknowledged as important determinants of the obesity epidemic of industrialized countries (Schmidt, 2004) (see also chapter 4).

Community Disruption and Social Isolation

Transport provides an important means of contact between family members, friends, and members of voluntary organizations and communities. At the same time, roadways and traffic act as a physical and psychological barrier to social contact. Whether the positive or negative social effects of transport dominate depends on both the volume of traffic and the geographical location of transport networks. In rural areas, transport is essential to maintaining social contact and in accessing facilities such as schools, shops, and community meeting areas. In urban neighborhoods, busy roadways and heavy traffic flows often act as barriers to community contact.

There is little information regarding the positive impact of motor vehicle transport on social networks, but some general issues can be identified.

- Facilitates social contact, especially in rural areas
- Enables people to reach places of work, education, and recreation, as the most common means of transport to school or work
- Facilitates access to various services in the community (shops, health services, sports facilities, etc.), which is particularly important in rural areas

Some of the negative issues are as follows:

- Social severance, the negative effect that roads and traffic have on social interaction within a community, for instance, when a road or a motorway cuts through a community, separating it into sections not easily accessible to one another; affects most those with limited mobility, such as children, the elderly, and people with disabilities
- Dominance of private cars, contributing to social inequalities, possibly increasing social isolation

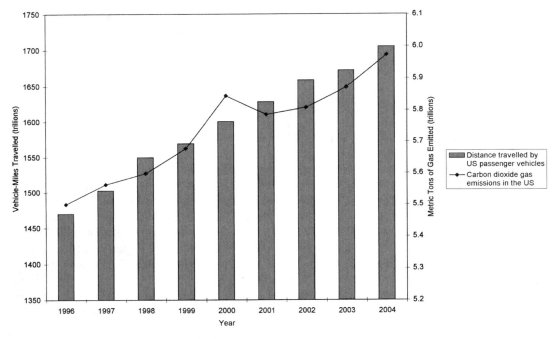

FIGURE 6.6. Distance Driven by Vehicles in the United States and Their Carbon Emissions, 1996–2004. *Source:* Energy Information Administration and Bureau of Transportation Statistics (2005).

by lack of car access, especially in areas with poor public transport

• Physical impact of roads and other transport facilities, with high rates of private vehicle usage leading to increased traffic volumes and creating pressure for the expansion of roadways

• Reliance on private vehicles, contributing to weaker public transport systems

ENVIRONMENTAL IMPACTS

Global Climate Change

Combustion of fossil fuels in motor vehicles produces carbon dioxide, the major greenhouse gas contributing to global climate change (IPCC, 2001). Vehicle emissions also include other chemicals, such as carbon monoxide, that may contribute to climate change (MacKenzie and Walsh, 1990). Transport emissions contribute approximately a third of the global greenhouse gases, but as they are increasing they pose a particular threat to achieving the aims of the Kyoto Protocol of the United Nations Framework Convention on Climate Change. Figure 6.6 shows

how these emissions are increasing in the United States more or less in parallel with the distance driven by motor vehicles.

The contribution to the greenhouse gases from different countries is often expressed in terms of "carbon emissions." Figure 6.7 indicates the great differences in carbon emissions per capita between developed and developing countries. As China and India develop economically and increase their energy consumption per capita and the rate of motor vehicle ownership, the carbon emissions per capita from these countries are likely to increase dramatically. In order to avoid damaging climate change, the total global carbon emissions have to be reduced. This can be achieved only by a reduction of carbon emissions in developed countries (figure 6.7), and the transport system has an important role to play in this (see also chapter 5).

In terms of climate change, there are already signs that the average temperature is increasing in many parts of the world (IPCC, 2001). Health impacts have started to be recorded (McMichael, 2002), and several likely effects are shown in chapter 5 (figure 5.2). Different geographic areas and population groups

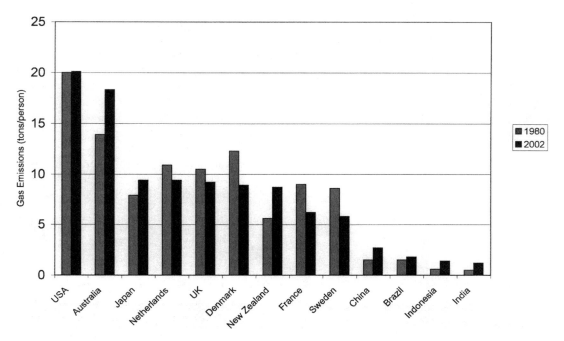

FIGURE 6.7. Carbon Emissions per Capita in Selected Countries, 1980 and 2002. *Source:* United Nations Development Program (2005).

will be affected in different ways, but it is likely that developing countries have the largest number of vulnerable people and that adaptations to climate change will be most difficult to implement there (IPCC, 2001).

Energy Use in Transport and Sustainable Development

Energy consumption in the transport sector is rising much faster than in other sectors. Petroleum is a nonrenewable resource, most of which has to be imported. This raises concerns about the world's continuing reliance on this energy source. The burning of fossil fuels causes greenhouse gas pollution, and its mining or extraction creates considerable local pollution problems. The rapidly rising price of a barrel of crude oil is an indication of the problems that oil dependency creates. The rapid increase of demand for motor vehicle fuels in countries such as China and India is one important reason for the oil price increase. Wars and hurricanes are other reasons. The oil supply situation is not sustainable, and it is becoming more and more urgent to reduce fossil fuel consumption in the transport system.

Walking, bicycling, and public transport plays an important role in developing sustainable means of travel. Because the improvement and protection of public health is the first principle of sustainable development (United Nations, 1993), all the detrimental health impacts of transport undermine sustainability. In addition, an energy inefficient and polluting transport system is in conflict with other principles of sustainable development.

Other environment stresses created by a motor-vehicle–based transport system is rainwater runoff from road surfaces and road sides, which are contaminated with the accumulated emissions from the vehicles. Heavy metals and polyaromatic hydrocarbons may be of particular interest (NZMFE, 1997). Other water and soil issues include loss of topsoil and waterway contamination during road construction, soil and water contamination from disposal of waste oil and tires, and increased storm-water runoff from sealed road surfaces.

Car manufacturing and repair also involve exposures to occupational hazards and local pollution. Petrol stations are some of the more contaminated sites in typical suburban areas, and filling petrol involves exposure to benzene (which is a common additive to petrol). Another example of health risks is the use of asbestos in brake linings, which exposes car mechanics to delayed health risks.

GLOBALIZATION AND TRANSPORT POLICY

Car reliance is operating as a pervasive and influential determinant of health in developed and developing countries around the world, with impacts across many domains of health. This is unsurprising given its fundamental role in globalization itself, in terms of both the uses of the automobile and also the powerful role of the automotive industry.

Transport and health policies are necessarily positioned within the agendas of broader global actors and national government agendas for social development. Economic concerns are usually given the most prominence in such decision making. However, it is clear in the case of transport at least that there is an interweaving of economic, social, environmental and health concerns. Transport and other policy decisions will inevitably affect all of these areas. Therefore, a more holistic and global sustainability perspective is required (UNEP, 2000).

In relation to transport planning, a multisectoral approach is emerging. The United Nations Economic and Social Commission for Asia and the Pacific called for a holistic vision in relation to the building of the Asian Highway Network (ESCAP, 2004): "Social, environmental and safety issues are often poorly addressed in traditional narrowly focused transport planning. . . . Environmental, social and health impact assessments are essential to reduce negative impacts that can impose costs several times greater than the direct cost of the transport services" (p. 15).

The holistic perspective of the economic, social, environmental, and health consequences of economic development and the role of transport within it must be guided by the principles of sustainable communities. Transport infrastructure lasts for many decades, and bad or good transport systems will last for a long time. In addition, the environmental and health impacts may take many decades to become apparent, which necessitates a forward-looking approach to impact assessments. The short-term wealth creation focus of the current globalization efforts is not a good base for the policies needed to develop health-promoting instead of health-threatening transport systems.

Within countries, urban design is a major factor in ensuring healthy and sustainable transport systems. A number of health promotion and environmental protection initiatives can be used as a bridge between the planning, health, and environment agencies within the community. Many localities already have programs addressing these multisectoral interests, such as "healthy cities," "eco-communities," and "sustainable communities." The promotion of a healthier transport system fits well into these programs (Laird et al., 2001).

Urban design is also the key to walkability, adoption of active transport, and use of public transport. City infrastructures are usually designed around car travel. This results in less funding available for cycling and walking trails and facilities. Providing infrastructure for fast-moving car-based travel can actively discourage active transport due to decreased safety for bike users and pedestrians and makes car travel a more appealing option (Mason, 2000). Denser residential areas with services (shops, schools, sporting facilities, etc.) located together, coined "mixed-use neighborhoods," plus good public transport linking these areas to places of employment, especially large employers or other significant "trip generators" (e.g., universities and hospitals), will aid efforts to promote active modes of transport (Vuchic, 1999; Koplan and Dietz, 1999).

CONCLUSIONS

Transport is an essential sector within a country's economic and social life. However, mobility is not synonymous with motor vehicle road transport. A car-reliant society causes more negative health and societal consequences than what is usually acknowledged. The principles and practices of economic globalization facilitate the development of a car-reliant society, and growing car ownership rates in developing countries show that the world is moving rapidly in this direction.

The various health impacts caused by the modern private motor-vehicle–based transport system includes car crash injuries, lung and heart effects of vehicle-related air pollution, disturbance and blood pressure effects of noise, reduced physical activity and associated obesity, and community disruption from major roads. In addition, greenhouse gases, climate change, and other environmental issues need to be considered. While there is a convincing and growing body of evidence on these effects, further research is required to fully quantify and understand them. Moreover, comprehensive assessments of the health impacts of transport systems and the value of interventions are essential.

The development of health-promoting transport systems relies on the introduction of a sustainability focus within economic policy, which provides support for health-promoting urban design and planning. Globalization efforts that rely on the "market" to find solutions to the social and health concerns is too limited. A broader approach to economic development and transport planning that fully takes into account the health issues will potentially ensure long-term gains in the health of populations in both developing and industrial countries. In other words, reducing car reliance is a global public good.

References

Alsop J, and Langley J (2001). Under-reporting of motor vehicle traffic crash victims in New Zealand. *Acc Anal Prev* 33: 353–359.

Andersen LB, Schnohr P, Schroll M, and Hein HO (2000). All-cause mortality associated with physical activity during leisure time, work, sports, and cycling to work. *Arch Int Med* 160: 1621–1628.

Australian Bureau of Statistics (2003). *Driving to Pluto and back: Australians drive 190 billion kilometers* (Media Release Cat. No. 9208.0) [online]. Canberra: Australian Bureau of Statistics. http://www.abs.gov.au/ausstats/abs@.nsf/0/FE55F1F116F73E16CA256D02000B40ED?Open

Beckmann J (2001). Automobility—a social problem and theoretical concept. *Environ Planning D: Soc Space* 19: 593–607.

Begg DJ, Langley JD, and Chalmers DJ (1990). Road crash experiences during the fourteenth and fifteenth year of life: an overview. *NZ Med J* 103: 174–176.

Berglund B, and Lindvall T (1995). *Community noise.* Archives of the Center for Sensory Research, Vol 2, Issue 1. Stockholm: Karolinska Institute.

Berlin JA, and Colditz GA (1990). A meta-analysis of physical activity in the prevention of coronary heart disease. *Am J Epidemiol* 132: 612–628.

Bostock L (2001). Pathways of disadvantage? Walking as a mode of transport among low-income mothers. *Health Soc Care Community* 9: 11–18.

Bradshaw YW, and Wallace M (1996). *Global inequalities.* Thousand Oaks, CA: Pine Forge Press.

Brinkley D (2003). *Wheels for the world.* London: Penguin Books.

Bromley RDF, and Thomas CJ (1993). The retail revolution, the carless shopper and disadvantage. *Trans Inst Br Geogr* 18: 222–236.

Bruhning E (1997). Injury and deaths on the roads: an international perspective. In: Fletcher T, and McMichael AJ, eds. *Health at the crossroads. Transport policy and public health.* Chichester: John Wiley, pp. 109–122.

Brunekreef B, and Holgate ST (2002). Air pollution and health. *Lancet,* 360: 1233–1242.

Bureau of Transportation Statistics (2005). *National transportation statistics, table 1-32: U.S. vehicle-miles.* U.S. Department of Transportation. http://www.bts.gov/publications/national_transportation_statistics/2005/html/table_01_32.html

Corvalan C, Briggs D, and Kjellstrom T (1996). Development of environmental health indicators. In: Briggs D, et al., eds. *Linkage methods for environmental health analysis.* Document WHO/EHG/95.26. Geneva: World Health Organization, pp. 19–54.

Davis, A (1999). *Active transport: A guide to the development of local initiatives to promote walking and cycling.* August 15. London: UK Health Education Authority. http://www.hda-online.org.uk/downloads/pdfs/activetransport.pdf

Davison, G (2004). *Car wars: How the car won our hearts and conquered our cities.* Crows Nest: Allen and Unwin.

Dowling R (2000). Cultures of mothering and car use in suburban Sydney: a preliminary investigation. *Geoforum* 31: 345–353.

Dupuy G (1999). From the "magic circle" to "automobile dependence": measurements and political implications. *Transp Policy* 6: 1–17.

ESCAP (2004) *ESCAP towards 2020.* Bangkok: United Nations Economic and Social Commission for Asia and the Pacific.

Egger G, and Swinburn B (1997). An "ecological" approach to the obesity pandemic. *BMJ* 315: 477–480.

Energy Information Administration (2005). *Emissions of greenhouse gases in the United States, 2004.* Report # DOE/EIA-0573(2004). Washington, DC: U.S. Department of Energy. http://ftp.eia.doe.gov/pub/oiaf/1605/cdrom/pdf/ggrpt/057304.pdf

Fisher G, Rolfe KA, Kjellstrom T, et al. (2002). *Health effects due to motor vehicle air pollution in New Zealand.* Technical Report. Wellington: Ministry of Transport.

Frank LD, Andresen MA, and Schmid TL (2004). Obesity relationships with community design, physical activity, and time spent in cars. *Am J Prev Med* 27: 87–96.

Freund P, and Martin G (1996). The commodity that is eating the world: the automobile, the environment, and capitalism. *Capit Nat Soc* 7: 3–29.

Galbraith K, ed. (2001). *Globalisation: Making sense of an integrating world.* London: Profile Books.

Galgali G, Beaglehole R, Scragg R, and Tobias M (1998). Potential for prevention of premature death and disease in New Zealand. *NZ Med J* 110: 7–10.

Hathway, T (2000). Planning local movement systems. In: Barton H, ed. *Sustainable communities.* London: Earthscan, pp. 216–229.

Hinde S, and Dixon J (2005) Changing the obesogenic environment: insights from a cultural economy of car reliance. *Transp Res D Transp Environ* 10: 31–53.

Hiscock R, Macintyre S, Kearns A, and Ellaway A (2002). Means of transport and ontological security: do cars provide psycho-social benefits to their users? *Transp Res D Transp Environ* 7: 119–135.

Hunt M (1989). *Synthesis of surveys on reaction to road traffic noise in New Zealand; a report to the Traffic Committee, Roads Research Unit, National Roads.* Wellington: National Roads Board.

Hygge S, Evans GW, and Bullinger M (2002). A prospective study of some effects of aircraft noise on cognitive performance in school children. *Psychol Sci* 13: 469–474.

Ingram G, and Liu Z (1998). *Vehicles, roads, and road use: Alternate empirical specifications.* Report PRWP-2036. Washington, DC: World Bank.

Ingram G, and Liu Z (1999). *Determinants of motorization and road provision.* Report PRWP-2042. Washington, DC: World Bank.

International Road Federation (2005). *World road statistics.* Brussels: International Road Federation.

IPCC (2001). *Climate change 2001.* Geneva: Intergovernmental Panel on Climate Change, World Meteorological Organization.

Jacobs G, Aeron-Thomas A, and Astrup A (2000). *Estimating global road fatalities.* TRL Report 445. Crowthorn, Berkshire, UK: Transport Research Laboratory.

Jensen M (1999). Passion and heart in transport—a sociological analysis on transport behaviour. *Transp Pol* 6: 19–33.

Kearns R (2001). The safe journeys of an enterprising school: negotiating landscapes of opportunity and risk. *Health Place* 7: 293–306.

Kenworthy JR (1997). Automobile dependence in Bangkok: an international comparison with implications for planning policies and air pollution. In: Fletcher T, and McMichael AJ, eds. *Health at the crossroads: Transport policy and public health.* Chichester: John Wiley, pp. 215–233.

Ker I, and Tranter P (2003). A wish called wander: reclaiming automobility from the motor car. In: Whitelegg J, and Haq G, eds. *Earthscan reader of world transport policy and practice.* London: Earthscan, pp. 105–113.

Kirdar U, ed. (1997). *Cities fit for people.* New York: United Nations Publications.

Kjellstrom T, and Corvalan C (1995). Framework for the development of environmental health indicators. *World Health Stat Q* 48: 144–154.

Kjellstrom T, Neller A, and Simpson R (2002). Air pollution and its health impacts: the changing panorama. *Med J Aust* 177: 604–608.

Kjellstrom T, van Kerkhoff, L, Bammer, G and McMichael, T (2003). Comparative assessment of transport risks: how it can contribute to health impact assessment of transport policies. *Bull World Health Organ* 81: 451–458.

Koplan JP, and Dietz WH (1999). Caloric imbalance and public health policy. *JAMA* 282: 1579–1581.

Kunzli N, Kaiser R, Medina S, et al. (2000). Public health impact of outdoor and traffic related air pollution: a European assessment. *Lancet* 356: 795–801. (see also, for a detailed report of methodology, Kunzli et al., 2000: http://www.euro.who.int/transport/HIA/20021107_3)

Laird P, Newman P, Bachels M, and Kenworthy J (2001). *Back on track: Rethinking transport policy in Australia and New Zealand.* Sydney: University of New South Wales Press.

Larssen S, Gram F, Hagen LO, Jansen H, Olsthoorn X, Aundhe RV, and Joglekar U (1996a). *URBAIR urban air quality management stratregy in Asia: Greater Mumbai report.* Washington, DC: World Bank.

Larssen S, Gram F, Hagen LO, Jansen H, Olsthoorn X, Lesaca R, Anglo E, Torres EB, Subida RD, and Fransisco HA (1996b). *URBAIR urban air quality management strategy in Asia: Metro Manila report.* Washington, DC: World Bank.

LTSA (1999). *The New Zealand transport survey.* Wellington: Land Transport Safety Authority.

LTSA (2000). *New Zealand pedestrian profile.* Wellington: Land Transport Safety Authority. http://www.ltsa.govt.nz/research/documents/pedestrian.pdf

LTSA (2002). *International comparison of death rates.* Wellington: Land Transport Safety Authority. http://www.ltsa.govt.nz/research/annual_statistics_2000/docs/international_table_1.pdf

Macintyre S, Ellaway A, Der G, Ford G, and Hunt K (1998). Do housing tenure and car access predict health because they are simply markers of income or self esteem? A Scottish study. *J Epidemiol Commun Health* 52: 657–664.

Macintyre S, Hiscock R, Kearns A, and Ellaway A (2001). Housing tenure and car access: further exploration of the nature of their relations with health in a UK setting. *J Epidemiol Commun Health* 55: 330–331.

MacKenzie JJ, and Walsh MP (1990). *Driving forces: Motor vehicle trends and their implications for global warming, energy strategies and transportation planning.* Washington, DC: World Resources Institute.

Mason C (2000). Transport and health: en route to a healthier Australia? *Med J Aust* 172: 230–232.

McMichael AJ (2002). Global climate change and health: an old story writ large. In: McMichael AJ, Campbell-Lendrum D, Ebi K, et al., eds. *Climate change and health: Impacts, adaptations and policy.* Geneva: World Health Organization, p. 1–17.

Mees P (2000). *A very public solution, transport in the dispersed city.* Melbourne: Melbourne University Press.

Miller D (2001). Driven societies. In: Miller D, ed. *Car cultures*. Oxford: Berg, pp. 1–34.

Mohan D, and Bawa PS (1985). An analysis of road traffic fatalities in Delhi, India. *Acc Anal Prev* 17: 33–45.

Morrison P, and Kjellstrom T (1987). A comparison of hospital admissions data and official government statistics of serious traffic accident injuries. *NZ Med J* 100: 517–520

Murray CJL, and Lopez AD (1996). *The global burden of disease*. Boston: Harvard University Press.

NZMFE (1997). *The state of New Zealand's environment*. Wellington: New Zealand Ministry for the Environment. http://www.mfe.govt.nz/publications/ser/ser1997/ser.zip

NZMFE (2002). *Environmental performance indicators: travel patterns to work*. Wellington: New Zealand Ministry for the Environment.

Ohm A, Lund SP, Poulsen PB, and Jakobsen S (2003). *Strategy for limitation of traffic noise—interim report 2* (in Danish). Working Paper No. 53. Copenhagen: National Environment Board.

Paterson M (2000). Car culture and global environmental politics. *Rev Int Stud* 26: 253–270.

Pope CA, Burnett RT, Thun MJ, et al. (2002). Lung cancer, cardiopulmonary mortality and long-term exposure to fine particulate air pollution. *JAMA* 287: 1132–1141.

Public Health Alliance (1991). *Health on the move: Policies for health promoting transport*. London: Public Health Alliance. http://www.stockport.nhs.uk/thsg/pages/onthemove-p1.pdf

Roberts I, Owen H, Lumb P, and MacDougall C (1996). *Pedalling health: Health benefits of a modal transport shift*. Unpublished paper.

Schmidt CW (2004). Sprawl: the new manifest destiny? *Environ Health Perspect* 112: A621–A627.

Scoggins A, Kjellstrom T, Fisher GW, Connor J, and Gimson NR (2004). Spatial analysis of annual air pollution exposure and mortality. *Sci Tot Environ* 321: 71–85.

Sheller M, and Urry J (2000). The city and the car. *Int J Urban Reg Res* 24: 737–757.

Statistics New Zealand (1996). *Census 1996*. Wellington: Statistics New Zealand.

Stiglitz J (2002). *Globalization and its discontents*. London: Penguin Books.

Sustrans (2001). *Healthy and active travel*. Bristol, UK: Sustrans National Cycle Network. http://www.sustrans.org.uk/downloads/9897FB_fh01.pdf

THE PEP (2004). Transport health and environment—Pan-European Project Homepage. Geneva: United Nations Economic Council for Europe. http://unece.unog.ch/the-pep/en/welcome.htm

Tiwari G (1997). Issues in planning for heterogeneous traffic: the case study of Delhi. In: Fletcher T, and McMichael AJ, eds. *Health at the crossroads: Transport policy and public health*. Chichester: John Wiley, pp. 235–242.

Tobias M, and Roberts MG (2001). Modelling physical activity: a multi-state life-table approach. *Aust NZ J Public Health* 25: 141–148.

Tunali O (1996). The billion-car accident waiting to happen. *World Watch* 9: 24–39.

UNDP (2005). *Human development report 2005*. New York: United Nations Development Program.

UNEP (2000). *Sustainable mobility*. Industry and Environment, Vol. 23, No. 4. Paris: United Nations Environment Program Division of Technology, Industry and Economics.

United Nations (1993). *Agenda 21*. New York: United Nations.

Urmetzer P, Blake D, and Guppy N (1999). Individualized solutions to environmental problems: the case of automobile pollution. *Can Public Policy* 25: 345–359.

Urry J (2000). *Inhabiting the car* [online]. Lancaster, UK: Department of Sociology, Lancaster University. http://www.comp.lancs.ac.uk/sociology/soc102ju.htm

U.S. EPA (1998). *Air quality standards*. Washington, DC: U.S. Environmental Protection Agency. http://www.epa.gov/oar/oaqps

van Kempen E, Kruize H, Boshuizen HC, et al. (2002). The association between noise exposure and blood pressure and ischemic heart disease: a meta-analysis. *Environ Health Perspect* 110: 307–317.

Vuchic VR (1999). *Transportation for livable cities*. New Brunswick, NJ: Center for Urban Policy Research, Rutgers, State University of New Jersey.

WHO (1997). *Health and environment in sustainable development*. Document WHO/EHG/97.8. Geneva: World Health Organization.

WHO (2000a). *Air quality guidelines for Europe*. 2nd ed. WHO Regional Publications, European Series No. 91. Copenhagen: World Health Organization Regional Office for Europe.

WHO (2000b). *A physically active life through everyday transport*. Copenhagen: World Health Organization Regional Office for Europe.

WHO (2002). *The world health report 2002*. Geneva: World Health Organization.

WHO (2004). *World report on traffic injury prevention*. Geneva: World Health Organization.

Widmer E (2002). Crossroads: the automobile, rock and roll and democracy. In: Wollen P, and Kerr J, eds. *Autopia: Cars and culture*. London: Reaktion Books, pp. 65–74.

Wollen P (2002). Introduction. In: Wollen P, and Kerr J, eds. *Autopia: Cars and culture*. London: Reaktion Books, pp. 10–19.

Wollen P, and Kerr J, eds. (2002). *Autopia: Cars and culture*. London: Reaktion Books.

World Bank (2000). *World development report*. Washington, DC: World Bank.

Worldwatch Institute (2003). *Cars barreling across the planet*. http://www.worldwatch.org/pubs/goodstuff/cars/

Chapter 7

Poverty and Inequality
in a Globalizing World

Ichiro Kawachi and Sarah Wamala

In the Richard T. Ely Lecture delivered at the American Economic Association meeting in 2003, the former deputy director of the International Monetary Fund Stanley Fischer characterized the often heated debate over globalization in the following way: "To listen to the debates in the terms each side paints the other, one might think that it is a discussion between Dr. Pangloss, who believed that all is for the best in the best of all possible worlds, and those who believe that the world is going to hell in a hand basket" (Fischer 2003, p. 5).

Although Fischer was quick to fault this characterization as "doubly misleading" (because the opposing viewpoints are seldom so polarized), it provides a good starting point for the frequently contradictory assessments that have been made by different camps about the global trends in poverty and inequality during the past two decades. On the one hand, we have the views of antiglobalization groups who marched in the streets of Seattle, Genoa, and Cancun, protesting that globalization has brought about an unprece-

dented increase in poverty and inequality throughout the world. Their claims have in turn been directly challenged by proglobalizers (Fischer among them), who assert that both poverty and inequality have fallen during the recent era of globalization (1980–2000). Even the experts often do not agree. By one estimate, the decline in global poverty has been so sharp that even the United Nations was unaware of it. According to Bhalla (2002), by the time the United Nations announced its Millennium Development Goals on poverty in 2000—to halve the proportion of people living on less than US$1 per day by 2015 (see chapter 14)—that goal had already been surpassed! So who is telling the truth?

The aim of this chapter is to describe trends in global poverty and inequality during the recent era of globalization. Providing a balanced account of what has happened requires navigating through a mine field of claims and counterclaims. In the first section, we review the evidence on global trends in poverty during the past two decades. In the second section, we examine the evidence on trends in income inequality. In the third section, we summarize the current debates concerning whether the forces of globalization—in particular, increased trade and the closer integration of developing countries into the global economy—are responsible for the observed trends in poverty and inequality. The final section will draw out some implications of globalization for the future of poverty and inequality in the world.

HAS POVERTY INCREASED OR DECREASED?

Before turning to a description of worldwide trends in poverty, we might well ask, what is the relevance of poverty to a book about globalization and health? The answer is straightforward. Poverty, no matter how it is defined or measured, presents a major obstacle to health and human development. Poverty, whether it occurs in the developing world or in rich countries, prevents people from having access to the basic goods and services necessary to sustain life. Poor people, no matter where they are, live shorter and sicker lives. We also hasten to add that people sickened by diseases such as malaria, HIV/AIDS and tuberculosis are also more likely to become stuck in a poverty trap (WHO Commission 2001; Subramanian, Belli, and Kawachi 2002). Although globalization per se cannot be directly credited (or blamed) for whatever has happened to poverty worldwide, the description of such trends is nevertheless a crucial piece of keeping the "score card" on the progress of the world during the most recent era of globalization. So what has been the record of poverty trends during the past two decades? Has it grown (as antiglobalization protestors claim), or fallen (as proglobalizers assert), or stayed the same?

The answer depends on where you happen to live in the world, as well as how the poor are counted. Different experts have come up with different numbers for the world's poor depending upon the data sources used to derive their estimates. The technical details of the alternative approaches to counting the world's poor need not detain us here,[1] because the different estimates yield a broadly consistent picture of the overall pattern of poverty trends during the past twenty years. We would characterize the pattern that has emerged as "the good, the bad, and the ugly" (with apologies to filmmaker Sergio Leone).

The good news is that there has been a sharp drop in the head count of citizens in developing countries living below the extreme poverty threshold (<US$1 per day). According to the latest estimates by the World Bank (Chen and Ravallion 2004), there were 390 million fewer people living in extreme poverty in 2001 (the latest year for which data are available) compared to twenty years earlier. The World Bank estimate, drawn from 454 household surveys covering ninety-seven developing countries (representing 93% of the population of the developing world), indicates that the poverty head count was cut in half, from 40% in 1981 to 21% in 2001 (table 7.1, figure 7.1). Champions of globalization frequently cite this statistic (Norberg 2003; Wolf 2004), adding that this represents the first episode in human history where such a sustained decline in poverty has been recorded.

The bad news, as also shown in table 7.1 (and figure 7.2), is that if we turn to a slightly less frugal measure of poverty—the World Bank's threshold of less than $2 a day (which experts somewhat euphemistically refer to as "moderate" poverty as opposed to "extreme" poverty)—there has been a pronounced "bunching" of poor people between the $1 and $2 per day threshold during the same period (Chen and Ravallion 2004). The bunching reflects poor people moving out of the less than $1 a day threshold into the $1–2 a day income range, as well as population growth in poor countries. As a consequence, there has been a net *increase* in the numbers of people living on less than $2 per day, from 2.4 billion in 1981 to 2.7 billion in 2001. Given the world's population of 6.4 billion, this means that roughly 40% of humanity still subsists on a living standard of less than $2 a day.

Finally, the ugly news is that the progress in poverty reduction has been extremely uneven across regions of the world (figure 7.3). The lion's share of poverty reduction in the developing world is attributable to the achievements of just one country, China, where 400 million citizens escaped the $1 per day threshold over the twenty-year period (and where roughly half of the decline occurred during the early 1980s). In other parts of the developing world, especially sub-Saharan Africa, there has been a sharp increase in the number of poor. Poverty also increased in Eastern Europe and Central Asia, as well as in Latin America and the Caribbean (figure 7.3). In 2001, there were still 1.1 billion people (or one in five of the developing world population) living below the

TABLE 7.1. Numbers of People Living on Less Than $1 and $2 per Day (in Millions)

	1981	1984	1987	1990	1993	1996	1999	2001
Living on Less Than $1 per Day								
East Asia	795.6	562.2	425.6	472.2	415.4	286.7	281.7	271.3
(China)	633.7	425.0	308.4	374.8	334.2	211.6	222.8	211.6
East Europe and Central Asia	3.1	2.4	1.7	2.3	17.4	19.8	29.8	17.6
Latin America	35.6	46.0	45.1	49.3	52.0	52.2	53.6	49.8
Middle East and North Africa	9.1	7.6	6.9	5.5	4.0	5.5	7.7	7.1
South Asia	474.8	460.3	473.3	462.3	476.2	461.3	428.5	431.1
Sub-Saharan Africa	163.6	198.3	218.6	226.8	242.3	271.4	294.0	315.8
Total	1,481.8	1,276.8	1,171.2	1,218.5	1,207.5	1,096.9	1,095.1	1,092.7
Living on Less Than $2 per Day								
East Asia	1,169.8	1,108.6	1,028.3	1,116.3	1,079.3	922.2	899.6	864.3
(China)	875.8	813.8	730.8	824.6	802.9	649.6	627.5	593.6
East Europe and Central Asia	20.2	18.3	14.7	22.9	81.1	97.4	112.3	93.5
Latin America	98.9	118.9	115.4	124.6	136.1	117.2	127.4	128.2
Middle East and North Africa	51.9	49.8	52.5	50.9	51.8	60.9	70.4	69.8
South Asia	821.1	858.6	911.4	957.5	1,004.8	1,029.1	1,039.0	1,063.7
Sub-Saharan Africa	287.9	326.0	355.2	381.6	410.4	446.8	489.1	516.0
Total	2,450.0	2,480.1	2,477.5	2,653.8	2,763.5	2,673.7	2,737.9	2,735.6

Source: Chen and Ravallion (2004). Reproduced with permission.

frugal threshold of $1 per day. Even the most optimistic experts have conceded that the "success [in reducing poverty] does not mean victory. The number of poor is still embarrassingly large" (Sala-i-Martin 2002b, p. 30).

In summary, both sides of the globalization debate have a point. The world witnessed a sharp decline in extreme poverty (the <$1 per day threshold) during

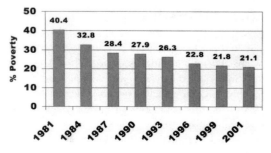

FIGURE 7.1. The Good News: Global Trends in Percentages of People Living on Less Than $1 per Day (1993 purchasing power parity). *Source:* Chen and Ravallion (2004). Reproduced with permission.

the most recent era of globalization. A large share of that decline was attributable to just two countries, China and India, which together account for 38% of world population and 60% of world's poor. On the other hand, half of the developing world still subsists on less than $2 per day and remains vulnerable to economic slowdowns. Moreover, the composition of poverty has changed dramatically. The number of poor people in sub-Saharan Africa has doubled during the past two decades. Although the region accounted for one in ten of the developing world's poor in 1981, it accounted for one in three of the poor by 2001. Thus, poverty in Africa remains worse than anywhere else in the world. As citizens in some parts of the world have risen above extreme poverty, many others have been left behind. This is also true for the transition economies of Europe and central Asia, which experienced sharp drops in income per capita in the 1990s (World Bank 2004).

As we have already intimated, globalization per se cannot be necessarily blamed (or credited) with worldwide trends in poverty. It is a fallacy to assume that just because globalization has increased while some social

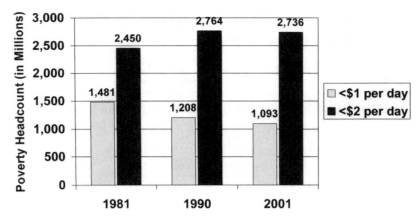

FIGURE 7.2. The Bad News: Long-Term Trends in the World's Poor. *Source:* Chen and Ravallion (2004). Reproduced with permission.

ill has worsened, the former must have caused the latter. As Bhagwati (2004) caustically noted:

> [The globalization debate] has gotten to an almost farcical level where if your girlfriend walks out on you, it must be due to globalization—after all, she may have left for Buenos Aires. These critics need to be asked, with a nod to Tina Turner's famous song "What's Love Got to Do with It?": what's globalization got to do with it? (Bhagwati 2004, p. 30)

Although attributing trends in poverty to globalization is a far more complex task than describing patterns and trends during the past twenty years, what is clear is that the eradication of poverty (as expressed in the first Millennium Development Goal) will require global action, particularly in the form of increased commit-

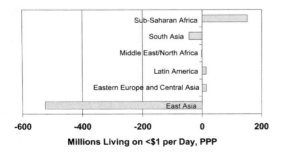

FIGURE 7.3. The Ugly News: Changes in World Poverty, 1981–2001. *Source:* Chen and Ravallion (2004). Reproduced with permission.

ments to official development assistance (ODA) and debt relief (Sachs 2005). We return to this point

HAS INEQUALITY INCREASED OR DECREASED?

A second yardstick for judging progress during the recent era of globalization is to turn to trends in income inequality. The relevance of income inequality for population health is that, all other things equal, a country or region with greater inequality in the distribution of incomes will have worse average health status than a country or region with a more egalitarian distribution of incomes (Kawachi and Kennedy 2002; Deaton 2003). The logic behind this prediction derives from the well-established concave relationship between individual income and achieved health status; that is, the curve is steeper at low levels of income and flattens out at higher levels of income. This is observed between individuals as well as between nations. A corollary of the concave relationship between income and health is that the more unequal the distribution of incomes (i.e., the more poor people there are in society), the lower the average health of that society relative to its per capita income.[2]

Inconveniently, empirical tests of the link between income inequality and aggregate health status have not yielded consistent or robust findings in cross-national studies across *rich* countries. However, as Angus Deaton (2003) noted in a recent survey of this field prepared for the World Health Organization

TABLE 7.2. Comparison of the Three Concepts of Inequality

	Unweighted International Inequality	Weighted International Inequality	"True" World Inequality
Main source of data	National accounts	National accounts	Household surveys
Unit of observation	Country	Country (weighted by its population)	Individual
Welfare concept	GDP or GNP per capita	GDP or GNP per capita	Mean per capita disposable income or expenditures
Within-country income distribution	Ignored	Ignored	Included

Source: Milanovic (2005). Reproduced with permission.

(WHO) Commission on Macroeconomics and Health, the relationship between income inequality and worse health is better supported among *developing* countries, particularly for indicators such as infant mortality.

What, then, does the evidence tell us about worldwide trends in income inequality during the recent era of globalization? The answer, as in the case of poverty, depends upon how inequality is conceptualized and measured.

There are three distinct ways of conceptualizing global inequality (Milanovic 2005). The first concept is cross-national inequality in their average national incomes. This concept takes each *country* as the unit of observation and compares average incomes (or gross domestic product [GDP]) per capita, ignoring population size. The second concept of inequality weights the comparison of income across nations according to their population size but ignores within-country distributions of incomes (i.e., the concept assumes that within each country there is a perfectly equal distribution of incomes). In other words, all Chinese are assigned the same level of income, and all Americans are assigned a higher (but equal) level of income based on national accounts data, and so on. Finally, the third concept of inequality attempts to calculate a "true" world distribution of income across *individuals* (compared to countries), based upon disposable income or expenditure data from country-specific household surveys. Under this concept, all the world's citizens are ranked from the poorest to the richest, and the distribution takes account of the number of poor Chinese as well as wealthy Chinese (as well as poor Americans and rich Americans). Table 7.2 (from Milanovic 2005) summarizes the distinctions between these three concepts.

According to Milanovic (2005), the first concept (unweighted cross-national inequality) answers whether nations are converging in terms of their average standard of living. The third concept ("true" world distribution of income) answers the question how *individuals* are doing in comparison with citizens in the rest of the world. The second concept (weighted cross-national inequality) is a halfway stage between the first and last concepts and is perhaps the least interesting concept. It deals with neither nations nor individuals but something in between (Milanovic 2005). So how do they compare?

Based on the first method of measurement (unweighted comparisons of average incomes across nations), inequality has been rising in the world for nearly two centuries. For example, according to the United Nations Development Programme (1999), which used this approach in its *Human Development Report 1999*, the 20% of the world's people in the richest countries in 1970 had twenty-three times the income of people in the poorest 20% of the world. By 1997, the richest 20% had seventy-four times the income of the poorest 20%. However, the United Nations figures have been faulted for exaggerating the between-country differences in incomes. According to critics, the United Nations comparison of national incomes is based upon conversion to a common currency (US$), using market exchange rates. The use of market exchange rates ignores the cheaper cost of living in poor countries, and critics contend that the spread of national average incomes is actually much less using purchasing power parity (PPP)–adjusted incomes (Sala-i-Martin 2002a). Nonetheless, the overall claim that inequality in national incomes has been rising is still supported by cross-country variance in PPP-adjusted incomes per capita. Over the past thirty years, rich countries have grown richer while the poorest countries have either stayed poor or slid backward (especially in sub-Saharan Africa) in terms of their per capita incomes. This pattern conforms to what the Harvard economist Lant Pritchett (1997) famously described as "divergence, big time." Others, such as Quah (1996), have suggested that the world distribution of income is characterized by a pattern of "emerging twin peaks," which refers to the observation that the world distribution of incomes in the 1960s and 1970s was unimodal but, over time, became progressively bimodal or "twin peaked," with the high-income club of countries that are members of the Organization for Economic Cooperation and Development (OECD) converging toward one peak, and the lower income countries settling toward a lower income level.

Does this mean that the world has become more unequal? Not according to dissenters, who maintain that it is misleading and inappropriate to judge global welfare by treating countries as the unit of observation without taking account of population size. This leads to the second approach to calculating inequality (cross-national comparisons of income weighted by population size), the motivation for which was forcefully stated by Sala-i-Martin (2002b):

[Estimating the extent of global inequality using each country as one data point] is sensible if one wants to analyze the success of individual country policies or institutions, and if we think of each country as performing an independent "policy experiment." However, it is not a good assumption if one wants to discuss global welfare: treating countries like China and Grenada as two data points with equal weights does not seem reasonable because there are about 12,000 Chinese citizens for each person living in Grenada. In other words, if income per capita in Grenada grows by 300% over a period of 20 years, the world distribution of individual income does not change by much because there aren't many Grenadians in the world. However, if income per capita in China grows at the same rate, then the incomes of one fifth of the world' citizens increase substantially and this has a great impact on global human welfare. (p. 1)

Following this logic, if one now weights each country's PPP-adjusted per capita GDP by its population size, a dramatic reversal is reached: international inequality actually *declined* during the past twenty years!

(Schultz 1998; Firebaugh 1999; Bourguignon and Morrison 2002). So which is true—is international inequality rising or falling? As lucidly explained by Milanovic (2005), the major contributors to the population-weighted decline in international inequality are China and India, two countries that achieved impressive increases in their *average* national incomes during the past twenty years. Since these two countries represent nearly 40% of the world's population, they have a correspondingly large impact on population-weighted estimates of cross-national comparisons. As Milanovic (2005) demonstrates, removing these two countries from the analysis results in a pattern of rising international inequality during the past two decades. Before we cry foul at this sleight of hand, however, it is important to point out the major (and possibly fatal) flaw in the population-weighted concept of inequality, namely, that it ignores within-country distributions of income (table 7.2). Notwithstanding their spectacular achievements in poverty reduction, both China and India have experienced steep increases in income inequality. This brings us to the final concept of inequality, the "true" world distribution of incomes.

The third way of measuring inequality is based upon estimating the distribution of incomes between persons rather than between countries. This method might be characterized as the "one person, one vote" approach, or what Prakash Loungani (2003, p. 22) humorously dubbed the "John Lennon definition of inequality because we're being asked to imagine that there are no countries."

Using the person-based measure of inequality has yielded conflicting accounts about what has been happening in the last twenty years (Bhalla 2002; Sala-i-Martin 2002b; Milanovic 2005). One of the more widely cited studies using this approach estimated the global distribution of income using yearly PPP-adjusted GDP per capita for 125 countries between 1970 and 1998 (Sala-i-Martin 2002b). Contrary to the "emerging twin peaks" described by Quah (1996), Sala-i-Martin (2002b) found a pattern of "vanishing twin peaks" in world incomes during the last two decades, with the emergence instead of a "world middle class." Instead of a pattern of "divergence, big time" described by Pritchett (1997), there has been "convergence, period" according to Sala-i-Martin's (2002b) estimates (*The Economist* 2002). Even in Sala-i-Martin's estimates, however, the long-term future of global inequality does not look cheery. If the worldwide growth rates 1980–1998 persist, global inequality will continue to decline until about 2015, after which it will again rise sharply, *unless growth in the African region starts to speed up* (Sala-i-Martin 2002b).

More significantly, however, Sala-i-Martin's methods have been sharply disputed by Milanovic (2005). The technical details need not detain us here, but the criticism boils down to absence of data. According to Milanovic (2005), Sala-i-Martin's estimates are an artifact of (a) the omission of countries with sharp increases in inequality post-1980 (e.g., Russia, Ukraine, Bulgaria); (b) extrapolation of within-country income distributions backward and forward in time (where data are missing 84% of the time), and assuming a constant distribution of income over a thirty-year period; and (c) assuming that everyone has the same income in cases where there are no data. When the "true" distribution of world income is calculated using reliable data (as Milanovic has done for the years 1988, 1993, and 1998), the trends indicate either no change over time, or even a slight rise in inequality during the ten-year period (Milanovic 2005).

To recapitulate, worldwide trends during the past twenty years suggest an increase in inequality using the benchmark of differences in average *national* incomes. On the other hand, if inequality is calculated among all of the world's people, we are left with a dispute between experts who claim that inequality has been falling (Sala-i-Martin 2002b) and others who question those results (Milanovic 2005). We may not know the true answer to the question about inequality among the world's people until better data are collected by each country, especially poor countries.

In the meantime, as Ravallion (2004) noted, "both sides of the globalization debate often use the term 'inequality' as though we all agree on exactly what that means. But we almost certainly don't agree" (p. 21). The factual claims made about global trends in inequality depend crucially on the conceptual position adopted by the observer to analyze "inequality." Sala-i-Martin (2002b) argues that ignoring the population sizes of countries leads to misguided judgments about global welfare. On the other hand, others like Milanovic (2003) have argued equally persuasively that (a) policies are typically implemented at the country level, (b) countries have borders and people do not move freely across them, and (c) countries are therefore relevant for making judgments about trends in inequality. In other words, it is cold comfort for a citizen of Lesotho living in direst poverty to be told that global inequality is falling because 400 million Chinese peasants escaped poverty during the last twenty years. Regardless of one's position on the measurement of inequality, perhaps the most important point to bear in mind is that "most readers of the popular press and the web sites reporting on this topic do not see the embedded value judgments in the facts presented to them" (Ravallion 2004, p. 22).

TRENDS IN WITHIN-COUNTRY INEQUALITY

So far, we have dwelt on the conundrums of estimating global inequality. However, a different approach to describing inequality over time is to examine the distribution of incomes among rich and poor people within individual countries. This is accomplished by standard summary measures of income distribution, such as the GINI coefficient, which is defined as half of the arithmetic average of the absolute differences between all pairs of incomes within a distribution, normalized on mean income. The GINI has a range from 0.0 (perfect equality) to 1.0 (perfect inequality). Using this measure, Cornia and Kiiski (2001) analyzed domestic trends in income inequality for seventy-three countries from the 1950s to the 1990s. They found that income inequality rose in forty-eight (59%) of the seventy-three countries analyzed. Only in nine (5%) of countries was there evidence of a decline in income concentration over time, while no trend was found for the remaining sixteen (36%) countries. The forty-eight countries that experienced an increase in inequality represented 47% of the world's population (Cornia and Kiiski 2001).

Looking to individual countries, there has been a marked surge in inequalities in wealthy countries such as the United States, the United Kingdom, Australia, and New Zealand that started in the 1980s and continues to the present time. Inequalities also increased in some poor countries, such as China and India (notwithstanding their achievements in poverty reduction), as well as many parts of Latin America (e.g., Brazil, Chile, Peru, and Venezuela). By contrast, inequalities do not seem to have increased markedly in Japan or Western European countries during the same period, most likely due to their labor market regulations, social welfare programs, and tax systems (Fischer 2003). Finally, in the former Soviet bloc, inequalities increased markedly following the transition to a market economy beginning in the 1990s (Fischer 2003).

All in all, within-country inequality seems to have been rising in many parts of the world. Even that conclusion, however, has been contested by some researchers (see, e.g., Dollar 2004). An important reason for the continuing disputes in this area relates to the issue of data quality. Outside of the wealthiest countries (covered by data sets such as the Luxembourg Income Study), reliable income inequality data are notoriously scarce. A widely used data set is the Deininger-Squire series maintained by the World Bank (Deininger and Squire 1996). These data contain GINI coefficients for more than 100 developing and developed countries spanning the period 1947–1994. Unfortunately, even in this data set, measurements are sparse for major regions of the world, including Africa, Latin America, and Asia. According to Galbraith (2002):

> A simple effort to compare changes from the 1980s to the 1990s—the decades for which the [World] Bank reports the *most* observations—shows no data for most of Africa, West Asia, and Latin America. And where observations exist, they are questionable: inequality falls for about half the countries in this exercise, in a decade marked by wide protests against rising inequality! (p. 15)

In an attempt to get around the scarcity of data on income inequality, some researchers have turned to the narrower concept of *wage* inequality (where wages are a subset of income). (Galbraith 2002; Freeman, Oostendorp, and Rama 2001) Where this has been done, the results indicate an unequivocal increase in inequality during the last two decades, which moreover cuts across both rich countries and poor countries (Galbraith 2002; Dollar 2004).[3]

IS GLOBALIZATION GOOD FOR POVERTY AND INEQUALITY?

As we have shown, judging recent trends in poverty and inequality is hardly a value-free exercise, and the pattern across the world does not provide unambiguous support for either the proglobalizer's or the antiglobalizer's position. A key issue is whether globalization per se is good or bad for poverty and inequality. The problem (as mentioned in chapter 1) is that there are many (loose) definitions of globalization in

the literature, and hence the question must be narrowed down to a testable hypothesis. In this section, we turn to the recent debate about whether openness to trade (which is a key aspect of *economic* globalization) can be linked to poverty and inequality.

One of the most widely cited studies on this question is the analysis by David Dollar and Aart Kraay (2004) of the World Bank. Originally circulated in draft form in October 2000, this paper seems to have become a lightning rod for people on both sides of the globalization debate. By September 2004, simply typing in the title of their paper, "Trade, Growth, and Poverty" on Google yielded more than 75,000 hits. In that study, the researchers identified a small group of developing countries ($n = 24$) that, in their judgment, had significantly opened up to foreign trade in the past twenty years. This group of "post-1980 globalizers" was selected on two criteria: (a) belonging to the top one-third of developing countries in terms of their growth in trade as a share of GDP between 1975–1979 and 1995–1997, and (b) belonging to the top one-third of developing countries based in reductions in the average tariff rate between 1985–1989 and 1995–1997. The list of countries defined by these criteria were not identical, though several populous countries made it on both lists, including China, India, Bangladesh, Thailand, Brazil, and Argentina. Dollar and Kraay then proceeded to compare the record of economic growth, poverty, and inequality among these globalizers to the remaining two-thirds of poor countries (the "nonglobalizers") in their sample ($n = 48$).[4]

Based on purely descriptive trends, the group of post-1980 globalizers appeared to have achieved a steady acceleration in their economic growth rate, measured by real per capita GDP growth, which rose from 1.4% per year in the 1960s, to 2.9% in the 1970s, 3.5% in the 1980s, and 5.0% in the 1990s. This rate of growth outperformed the rich countries of the world, which actually saw steady declines in growth from a high of 4.7% in the 1960s to 2.2% by the 1990s. The worst performance was recorded among the nonglobalizing poor countries, where growth rates fell from a high of 3.3% per year during the 1970s to only 1.4% by the 1990s (Dollar and Kraay 2004).

Turning to the relationships between trade openness and poverty and inequality, Dollar and Kraay went on to make two additional observations. First, when changes in trade openness (measured by the average annual change in the trade:GDP ratio) was plotted against average annual change in the GINI coefficient, they found no systematic relationship between the two variables (correlation coefficient, 0.036) within their data set spanning more than 100 developed and developing countries. Dollar and Kraay acknowledged that several individual countries among the "globalizers" have, in fact, experienced an increase in inequality, such as China (where the GINI rose from 32 in the early 1980s to 40 by the mid-1990s). However, they attributed these shifts in income distribution to factors far removed from openness to international trade, such as domestic liberalization, restrictions on internal migration (in the case of China), and agricultural policies.

The second key finding of Dollar and Kraay is that the combination of increases in growth and little systematic change in inequality among the globalizers lifted millions out of poverty. In particular, they made their now famous contention that the incomes of the poor (those in the bottom quintile of the income distribution) on average rose "one-for-one" with average incomes. In other words, the poor benefited "proportionately" from rising national incomes brought about by trade openness. This is a particularly striking claim, given the widespread perception that trade has distributional consequences—that is, there are winners and losers, at least in the short term. But according to Dollar and Kraay, there is no tendency for the losses to be concentrated among the poor.

Taken together, the claims made by Dollar and Kraay amount to a ringing endorsement of one of the chief forces behind globalization: the greater economic integration of the world through trade openness. Their findings have since been repeated by popular accounts defending globalization (Norberg 2003; Wolf 2004). The mantra runs as follows: liberalizing trade accelerates growth, thereby diminishing the income gap between rich and poor countries (while leaving unchanged within-country inequality) and, at the same time, helps poor countries to lift millions out of poverty. In their words, "the real losers from globalization are those developing countries that have not been able to seize the opportunities to participate in the process" (Dollar and Kraay 2001, p. 6).

Have Dollar and Kraay got it right? At the very outset of their widely cited study, Dollar and Kraay confidently assert that "openness to international trade accelerates development: this is one of the most widely held beliefs in the economics professions, one of the few things on which Nobel prize winners of

both the left and right agree" (Dollar and Kraay 2004, p. F22). However, beyond this generalization, many disagreements and uncertainties remain concerning the optimal combination of liberalizing policies that promote growth. Trade liberalization policies differ in their speed, the level of openness achieved at the end, and the pattern of protections that are retained (Nye, Reddy, and Watkins 2002). Indeed, skepticism has been expressed about even the ability of cross-national comparisons to reveal a causal connection between trade liberalization and economic growth (Rodriguez and Rodrik 2000). Nor has Dollar and Kraay's study and conclusions escaped critical scrutiny, and we proceed now to summarize the major points of contention that have followed in the wake of their seminal analysis. These criticisms can be grouped under the categories of concern about reverse causation, inappropriate measurement, omitted variable bias, and the existence of competing notions of inequality that might affect our judgment about how trade affects welfare.

Reverse Causation

The first category of concern is about the difficulty of establishing a correct causal sequence between trade openness and growth. It is widely accepted that the relationship between these two variables can be bidirectional; that is, trade openness may promote growth, but equally plausibly, growth in incomes can stimulate trade. For example, as national incomes rise, so does import demand. Rising incomes also stimulate demand for domestic products, enabling firms to capitalize on economies of scale to boost export capacity (Nye, Reddy, and Watkins 2002).

In their analysis, Dollar and Kraay attempted to address the problem of reverse causality by using an econometric technique for which the results are less likely to reflect bias from this source. Using this approach, they still found a statistically significant effect of trade on growth: an increase in trade as a share of GDP of twenty percentage points increased growth by between 0.5 and 1 percentage point each year. Nevertheless, critics maintain that a closer examination of individual (and influential) countries in their group of "globalizers" tells a different story. For example, Rodrik (2000) points out that in both India and China, the main trade reforms took place about a decade *after* the onset of higher growth. In China, growth was jump-started in the late 1970s with *domestic* reforms, notably the "household responsibility" system of production. Trade liberalization was introduced only in the second half of the 1980s and focused at first on *export* liberalization. Import liberalization was gradually introduced in the 1990s, only after growth had already taken off (Rodrik 2000).

In India, growth rates accelerated in the early 1980s, but serious trade reform did not begin in earnest until 1991–1993. Moreover, both India and China continue to maintain some of the highest trade protections in the world; that is, they had higher tariffs and nontariff barriers to trade at the end of the 1990s than did many other countries with open trade regimes.

The contentious nature of the relationship between trade and growth is underscored by Cornia's (2001) assessment that countries such as China achieved their high growth, dramatic improvements in health status, and integration into the world economy "through a mixture of outward orientation and unorthodox policies such as high levels of tariff and non-tariff barriers, public ownership of large segments of banking, patent and copyright infringements and restrictions on foreign capital flows" and that "by following a highly unorthodox two-track economic policy, (they) violated practically every prescription of the orthodox model" (Cornia 2001, p. 839).

Inappropriate Measurement

The second cogent criticism of Dollar and Kraay focuses on their choice of variables to measure "trade openness." As pointed out by Rodrik (2000), what we are really interested in identifying is the causal effect of trade *policy* on growth, poverty, and inequality. Unfortunately, "trade volume as a percentage of GDP" is not the same as trade policy. The problem is that trade volume is an endogenous variable; that is, it is influenced by several other variables, such as the size of the country, geography (proximity to routes of transport), and the quality of domestic institutions, that have little to do with the policy decisions of nations to open their borders to trade. Worse, if these other variables (e.g., geography) simultaneously determine growth (as some studies suggest; see Sachs 2001), then we have an omitted variable bias (see below). In some instances, temporal *changes* in trade volume may be simply an artifact of the cessation of domestic turmoil or conflict (e.g., seems to be the case for such countries as Rwanda and Haiti, which

ended up in the group of Dollar and Kraay's "post-1980 globalizers").[5]

Omitted Variable Bias

The third problem identified by critics of Dollar and Kraay is that of omitted variable bias. Dollar and Kraay (2004) acknowledged that many countries that liberated trade often simultaneously embarked on other domestic reforms, such as investments in domestic infrastructure (e.g., improved transportation routes, marketing). To the extent that these "third variables" also stimulate trade and growth, their omission in cross-country regression studies can lead to a spurious correlation between trade and growth. Dollar and Kraay attempted to address this issue by using decade-over-decade changes in countries' trade volumes (which, they argued, removes the spurious influence of geography on trade and growth), as well as including measures of the stability of monetary policy, financial development, and political instability in their regression models. Critics of Dollar and Kraay contend, however, that even these technical fixes may not have overcome omitted variable bias.[6]

Competing Concepts of Inequality

The fourth and final critique of Dollar and Kraay focuses on their claim that growth is not systematically associated with rising levels of inequality. However, as Ravallion (2004) points out, this claim rests on a specific concept of "inequality" that not everyone may subscribe to. Specifically, Dollar and Kraay are referring to the effects of trade and growth on "relative inequality," which depends on the ratios of individual incomes to the mean. In other words, if all incomes rise by the same proportion, then relative inequality remains unchanged.[7] However, many people prefer to think about inequality in *absolute* terms, which depends on the absolute differences in levels of living. In the simple example that Ravallion (2004) provides, consider an economy with just two households with incomes $1,000 and $10,000. If both incomes double, then relative inequality (e.g., as measured by the GINI) will remain the same. On the other hand, the absolute difference in their incomes has doubled, from $9,000 to $18,000. Ravallion (2004) goes on to add:

These value judgments about what inequality means have considerable bearing on the position one takes in the globalization debate. Finding that the share of income going to the poor does not change on average with growth does not mean that "growth raises the incomes (of the poor) by about as much as it raises the incomes of everybody else" (*The Economist*, May 27, 2000, p. 24). Given existing inequality, the income gains to the rich from distribution-neutral growth will of course be greater than the gains to the poor. In the above example of two households, the income gain from growth is 10 times greater for the high-income household. To say that this means that the poor "share fully" in the gains from growth is clearly a stretch. And the example is not far fetched. For the richest decile in India, the income gain from distribution-neutral growth will be about four times higher than the gain to the poorest quintile; it will be 15–20 times higher in Brazil or South Africa. (Ravallion 2004, p. 6)

In summary, the available evidence on the effects of trade on growth, poverty, and inequality is mixed. The evidence does not provide strong vindication for the proglobalizers' view that open trade policies have been the primary determinants of growth and poverty reduction in developing nations. On the other hand, nor does the evidence support the antiglobalizers' contention that trade liberalization is primarily responsible for growing inequalities between and within countries. While autarchy is not a desirable option for developing countries (in the sense that no country has yet developed successfully by turning its back on international trade), neither is unchecked openness to trade. There is no one-size-fits-all prescription for how countries ought to go about integrating into the global economy (Cornia 2001).

A sustainable solution to the problems of persistent poverty and inequalities requires a broader set of prescriptions than opening a country's borders to trade or reforming the international trade regime. The solutions must also involve effective reforms of *domestic* policies such as social protections for the unemployed and food insecure, as well as improving access to health care and education.

THE FUTURE OF POVERTY AND INEQUALITY IN THE WORLD

As we have tried to show, the role of globalization in inequality and poverty reduction remains hotly contested. There are fundamental disagreements about even the descriptive pattern of worldwide trends in poverty and inequality during the last twenty years. Do we inhabit a world in which all is for the best in the best of all possible worlds, or is the world going to hell in a hand basket? While the truth lies in neither of these extremes, fundamental differences in value judgments (e.g., concerning the conceptualization of inequality) added to the limitations of existing data suggest that the globalization debate is unlikely to die down any time soon.

In this concluding section, we turn to highlight two issues bearing on the future of global poverty and inequality. The first relates to the need for broadening the concept of poverty. The second relates to the opportunities for reducing global poverty and inequality through collective global action.

Throughout this chapter we have used the income concept of poverty. Following the practice of most international poverty researchers, we have defined poverty as the lack of income (or of consumption). However, this is clearly not the only definition of poverty that people subscribe to. Just as money does not describe the sum total of human lives, so, too, poverty cannot simply refer to the lack of income (United Nations Development Programme 1996). Amartya Sen pioneered the conceptualization of poverty as a "capability failure," by which he means the absence of capabilities needed to achieve minimal functioning within a given society (Sen 1999). Such capabilities include not only sufficient income to purchase food, clothing, and shelter but also basic education, the rights to political participation, the respect of others, and even good health status. To wit, though we earlier described income poverty as one of the *inputs* to health, the capability approach treats the lack of good health as part of the *definition* of poverty. When the concept of poverty is broadened in this way, it becomes clear that the world's poor are doubly disadvantaged, not only because of lower income, but also because of their limited health achievement.

According to WHO, about 56 million deaths occurred worldwide in 2000, of which 10.9 million (20%) were deaths among children younger than five years of age (WHO 2001). Of these 10.9 million deaths, 99.3% occurred in developing countries. Developing countries also share a disproportionate burden of premature deaths at young adult ages (fifteen to fifty-nine years of age). Just over 30% of all deaths in developing countries occur at these ages, compared with 15% in richer countries. By contrast, 70% of deaths in developed countries occur beyond seventy years of age (Bonita and Mathers 2003).

While global life expectancy has continued to rise over time, the improvement in *average* life expectancy hides the widening gaps between and within countries. Specifically, life expectancy at birth currently ranges from 81.4 years for women in the established market economies of Western Europe, North America, Japan, Australia, and New Zealand, down to 48.1 years for men in sub-Saharan Africa (Bonita and Mathers 2003). While mortality rates have declined markedly for specific causes of death (e.g., coronary heart disease) in wealthy countries, other regions of the world have witnessed equally spectacular reversals in life expectancy. For example, between 1991 and 1994, life expectancy at birth in the former Soviet republics fell by four years for males and by 2.3 years for females (McKee 2001). Life expectancy for Russian men improved slightly between 1994 and 1998 but declined significantly again in the next three years (Bonita and Mathers 2003). Worldwide, about 37 million people are currently living with HIV/AIDS, of whom 95% reside in developing countries. The impact of HIV/AIDS has been catastrophic in sub-Saharan Africa, where the United Nations Development Programme (2002) has projected that between 2000 and 2005, the decline in life expectancy due to the disease will amount to thirty-four years in Botswana, twenty-six years in Zimbabwe, nineteen years in South Africa, and seventeen years in Kenya.

While the devastating Boxing Day tsunami disaster in the Indian Ocean is estimated to have killed upward of 300,000 (mostly poor) people, the worldwide media attention it received needs to be placed within the context of the daily toll of deaths caused by extreme poverty, most of which goes unnoticed. As Jeffrey Sachs (2005) asks us to imagine, *every* morning our newspapers could report, "More than 20,000 people died yesterday of extreme poverty— 8,000 children from malaria, 5,000 adult of tuberculosis, and 7,500 young adults of AIDS." Such statistics give added poignancy to the uneven progress of poverty reduction that we described above.

The goal of adopting an expanded conceptualization of poverty is not to combine the different aspects (e.g., income and health status) into a single measure. Rather, to quote Deaton (2004): "If we confine ourselves to income-based measures, we risk missing important features of poverty. For example, a govern-

ment that raises taxes to pay for better public services, or better public health, may *increase* income poverty, while reducing poverty more broadly" (p. 12, emphasis original). In other words, the capability-based approach to poverty reminds us that government policies to combat poverty need to do more than raise the incomes of the poor; they must also enhance the *capabilities* of the poor to function in society by providing them with access to education, health care, and public health programs. As discussed in chapter 14, recent developments in poverty reduction plans (required by the international financial institutions as a condition of receiving loans) have begun to address the multidimensional nature of poverty, although progress remains slow and painfully uneven.

An important lesson from development is that a country does not have to be rich in order to deliver basic education or health to its poorest citizens. Caldwell (1986) and Sen (1999) have pointed to the examples of low-income countries such as Costa Rica, Sri Lanka, the Kerala region of India, and China (before its economic reforms) as having achieved a level of average life expectancy that outperforms far richer countries such as Brazil, South Africa, and Gabon. The former countries delivered a high level of health to their citizens through what Sen (1999) called "support-led policies," including investments in education, health care, and other relevant social arrangements. In short, the health of nations is not exclusively determined by their level of economic development, but equally importantly by factors such as their domestic policies and priorities, patterns of social spending, and equality of income distribution (Kawachi and Kennedy 2002).

That is not to suggest for a moment, however, that poor countries should be left to pull themselves up by their shoestrings. Poverty eradication also requires global collective action because it is a global public good:

> Societies everywhere gain from poverty reduction, especially in a globalizing world, not just because of the moral imperative, but because of the negative externalities associated with poverty—such as conflict and violence, the spread of communicable diseases, illegal immigration, and pressures on the environment. (World Bank 2000, p. 11)

Indeed, the major emerging global threats to public health highlighted throughout the rest of this book[8] have their origins in the persistent poverty and inequality across major regions of the world.

One of the foremost priorities in mobilizing global collective action to combat poverty is to expand debt relief and debt cancellation (see chapter 17). At present, many developing countries expend a crippling proportion of their current exports to repaying loans from rich countries. Without debt forgiveness, it is doubtful that these countries will ever climb out of poverty. Unfortunately, under present arrangements, debt relief is only available to the poorest of the poor countries (Stiglitz 2002). A number of countries with high rates of poverty, such as Indonesia and Argentina, are considered too "well off" to qualify.

ODA, or foreign aid, is an additional avenue for global collective action to combat poverty (Sachs 2005). Here also, the actions by rich countries have fallen woefully short (see chapter 17). Foreign aid by rich countries (as a percentage of their GDP) actually *fell* from 0.33% to 0.22% over the period 1990–2000 (Sachs 2005). Despite the longstanding commitment by rich governments to raise their level of foreign aid to a 0.7% level (as a proportion of their national income), the United States, along with the majority of other rich countries, has a long way to go to meet this target. Current levels of foreign aid provided by the U.S. government amount to a paltry 0.15% of GDP, the lowest of the OECD countries.[9]

The Center for Global Development and *Foreign Policy* magazine annually publish their Commitment to Development Index (Center for Global Development 2004), which ranks twenty-one rich nations on a variety of government actions to help poor countries. Although details of how the index is constructed are debatable (e.g., it rewards governments for taxing their citizens less—on the grounds that this leaves more money in private hands for charity!), the United States nonetheless ranked twentieth out of twenty-one countries in foreign aid in 2004, one place ahead of Japan. Nor does private giving make up the shortfall (despite public perceptions to the contrary) (Center for Global Development 2004).

The extent of inequality in the world now is such that it represents an unprecedented opportunity for redistribution. The United Nations Development Program (1999) pointed out that the assets of the three richest individuals in the world amount to more than the combined gross national product (GNP) of the poorest thirty-five countries of the world, while the assets of the 200 richest people (who are annually named by *Forbes* magazine) amount to more than the combined incomes of 41% of the world's poorest people. It has been estimated that an annual contribution of just 1% of the wealth of the richest 200 people could provide universal access to primary education for all the world's children (which would cost about $7–8 billion).

A striking illustration of global inequality (and the opportunities for redistribution) was highlighted during the summer of 2003, when U.S. President George W. Bush visited Africa to pledge more foreign aid and increased funding for AIDS treatment. Coinciding with his visit, the economist Jeffrey Sachs wrote an editorial to the *New York Times* pointing out that the top 400 Americans earned an average income of $174 million *each* in 2000. Their combined income of $69 billion amounted to more than the combined incomes of the 166 million people living in four of the countries that the President Bush visited in sub-Saharan Africa during July 2003—Nigeria, Senegal, Uganda, and Botswana. The combined incomes of the 400 richest Americans is also more than 2.5 times the $27 billion that the WHO Commission on Macroeconomics and Health estimates will be needed to support a global fund to prevent 8 million deaths from AIDS, tuberculosis, and malaria in poor countries (WHO 2001). Given the size of the economy, the U.S. share of that $75 billion fund should be about $8 billion. But in reality, even with the U.S. President's Emergency Plan for AIDS Relief, the country was projected to give only about $1 billion in 2004 (Sachs 2003).

To put these numbers into perspective, the taxes paid by the top 400 income earners in America was slashed from 30% in 1995 down to less than 18% in 2003 as a result of the successive tax cuts introduced by President Bush. If the top 400 individuals donated their tax savings to the world's poor instead of pocketing their windfall, their gift would amount to $7 billion—or 88% of contribution toward the global fund needed from the United States (Sachs 2005).[10]

The level of ODA required for meeting the United Nations Millennium Development Goals (see chapter 14) is even more ambitious than the target set by the WHO Commission on Macroeconomic and Health. According to the United Nations Millennium Development Project, the price tag for scaling up basic needs to meet the Millennium Development

Goals for all developing countries will be $135 billion in 2006, rising to $195 billion by 2015 (in 2003 US$). While this may seem like a lot of money, in fact it amounts to between 0.44% and 0.54% of rich-world GNP each year during the coming decade; that is, the Millennium Development Goals can be financed *within* the bounds of ODA targets (0.7% GNP) that rich countries have *already* promised (Sachs 2005).

The future of poverty, inequality and human development across the planet will thus depend upon the effectiveness of global collective action, as well as the ability of international and domestic institutions to deliver the supposed benefits of globalization to the millions who have so far been left behind.

Notes

1. An important difference in the estimates occurs depending on whether the analysts have relied on national accounts data (i.e., macro-level data such as gross national product), or on estimates from nationally representative household surveys. For technical discussion and debate on these issues, see Deaton (2004).

2. Some researchers (including us) have advanced an additional hypothesis, namely, that the degree of income inequality in society per se is detrimental to population health (see Wilkinson 1996; Kawachi, Kennedy, and Wilkinson 1999; Kawachi and Kennedy 2002; Subramanian and Kawachi 2004), although the empirical findings on this hypothesis have been contested (see Deaton 2003). However, even if income inequality has no direct effect on health, the nonlinear relationship of individual income to health implies that redistribution toward the poor will improve average health (because their gains will more than offset any loss of health among the rich).

3. Although Dollar (2004) argues that because wage earners are typically a small fraction of the population in most poor countries, there is not a necessary relationship between higher wage inequality and higher *income* inequality in the developing world. Among rich countries, where most people are wage earners, higher age inequality is likely to translate into higher income inequality.

4. The authors set aside the members of the rich club of twenty-four OECD countries, as well as countries that they deemed "early" (i.e., pre-1980) globalizers—Hong Kong, Singapore, South Korea, Taiwan, and Chile.

5. Rodrik (2000) has also pointed out that the choice of a different base year for defining "globalizers" results in murkier conclusions about growth. For example, he notes that Dollar and Kraay (2004) used different base years to define globalizers based on trade volume (1975–1979 to 1995–1997) and tariff cuts (1985–1989 to 1995–1997). When he defines globalizers based upon a consistent set of years (1980–1984 and 1995–1997), Ro-

drik obtains a different set of countries, as well as a suggestion of a slowdown in growth in the 1980s and 1990s compared to the 1960s and 1970s.

6. For example, Dollar and Kraay (2004) suggest that their focus on the relationship between changes in trade volumes and changes in growth rates allows them to control for the effect of fixed factors such as geography and the quality of domestic institutions that affect trade volumes. However, as Nye, Reddy, and Watkins (2002) have pointed out, the effect of omitted country-specific factors that *do* change over time (and that influence both growth and trade) will still be misattributed to trade by this procedure.

7. This is tied to the axiom of "scale invariance" in inequality measurement (Sen 1997), whereby measures of inequality, such as the GINI, do not increase simply because everyone's incomes increase by the same amount.

8. See chapter 2 on communicable diseases, chapter 5 on global climate change, chapter 9 on population displacement, and chapter 18 on military spending.

9. By contrast, Scandinavian countries rank among the most generous givers (Norway, 0.92% of gross national income; Denmark, 0.84%; Sweden, 0.70%). The United States was not always so stingy. During the days of the Marshall Plan, the country spent 1–2% of GDP on aid.

10. Some private individuals have, in fact, turned to philanthropy on a global scale. For example, when Microsoft Corporation paid out a one-time cash dividend to its shareholders in the summer of 2004, Microsoft's chairman, William H. Gates III, personally stood to gain $3.35 *billion*. He announced that he would donate his windfall to charitable causes.

References

Bhagwati J (2004). *In Defense of Globalization*. New York: Oxford University Press.

Bhalla S (2002). *Imagine There's No Country: Poverty, Inequality, and Growth in the Era of Globalization*. Washington, DC: Institute for International Economics.

Bonita R, and Mathers CD (2003). Global health status at the beginning of the twenty-first century. In: R Beaglehole and R Bonita (eds.). *Global Public Health: A New Era*. Oxford: Oxford University Press, pp. 24–53.

Bourguignon F, and Morrisson C (2002). Inequality among world citizens: 1820–1992. Am Econ Rev 92(4):727–744.

Caldwell, JC (1986). Routes to low mortality in poor countries. Pop Dev Rev 12(2):171–220.

Center for Global Development. (2004). Ranking the rich: the 2004 CGD/FP Commitment to Development Index. Foreign Policy, May. http://www.cgdev.org/rankingtherich/home.html.

Chen S, and Ravallion M (2004). How Have the World's Poorest Fared since the Early 1980s? Washington,

DC: World Bank Research for Poverty, Development Research Group. http://www.worldbank.org/research/povmonitor/MartinPapers/How have the poorest fared since the early 1980s.pdf.

Cornia GA (2001). Globalization and health: results and options. Bull World Health Org 79:834–841.

Cornia, GA, and Kiiski S (2001). Trends in Income Distribution in the Post World War II Period: Evidence and Interpretation. Paper No. 2001/89. Helsinki, Finland: United Nations University/World Institute for Development Economics Research Discussion. http://www.wider.unu.edu.

Deaton A (2003). Health, inequality, and economic development. J Econ Lit 41:113–158.

Deaton A (2004). Measuring Poverty. Princeton, NJ: Princeton University Research Program in Development Studies. www.wws.princeton.edu/Erpds/downloads/deaton_povertymeasured.pdf.

Deininger K, and Squire L (1996). A new data set measuring income inequality. World Bank Econ Rev 10:565–591.

Dollar D (2004). Globalization, Poverty, and Inequality since 1980. Policy Research Working Paper 3333. Washington, DC: World Bank.

Dollar D, and Kraay A (2001). Trade, growth, and poverty. Finance Dev 38(3):1–6.

Dollar D, and Kraay A (2004). Trade, growth, and poverty. Econ J 114(493):F22–F49.

The Economist (2002). Convergence, Period. July 18. http://www.columbia.edu/~xs23/papers/worldistribution/Economist.htm.

Firebaugh G (1999). Empirics of world income inequality. Am J Sociol 104:1597–1630.

Fischer S (2003). Globalization and its challenges. Richard T. Ely lecture. Am Econ Rev 93(2):1–30.

Freeman R, Oostendorp R, and Rama M (2001). Globalization and Wages. Mimeo. Washington, DC: World Bank.

Galbraith JK (2002). A perfect crime: inequality in the age of globalization. Daedalus, Winter, 11–25.

Kawachi I, and Kennedy BP (2002). The Health of Nations. Why Inequality Is Harmful to Your Health. New York: New Press.

Kawachi I, Kennedy BP, and Wilkinson RG (1999). The Society and Population Health Reader. Vol. 1. Income Inequality and Health. New York: New Press.

Loungani P (2003). Inequality: now you see it, now you don't. Finance Dev, Summer, 22–23.

McKee M (2001). The health consequences of the collapse of the Soviet Union. In: D Leon and G Walt (eds.). Poverty, Inequality and Health. An International Perspective. Oxford: Oxford University Press, pp. 17–36.

Milanovic B (2003). The two faces of globalization: against globalization as we know it. World Dev 31(4):667–683.

Milanovic B (2005). Worlds Apart. Measuring International and Global Inequality. Princeton, NJ: Princeton University Press.

Norberg J (2003). In Defense of Global Capitalism. Washington, DC: Cato Institute.

Nye HLM, Reddy SG, and Watkins K (2002). Dollar and Kraay on "Trade, Growth, and Poverty": A critique. New York: Columbia University. http://www.newschool.edu/cepa/papers/workshop/reddy_030419.pdf.

Pritchett L (1997). Divergence, big time. J Econ Perspect 11(3):3–17.

Quah D (1996). Twin peaks: growth and convergence in models of distribution dynamics. Econ J 106(437):1045–1055.

Ravallion M (2004). Competing Concepts of Inequality in the Globalization Debate. Policy Research Working Paper 3243. Washington, DC: World Bank. http://econ.worldbank.org/files/34170wps3243.pdf.

Rodriguez F, and Rodrik D (2000). Trade policy and economic growth: a skeptic's guide to the cross-national evidence. In: BS Bernanke and K Rogoff (eds.). NBER Macroeconomics Annual 2000. Cambridge, MA: MIT Press, pp. 261–325.

Rodrik D (2000). Comments on "Trade, Growth, and Poverty" by D. Dollar and A. Kraay. http://www.ksghome.harvard.edu/~.drodrik.academic.ksg/Rodrik on Dollar-Kraay.pdf.

Sachs J (2001). Tropical Underdevelopment. Working Paper 8119. Cambridge, MA: National Bureau of Economic Research.

Sachs J (2003). Editorial. New York Times. July 9.

Sachs JD (2005). The End of Poverty. Economic Possibilities for Our Time. New York: Penguin Press.

Sala-i-Martin X (2002a). "The Disturbing Rise" of Global Income Inequality. Working Papers No. 8904. Cambridge, MA: National Bureau of Economic Research.

Sala-i-Martin X (2002b). The World Distribution of Income (Estimated from Individual Country Distributions). Working Paper No. 8933. Cambridge, MA: National Bureau of Economic Research. http://www.nber.org/papers/w8933.

Schultz TP (1998). Inequality and the distribution of personal income in the world: how it is changing and why. J Pop Econ 11(3):307–344.

Sen A (1997) On Economic Inequality. 2nd ed. Oxford: Clarendon Press.

Sen A (1999). Development as Freedom. New York: Alfred A. Knopf.

Stiglitz JE (2002). Globalization and Its Discontents. New York: W.W. Norton and Co.

Subramanian SV, Belli P, and Kawachi I. (2002). The macro-economic determinants of health. Annu Rev Public Health 23:287–302.

Subramanian SV, and Kawachi I (2004). Income inequality and health. What have we learned so far. Epidemiol Rev 26:78–91.

United Nations Development Programme (1996). Human Development Report 1996. New York: Oxford University Press.

United Nations Development Programme (1999). *Human Development Report 1999*. New York: Oxford University Press.

United Nations Development Programme (2002). *Human Development Report 2002*. New York: Oxford University Press.

WHO (2001). *World Health Report 2001*. Geneva: World Health Organization.

WHO Commission on Macroeconomics and Health (2001). *Macroeconomics and Health: Investing in Health for Economic Development*. Geneva: World Health Organization.

Wilkinson RG (1996). *Unhealthy Societies: The Afflictions of Inequality*. London: Routledge.

Wolf M (2004). *Why Globalization Works*. New Haven, CT: Yale University Press.

World Bank (2000). Poverty in an Age of Globalization. Mimeo. Washington, DC: World Bank.

World Bank (2004). *World Development Indicators*. Washington, DC: World Bank.

Chapter 8

The Consequences of Economic Globalization on Working Conditions, Labor Relations, and Workers' Health

Christer Hogstedt, David H. Wegman, and Tord Kjellstrom

Globalization has led to an integration of national economies into a world economy where the dominant themes are economies of scale and competition between nations and enterprises for the most cost-efficient production of goods and services. As we will show in this chapter, working conditions and occupational safety and health (OSH) are vulnerable in the globalized market-based economic system. This system—promoted by institutions such as the World Bank, International Monetary Fund (IMF), World Trade Organization, and transnational corporations—involves the relaxation of wage controls, union protections, and workplace standards (frequently promoted under the guise of "flexible labor markets").

In order to prevent a "race to the bottom" in workers' health protection, a sustained effort is required from international agencies, trade unions, and consumer organizations to monitor the OSH performance in countries and enterprises. Published systematic evaluations of OSH conditions before and after globalization are not common, but analysis and reviews of the general trends by agencies in the field indicate the risks at hand.

A further consequence of globalized markets is the increasing global division of labor, with exports of "dirty and hazardous" work to developing countries. In order to avoid repeating the same sad experience of occupational diseases as documented in developed countries, available knowledge about safer and cleaner technologies needs to be applied in developing countries. Long working hours, deficient protection against known hazards, and poor social support systems are common hazards in the export processing zones (EPZs) and in other production units encouraged by globalization. National OSH legislation is often not applied in the EPZs in order to make the costs of production low. On the other hand, the OSH conditions in other enterprises in the country may be even worse due to lack of enforcement of legislation and lack of awareness of OSH issues. Women and child workers are particularly vulnerable. Globalization of communication systems, however, has created new avenues for information about poor conditions to be publicized and for union and consumer campaigns to improve the conditions.

The globalized market-based economic system with a minimum of regulations and its aim of "flexible" working conditions and nonunionized labor creates job insecurity in both developed and developing countries. Globalization without policies and systems to ensure appropriate social support for people affected by these insecurities creates health risks through stress.

Overall, it is not global integration of economies and cultures in itself that is a health threat, but the way that globalization is carried out: with or without proper OSH and social support systems in place. In this chapter we highlight the health risks of globalization without preventive systems and make reference to the international efforts to ensure effective worker protection programs are in place. The improved global information and communications systems create new opportunities for occupational health advocacy that can help bring about such programs.

GLOBAL WORKFORCE AND WORK ORGANIZATION TRENDS

As the world population has increased, so has the workforce, and therefore, OSH is of importance to more people than ever. The potential workforce is often estimated as the proportion of the total population that is in the range of fifteen to fifty-nine years of age. The changing demographics of the world means that this proportion is increasing in developing countries, while it is decreasing in developed countries. In the former, the size of the child population has been large (though diminishing), while in the latter the size of the elderly population is rapidly increasing. However, many people outside this age range are actively working. The group above sixty years of age includes a considerable proportion of working people in many countries, while the fifteen- to nineteen-year-olds are increasingly going to school. Furthermore, the participation of women in the employed workforce has increased over time in most countries, depending on social, cultural, religious, and other customs (ILO, 2002b).

It is important to think beyond the "standard" workforce when considering globalization and work. In traditional societies, everyone who is able-bodied participates in family and community activities that are required to maintain and build the community. In these settings, work is not an isolated element from other aspects of daily living, such as child rearing, cooking, and other family activities. The amount of work carried out is limited to what is seen as necessary for the survival and consolidation of the community.

OSH hazards can be of great importance to the health of these people but are often overlooked or ignored by authorities concerned with worker health because the concept of "work" is not applied to these activities. As globalization brings industrial development, new structures of "employment" in traditional agricultural societies will exacerbate this division between "work" and other family and societal activities

In theory, the global workforce encompasses every able-bodied adult. In practice, however, international statistics (ILO, 2002b) only refer to the "economically active population," which is described by age and sex group in a International Labour Organization publication (ILO, 2002b) and in the online LABORSTA database (ILO, 2003b). Of the 3 billion people in the world in 1960 (916 million + 2,104 million; table 8.1), 1.4 billion were considered economically active (411 million + 966 million; table 8.1), and in 2000 these numbers had increased to 6.1 billion and 2.9 billion, respectively (table 8.1) (ILO, 2003b).

If focus is restricted to those economically active, the "activity rate" measures the proportion of the total population that is involved in "economic activities." Overall, it has increased slightly (from 45% to 49%), but more important changes have taken place at the lower and upper ends of the age spectrum for men, and in the middle range of ages for women (ILO, 2002b). The activity rate among men has gone down considerably below twenty-five years of age and above fifty years of age, while among women there has been a significant increase in the activity rate from 60% to 70% in the age range of twenty-five to sixty years.

One of the key differences in activity rates between developed and developing countries is the very high economic activity rate among children and young people in developing countries. In developed countries, with the exception of the United States, the economic activity rates for children under age fifteen is now almost zero, and one can assume that almost all of them are instead studying at school. The rate for fifteen- to nineteen-year-olds has decreased from about 50% to 30% since 1960. In less developed regions reductions of economic activity rates among

TABLE 8.1. Total Population and Economically Active Population in More and Less Developed Regions

	1960	1970	1980	1990	1995	2000
More Developed Regions (total)[a]						
Population/Millions						
Both sexes	916	1,008	1,083	1,148	1,174	1,191
Men	439	486	524	558	571	579
Women	477	522	559	591	603	612
Economically Active Population/Thousands						
Both sexes	411	463	523	566	584	601
Men	258	280	305	320	327	332
Women	152	182	218	246	257	269
Less Developed Regions (total)[b]						
Population/Thousands						
Both sexes	2,104	2,683	3,347	4,106	4,488	4,865
Men	1,071	1,365	1,705	2,091	2,282	2,472
Women	1,033	1,317	1,642	2,015	2,206	2,394
Economically Active Population/Thousands						
Both sexes	966	1,192	1,528	1,932	2,136	2,347
Men	616	750	945	1,181	1,296	1,415
Women	350	442	583	751	840	931

[a]More developed regions comprise Northern America, Japan, Europe, and Australia–New Zealand. [b]Less developed regions comprise all regions of Africa, Latin America and the Caribbean, Asia (excluding Japan), Melanesia, Micronesia, and Polynesia.

Source: ILO (2003b).

children are also taking place, albeit more slowly. Child labor remains an important issue in developing countries.

Major changes in the workforce composition by type of economic activity have taken place during recent decades, and economic globalization has only accelerated these changes. Agriculture has been, and remains, the primary workplace for the majority of people in developing countries (reduced from 80% in 1960 to 60% in 2000; ILO, 2003b). Health hazards of traditional agriculture include vector-borne diseases, injuries, and, increasingly, pesticide poisoning. Other primary industries, such as mining and forestry, also pose high risks for occupational injuries and diseases (ILO, 2003b).

Industrialization comes with increasingly sophisticated technologies, which in turn leads to marked changes in the OSH issues of concern. Globalization has led to a shift of manufacturing from the affluent to the developing countries, with concomitant shifts in workforce composition. These industries bring with them new potential hazards (Fustukian et al., 2002).

Injuries, ergonomic hazards, exposure to physical and chemical agents, and an increasing work pace are the main problems in manufacturing industries, while pesticides, organic dusts, heavy physical work, biological factors, and injury hazards are the occupational health hazards of modern agriculture. Globalization can intensify hazardous exposures for workers in developing countries. A number of studies show that in the worst cases, 50–100% of the workers in some hazardous industries in developing countries may be exposed to levels of chemical, physical, or biological factors that exceed the occupational exposure limits applied in industrial countries (WHO, 1995).

The latest wave of change also includes major growth of service industries, again accelerated by globalization. This is long evident in the more developed regions and is now an emerging trend in the less developed regions. The consequence for the latter is that, while the "old" occupational health problems still persist, "new" hazards have also emerged. During the last decade, many administrative functions that used to be based in the home country of corporations, for example, accounting, call centers, and data management, have been outsourced to subcontractors in developing countries providing local employment there for people trained in information technology and related fields. These workplaces may be seen as rather benign from an OSH point of view, but new hazards are eventually uncovered, such as musculoskeletal disorders from repetitive and forceful movements and stress-related diseases.

The reduced influence of trade unions in recent decades has contributed significantly to the character of globalized economies. Many corporations and governments have made efforts to limit trade union membership and involvement in work organization and OSH matters. The result is a workplace environment where individual rather than collective concerns and actions are emphasized. Competition rather than collaboration is the basis of daily work life. The "winners" are given privileges and higher salaries and are hailed as examples to emulate for the majority, while "losers" are kept at lower incomes and told to try harder. Losing one's job becomes a more frequent crisis, as restructuring and downsizing are carried out to protect "shareholder value." In fact, share prices of corporations invariably go up when announcements are made of substantial reductions of the workforce. Unemployment, at least temporary, has become a "normal" occurrence, and macroeconomic models build in a 5% unemployment rate as "ideal." The social and health impact at the population level of unemployment needs to be built into the models in order to take full account of the costs to society.

At the country level, the proportion of the population that is economically active and the distribution according to sector can change dramatically over time due to changes in the general economic situation influenced by the forces of globalization. Unemployment varies in conjunction with these changes. An example is the dramatic crisis in Thailand (box 8.1), where the liberalization of capital markets (making it easy to exchange Bhat with other currencies) led to significant effects on employment. A root cause of such dramatic changes often appears to be premature liberalization of a country's financial sector and foreign exchange regulations. It is important to note that these types of changes are among the "pillars" for growth encouraged by the IMF (see chapters 7 and 13).

EXPORT PROCESSING ZONES

EPZs are an important feature of globalization (ILO, 2002c). The ILO defines an EPZ as an "industrial

Box 8.1 – Workforce Changes in Thailand in Conjunction with the Bhat Crisis in 1997

In the early 1990s, the government of Thailand was encouraged by the IMF to liberalize its financial sector and make the local currency, the Bhat, freely convertible on international financial markets. By 1997, investors lost confidence in the Bhat, and the currency rapidly lost value. In Thailand, companies dependent on foreign exchange had to pay much more for it. Some companies could not pay back their loans, and general economic trouble emerged. This led to employers shedding staff (downsizing) and an increase of unemployment. The number employed was reduced for the first time in a long series of years, and for men in the construction industry the loss of employment from 1997 to 1998 was particularly dramatic: approximately one-third of workers lost their jobs. Many men who had been working in construction or manufacturing went back to agricultural work, from where they had come some years earlier.

Source: Stiglitz (2002), and ILO (2003b).

---

zone with special incentives set up to attract foreign investors, in which imported materials undergo some degree of processing before being re-exported" (p. 1). Imported materials may include electronic data or telephone conversations, thus making it possible to include call centers and data services in an EPZ. The incentives to the investors may include exemptions from customs duties and preferential treatment with respect to various fiscal and financial regulations.

These zones are intended to attract foreign investment for production facilities that process imported materials into final exported products. Depending on their purpose, they have been called various names, such as free trade zones, special economic zones, bonded warehouses, free ports, and *maquiladoras* (primarily along the U.S.–Mexico border). In many cases, EPZs are specifically exempt from key national regulations on working conditions and OSH.

The North American Free Trade Agreement (NAFTA) provides an example of how globalization efforts have relegated the concerns of OSH to the margin. During debate in the United States on ratification of NAFTA, labor union demands led to the establishment of the North American Agreement for Labor Cooperation (NAALC) as a side agreement,

TABLE 8.2. ILO Estimates of the Development of EPZs

	1975	1986	1995	1997	2002
Countries with EPZs	25	47	73	93	116
Number of EPZs	79	176	500	845	3000
Total employment in EPZs (millions)	NA	NA	NA	22.5	37
In Chinese EPZs	NA	NA	NA	18	30

NA = estimate not available.

Source: ILO (2002c).

the first instance in which the United States had negotiated an agreement dealing with labor standards to supplement an international trade agreement. NAALC was designed to protect labor organizing and worker health and safety. An evaluation of the effectiveness of this agreement in 2004 concluded that, although the NAALC has exposed violations of worker health and safety regulations, it has failed to protect workers' rights to safe jobs (Delp et al., 2004). EPZs, therefore, present a particular concern with respect to adequate attention to OSH.

A list of priorities for improving social and labor conditions in the EPZs established by ILO (2002c) highlights the problems that may arise:

- Labor standards: Internationally or nationally established standards for work hazard exposures should be applied to EPZs and strongly enforced.
- Labor-management relations: The right to join a union and for the union to be actively involved with working conditions should be applied in EPZs. Collective bargaining and tripartite negotiation mechanisms should be established.
- Human resources development: General education and job skills training should be a key aspect of EPZ operations, in order to broaden the future job opportunities for workers and to upgrade the level of production toward more advanced technologies. This includes retraining of workers as production methods change.
- Wages and working conditions: Remuneration packages should be fair and contribute to an improved living standard for the workers. Working hours is a particular problem to monitor to ensure that excessive demands are not created on the workers. This is of particular importance for women. Safety issues concerning night work need to be resolved. Another issue in tropical countries is the impact of extreme heat on workers.
- Social infrastructure: This includes adequate

and sanitary accommodation, safe and reliable transportation, educational and recreational facilities, health centers, and childcare facilities. In addition, pension and other social security measures should be provided to the EPZ work force.

EPZs are an important aspect of foreign direct investment, and they have grown in number and taken on ever more diverse economic activities. They began as assembly factories and labor-intensive processing of materials that were designed to take advantage of low salaries in developing countries. More recent zones include finance operations, technology and science centers, logistics and transport centers, and tourist resorts (ILO, 2002c). The dramatic growth of EPZs and the number of workers involved are shown in table 8.2.

An analysis for China shows the potential impact that EPZs may have on the workforce distribution. Between 1990 and 2000, the economically active population in China increased by about 80 million people (ILO, 2002b). The industrial manufacturing field in China had 83 million economically active (employed) in 1999 (ILO, 2002b). The 30 million people in EPZs (table 8.2) thus amounts to about one-third of the ten-year growth in employment in China or a third of the whole industrial manufacturing workforce.

The effect on employment of the EPZs in China and other Asian countries has been of particular importance for young women, who gain entry into the formal labor market through these jobs, often with better wages than in agriculture or domestic service. This is for many a positive aspect of EPZs. However, poor work environments and work practices have been a common concern (Fustukian et al., 2002). This has included lack of proper accommodation for women workers (ILO, 2002c) and the creation of social "ghettos" in barrack-style living quarters. In addition, pregnancy testing to avoid hiring women (who will need maternity leave) promotes gender discrimination (ILO, 2002c). Framework agreements between a few multinational corporations and international union federations have played an important role in addressing these negative factors and in upgrading the working conditions. In addition, pressure on high-profile companies (e.g., Nike) has encouraged important improvements in the working environment and conditions in their factories in EPZs.

The positive and negative aspects of EPZs have been discussed in recent years. For instance, a report by a South African nongovernmental organization (NGO), the International Labour Resource and Information Group, suggests that four countries surveyed (South Africa, Zimbabwe, Tanzania, and Namibia) had enjoyed little benefit (Khan, 2002). A number of potential EPZ sites had been identified in the countries, but few were actually operational, and the cost per job created was extremely high. In Zimbabwe, fewer than half of 138 planned EPZs were operational. In Namibia, 25,000 new jobs were predicted, but only 370 were documented. In Tanzania, only 500 of 7,000 expected jobs had materialized. The report concludes that industrialization based on exports is not a good development strategy for the African region.

A similar critique of EPZs in Eastern Europe (Vaknin, 2003) indicates that these zones without taxes, low customs duties, and "flexible" labor rules are growing rapidly in the former Soviet Union states. They provide a form of hidden export subsidies and have become major centers of money laundering, parallel imports of counterfeit goods, and illegal reimportation of merchandise destined for other countries. Governments are becoming concerned about these practices, and restrictions are now being placed on them.

TRADITIONAL SUBSISTENCE WORK AND THE INFORMAL SECTOR

The boundary between "work" and other household tasks is fluid in traditional settings. Each task involves health hazards. For instance, indoor cooking with wood, coal, agricultural waste or cow dung exposes the cook (usually a woman) and young children in her care to very high levels of indoor air pollution (Sims, 1994). Levels of particulate matter and carbon monoxide up to 100 times higher than what is mea-

sured outdoors in polluted areas have been reported. As many as 500 million women and children may be exposed to these conditions (WHO, 1997), and the health implications in terms of acute respiratory infections for children and chronic obstructive lung diseases and mortality for the women are very large ($\sim$ 2.5 million deaths/year; WHO, 1997).

Daily collection of water and firewood make up the other chores that create a high work load, especially for women (Sims, 1994). Increasing population density and meteorological conditions (e.g., droughts) make these chores more and more cumbersome for many people. Opportunities for exposure to insect and snake bites are high in wood collection activities in tropical areas, while fresh water collection creates risks of schistosomiasis from water contact (Sims, 1994). To the extent that globalization reduces the number of people involved in these jobs and associated hazardous exposures, it may have a positive impact on health.

However, the effects of globalization on traditional farming include the increasing use of pesticides in family farms with few, if any, safety precautions (box 8.2). In addition, pressures to produce foodstuffs and other agricultural produce for export extend plantation farming practices, with associated high use of pesticides. This process may also result in a reduction of the production of local food for family consumption and associated development of malnutrition.

Agriculture has a central economic role in most developing countries, not only because food production is a key element in survival at the community level, but also because cash crops are seen as a way to economic development. These crops include directly edible plants and fruits, as well as coffee beans, palm oil, and inedible cotton and flowers. Developing countries are encouraged (or forced through "structural adjustment" policies) to establish new agricultural production at a very intensive level (industrialized agriculture), which uses larger amounts of fertilizers and pesticides than does traditional agriculture (London et al., 2002). The pesticides used may involve those that have been banned or severely restricted in high-income countries, and the risk of occupational poisoning as well as the use of these pesticides for suicides has increased (London et al., 2002). Women often work longer hours than men, their work tasks bring them into more contact with pesticides, and their exposure may occur during food preparation and other household tasks. The risk of poisoning for women may

Box 8.2 – Pesticide Use in Vietnam after Market "Reforms" of Family Farming

The *Doi Moi* policies of privatization of formerly communally owned farms can be seen as a consequence of globalization on national policies in Vietnam. *Doi Moi* was established during the 1990s. One feature of the new order was that pesticides became available in local shops with scant attention to safety information and precautions. This led to a rapid increase of severe pesticide poisonings. In the previous communal farming situation, specially trained staff would provide pesticides and carry out the spraying. After *Doi Moi*, individual farmers were made responsible for this work, with disastrous effects. Pesticide containers would be stored in the cooking areas. Children could be exposed inadvertently, and leaking containers could contaminate food preparation surfaces. The hazards were often poorly understood by the farming family members, and protective equipment was not used. Overuse of pesticides occurred, because the merchants encourage the notion that "more is better." After more than ten years of *Doi Moi*, the Ministry of Health is considering ways to bring back specialized pesticide spraying staff.

Source: Personal communications from staff in the Ministries of Health and Agriculture, Hanoi, 2001.

---

therefore be higher than for men, and in addition, they are more vulnerable to certain reproductive effects than are men (London et al., 2002).

The informal sector includes small-scale industrial and service enterprises that emerge with economic development from traditional household work activities. These jobs often involve heavy workloads, poor safety precautions, and long working hours. Work usually takes place in an environment that seldom meets safety standards. Family members of the entrepreneurs and workers, including children, pregnant women, and elderly people, share the work in these small-scale enterprises, such as home industries, small farms, and cottage industries.

CHILDREN AS WORKERS

The problems of the informal sector are compounded by the fact that many of its jobs are carried out by women and children. The low status of women in many societies means that scant attention is paid to the conditions under which their work is carried out (London et al., 2002; see also chapter 10). Similarly, when it comes to child labor, concerns about work hazards receive low priority. Children are powerless to influence their own working environment and are completely dependent on adults for their protection. ILO is mounting a major campaign to change attitudes and practices (see box 8.3).

Child labor presents a problem in most developing and in some industrialized nations. It is not specifically an effect of globalization, but it may be exacerbated by the commercial pressures of globalization. A cross-sectional analysis of data on trade openness and child labor in a number of developing countries concluded that globalization may possibly reduce child labor (Cogni, 2003), but the report also pointed out the critical role of domestic policies to address the problem. Children of the poor in developing countries are treated as a necessary part of the economy in roles that range from employment in enterprises important to economic development to those essential to the survival of the family (Forastieri, 1997; Fassa et al., 2000). Globalization forces countries and enterprises in many industries to compete to achieve the lowest possible labor costs, and child labor is cheap labor. Children's work duties compete directly with the primary importance of childhood as a time for education and development. ILO estimates that more than 350 million children worldwide are economically active, more than half of whom are younger than fifteen (ILO, 2002f). A combination of better working conditions for adults and effective support for parents to send their children to school would be the best way to reduce child labor.

Despite the consequences of child labor, government attention to these hazards is often minimal, and very few countries prohibit child labor. Internationally, the most common regulations address mining (101 countries), while child labor is most common in agriculture, and only fourteen countries have regulations prohibiting even selected tasks (Fassa, 2003). Domestic regulations and their proper enforcement are a necessary part of development efforts linked to global markets if the promise represented by youth is to be protected. An experimental program in Brazil (Programa de Erradicacao do Trabalho Infantil) was introduced in rural Brazil in 1996. The program lengthened the school day and provides an income subsidy to low-income families who participate. Examination of the program impact suggests

Box 8.3 – ILO Child Labor Convention

In the context of ILO Convention concerning the Prohibition and Immediate Action for the Elimination of the Worst Forms of Child Labor (Convention 182, 1999), the ILO has carried out 38 rapid assessments of the most egregious forms of child labor. The investigations explored very sensitive areas including illegal, criminal, and immoral activities. More specifically, they focused on the topics of children in bondage; child domestic workers; children engaged in armed conflict; child trafficking; drug trafficking; hazardous work in commercial agriculture, fishing, garbage dumps, mining, and the urban environment; sexual exploitation; and working street children. The studies used the ILO/UNICEF rapid assessment methodology on child labor, which balances statistical precision with qualitative analysis and aims to provide policy makers with insights into the magnitude, character, causes, and consequences of the worst forms of child labor quickly and at low cost. In addition to the thirty-eight rapid assessment reports resulting from this project, two reports on child domestic workers based on national statistics from Brazil and South Africa were produced. The purpose of the national reports is to provide an in-depth analysis of child domestic workers—a widespread yet hidden form of child labor—at the country level. It is hoped that these reports will raise awareness and promote the urgency of preventing more children from entering the worst forms of child labor.

Source: ILO (2002f, 2004a).

---

that it led to improved academic performance and lowered child labor among participating families (Lund, 2001). Other experiments in Brazil, such as Bolsa Escola, provide evidence that government commitment to reducing child labor can be implemented by addressing poverty, one of the primary determinants.

BONDED LABOR AND TRAFFICKING

Many other work arrangements and work situations are associated with particular health risks. These include bonded labor, actual slavery (still existing in certain countries under different names), and traffick-

ing (Stellman, 1998, section 24.9). It has been estimated that globally there are around 25 million people working under these conditions (Bales, 2004). Each situation poses its own hazards, and because of the sometimes illegal nature of these work arrangements, it is very difficult to undertake any OSH activities for those affected apart from eliminating the work arrangement itself.

A group of workers with particular health risks are prostitutes or "sex workers" (Stellman, 1998, sections 96, 49). Women are mainly involved, but male prostitution and child prostitution are increasing concerns. In recent years, their health protection needs have become more widely discussed as a result of the global HIV/AIDS epidemic and the need to engage sex workers in prevention efforts. Sexually transmitted disease is not the only health problem these workers face. Violence from clients and pimps is a daily threat. Prostitution is also closely linked to drug abuse, itself stemming from the conditions of mental and social deprivation among sex workers. Some drug abusers also use prostitution as a source of income for their habits. Globalization of travel and tourism has enabled the growth of "sex tourism," which has created an expanded and lucrative market for prostitution.

"Trafficking" in young women, girls, and boys, who become virtual slaves for sex services, has received increasing attention in recent years (Bales, 2004). It is facilitated by low-cost air travel and global outreach of organized crime. Differences in ethical and legal standards concerning prostitution in different countries make it difficult to develop a coherent international approach to deal with the problem. The globalization of the sex industry is also facilitated by the Internet, which makes it easy for clandestine services to be established and advertised while its actual physical location is moved as required.

MIGRANT WORKERS

Migration of people between countries and within countries is a longstanding issue. Wars, environmental degradation, and other cataclysms have led to decisions by large population groups to move throughout history. The distribution of nationalities within Europe was shaped by such mass migrations. The slave trade was another phenomenon that moved populations from Africa to America. Modern migrants can be divided into economic migrants, usually voluntary; displaced persons and refugees; and trafficked individuals (see also chapter 9).

In recent decades migration has again been expanded due to active recruitment of workers from one country to another, for example, the "guest worker" phenomenon in Germany and Switzerland. Some Middle Eastern countries also have recruited workers systematically from abroad, for example, domestic workers in Saudi Arabia and Kuwait from the Philippines or India. Major internal economic migration to EPZs occurs, for instance, in China. Globalization, through increased possibilities for long-distance travel, has accelerated these flows of people. As manufacturing facilities are established by Western multinational corporations in EPZs of developing countries, the need for "guest workers" from abroad has reduced while internal migration has increased. On the other hand, highly skilled workers (as well as service workers) from developing countries are sought after by industrial countries in order to fill "gaps" in the workforce. Such gaps are often the consequence of demographic aging in developed countries, which have been experiencing a long-term decline in the economically active segments of their population.

Health care personnel represent an important group of economic migrants, as the increasing ranks of elderly in rich countries lead to increased demand for health care and services. One negative consequence of migration from developing to developed countries is the "brain drain" from developing countries who can ill afford to lose these highly trained people (Aiken et al., 2004). In some developing countries, for example, the Philippines, the training of nurses is at levels high above national demands, as these nurses can obtain jobs in developed countries or the Middle East. Their remittances contribute significantly to the "export" income of the Philippines. However, their health care skills are not being used to improve health in their home country.

Many economic migrant workers end up having to take the jobs that local people do not want, which often involve more occupational hazards (Stellman, 1998, section 24.9; Landrigan et al., 1998). The wages and other conditions (e.g., working hours) are also likely to be worse than for the "regular" work force. Access to health services may be more limited. All of these factors create more health risks than in usual work situations.

Migration inside countries can be driven by systematic efforts to concentrate new industries in "border zones" or EPZs with lower taxes, lower (or often absent) occupational health regulation protection for workers, and other limitations on workers' health conditions. In Latin America, these industries are often *maquiladoras* that carry out only the labor-intensive parts of the production while the actual product is sold from a developed country base. Migrant workers often have to leave their families when they migrate for work, leading to social isolation, poor living conditions, and other social health risks. These include alcohol abuse, sexually transmitted diseases, and violence (Landrigan et al., 1998).

HAZARDS IN THE NEWLY EMERGING WORKPLACES

Detailed information on specific occupational exposures in different work situations can be found in a number of recent textbooks and reference volumes (e.g., Stellman, 1998; Herzstein et al., 1998; Levy and Wegman, 2000). We briefly refer here to some key issues concerning hazards of importance in globalizing economies.

It is important to point out that some of the changes in workforce structure in developing countries as a consequence of globalization may lead to less dangerous workplaces and reductions of exposures to the hazards listed here. In addition, investments in new workplaces can be used to introduce new and safer technologies. OSH professionals are in good positions to monitor developments and to make hazards known to employers, regulators, and decision makers.

Mechanical Factors

Unshielded machinery, unsafe structures at the workplace, and unprotected tools are among the most prevalent hazards in both industrial and developing countries. Globalization has contributed to the export of hazardous machinery to developing nations when the original owners in developed countries upgrade to safer and more efficient equipment. Occupational injury hazards are particularly common in developing countries (Kjellstrom et al., 1992; Takala, 1999), and most of these injuries could be prevented by improving machinery, working practices, and safety systems (Kogi et al., 1989).

Chemical Hazards

These are an increasingly important concern when countries develop new industries as a consequence of globalization. About 100,000 different chemical products are currently in use in work environments, and the number is increasing constantly (International Program on Chemical Safety, 1999). Globally, the most common chemicals of concern include lead, organic solvents, and pesticides. Pesticide exposure is a major chemical hazard in developing countries, where personal protection is particularly difficult, and alternative preventive means need to be implemented (Wesseling et al., 1997). Often, there are alternative less toxic methods of pest control available (box 8.4).

The export to developing countries of agrochemicals that have been banned in developed countries, due to high human toxicity or ecotoxicity, is an important OSH concern. An analysis of exports from the United States of highly toxic, banned, or never registered pesticides (Smith and Root, 1999) showed that 14 tons per day were exported to developing countries. The receiving countries usually have very limited resources for the development of effective national regulations concerning pesticide safety and for enforcement of such regulations. One approach to overcoming these deficiencies is the voluntary code of conduct for the chemical industry under the auspices of the Food and Agriculture Organization of the United Nations (FAO) (box 8.4).

Many other chemical exposure situations that are now "history" in developed countries have been shifted to developing countries. The concept of "export of hazard" is well established, and in some cases, whole factories using out-of-date technologies have been moved from developed countries to developing countries (LaDou, 1999). This is an aspect of globalization that poses a particular barrier to the effective development of OSH in developing countries. One example of such a hazard is the use, in developing countries, of highly toxic solvents in glues utilized in shoe manufacturing and other industries (see box 8.5).

Occupational Dust Diseases

These are a common and increasing concern in developing countries, due to the growth of mining and quarrying industries in these regions. Estimates from epidemiological studies have indicated that many thousand silicosis cases are found each year in China

Box 8.4 – Alternative Pesticides

Toxic chemical pesticides have important applications when insects, fungi, and plant diseases seriously reduce the yield of harvests. However, on average, the enhanced yield from use of chemical pesticides is often exaggerated by the manufacturers of pesticides, and other methods of pest control can often maintain the yield at 90% or more of the yield achieved using chemicals (WHO, 1990). One way of reducing toxic chemical pesticide use is to apply integrated pest management (FAO, 2003a) techniques. These combine careful monitoring of the pests on plants with programmed low-intensity use of chemicals, if required. The integrated pest management approach also uses carefully designed "companion planting," which works because different insects are attracted to or repelled by different plants. For example, careful mixture of maize and grass planting in Kenya increased the maize yield by 30% (Radford, 2003).

Another important way of reducing pesticide poisonings is for farmers to use the least toxic pesticide that does the job intended and to use the precautions required for each specific pesticide. A voluntary code of practice developed by FAO and international chemical industry organizations (FAO, 2003b) is intended to ensure that appropriate hazards and safety information is provided through all stages of production, shipment, wholesale, retail, and application of pesticides. Local OSH professionals can use this code of practice to request needed information from pesticide manufacturers and importers.

Other means of ensuring that the information reaches the users of the pesticides include, for example, Non-Governmental Organization Pesticide Information centers (Razak et al., 1998) and official poison control centers.

---

alone (He, 1998), and the situation in other countries with many mines (e.g., India) is likely to be similar. Asbestos exposure is an ongoing problem, even though all developed countries have placed severe restrictions on the use of asbestos and some countries (e.g., Sweden and Australia) have banned its use altogether. In spite of the high occupational health risks of asbestos use, a number of developing countries continue to use asbestos in production of fiber-cement building products (e.g., roof panels) and brake linings (e.g., China, Vietnam, Indonesia, and

Box 8.5 – Replacing Hazardous Solvents with Less Toxic Alternatives

Organic solvents are some of the more toxic compounds widely used in industry, primarily in glues, paints, and cleaning fluids (e.g., for cleaning oil and metal grease). Benzene was one of the first solvents used in workplaces, but it is highly toxic and carcinogenic (leukemia) and has now been eliminated from routine use in industrial countries. It is still used in some developing country shoe factories, and the hazards for the workers are high. The multinational Nike shoe factory was embarrassed some years ago by the finding that their subcontractors (usually Korean- or Taiwanese-owned factories in other countries, e.g., Vietnam) were using benzene-containing glues. The establishment of production in Vietnam using obsolete and dangerous technology is another aspect of globalization. When union- and consumer-led campaigns publicized the serious OSH concerns, Nike ordered a change to water-based glues and implemented other OSH improvements to avoid further embarrassment. However, other shoe factories in Vietnam, many of them owned by the Vietnamese government and producing shoes for export, were still using the very toxic glues in 2002 (T. Kjellstrom, unpublished observation). Union and consumer vigilance could make a difference here too.

Brazil). Safer alternatives do exist and are used in all developed countries (London Hazards Centre, 2004). In many developing countries, either it is too early to be able to record an increase of asbestos-induced mesothelioma and lung cancer (due to the long latency), or the data for surveillance simply do not exist. Some information from Hanoi provides an indication of what may be on the horizon, after 30 years' delay, in comparison with Australia, Sweden, and New Zealand (figure 8.1).

The mesothelioma mortality rate has risen dramatically during recent decades in the three industrial countries. The Hanoi data appear to follow a similar rising pattern, but with a twenty-year lag. There are 7,000 asbestos-cement product manufacturing workers in Vietnam, and many more construction workers who use the products in their daily work (Vietnam Ministry of Health, unpublished data).

Biological Hazards

Biological hazards of various kinds, including viruses, bacteria, parasites, fungi, molds, and organic dusts, are common causes of occupational diseases in developing countries (WHO, 1995). Hepatitis B, hepatitis C, and tuberculosis infections occur particularly among health care workers. Global spread of improved health care methods and technology would assist in controlling these occupational diseases, but the lack of resources allocated to health services in many developing countries poses a barrier to such OSH improvements. Vector-borne tropical diseases common in the general population of many developing countries, such as malaria and schistosomiasis, are likely to be a particular risk for agricultural, forestry, and other outdoor workers.

Physical Stressors

Stressors of concern include noise, vibration, radiation, and climate conditions (WHO, 1995; Stellman, 1998). An issue that has not received much attention is the effect of high temperature and humidity on people's ability to work both in traditional and modern occupations. This is of particular importance in tropical climates, where temperatures and humidity levels in the work environment are already within the "danger zone." Global warming will exacerbate this hazard in many parts of the world (see chapter 5). Heavy work is difficult to maintain at temperatures above 26°C if the humidity is also high (Intergovernmental Panel on Climate Change, 2001). The effect on workers will be increased heat stress and lower productivity. The latter may be seen as a problem for employers, but in fact the workers end up paying for the consequences by enduring longer work hours to meet production targets (box 8.6).

Psychological Stress

Globalization has created a new emphasis on "flexibility" of working conditions and "competitiveness" between enterprises and countries, which has led to increased pressure on workers and employees at all levels to work harder and faster (Fustukian et al., 2002). The type of work organization and management of workplaces that goes with the current form of globalization creates uncertainty within a very

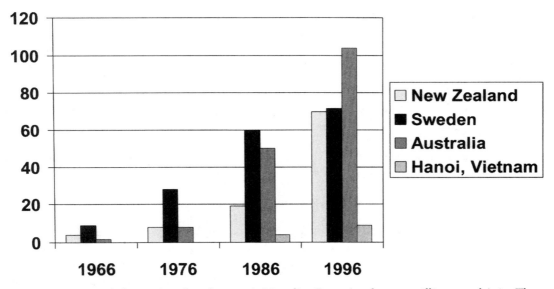

FIGURE 8.1. Mesothelioma (or pleural cancer) Mortality Rates (crude, per million people) in Three Countries and Hanoi City at Different Times. *Source:* T. Kjellstrom, unpublished data, based on national death statistics and data for Hanoi from an unpublished report by the Vietnam Ministry of Health.

Box 8.6 – Heat and Work in Vietnam

A shoe factory in Haiphong, Vietnam, employs 2,900 young women producing sports shoes for European markets. In Haiphong, it is very hot (30–38°C) inside the factory in the summer but relatively cool (15–20°C) in the winter. The factory is not air-conditioned, and during the summer the workers have to work longer hours to maintain the daily production quota. Typical working days in the winter and summer are listed below. The workers have to work at least an hour longer and have to spend at least two hours longer at the workplace on hot summer days than in the winter, because heat load increases time needed to reach the production target.

Winter
7:30 start work
10:00–10:15 break
11:30–12:30 break
15:00–15:15 break
Finish at about 18:00 (when production target reached; same target in winter and summer)

Summer
6:30 start work
10:00–10:30 break

11:30–13:00 break (employer provides complimentary bean soup)
15:00–15:30 break
Finish later at about 19:00 because of heat

Source: Tord Kjellstrom, unpublished observation.

---

competitive environment in both developed and developing countries (Eckersley, 2004). Long working hours and less flexibility for workers to adapt their workload and working hours to their needs, such as family needs, have become the norm.

UNEMPLOYMENT AS A HEALTH HAZARD

Lack of income and status due to unemployment or underemployment is another important health hazard, particularly in countries where social security systems are poorly developed (Levy and Wegman, 2000; ILO, 2002a). ILO estimates that the number of people unemployed or underemployed in the world today exceeds 800 million. The implementation of "flexible" labor market principles has led to a rapid increase in the number of part-time workers. For many homemakers with young children, a part-time job is often the only solution to entering the labor market, but the limited income this generates may not be sufficient for the family's needs. Affordable childcare is a key issue linked to women's entry into the labor market. Part-time work may represent an aspect of underemployment, which can have similar adverse impacts on workers' health as unemployment.

Globalization has had particular impacts on employment in the public sector. In some countries, restructuring of the public sector to create more meaningful output at reasonable cost has been a good thing. However, the neo-liberal form of globalization incorporates a general notion that public services are always inefficient, that taxes should be reduced (thus taking away the resources from the public sector), and private enterprise would do a better job of providing water, electricity, mass transport, and so forth. A number of examples are available of how privatization of public services has created more problems than the systems it replaced. Cuts in the public health sector, often demanded by the IMF as part of structural adjustment programs in heavily indebted countries (Stiglitz, 2002), has adversely affected the availability of health services (see chapter 13).

THE OCCUPATIONAL BURDEN OF DISEASE AND INJURY

Measuring the burden of occupational disease and injury, globally, regionally, nationally, and locally, has become increasingly important in a world where quantification and cost–benefit analysis is becoming a necessity. The disability-adjusted life year (DALY) metric provides an integrated picture of mortality and morbidity (Murray and Lopez, 1996) and has been widely applied in recent years, primarily because the World Bank, and later the World Health Organization (WHO), provided major financial support for its development and application in major international reports (World Bank, 1993; WHO, 2002; see also chapter 11).

In order to quantify the contribution of occupational health hazards to the global burden of disease and injury, a detailed review of available data and epidemiological studies was undertaken for the World Health Report (WHO, 2002). Five major occupational hazard groups were selected for which mean-

ingful quantifications could be made (WHO, 2002). WHO recognized that this approach produces a lower bound estimate of the global occupational burden of disease because it excludes many known causes of disease where adequate quantitative data are missing. Burden estimates were made for work-related risk factors for injuries, work-related carcinogens, selected airborne particles, work-related ergonomic stressors, and work-related noise.

Overall, it was estimated that about 1.6% of all DALYs were due to these occupational hazards (table 8.3). The WHO calculations placed the lower bound estimate at 709,000 occupational deaths globally. However, the DALY numbers for occupational injuries in table 8.3 may be more than three times underestimated. The most recent estimate by ILO (2002e) gives a much higher figure, 2 million deaths, with a range from 1.92 to 2.33 million. Neither estimate gives adequate consideration to the impact of work in the informal sector or work risks in the home environment. Thus, an upper bound estimate would be even higher.

Other important occupational hazards were excluded, such as pesticides, heavy metals, infectious organisms, agents causing occupational asthma or chronic pulmonary disease, and stress at work causing increased cardiovascular diseases (WHO, 2002). Pesticides alone cause major public health impacts (WHO, 1990): each year, about 700,000 acute unintentional pesticides poisonings, 770,000 chronic poisonings, and 12,000 deaths occur. Population increase alone may have increased the death toll by 16,000 in the year 2000. ILO (2002e) estimates more than 500,000 deaths caused by work-related cardiovascular diseases. Similar calculations for other work-related diseases excluded from the WHO (2002) calculations would increase the total DALYs significantly.

Improvements in the health status of populations depend on improvements in adult health. The reduction of infant and child mortality goes hand in hand with the lengthening of average life span (Rosling, 2003). However, one of the most important inputs to good child health is good health (and survival) of the child's parents (Feachem et al., 1992), and to achieve good adult health, a decent quality of working environment and OSH practices are paramount.

The burden of occupational disease and injury can also be expressed as economic losses (WHO, 1999; updated figures become available at regular intervals at the WHO website):

TABLE 8.3. Burden of Disease and Injury from Occupational Hazards, Whole World, 2000: DALYs (Thousands) and Percentages

Occupational Hazard	World, Both Sexes		World, Males		World, Females	
	DALYs	%	DALYs	%	DALYs	%
Total, DALYs	1,467,257	100	768,131	100	699,126	100
Injury factors	13,124	0.89	12,070	1.57	1,054	0.15
Carcinogens	1,420	0.10	1,137	0.15	283	0.04
Air pollutants	4,346	0.30	4,079	0.53	267	0.04
Ergonomic factors	819	0.06	486	0.06	333	0.05
Noise	4,151	0.28	2,788	0.36	1,363	0.19
Occupational hazards, total	23,860	1.63	20,560	2.67	3,300	0.47

Source: WHO (2002).

- The global economic losses resulting from work-related diseases and injuries (including the value of lost work days) amounted to approximately 4% of the world's gross world product (US$31,000 billion in the year 2000), or US$1,200 billion.
- In 1992, the *direct* cost paid out in compensation for work-related diseases and injuries in European countries reached 27 billion Euros (US$30 billion).
- In 1992, total *direct and indirect* costs associated with work-related injuries and diseases in the United States were estimated to be US$171 billion (or about 3% of the total gross domestic product in the United States), surpassing the costs of AIDS and on a par with those of cancer and heart disease.

GLOBAL GOVERNANCE ORGANIZATIONS WITH OSH RESPONSIBILITIES

The most important agencies dedicated to improving OSH at international level are ILO and WHO. Civil society representing stakeholders for OSH issues also has an important place in modern governance. These stakeholders include employers, workers and their organizations, health services, insurance companies, consumer organizations, and the community at large.

The ILO, based in Geneva, Switzerland, is a member of the United Nations family of organizations, whose special mandate is the promotion of safe and decent work in all countries. ILO is the only organization in the United Nations family that has a tri-partite structure: governments, employers, and workers. ILO promulgates conventions and recommendations (ILO, 2004a), which set minimum standards of basic labor rights. To be effective, those standards must be ratified by the member states and implemented in a systematic way. Ratification often involves legislative changes in both developed and developing countries, but many parliaments are reluctant to carry out such changes.

Two international conventions (convention 148 in year 1977, convention 151 in 1981) and their accompanying recommendations (recommendations 156 and 164, respectively) provide for the adoption of national OSH policies and describe the actions needed at national level and at enterprise level to promote OSH and to improve the working environment. A number of conventions deal with specific industries, for example, agriculture, construction, and mining, while others deal with specific hazards, for example, chemicals, asbestos, and radiation (ILO, 2004a).

The International Safety and Health Information Centre is a worldwide ILO service dedicated to the collection and dissemination of information on the prevention of occupational accidents and diseases. It is one of the key sources of practical advice for OSH practice in developing countries.

A new "umbrella" policy for the ILO work on working conditions and OSH was launched in 1999. Called "Decent Work," it was the result of internal soul searching in ILO about ways in which the organization could respond to globalization. It was based on the ILO Declaration on Fundamental Principles and Rights at Work (ILO, 1999), also called the

"Social Declaration." The goal for Decent Work is not just the creation of jobs, but the creation of jobs of acceptable quality.

Another ILO initiative, which may assist in the development of better occupational health protection in agriculture and industry during the economic development of less affluent countries, is the establishment of the ILO World Commission on the Social Dimension of Globalization (ILO, 2002a, 2002d, 2003a, 2004b). The commission's goals were to make globalization more attuned to human needs, particularly in the area of work and employment. The dialogue between different stakeholders in globalization has aimed to bring clarity to the issues in a nonconfrontational atmosphere. Strong statements about the needs for protection of the social aspects of work were made by the commission (ILO, 2004b), but unless this is backed by enforceable guidelines, the "race to the bottom" for social protection and OSH may still occur.

The WHO is another United Nations–associated organization with its headquarters in Geneva, Switzerland. All countries' ministries of health are "members" of this organization, which also has official relations with certain intercountry organizations, such as the European Union, and with NGOs, such as the International Commission on Occupational Health (ICOH), international trade unions, and certain business organizations (see chapter 16). Its agenda encompassed all health issues, including OSH. Traditionally, in many countries, occupational safety (with a focus on injuries) has been the concern of the ministries of labor, while occupational health (with a focus on the prevention of occupational diseases) has been the concern of the ministries of health. Increasingly, developed countries have centralized all work-related health and safety issues under ministries of labor (or equivalent) through new OSH legislation (e.g., United Kingdom, Sweden, Australia). In many developing countries the ministry of health still has an occupational health role, and it is vital for them the link to the WHO's programs.

As with all other WHO activities, occupational health activities occur at the global level and at the regional and national level, the latter being implemented by the six regional offices (in Copenhagen; Washington, DC; Alexandria, Egypt; Delhi; Brazzaville, Congo; and Manila). The regional activities in Europe are focused on capacity building in Eastern Europe and the newly independent states of the former Soviet Union. The American region develops training and intraregional collaboration primarily for Latin America.

One important means of implementing country programs, particularly in relation to training and technical/scientific collaboration, is the engagement of the WHO Collaborating Centers in Occupational Health (about 40 in different parts of the world). These are usually national research and training institutions that have substantial staff resources and experience in carrying out investigations and capacity building in this field. The centers have regular joint meetings to evaluate and plan the global activities.

In addition, there are international collaborative programs on specific issues between different United Nations and other agencies, for instance, in the field of chemical safety. The International Program on Chemical Safety is a collaborative effort between the United Nations Environment Program, WHO, and ILO, which was started in 1976. It has produced a large number of reports and advisory booklets on the hazards of specific chemicals and promoted training in many developing countries. In order to develop a stronger policy impact of the international chemical safety work, the International Forum on Chemical Safety was started in 1994 with about 100 member states. A third collaborative mechanism is the Interorganization Programme for the Sound Management of Chemicals, which also includes FAO, the United Nations Industrial Development Organization, and the Organization for Economic Cooperation and Development (OECD).

INTERNATIONAL TRADE UNION ORGANIZATIONS AND NGOS

Trade unions are important organizations for the implementation of good OSH practices at the local and national level. To support these efforts, trade union federations at international level have developed their own information, training, and action programs. The key player is the International Conference of Free Trade Unions (ICFTU), but there are several large specialized associations of this type (sometimes called the "trade secretariats") with their own OSH activities for member unions at the country level, for example, the International Metalworkers Federation; International Chemical, Energy, Mine and General Workers Federation; International Union of Food and Allied Workers; International Transport Workers Federation; Public Services International (PSI); and so forth.

The focus of the OSH work is different in each organization. For instance, in the International Metalworkers Federation, much of the effort has been devoted to developing and implementing framework agreements with large multinational corporations (e.g., the large car manufacturers), which include all aspects of working conditions. This has ensured that, for metalworkers, OSH issues are not isolated from mainstream union activities. The International Chemical, Energy, and Mining Workers Federation has placed a lot of emphasis on chemical safety activities and the support of protective safety guidelines for the use of specific chemicals, while the Public Services International has focused on the protection of public services including those that provide national OSH activities by governments.

It should also be pointed out that large trade unions in certain industrial countries have traditionally been very active in supporting OSH activities in developing countries. In Sweden, the combined union international cooperation program (LO-TCO joint program) has supported training and union strengthening programs in this field in a number of other countries. In the United States, the United Auto Workers; the Laborers Union; the Paper, Allied-Industrial, Chemical and Energy International Union; and the central union (AFL/CIO) have all been actively involved in international OSH work, as have unions in Canada, Australia, and the United Kingdom. It is notable that the important benefits of labor unions in promoting safe and healthy working conditions are largely absent from developing nations due to the low proportion of organized workers in most of these nations.

Large international professional organizations are also involved in OSH and have played an important role. These include the International Commission on Occupational Health (ICOH) and the International Occupational Hygiene Association (IOHA). ICOH has 2,000 individual members, primarily in the occupational medicine profession, and works through a number of specialized scientific committees. IOHA is an affiliation of more than twenty national occupational hygiene organizations with around 20,000 members.

Business organizations and other business-friendly NGOs are also active in encouraging better OSH practice in corporations. The World Business Council for Sustainable Development is one of the more important organizations (WBCSD, 2004), and discussions about alternative economic development paths have also been on the agenda at the World Economic Forum in Davos.

THE IMPACT OF MAJOR GLOBAL CONFERENCES ON OSH

The United Nations Conference on Environment and Development in Rio 1992 (Earth Summit) adopted Agenda 21 (United Nations, 1993) with a section highlighting the increased role of workers and trade unions. Among the activities to be implemented by the year 2000 mentioned in this section were the following:

- To promote the right to establish trade unions
- To promote ratification of relevant ILO conventions
- To establish mechanisms with bi- or tripartite composition for safety, health, and sustainable development
- To increase the number of treaties on environment issues between the labor market partners
- To reduce the number of work accidents and occupational diseases and to improve the statistical reporting of those
- To increase training for employees, particularly in OSH

In a report on progress in OSH since the Earth Summit, the ICFTU (2002) drew some pessimistic conclusions with an optimistic note on the role of trade unions: almost ten years after the United Nations Earth Summit in Rio de Janeiro, governments have yet to adopt effective measures for worldwide action to counter the alarming pace of environmental degradation. At the same time, the pressures of increased competition and budget cuts are leading to a steady erosion of existing health and safety standards and programs. However, trade unions are taking a leading role in fighting these trends by extending OSH rights into the wider arena of environmental protection and forging new alliances with environmental NGOs. A five-year evaluation of the results of the Earth Summit highlighting the importance of workplace hazards for the implementation of Agenda 21 and for health development was emphasized by WHO (1997).

To address health and social deprivation issues, a meeting of the United Nations in 2001 developed the Millennium Development Goals for poverty reduction, hunger, water and sanitation, education, and communicable disease control (United Nations, 2004) (see chapter 16). These goals do not directly touch upon the conditions of working life, but if achieved by 2015, they will create better living conditions for many of the poorest people who are most affected by hazardous working and living conditions. The lack of specific goals for working conditions and OSH reflects a notion that OSH hazards contribute a minor part of the global burden of disease and injury (which is erroneous, as discussed above) and the notion that adult health is lower priority than child health. However, workers affected by working environment hazards are often powerless to change their conditions, and in the end the health of parents will affect their children's health (Feachem et al., 1992).

The most recent major global conference on development issues was the World Summit on Sustainable Development in Johannesburg in 2002 (United Nations, 2002). It became a controversial affair, as large industrial countries focused their efforts on turning this conference into a forum to discuss trade liberalization issues of importance to them, while developing countries focused on the general imbalance of resources between industrial and developing countries. The impact of trade regulation changes on developing countries and the lack of aid were other issues of disagreement. The conference did not specifically deal with OSH issues, but the result of general development and trade policies will undoubtedly affect OSH.

Finally, the war on Iraq in 2003 is likely to undermine the stated intentions from the World Summit on Sustainable Development, the Millennium Goals, and Agenda 21, by causing countries to divert development aid funds to the "rebuilding Iraq" activities.

GLOBAL RESEARCH NEEDS
FOR OSH

Health research worldwide is characterized by the 10/90 phenomenon: only 10% of health research efforts are devoted to the 90% of the global burden of disease that primarily affect poor peoples, including much of the occupational burden of disease (Hogstedt, 2002). Occupational health research is an important step toward reducing health inequalities, and calls have been made at different occupational health conferences to incorporate occupational health evidence into the requirements for environmental impact assessment of loans and other investments in workplaces in developing countries (Hogstedt, 2002).

The OSH research needs at local levels are driven to a great degree by the "body-count mentality": in order to be taken seriously by local politicians and OSH personnel, OSH hazards that are known to have had major health impacts in other countries must be shown to have the same major impacts in local workplaces. One such example is the absence, during the 1970s, of asbestos cancer prevention in New Zealand, where local cancer research was not yet available, yet despite there being available publications from the United States and United Kingdom in which the risks of asbestos had already been documented. Prevention efforts in New Zealand started in earnest only after asbestos cancer cases were documented locally (Kjellstrom, 2004). We believe that the precautionary principle should be applied to OSH hazards and that effective prevention policies should be initiated before cancer cases occur.

Another area of research in developing countries that is of importance for making a difference to OSH is the systematic study of the impact of different preventive interventions applied to the local context. This would create a record of what works and what does not and would create important "ammunition" in the ongoing discourse about how to get positive OSH outcomes from globalization.

At the global level, research directed at a more refined analysis of the importance of OSH to global health—particularly the burden of disease and injury—is of vital importance. Such analysis would help to put OSH on the agenda for more general health policies, as well as raise the profile of OSH within the health sector.

In order to develop these areas of research and to provide researcher training, the role of national institutes of OSH is critical. A number of countries, both developing and industrial, have institutions with expertise in different areas. Many of these institutions are participants in the WHO network of collaborating centers, which include rich countries as well as industrializing countries such as Mexico, China, India, Vietnam, Egypt, Thailand, and South Africa. In industrial countries, some of the institutes have long experience of supporting research activities in developing countries, particularly institutes in Finland (FIOH), Sweden (NIWL), Denmark (DIOH), Singapore, and the United States (National Institute of Occupational Safety and Health). In the United States, a special program for collaborative research training through the Fogarty International Center at the U.S. National Institutes of Health has been established. An example of the collaboration between Sweden and Nicaragua and Costa Rica has been described in detail (Hogstedt et al., 2001). Another recent example is the new program on Health and Work in Central America (SALTRA).

CONCLUSIONS: CHALLENGES FOR OSH IN AN ERA OF GLOBALIZATION

Globalization with appropriate concern for its social dimensions can be a major force for the positive development of OSH. If ILO conventions and recommendations were accepted as minimum standards in all countries, any competitive advantage stemming from poor labor standards in a particular country would be eliminated. Improved information access through globalization of communications can make it easier for local stakeholders to make their views known when specific OSH issues are debated. Global agreements about banned chemicals and technologies, and other ways to improve OSH at the local level, can be more easily enforced in a globalized system of development.

No comprehensive studies have been carried out that directly study the effects of globalization on working life and related health effects. Most information is based on indirect evidence, aggregated data, or case reports. The lack of systematic comparative studies on the situation before and after the era of globalization (or between work situations in countries or corporations within more or less globalized economies) makes it difficult to quantify or predict the positive and negative effects with any precision. Considering the enormous significance of the effects of globalization on working life, there is an urgent need for more and better studies of these issues.

Specific national or local priorities for OSH need to be considered. The degree of influence of globalization will also vary depending on the context. What is important in one country is not necessarily important in another, because of different types of occupations being prominent, different geographic conditions, or the different development context of the country. At an early development level, traditional work in primary industries dominates. As a country develops economically, industrial work and the service sector usually expand, and the proportion of people working in such industries as agriculture and mining diminishes. At the global level, approximately half of the population (3 billion people) still live in traditional subsistence conditions. For them, the occupational health impact of the changes related to development is enormous. This impact can be positive as traditional hazards diminish, but poor implementation of development can lead to new health risks.

Globalization carried out in a people-centered manner can create improvements in living and working conditions in those areas of the world and those population groups that suffer from social and economic deprivation, as well as from preventable health problems. Such globalization can make use of modern scientific knowledge and available technologies to improve quality of life for the billions of people living in poverty. However, it has to take into account the cultural and social conditions of each community, so that a standardized "Western way of life in a global setting" does not come to be viewed as the only path toward a better life (Eckersley, 2004).

People-centered globalization will depend on resource transfer from the affluent societies to the less affluent ones. This was already accepted in 1970 as a principle for international cooperation within the United Nations, when the benchmark for "foreign aid" was set at 0.7% of the gross domestic product of affluent countries. Only a handful of countries ever achieved this (including Norway, Sweden, and Denmark), and the average for all OECD countries has never risen above 0.33% (see chapter 17).

Another major challenge, which all countries will have to deal with eventually, is the aging of the population and the consequent adaptation of work and how it is organized in a population with large numbers of "elderly" people. This is not an effect of globalization as such, but this demographic development certainly goes hand in hand with the trends of globalization. It will create expanded needs for social security systems and changes in workplaces and workforce utilization that will affect OSH. In addition, an aging workforce may be particularly affected by the stress involved in more rapid work pace and more rapid change of work content and technologies. The ultimate effects could be "burnout" and other stress-induced conditions.

Occupational diseases and injuries are essentially preventable. The approaches to prevention include developing awareness of OSH hazards among workers and employers, assessing the nature and extent of hazards, and introducing and maintaining effective control and evaluation measures (Levy and Wegman, 2000). These measures involve employers and workers within each local workplace. To make this happen efficiently, external involvement is needed. This can range from encouragement by appropriate individuals or agencies outside the specific workplace to promulgate rigorous enforcement of OSH regulations at a national level. International or global policies, statements, and guidelines are also crucial to facilitate good OSH development at the local level.

References

Aiken LH, Buchan J, Sochalski J, Nichols B, Powell M (2004). Trends in international nurse migration. *Health Affairs* 23: 69–77.

Bales K (2004). *Disposable people: new slavery in the global economy*. 2nd ed. Berkeley: University of California Press.

Cogni A (2003). Globalization can help reduce child labour. *CESifo Econ Stud* 49: 515–526.

Delp L, Arriaga M, Palma G, Urita H, Valenzuela A (2004). *NAFTA's labor side agreement fading into oblivion? An assessment of workplace health and safety cases*. Los Angeles: UCLA Center for Labor Research and Education Institute of Industrial Relations.

Eckersley R (2004). *Well and good. How we feel and why it matters*. Melbourne: Text Publishing.

FAO (2003a). *Social dimensions of integrated production and pest management—a case study in Mali*. Rome: Food and Agriculture Organization of the United Nations. http://www.fao.org/sd/2003/PE0501_en.htm

FAO (2003b). *International code of conduct on the distribution and use of pesticides*. Rome: Food and Agriculture Organization of the United Nations. http://www.fao.org/DOCREP/005/Y4544E/Y4544E00.HTM

Fassa AG (2003). *Health benefits of eliminating child labour*. Geneva: International Labour Office.

Fassa AG, Facchini LA, Dall'agnol MM, Christiani DC (2000). Child labor and health: problems and perspectives. *Int J Occup Environ Health* 6: 55–62.

Feachem RGA, Kjellstrom T, Murray CJL, Over M, Phillips MA (eds.) (1992). *The health of adults in the developing world*. Oxford: Oxford University Press.

Forastieri, V (1997). *Children at work: Health and safety risks*. Geneva: International Labour Office.

Fustukian S, Sethi D, Zwi A (2002). Workers health and safety in a globalising world. In: Lee K et al., eds. *Health policy in a globalizing world*. Cambridge: Cambridge University Press, pp. 208–228.

He F (1998). Occupational medicine in China. *Int Arch Occup Environ Health* 71: 79–84.

Herzstein JA, Bunn WB, Fleming LE, Harrington JM, Jeyaratnam J, Gardner IR (eds.) (1998). *International occupational and environmental health*. St. Louis, MO: Mosby.

Hogstedt C (2002). Research needs and priorities for work in the global village. In: Rantanen J et al., eds. *Work in the global village*. People and Work Research Report No. 49. Helsinki: Finnish Institute of Occupational Health, pp. 128–136.

Hogstedt C, Ahlbom A, Aragon A, Castillo L, Kautsky N, Liden C, Lundberg I, Tedengren M, Thorn A, Wesseling C (2001) Experiences from longterm research cooperation between Costa Rican, Nicaraguan and Swedish institutions. *Int J Occup Environ Health* 7: 130–135.

ICFTU (2002). *Report on outcomes of the Earth Summit*. Brussels: International Council of Free Trade Unions. http://www.icftu.org/focus.asp?Issue=ohse&Language=EN

ILO (1999). *ILO Declaration on fundamental principles and rights at work. The "Social Declaration."* Geneva: International Labour Office. http://www.ilo.org/dyn/declaris/DECLARATIONWEB.INDEXPAGE

ILO (2002a). *ILO activities on the social dimension of globalization: Synthesis report*. Geneva: International Labour Office. http://www.ilo.org/public/english/wcsdg/globali/synthesis.pdf

ILO (2002b). *Yearbook of labour statistics*. Geneva: International Labour Office.

ILO (2002c). *Export Processing Zones*. Geneva: International Labour Office. http"//www.ilo/public/english/dialogue/sector/themes/epz.htm

ILO (2002d). *Facts and figures on globalization*. Document from the World Commission on the Social Dimension of Globalization, August 4. Geneva: International Labour Office. http://www.ilo.org/public/english/wcsdg/globali/facts.pdf

ILO (2002e). *Global estimates of occupational mortality from injuries and diseases*. Geneva: International Labour Office. http://www.ilo.org/public/english/protection/safework/accidis/globest_2002/dis_world.htm

ILO (2002f). *Every child counts: New global estimates on child labor*. Geneva: International Labour Office.

ILO (2003a). World Commission on the Social Dimension of Globalization. Geneva: International Labour Office. http://www.ilo.org/public/english/wcsdg/index.htm

ILO (2003b). *LABORSTA, the labour statistics database operated by the ILO Bureau of Statistics*. Geneva: International Labour Office. http://laborsta.ilo.org/

ILO (2004a). *List of ILO conventions and recommendations*. Geneva: International Labour Office. http://www.ilo.org/public/english/protection/safework/standard.htm

ILO (2004b). *Final report of the ILO Commission on the Social Dimension of Globalization.* Geneva: International Labour Office.

Intergovernmental Panel on Climate Change (2001). *Third assessment report.* Geneva: World Meteorological Organization.

International Program on Chemical Safety (1999). *Principles for assessment of risks to human health from exposures to chemicals.* Environmental Health Criteria No. 210. Geneva: World Health Organization and International Programme on Chemical Safety.

Khan F (2002). Africa benefits little from export zones—report. *WOZA J*, April 22. http://www.woza.co.za/apr02/export22.htm.

Kjellstrom T (2004). The epidemic of asbestos diseases in New Zealand. *Int J Occup Environ Health* 10: 212–219.

Kjellstrom T, Koplan JP, Rothenberg RB (1992). Current and future determinants of adult ill health. In: Feachem RGA, Kjellstrom T, Murray CJL, Over M, Phillips MA, eds. *The health of adults in the developing world.* Oxford: Oxford University Press, pp. 209–260.

Kogi K. Phoon W-O, Thurman JE (1989). *Low-cost ways of improving working conditions: 100 examples from Asia.* Geneva: International Labour Office.

LaDou J (1999). DBCP in global context: the unchecked power of multinational corporations. *Int J Occup Environ Health* 5: 151–153.

Landrigan PJ, Costa Dias E, Sokas RK (1998). Vulnerable populations. In: Herzstein JA, Bunn WB, Fleming LE, Harrington JM, Jeyaratnam J, Gardner IR, eds. *International occupational and environmental health.* St. Louis, MO: Mosby, pp. 531–542.

Levy BS, Wegman DH (eds.) (2000). *Occupational health: Recognizing and preventing work-related disease and injury.* 4th ed. Boston: Little, Brown.

London L, de Grosbois S, Wesseling C, Kisting S, Rother HA, Mergler D (2002). Pesticide usage and health consequences for women in developing countries: out of sight, out of mind. *Int J Occup Environ Health* 8: 46–59.

London Hazards Center (2004). *Asbestos alternatives.* London: London Hazards Center. http://www.lhc.org.uk/members/pubs/factsht/59fact.htm.

Lund L (2001). They call it a revolution: Brazil's program to eradicate child labor attacks poverty at its roots with unexpected results. *Spectrum*, winter, pp. 5–7.

Murray CJL, Lopez AD (1996). *The global burden of disease.* Boston, MA: Harvard School of Public Health, World Bank, World Health Organization.

Radford T (2003). Perfect maize, in three simple steps. *Guardian Wkly*, October 16–22.

Razak DA, Latiff AA, Majid MIA, Awang R (1998). Case study: Malaysian information service on pesticide toxicity. In: *Encyclopaedia of Occupational Health and Safety*, Vol. 1, section 22.15. Geneva: International Labour Organization.

Rosling H (2003). *World health chart.* Stockholm: Department of International Health Care, Karolinska Institute. http://www.whc.ki.se/index.php

Sims J (1994). *Women, health and environment: An anthology.* Document WHO/EHG/94.11. Geneva: World Health Organization.

Smith C, Root D (1999). The export of pesticides: shipments from US ports, 1995–1996. *Int J Occup Environ Health* 5: 141–150.

Stellman JM (ed.) (1998). *Encyclopaedia of occupational health and safety.* 4th ed. Vols. 1–4. Geneva: International Labour Organization.

Stiglitz J (2002). *Globalization and its discontents.* London: Penguin Books.

Takala J (1999). Global estimates of fatal occupational accidents. *Epidemiology* 10: 640–646.

United Nations (1993). *Agenda 21.* New York: United Nations.

United Nations (2002). *World summit on sustainable development.* New York: United Nations. http://www.johannesburgsummit.org/

United Nations (2004). *The United Nations Millennium Development Goals.* New York: United Nations. http://www.un.org/millenniumgoals/

Vaknin S (2003). *Processing the export zones.* United Press International. http://www.upi.com/view.cfm?StoryID=20030210-012415-8430r.

WBCSD (2004). *Activities of the WBCSD.* New York: World Business Council for Sustainable Development. http://www.wbcsd.ch/templates/Template WBCSD4/layout.asp?MenuID=1

Wesseling C, McConnell R, Partanen T, and Hogstedt C (1997). Agricultural pesticide use in developing countries: health effects and research needs. *Int J Health Serv* 27: 273–308.

WHO (1990). *Public health impact of pesticides used in agriculture.* Geneva: World Health Organization.

WHO (1995). *Global strategy on occupational health for all: The way to health at work.* Recommendations of the Second Meeting of the WHO Collaborating Centres in Occupational Health, October 11–14, Beijing, China. Geneva: World Health Organization.

WHO (1997). *Health and environment in sustainable development. Five years after the Earth Summit.* Document WHO/EHG/97.8. Geneva: World Health Organization.

WHO (1999). *Occupational health.* Fact Sheet No. 84. Geneva: World Health Organization.

WHO (2002). *World health report 2002.* Geneva: World Health Organization.

World Bank (1993). *World development report 1993.* Washington, DC: World Bank.

Chapter 9

Population Movements

Pascale Allotey and Anthony Zwi

A consequence of globalization has been the unprecedented increase in the movement of people, within and across national borders, between regions, and globally. The International Organization for Migration (IOM) estimates that about 3% of the world's population (175 million people) are residing outside their country of birth (IOM 2003a), a figure that has doubled over a period of three decades. Migration is motivated by a range of factors, but in broad terms, it is characterized, on the one hand, by voluntary migration in search of better opportunities and, on the other, by forced migration resulting from violence, persecution, and environmental disasters. Between these is a spectrum of experiences reflecting complex interacting forces that not only affect the extent and characteristics of agency in the decision to migrate but also have long-term health implications for those involved.

These complexities present one of the greatest challenges to public health today. The evolution of the discipline has been based on factors affecting individuals, their environment, and the interaction of these within a social, political, and cultural context. Public health practitioners engage with governments and political processes, challenging the state to provide and facilitate the development of the physical and social infrastructure necessary to promote and maintain the public health of its citizens. Within this framework and the boundaries of its predictability, the principles and practice of public health can be informed by an evidence base that guides, among other things, a "rational" allocation of health and welfare resources.

However, increasing migration has resulted in governments questioning their obligations toward noncitizens resident within their borders (Tiburcio 2001; Ghosh 2003a, 2003b). There is increasing differentiation between the rights and entitlements of citizens and noncitizens (Richmond 1994; ICHRP 2000; Taran 2000; de Bousingen 2002). This notion of the "deserving and undeserving" citizen takes precedence over general approaches to public health practice. In restricting the access of goods and services to noncitizens, states sanction the "othering" of subsections of the population and promote marginalization and the establishment of underclasses. These are known to lead to poor health outcomes. Under these circumstances, the challenge to public health practice is to engage more directly with political processes.

The resistance to in-migration is targeted at particular groups and depends largely on the category under which migrants arrive. It is closely related to two key features: the ability of the migrant to be self-supporting and independent of the public purse, and the degree to which the host population perceives their degree of choice in accepting the new migrant into the community. For migrant populations, the degree to which they have a choice in their decision to migrate is often blurred, given that they are subject to so many competing pressures and influences.

In this chapter, we present an analysis of migration and health with a focus on a broadly defined concept of forced or "compelled" migration. We highlight the influence of structures created through globalization on the level of agency of mobile populations. We argue that globalization has had a paradoxical effect on migration and the health particularly of the migrating populations. The primary focus of the discussion is on the ethical and humanitarian challenges presented by the "othering" of migrant groups. These issues are often regarded as outside the purview of public health because of the lack of an "evidence" base (for discussion, see Susser 1993; Rothman, Adami et al. 1998; Susser and Susser 1999) but nonetheless need to be explored to address the vulnerabilities created by globalization (Beaglehole and Bonita 1997).

CATEGORIES OF MIGRATION

The migration literature refers broadly to two main categories of migrants, economic or voluntary and forced or involuntary migrants (Castles 2003). These are broad categories, often ill-defined and blurred at their point of overlap. The classifications are nonetheless important because the political and legal definitions of the designated categories determine aspects of the journeys undertaken in the process of migration, the resulting exposure to health risks, and, in the country of settlement, entitlements and access to goods and services such as health care. The categories

also indicate the preparedness of host communities to accept and accommodate the new comers as part of their community (Walzer 1981; Reidpath, Chen et al. 2004).

Voluntary Migrants

Voluntary or economic migrants are those who migrate largely for reasons that relate to employment, opportunity, and family. They range from the few who take over multimillion dollar corporations, to professionals in the health, business, and information technology sectors, to the much larger numbers who engage in low-wage labor. The latter overlaps with various forms of forced migration, including those who have to seek employment opportunities elsewhere because of economic failures and high unemployment at home. For many from poorer economies, migration provides opportunities to improve their financial situation and invest in a better future for themselves and their families (Jasso, Rosenzweig et al. 2003). The International Labor Organization estimated that, in 2000, 130 million people were working as migrants compared to 75 million in 1965 (ILO 2000).

Voluntary migration is ideally regulated through procedures determined by national departments responsible for immigration. In broad terms, decisions are made at the state level about the quota of immigrants for any particular year, based loosely on national priorities for the skilled workforce and a population policy for the desired demographic targets and the distribution of the population across the nation. For these migrants, any negative impact they may have on the welfare system is weighed against a broader contribution to the economy and social fabric of the receiving community (Weiner 1996).

The rights and entitlements of immigrants in a receiving country are also regulated by states' authorities. While basic human rights are universal and nonderogable, that is, they are core rights that are not negotiable and that cannot be suspended, the recognition of the human rights of aliens or noncitizens as opposed to citizens has, in recent years, been subject to narrow interpretation (Tiburcio 2001; Ghosh 2003a, 2003b). For instance, protection against racial and ethnic discrimination in the workplace (ILO 1999), poor occupational health standards, and poor access to health care, education, and housing (Ghosh 2003a) are often raised as problems faced by the low-paid migrant workforce usually required for "3D" (dirty, demanding, and dangerous) jobs (UNESCO 2003).

The International Convention on all Migrant Workers and their Families addresses many of the issues related to the vulnerability of different groups of migrants. To date, however, it has been ratified by only 20 countries (Ghosh 2003b).

Women and Migration

An important change in the demographic profile of voluntary migrants is the increase in the numbers of women migrating as potential participants in the labor market and principal breadwinners for their families and not just as family members of a principal breadwinner (IOM 2003a). Based on data from 1990, the United Nations estimated that females accounted for 48% of migration (IOM 2003d). However, the ratio of women to men migrating may be almost double in some countries. In Nepal for instance, the ratio was 251 women to every 100 men[1] (IOM 2003d).

On the one hand, the "feminization of migration" demonstrates the positive outcomes of globalization for women. More women from poorer developing countries have been able to obtain paid employment and have the opportunity to travel and become economically and socially independent of cultures that can be repressing. The increased availability of affordable migrant providers of care for young children, elderly parents, and disabled relatives has also enabled women in wealthier countries to join or remain in the work force (Ehrenreich and Hochschild 2004). On the other, the exposure of women to poor employment conditions highlights the potential vulnerabilities that need to be reflected in a system that is able to respond appropriately to the gender implications of migration (Staab 2004). The poor conditions for a very large domestic work force of women from poorer to wealthier countries (e.g., between South and North America, or Asian to Middle Eastern countries) as well as within countries (rural to urban areas) and between lower income countries (within the Asia Pacific region) have generated a large body of literature (Dankelman, Davidson et al. 1988; World Bank 1995; Zlotnik 1998; Taran 2000; Agustin 2003; Ghosh 2003a). With lack of knowledge about their rights and entitlements, they fail to present for health care when it is needed with poor longer term consequences. Poor health is also intertwined with the adverse social, economic, and institutional factors that characterize low-wage earners and their families. Sexually transmitted infections and being subject to gender-based violence are two important adverse findings.

There is some concern about the negative impact on families of women migrating for work. While their independence may have positive outcomes for them as individuals, there are implications to the change in the family dynamics with families left behind and to the evolution of relationships with husbands and children. In addition, their absence may create a care deficit for their children and disabled or elderly relatives—a role that many fill for other women in wealthier countries (Ehrenreich and Hochschild 2004). The resulting breakdown of their families further provides the motivation for their family members to emigrate.

Forced Migrants

Forced migrants are generally described as those who have no choice in the decision to leave their homes and move because of an imperative to secure their own survival. Refugees are persons outside their country of origin and who for demonstrable reasons can no longer rely on their governments to protect their human rights. The 1951 Convention and 1967 Protocol on the Status of Refugees provide the foundations in international and refugee law for the protection and the rights of refugees. In acknowledgment of the serious human rights violations and vulnerability, member states of the United Nations that have ratified the convention and protocol undertake to protect refugees. They also agree to respect the principle of non-*refoulement*, that is, not to return a refugee to the country from which they fear persecution. The acceptance of refugees is argued on the basis of the moral claims of refugees and the humanitarian obligations countries assume in ratifying the relevant international instruments.

Assuming a relatively uncomplicated world, voluntary and forced migrants as described above would not present major obstacles to state authorities and standard migration procedures—as long as they possessed appropriate documentation to support their legitimacy. Voluntary migration would be in response to a receiving country's projected needs for immigration and forced migrants would enable the demonstration of largesse, humanitarianism, and global citizenship. However, as highlighted above, a dichotomous classification of motivation for migration fails to reveal the complex and powerful forces in operation. From the broader context of globalization, the dynamics of forced migration result from a range of distal factors interacting to compel emigration.

COMPELLED EMIGRATION IN THE CONTEXT OF GLOBALIZATION

The gains produced by uniform regulatory environments, transnational corporations, and trade agreements have opened up new opportunities, economic growth has accelerated, and standards of living have improved for many. However, the benefits of these changes have been unequally distributed with advantages unevenly spread within a small number of countries (Annan 2000a). The rapid changes that have occurred in the last 10 years include a reduction in social welfare safety nets and greater vulnerability of groups marginalized through poverty, ethnicity, and other social factors, including migration status. Extreme poverty that threatens survival and sustenance has been described as hindering the fulfillment of economic, social, and cultural rights (WHO 2003). Failing the amelioration of the structural determinants of these disadvantages, mobility toward relatively wealthier communities and countries, even for low-paid unskilled labor, is arguably a necessity and an important response to the global labor market (Ghosh 2003b; IOM 2003d; Pritchett 2003). The demand for cheap labor clearly exists.

The inequalities brought about by globalization have also been linked with the loss of long-held traditional mores, cultures, and practices because the global market has shown little consideration for shared social objectives (Annan 2000a). So while globalization may have reduced the need for territorial annexation and cross border conflict (Annan 2000b), for instance, the unequal distribution of limited resources has had an impact at a local level. Inequalities have precipitated long-dormant tensions, civil strife, generalized violence, and armed internal conflict (Lipschutz and Crawford 1999). Wars today are usually characterized by low intensity but often protracted internal insurgencies. Over the last decade, Asia and Africa have consistently recorded over 15 armed conflicts every year; medium- to high-intensity conflicts have persisted in the Middle East (WHO 2002). With the opening of markets and removal of

limitations on the sale of small arms, insurgents no longer need to be particularly well organized or wealthy to gain access to weapons (Lumpe 2000). In many conflicts, the combatants have neither a clear political allegiance nor an idea of who represents the enemy. Civilians have become the targets for negotiating political agendas and are no longer protected by the "rules of engagement." In recent larger scale wars such as in Iraq and Afghanistan, armed strikes have occurred within cities, with little distinction made between military targets and residential areas. The proportion of civilians affected by conflict continues to be extremely high despite the availability of more sophisticated, high-precision weapons. In addition, low technology such as machetes in Rwanda and terror and plunder in Darfur in western Sudan continue to be very effective mechanisms for genocide. Recent internal conflicts have claimed in excess of 5 million lives (Murray, King et al. 2002). These numbers are reflected in the case load of asylum seekers fleeing conflict but who do not meet the criteria for refugee status under the convention (UNHCR 2000).

Direct deaths from complex humanitarian emergencies rank in the top 12 most common causes of death worldwide, and projections are for them to become the eighth most common cause by 2020 (Murray, King et al. 2002). Health risks inevitably increase for these populations, who often have preexisting poor health due to the multiple disadvantages that also make them vulnerable to conflict. For instance, a significant proportion of infectious disease epidemics occur in unstable countries, typically with high rates of mortality (Zwi 1996).

There have been numerous indirect health effects of recent conflicts that create challenges for consistency of measurement of morbidity and mortality in these situations. While injury and fatality from direct trauma are easier to ascertain, deaths that result from malnutrition, infectious diseases, dangerous journeys, and unhealthy conditions in refugee camps are more difficult to classify. The highest mortality is in children, but women are also particularly vulnerable. Consistent reports of rape, sexual exploitation, and sexual abuse suffered by women account for high rates of sexually transmitted diseases and a range of reproductive and mental health conditions. The women-at-risk category was created by the United Nations High Commissioner for Refugees (UNHCR) specifically in recognition of the inordinately high risk faced by women in displaced populations who are without the "protection" of a male family member (Manderson, Kelaher et al. 1998; Bartolomei, Pittaway et al. 2003).

At the same time, with increased availability of information, there has been a globalization of rights: a wider global awareness of human rights issues (Bengoa 1997). When individuals can no longer rely on their nation-states to protect their human rights, there is a greater tendency to either seek refuge with other states that recognize and protect the rights of individuals or seek protection from the international system responsible for the implementation of universal norms (Adelman 1999). For example, arguments are now presented by human rights activists for the international protection of women and girl children at risk of female genital cutting (Copelon 2000; Kelley 2001) or Chinese couples in breach of their government's one-child policy.

Other poorly recognized causes of forced displacement include development projects funded through bilateral and multilateral agreements and natural and man-made environmental disasters. These often leave survivors without homes or livelihoods. The World Bank estimates that approximately 10 million people are displaced from their homes every year to accommodate development projects alone (McDowell 1996; Cernea and McDowell 2000). The Three Gorges Dam across the Yangtze displaced more than a million people and has been associated with poor health conditions and a resurgence of endemic infections (Sleigh and Jackson 1998). Although displacees under these situations may have access to some international aid, they are not eligible for official international protection.

The net effect of these factors on population movements is an osmotic force that draws people from countries with a lower concentration of wealth and opportunity, to richer ones, and from poorer rural areas to wealthier urban ones. A similar process is created by complex humanitarian emergencies resulting from internal conflicts and other disasters, which encourage the movement of people away from their regions to seek asylum or livelihoods in more stable, towns, regions, and countries. Annual requests for asylum in Western Europe, Australia, Canada, and the United States increased more than eightfold over the ten-year period from 1983 to 1993, from fewer than 100,000 to more than 800,000 (Castles 2003), reflecting the increase in conflict and instability in the countries of origin of the asylum seekers. It is also

noteworthy that the movement is multidirectional and not only toward countries in the "north." Almost half (45%) of the volume of migration occurs between countries of relatively similar levels of economic development (UNESCO 2003). Similarly two-thirds of refugees reside in neighboring developing countries and do not seek to resettle in the wealthier, northern nations (Allotey and Reidpath 2003).

The Resistance to Migration

The direction of migration is countered by an increasingly impermeable barrier representing the reluctance of host countries to accept migrants particularly from poorer countries. Most countries have introduced stringent procedures for immigration, with a requirement to demonstrate financial independence or a legitimate means of ensuring livelihoods outside the state-provided (where applicable) social welfare safety net. In recognition of the global market demands for migrant labor, some countries have tried to control labor migration through programs such as the guest worker programs in Europe and Japan, to enable *temporary* employment-related settlement. In addition, penalties are imposed on employers who employ illegal migrant workers. Whether actively applied or not, this thrusts illegal workers into the background and reduces their access or willingness to access goods and services. There is no evidence that these measures have reduced the potential flows in search of employment and opportunities (Cornielius 1992).

The criteria for selection of "acceptable" migrants often result in a level of selectivity that arguably reflects preferences on the basis of race, ethnicity, or religion (Weiner 1996). However, it is ultimately the sovereign right of states to determine who can enter their borders.

There always has been and always will be some resistance to immigration. Accepting immigrants necessarily entails the sharing of resources, which in some countries may already be stretched. Migrants are often prepared to work for lower wages that may disrupt the existing labor market, and when the migrating groups are from different cultures, they may present a perceived threat to the existing culture and way of life.

To many, resisting these threats through closed borders appears reasonable (Weiner 1996). Indeed academics like Michael Walzer (1983) argue the morality of maintaining a particular way of life and sense of identity as a stable feature of human life, even at the cost of refusal of potential immigrants (Walzer 1983). By this argument, the obligations governments have toward their citizens are much greater than toward those who do not belong to the community. An international social survey showed that most people take this position and would resist any migration rate higher than 10% (Mayda 2002).

More recent arguments for restricted immigration have focused on the strong need to maintain security, stability, and sovereignty through border control. Terrorist activities across the globe have heightened the suspicion and general antipathy toward nonnationals and immigrants. The media has had a significant role in both reporting and, to a large extent, influencing the debate and, ultimately, governments' policies on migration (O'Shaughnessy 1999). The availability of information through the media has been one of the key successes of globalization, but despite the claim to convey objective news and information, the public interest role of the media often stands in conflict with the need to engage and hold audiences (Mares and Allotey 2003). Audiences in homes worldwide have been witness to confronting vivid images of armed conflict, ethnic and communal violence, human suffering, and vulnerability (Mares and Allotey 2003). Mares and Allotey (2003) highlight the contradictory reactions to images that largely reflect similar stories: the shared anxiety with and support for the solo English adventurer awaiting rescue in the capsized hull of a state-of-the-art yacht versus the antipathy, fear, and aggression toward a boatload of Afghan asylum seekers risking their lives in an unseaworthy vessel in a bid for protection (Mares and Allotey 2003). In a similar twist, the same media that reported the arrival of temporary evacuees from Kosovo to Australia in 1999 with unrestrained generosity described them as ingrates for not showing "beggars gratitude" when they protested about the condition of their residential facilities, and then as pariahs when many expressed a reluctance to return due to fears of continued persecution (Mares 2001).

Coverage in the Western media of the large numbers of those affected by disasters, conflicts, and violence is relatively limited and usually biased. The narrative technique elicits sympathy as long as those affected remain in distant lands. Sympathy is rapidly lost when the vulnerable victims show tenacity and temerity to reach the borders of receiving countries. When they seize agency and seek to get their stories

in the media, the clampdown is rapid and severe. In addition, the media focus on the demonization of insurgents (to the exclusion of critical analyses of possible causes of uprising) has been adeptly generalized to larger groups of migrants particularly from less developed countries who do not arrive under an authorized migration program (Gaita 2001; Manne 2001). Using voter reaction as a proxy for general community views on migration, it is clear that these views resonate with a significant majority of the population (Zelinka 1996; Mateen and Titemore 1999; McMaster 2001; de Bousingen 2002; Glèlè-Ahanhanzo 2002; Mares 2002; Ghosh 2003b; Mares and Allotey 2003; WHO 2003). The rise in xenophobia is demonstrated by the wave of anti-immigration sentiment across most of Europe, North America, and Australia (Allotey 2004). Even countries in Africa that have traditionally accepted the greatest proportion of asylum seekers fleeing from political unrest in neighboring countries are beginning to tire of playing host to neighbors in distress (Vas Dev 2003). In addition, donor fatigue, present for the last few years and manifesting as declining commitment to development assistance, limits the commitment to support others less fortunate.

Countering the Resistance

The sheer numbers of those "compelled" to emigrate and of asylum seekers have overwhelmed the international protection system and the goodwill that states feel they have the capacity to provide. There has also been some "abuse" of the humanitarian protection system by those who do not meet the strict refugee criteria and are regarded as economic migrants (Allotey 2004). Rather than deter potential migrants, however, restrictive immigration has resulted in an increase in undocumented and irregular forms of migration that circumvent the legal procedures instituted to regulate movements across borders. Human trafficking and smuggling are a major form of people movements today. Trafficking and people smuggling are recognized as high-return, low-risk endeavors that appeal to major, transnational organized crime.

Irregular Migration

Trafficking involves the illegal trading and movement of mostly (but not exclusively) women and children in economically exploitative situations often taking advantage of the sociocultural undervaluing of women and girls. Those trafficked are usually expected to engage in forced domestic labor, sex work, false marriages, and indentured labor. There is an increasing market in the sex industry supported through tourism and a market in children trafficked for adoption (UNICEF 2004).

Trafficking is not new, and many countries have significant populations of the descendants of people who were originally trafficked as slaves. However, centuries after the abolition of the slave trade, people trafficking is on the increase. A recent IOM study revealed that at any one time there are an estimated 15–30 million irregular migrants worldwide. Of this total, the best estimates provided by the U.S. Department of Justice are between 2 million and 7 million women and children (IOM 2001). The numbers of irregular migrants and trafficked persons are likely to remain significantly underreported, and while reliable statistics are kept on the arrest and detention of unauthorized migrants at borders and on arrests of traffickers, these figures account for a small fraction of the overall problem (IOM 2003b).

People smuggling is defined by the United Nations 2000 Protocol against Smuggling of Migrants by Land, Sea, and Air as "the procurement, in order to obtain, directly or indirectly, a financial or other material benefit, of illegal entry of a person into a State Party of which the person is not a national or permanent resident" (United Nations 2000a, Article 3, section a). Unlike trafficking, people smuggling reflects a commercial rather than exploitative transaction, although like most illegal transactions it is difficult to argue that the partners are equal. Smuggled migrants are usually "economic" migrants or asylum seekers who for various reasons may not have access to or may have been refused the authorized migration or international protection systems.

In reality, the difference between these forms of movement is blurred. Trafficking and smuggling may present the only opportunities individuals or families have to lift themselves out of economic hardship (Schaeffer 2003). There is vigorous debate between protection and legislative bodies, on the one hand, and advocates for those who exercise their agency and "choose" to enter into the above arrangements, on the other (Doezema 1998). One of the largest studies of brothel workers conducted in Israel showed that out of 45 women labeled as trafficked, 64% reported that

they had been sold with their consent, preferring to be described as *transferred* from another country. While they had not anticipated the risks and poor work conditions, 89% reported that they engaged in prostitution of their own volition and knew what was expected when they left their countries of origin, mostly Eastern Europe (Cwikel, Ilan et al. 2003).

Under international law, smuggling is considered a crime against the state; trafficking is a crime against the person. This is an important distinction because on apprehension, the smuggled person, as a party to an illegal transaction, is considered a criminal. Notwithstanding the crime, smuggled persons are entitled to be treated with dignity and, in the event of detention, under the provisions of the Geneva Convention (United States Committee on Refugees 2003). A trafficked person, under international law, however, is considered a victim of coercion, abduction, fraud, or deception. Under these circumstances, consent is regarded as lacking or defective and, consequently, irrelevant (United Nations 2000a, Article 3, section a). States that are party to the Protocol to Prevent, Suppress and Punish Trafficking in Persons (United Nations 2000b) are therefore mandated to provide temporary or permanent protection to trafficked persons (Article 18, section 1). That notwithstanding, many countries do not distinguish between the circumstances of irregular and undocumented migrants (Cwikel, Ilan et al. 2003), and trafficked persons are just as likely to end up in detention centers. The conditions under which they are detained remain a constant source of concern to groups such as Amnesty International and Human Rights Watch (Human Rights Watch 2002).

In addition to issues of sovereignty and security, there are obvious health and humanitarian reasons that demand a global response to trafficking and people smuggling. The journeys of smuggled and trafficked persons are often fraught with danger in order to circumvent legal controls. Over a one-year period (1999–2000), the IOM obtained reports of 435 deaths that included drowning in unseaworthy vessels, attacks from pirates, suffocations in containers and vehicles, prolonged exposure to heat or cold, or injury from the traffickers (Migration and Health 2000a). In a single incident, more than 350 people drowned when their ship sank in an attempt to seek asylum in Australia on October 19, 2001. There are frequent reports of drowning off the Mediterranean Coast as people try to enter Europe (IOM 2003b). Approximately 400,000 people a year undertake these high-risk journeys to enter the European Union illegally (O'Kelly 2001).

The potential for exploitation and human rights violations through these illegal avenues is necessarily high because of the lack of legal status of the people being smuggled or trafficked. Because they have to pay back a debt or are indentured to traffickers and smugglers, undocumented migrants frequently find themselves confined to sweatshops or factories or forced into prostitution or begging. HIV rates in women trafficked for prostitution are at least as high as the rates among prostitutes in general (Gender Matters Quarterly 1999), for instance, 31% in Mandalay, Burma, and 44% in Phnom Penh, Cambodia, collected from centers for sexual tourism and trafficking (Gender Matters Quarterly 1999). Where sex workers are organized for their own protection, infections have been found to be better controlled compared to prostitution controlled by organized crime (Gender Matters Quarterly 1999).

Some undocumented migrants may have preexisting illnesses endemic in their countries of origin and show disease patterns reflective of poverty, undernutrition, lack of education, and other social determinants of health (Gushulak and MacPherson 2000). Where diseases are acquired in transit, there is little access to health care en route (Migration and Health 2000b). Access to legal assistance and medical care is limited, if available, and ill health is less effectively managed in undocumented migrants than in host communities (Johnston 2003).

The risks involved are related not only to poor travel conditions but also to the potential for human rights abuses when detained by the authorities in some of the transit countries or on arrival in the destination country. Amnesty International and Human Rights Watch document inhumane overcrowded conditions in which undocumented migrants are kept in a number of countries (WHO 2003). Reviews of conditions in immigration detention centers including in Australia are not dissimilar and in particular highlight the mental health effects of detention on children (Bhagwati 2002; Pittaway and Bartolomei 2003; HREOC 2004). For those fleeing war, and victims of trafficking, preexisting trauma related to the conflict experience has been exacerbated by the experience of detention (Silove, McIntosh et al. 1993; Silove, Curtis et al. 1996; Silove, Steel et al. 2000, 2001; Silove 2002). Mental health distress is highlighted by the frequently reported incidents of hunger

strikes and self-harm, such as lip stitching and suicide attempts (Sultan and O'Sullivan 2001).

Detention as a policy for irregular migration has become so successful that it has supported the burgeoning of a transnational industry in the provision of detention facilities and services. Not only is the management of detention centers contracted out to private companies, but also the provision of minimum basic services required by detainees such as food and health care is tendered out for competitive bidding (ADIMIA 2004). For private security companies, protection of the human rights of the detainees is secondary to the financial benefits of entering into such a contract with state governments. For state governments, the privatization of detention centers affords "moral immunity" from questions that arise from bodies monitoring human rights violations about the treatment of those in detention (HREOC 2004).

Other policies designed to deter potential irregular immigrants include severely restricting the rights and entitlements of asylum seekers in detention and following their release, even when they are determined to have a genuine claim for refugee status. Temporary protection is offered requiring regular review of conditions in the countries of origin to determine the appropriateness of repatriation. The state of limbo has the effect of further prolonging the disruption created by the conflict or the trigger that forced the migration in the first place. Temporary protection in itself does not breech international obligations; many host countries have granted temporary protection to large groups of asylum seekers in humanitarian crisis situations. Temporary "safe haven" granted by the Australian government to the large numbers of Kosovar Albanians in 1999 fleeing ethnic cleansing provides a case in point (Smith and Harvey 2003). However, in its policy, Australia has set a precedent in according temporary protection to individuals who have undergone the rigorous screening to establish their refugee status. These policies are designed to discourage potential asylum seekers from considering Australia as an easy destination country (McMaster 2001, 2002; Mares 2002).

In the United Kingdom, restrictive welfare policies toward undocumented asylum seekers have been extended to create markers for stigmatization. Asylum seekers were issued vouchers instead of money for purchases redeemable in designated supermarkets. Furthermore, a ban was placed on the accessibility of "leisure" goods such as tobacco and alcohol with vouchers. They were subject to compulsory dispersal to separate them from the mainstream community and were restricted in access to employment and housing (Bloch and Schuster 2002; Sales 2002).

THE CHALLENGES FOR PUBLIC HEALTH

The traditional focus on classical communicable disease screening prearrival or on arrival for infectious tuberculosis, intestinal parasites, sexually transmitted diseases, malaria, and, more recently, HIV (Migration and Health 200b) remains critical. There is no denying that travel and migration have helped to spread contagious diseases. Indeed, communicable diseases have been the target of media stigmatization of asylum seekers, encouraging fear of contagion from exotic diseases (Mares and Allotey 2003).

It is clear, however, that the health issues from a population perspective are more complex than just communicable disease control. Migration can proffer both advantages and disadvantages to the health of migrants, host populations, and people remaining in the countries of origin. Recent epidemiological studies of migrants, diasporas, and the healthy migrant effect have contributed to the understanding of the complex effects of social determinants such as race and ethnicity on health outcomes. We also have a better understanding of the interactions between genetics, place of birth, environment, and country of residence factors (David and Collins 1991; Geronimus 2002; McKay, Macintyre et al. 2003).

The health advantages, particularly of voluntary migrants, are lost with increasing period of residence as their health profiles begin to mirror that of the host population. In addition, the indicators for the healthy migrant effect do not take into account the sometimes deleterious psychosocial effects of the broader societal context in the country of resettlement. The well-being of individuals is strongly associated with some degree of stability and predictability in social relations as well as the physical environment. Resettling populations have to cope with the challenge of adapting to new societies, disruption of social and cultural connections, discrimination, and xenophobia (de Bousingen 2002). Research consistently demonstrates poorer mental and emotional health and well-being in many migrant groups (de Bousingen 2002; McKay, Macintyre et al. 2003; UNESCO 2003; WHO 2003).

Access to health services clearly depends on legal status even though states have a legal responsibility for the health of those within their jurisdiction. Guest workers on temporary residence permits for instance would not have access to health insurance or universal health coverage schemes. They also tend to be low wage earners, and the cost of health care can therefore be prohibitive. A study in the United States found that three-quarters of a sample of Hispanic workers did not have access to health insurance, a quarter were at high risk for heart disease, but only 7% were covered by government-sponsored health care (Hanson 2002). As highlighted above, the situation is often worse for irregular migrants.

Detailed discussions on the health of receiving populations and those in countries of origin are beyond the scope of this chapter. However, the implications of increasing social disharmony in receiving countries are important to highlight in the context of increasing xenophobia. The restriction of resources to sections of a population does have consequences for the mainstream, and this has been demonstrated historically through policies that have disenfranchised indigenous groups (Rowse 1992; Mooney 2002) and racial minorities (Reidpath 2003).

There are other important public health effects of global movements. Movements of refugees and internally displaced populations can improve the health status of communities in proximity to temporary settlement and camps. There is evidence of improved health as a result of access to the increased injection of resources through international assistance and health services (Toole and Bhatia 1992; Toole, Waldman et al. 2001; Toole 2003).

The brain drain is a major concern in global movements, particularly its effects on the health sector. Populations in sending countries clearly benefit from remittances sent by émigrés. The World Bank (2003) identifies a number of countries for which remittances provide the second highest source of foreign income. However, the countries of origin are also disadvantaged by reduction in professional capacity. Developing country governments in countries such as the Philippines invest in building the capacity of the health workforce, an investment that is lost to such countries as the United States (Buchan and Sachalski 2004). For countries with a lack of quality training facilities, the loss of personnel results from potential trainees leaving to seek educational opportunities elsewhere and then taking advantage of better work conditions than would be available in the country of origin (Saravia and Miranda 2004).

A further consequence of the brain drain in the health sector is the effect on the cost of health services. The higher demand and limited supply of health professionals who remain in their countries of origin make the increase in health care costs almost inevitable. In addition, greater incentives for employment in the private health sector encourage movement of qualified staff from cheaper, subsidized public health systems to private facilities that offer better quality service and superior infrastructure but beyond the price range of the majority of the population.

CONCLUSION

The majority of people moving are doing so to counter poverty, lack of opportunities, conflict, exploitation, and environmental circumstances beyond their control. A significant change in the trends in population movement is unlikely (IOM 2003c) even though it is clear that many of the public health challenges result from the tensions between the desire or need migrate and the willingness of host countries to accept open migration as a viable policy. It has been argued that free migration, open borders, and automatic conferring of citizenship rights on individuals seeking a new life would threaten public health, stretch social and welfare services to the limit, and create politicide (see Carens 1979, 1992, 1996; Singer and Singer 1988; Weiner 1996). However, agreements on open borders as an economic consideration appear to have been reasonably successful within regions such as the European Union and the Economic Community of West African States. Limited restrictions occur among countries of the Organization for Economic Cooperation and Development, with visa waiver schemes for some degree of movement between countries. However, extending these agreements to include poorer nations and redress some of the disadvantage caused through globalization changes the argument to a moral one and is more complicated to address without political will.

It is clear that the response needs to be global. The control of emigration and immigration needs to be a joint responsibility of both sending and receiving countries. The reasons for emigration need to be tackled as vigorously as the efforts to control the borders in receiving countries. This means addressing the causes of instability and poverty, human rights abuses, and marginalization. It also requires addressing social as well as economic agendas in various bilateral and multilateral agreements.

Coordinating immigration polices and addressing humanitarian responses uniformly is also critical. Even within regions, policies for receiving and supporting refugees and asylum seekers differ. Any single country that opens up its borders to open migration does indeed run the risk of being overrun in a world where there are vast inequalities, a range of repressive regimes and a heterogeneity of cultures, health status, levels of wealth, and education.

The current focus on deterrence through punitive and marginalizing policies for migrants already in host countries is reactive and counterproductive, and the effects on social exclusion are already being documented (Sales 2002). In addition, these policies are often in direct conflict in their effect, if not in intent, with strategies to protect migrants, also coordinated through globalized responses of the United Nations organizations.

Finally, for public health to be effective, universal access is required. Health policy cannot be implemented within a context that actively excludes sections of the population who by definition may require greatest access to health promotion and health care.

Note

1. Note that, in some countries, the higher percentage of women reflects trafficking rather than voluntary migration. This is discussed in greater detail later in the chapter.

References

Adelman, H. (1999). Modernity, globalization, refugees and displacement. In: *Refugees: Perspectives on the experience of forced migration*. A. Ager, ed. London, Pinter: 83–110.

Agustin, L. (2003). Forget victimization: granting agency to migrants. *Development* 46(1): 30–36.

Allotey, P. (2004). Refugee health. In: *Encyclopedia of medial anthropology: Health and illness in the world's cultures*. C. R. Ember and M. Ember, eds. New York, Kluwer Academic/Plenum Publishers, 1: 191–197.

Allotey, P., and D. Reidpath (2003). Refugee intake: reflections on inequality. *Aust N Z J Public Health* 27(1): 12–16.

Annan, K. (2000a). Freedom from fear. In: 'We the peoples': The role of the United Nations in the 21st century. *Report of the UN Secretary General to the Millennium Assembly.* New York, United Nations: 43–53.

Annan, K. (2000b). Globalization and governance. In: *'We the peoples': The role of the United Nations in the 21st Century. Report of the UN Secretary General to the Millennium Assembly.* New York, United Nations: 9–17.

ADIMIA (2004). Unauthorised arrivals and detention. Information paper. Canberra, Australian Department of Immigration and Multicultural and Indigenous Affairs.

Bartolomei, L., E. Pittaway, et al. (2003). Who am I? Identity and citizenship in Kakuma refugee camp in Northern Kenya. *Development* 46(3): 87–93.

Beaglehole, R., and R. Bonita (1997). *Public health at the crossroads: Achievements and prospects.* Cambridge, Cambridge University Press.

Bengoa, J. (1997). *The relationship between the enjoyment of human rights, in particular economic social and cultural rights and income distribution. E/CN.4/Sub.2/1997/9.* Geneva, United Nations High Commissioner for Refugees.

Bhagwati, P. (2002). Detention centres in Australia. Geneva, United Nations High Commissioner for Human Rights.

Bloch, A., and L. Schuster (2002). Asylum and welfare: contemporary debates. *Crit Soc Policy* 22(3): 393–413.

Buchan, J., and J. Sachalski (2004). The migration of nurses: trends and policies. *Bull World Health Organ* 82(8): 587–594.

Carens, J. (1979). Aliens and citizens: the case for open borders. *Rev Politics* 49(2): 251–273.

Carens, J. (1992). Migration and morality: a liberal egalitarian perspective. In: *Free movement: Ethical issues in transnational migration of people and money.* B. Barry and R. Goodin, eds. University Park, Pennsylvania State University Press.

Carens, J. (1996). Realistic and idealistic approaches to the ethics of migration. *Int Migr Rev* 30(1): 156–170.

Castles, S. (2003). The international politics of forced migration. *Development* 46(3): 11–20.

Cernea, M. M., and C. McDowell, eds. (2000). *Risks and reconstruction: Experiences of resettlers and refugees.* Washington, DC, World Bank.

Copelon, R. (2000). Gender crimes as war crimes: integrating crimes against women into international criminal law. *MCGill Law J* 46: 217–240.

Cornielius, W. (1992). *Controlling illegal immigration: A global perspective. The case of Japan.* San Diego, Center for U.S.–Mexican Studies, University of California–San Diego.

Cwikel, J., K. Ilan, et al. (2003). Women brothel workers and occupational health risks. *J Epidemiol Commun Health* 57(10): 809–815.

Dankelman, I., J. Davidson, et al. (1988). *Women and environment in the third world: Alliance for the future.* Wolfeboro, NH, Earthscan Publications in association with the International Union for Conservation of Nature and Natural Resources; distributed in the United States by Longwood Publishers Group.

David, R. J., and J. W. J. Collins (1991). Bad outcomes in black babies: race or racism? *Ethn Dis* 1: 236–244.

de Bousingen, D. D. (2002). Health issues and the rise of Le Pen in France. *Lancet* 359(May 11): 1673.

Doezema, J. (1998). Forced to choose: beyond the voluntary v. forced prostitution dichotomy. In: *Global sex workers: Rights, resistance, and redifinition.* K. Kempadoo and J. Doezema, eds. New York, Routledge: 34–50.

Ehrenreich, B. and A. R. Hochschild, eds. (2004). *Global woman: Nannies, maids, and sex workers in the new economy.* New York, Metropolitan Books.

Gaita, R. (2001). Terror and justice. *The best Australian essays 2001.* P. Craven, ed. Melbourne, Black Inc.: 19–36.

Gender Matters Quarterly (1999). Women as chattel: The emerging global market in trafficking. 1(February): 1–8.

Geronimus, A. (2002). Black-white differences in the relationship of maternal age to birthweight: a population-based test of the weathering hypothesis. In: *Race, ethnicity, and health: A public health reader.* T. LaVeist, ed. San Francisco, Jossey-Bass: 213–230.

Ghosh, B. (2003a). *Elusive protection, uncertain lands: Migrants' access to human rights.* Geneva, International Organization for Migration.

Ghosh, B. (2003b). The human rights of migrants: strategies for moving forward. *Development* 46(3): 21–29.

Glèlè-Ahanhanzo, M., (2002). *Racism, racial discrimination, xenophobia, and all forms of discrimination: Mission to Australia.* Geneva, United Nations Economic and Social Council, Commission on Human Rights: 1–64.

Gushulak, B., and D. MacPherson (2000). Health issues associated with the smuggling and trafficking of migrants. *J Immigr Health* 2: 67–78.

Hanson, P. (2002). Migrant farmers suffering in silence. *Hisp Outlook Higher Educ Ethnic News* 12(17): 28.

HREOC (2004). *The last resort? National inquiry into children in immigration detention.* Sydney, Human Rights and Equal Opportunity Commission.

Human Rights Watch (2002). *Human Rights Watch world report 2003.* New York, Human Rights Watch.

ICHRP (2000). *The persistence and mutation of racism.* Geneva, International Council for Human Rights Policy.

ILO (1999). *Migrant workers: Report of the ILO 87th Session.* Geneva, International Labor Organization.

ILO (2000). *Globalization may increase number of migrant workers.* London, International Labour Organization.

IOM (2001). New IOM figures on the global scale of trafficking. *Traffick Migr* 23(spec issue April): 1–6.

IOM (2003a). Approaches to and diversity of international migration. In: *World migration 2003. Managing migration. Challenges and responses for people on the move.* Geneva, International Organization for Migration: 4–24.

IOM (2003b). Eighty-sixth session. Trafficking in persons: IOM strategy and activities. Geneva, International Organization for Migration: 1–11.

IOM (2003c). Ways to curb the growing complexity of irregular migration. In: *World migration 2003. Managing migration. Challenges and responses for people on the move.* Geneva, International Organization for Migration: 58–70.

IOM (2003d). *World migration 2003. Managing migration challenges and responses for people on the move.* Geneva, International Organization for Migration.

Jasso, G., M. R. Rosenzweig, et al. (2003). The earnings of US immigrants: world skill prices, skill transferability and selectivity. Economics Working Paper Archive 0312007: 1–42.

Johnston, V. (2003). Mobilizing the chattering classes for advocacy in Australia. *Development* 46(3): 75–80.

Kelley, N. (2001). The convention refugee definition and gender based persecution: a decade's progress. *Int J Refugee Law* 13(4): 559–568.

Lipschutz, R., and B. Crawford (1999). 'Ethnic' conflict isn't. Policy Brief No. 2, March 1995, Institute on Global Conflict and Cooperation. Reprinted in: *Globalization and conflict.* L. E. Sneden, ed. Dubuque, IA, Kendall Hunt: 189–193.

Lumpe, L., ed. (2000). *Running guns: The global black market in small arms.* London, Zed Books.

Manderson, L., M. Kelaher, et al. (1998). "A woman without a man is a woman at risk: women at risk in Australian humanitarian programs." *J Refug Stud* 11(3): 267–283.

Manne, R. (2001). Exclusionary nationalism. In: *The best Australian essays 2001.* P. Craven, ed. Melbourne, Black Inc.: 54–62.

Mares, P. (2001). A safe haven? In: *Borderline: Australia's treatment of refugees and asylum seekers.* Sydney, University of New South Wales Press: 162–184.

Mares, P. (2002). *Borderline.* Sydney, University of New South Wales Press.

Mares, P., and P. Allotey (2003). Controlling compassion: the media, refugees and asylum seekers. In: *The health of refugees: Public health perspectives from crisis to settlement.* P. Allotey, ed. Melbourne, Oxford University Press: 212–227.

Mateen, F., and B. Titemore (1999). The right to seek asylum: a dwindling right? *Brief, Centre Hum Rights Hum Law* 2(2): 1

Mayda, A. M. (2004). Who is against migration? A cross-country investigation of individual attitudes toward immigrants. Institute for the Study of Labor (IZA), Discussion Paper 1115: 1–59.

McDowell, C., ed. (1996). *Understanding impoverishment: The consequences of development displacement.* Providence, RI, Beghahn Books.

McKay, L., S. Macintyre, et al. (2003). *Migration and health: A review of the international literature.* Glasgow, Medical Research Council.

McMaster, D. (2001). *Asylum seekers: Australia's response to refugees.* Melbourne, Melbourne University Press.

McMaster, D. (2002). Refugees: where to now? White Australia to Tampa: the politics of fear. *Acad Soc Sci Aust* 21: 3–9.

Migration and Health (2000a). Infections in mobile populations: which are more important? No. 3: 1–3.

Migration and Health (2000b). Trafficking of migrants—hidden health concerns. No. 2: 1–3.

Mooney, G. (2002). Public health, political morality and compassion. *Aust N Z Public Health* 26(3): 201–202.

Murray, C., G. King, et al. (2002). Armed conflict as a public health problem. *BMJ* 324(9 February): 346–349.

O'Kelly, B. (2001). Gardai face difficulty in enforcing illegal immigrants act. *(Ireland) Sunday Business Post on-line.* December 10. http://archives.tcm.ie/businesspost/2001/12/16/story57529728.asp

O'Shaughnessy, M. (1999). *Media and society.* Melbourne, Oxford University Press.

Pittaway, E., and L. Bartolomei (2003). Double jeopardy: children seeking asylum. In: *The health of refugees: Public health perspectives from crisis to settlement.* P. Allotey, ed. Melbourne, Oxford University Press: 93–103.

Pritchett, L. (2003). *The future of migration: Irrestible forces meeting immovable ideas. The future of globalization: Explorations in light of the recent turbulence.* New Haven, CT, Yale University, Center for the Study of Globabization.

Reidpath, D. (2003). Love thy neighbour, its good for your health. *Soc Sci Med* 57: 253–261.

Reidpath, D. D., K. Chen, et al. (2004). He hath the French pox: stigma, social value, and social exclusion." *Soc Health Illness* 27(4): 468–489.

Richmond, A. (1994). *Global apartheid: Refugees, racism, and the new world order.* Oxford, Oxford University Press.

Rothman, K. J., H. O. Adami, et al. (1998). Should the mission of epidemiology include the eradication of poverty? [see comment]. *Lancet* 352(9130): 810–813.

Rowse, T. (1992). The Royal Commission, ATSIC and self-determination: a review of the Royal Commission into Aboriginal deaths in custody. *Aust J Soc Issues* 27(3): 153–172.

Sales, R. (2002). The deserving and the undeserving? Refugees, asylum seekers and welfare in Britain. *Crit Soc Policy* 22(3): 456–478.

Saravia, N. G., and J. F. Miranda (2004). Plumbing the brain drain. *Bull World Health Organ* 82(8): 608–615.

Schaeffer, R. K. (2003). *Understanding globalization. The social consequences of political, economic and environmental change.* Lanham, MD, Rowman and Littlefield.

Silove, D. (2002). The asylum debacle in Australia: a challenge for psychiatry. *Aust N Z J Psychiatr* 36(3): 290–296.

Silove, D., J. Curtis, et al. (1996). Ethical considerations in the management of asylum seekers on hunger strike. *JAMA* 276(5): 410–415.

Silove, D., P. McIntosh, et al. (1993). Risk of retraumatisation of asylum-seekers in Australia. *Aust N Z J Psychiatr* 27(5): 606–612.

Silove, D., Z. Steel, et al. (2001). Detention of asylum seekers: assault on health, human rights, and social development. *Lancet* 357: 1436–1437.

Silove, D., Z. Steel, et al. (2000). Policies of deterrence and the mental health of asylum seekers. *JAMA* 284(5): 604–611.

Singer, P., and R. Singer (1988). The ethics of refugee policy. In: *Open Borders? Close societies? The ethical and political issues.* M. Gibney, ed. Westport, CT, Greenwood Press: 111–130.

Sleigh, A., and S. Jackson (1998). Public health and public choice: dammed off at China's Three Gorges? *Lancet* 351(9114): 1449–1450.

Smith, M., and B. Harvey (2003). Operation safe haven: health service delivery to temporary evacuees. In: *The health of refugees: Public health perspectives from crisis to settlement.* P. Allotey, ed. Melbourne, Oxford University Press: 139–155.

Staab, S. (2004). *In search of work: International migration of women in Latin America and the Caribbean.* Santiago, Women and Development Unit, United Nations Economic Commission for Latin America and the Carribean.

Sultan, A., O'Sullivan, K. (2001). Psychological disturbances in asylum seekers held in long term detention: A participant observer account. *Med J Aust* 175: 593–596.

Susser, M. (1993). Health as a human right: an epidemiologist's perspective on the public health [see comment]. *Am J Public Health* 83(3): 418–426.

Susser, M., and E. Susser (1999). Preserving public health values [comment]. *Epidemiology* 10(2): 204–205.

Taran, P. A. (2000). Human rights of migrants: challenges of the new decade. *Int Migr* 38(6): 7–51.

Tiburcio, C. (2001). *The human rights of aliens under international and comparative law.* The Hague, Nijhoff.

Toole, M. (2003). The health of refugees: an international public health problem. In: *The health of refugees. Public health perspectives from crisis to settlement.* P. Allotey, ed. Melbourne, Oxford University Press: 35–53.

Toole, M. J., and R. Bhatia (1992). A case study of Somali refugees in Hartisheik A camp, eastern Ethiopia: health and nutrition profile, July 1988–June 1989. *J Refug Stud* 5: 313–326.

Toole, M. J., R. J. Waldman, et al. (2001). Complex humanitarian emergencies. In: *Textbook of international public health: Diseases programs, systems, and policies.* M. Merson, R. Black, and A. Mills, eds. Gaithersburg, MD, Aspen Publications: 439–513.

United Nations (2000a). *Protocol against the smuggling of migrants by land, sea, and air: Supplementing the United Nations Convention Against Transnational Organized Crime.* Geneva, United Nations.

United Nations (2000b). *Protocol to prevent, suppress, and punish trafficking in persons, especially women and children: Supplementing the United Nations Convention Against Transnational Organized Crime.* Geneva, United Nations.

UNESCO (2003). *Information kit on the UN Convention on Migrants' Rights.* Geneva, United Nations Educational, Scientific, and Cultural Organization.

UNHCR (United Nations High Commissioner for Refugees) (2000). *The state of the world's refugees: Fifty years of humanitarian action.* New York, Oxford University Press.

UNICEF (2004). *Trafficking in human beings, especially women and children.* Florence, Italy, UNICEF Innocenti Research Centre.

United States Committee for Refugees (USCR) (2003). Trafficking in persons: a country by country report on a contemporary form of slavery. *Refugee Rep* 24(7): 11–14.

Vas Dev, S. (2003). Asylum in Africa: the emergence of the reluctant host. *Development* 26(3): 113–118.

Walzer, M. (1981). The distribution of membership. In: *Boundaries: National autonomy and its limits.* P. G. Brown and H. Shue, eds. Totowa, NJ, Rowman and Littlefield: 1–35.

Walzer, M. (1983). *Spheres of justice: a defense of pluralism and equality.* New York, Basic Books.

Weiner, M. (1996). Ethics, national sovereignty, and the control of immigration. *Int Migr Rev* 30(1): 171–197.

WHO (2002). *World report on violence and health.* Geneva, World Health Organization.

WHO (2003). *International migration, health and human rights.* Health and Human Rights Publ. Ser. No. 4. Geneva, World Health Organization.

World Bank (1995). *Workers in an integrating world: World development report.* Oxford, Oxford University Press.

World Bank (2003). *World Bank, global development finance.* New York, World Bank.

Zelinka, S. (1996). *Understanding racism in Australia.* Canberra, Human Rights and Equal Opportunities Commission, Australian Government Publishing Service.

Zlotnik, H. (1998). "International migration 1965–96: an overview." *Popul Dev Rev* 24(3): 429–468.

Zwi, A. B. (1996). Numbering the dead: counting the casualties of war. In: *Defining violence: Understanding the causes and effects of violence.* H. Bradby, ed. Aldershot, Avebury Press: 99–124

Chapter 10

Globalization and Women's Health

Sarah Wamala and Ichiro Kawachi

No society treats its women as well as its men, whether measured by gender gaps in economic activity, educational attainment, or political representation (United Nations Development Programme [UNDP] 1995). Although women typically live longer than men, they also report worse health status and a higher prevalence of morbidity. According to calculations made by the World Health Organization, the female advantage in life expectancy is decreased by between 10% and 20% once we take into account the life years "lost" due to disability (Bonita and Mathers 2003). Moreover, demographers note a substantial imbalance in the population ratios of women and men in certain regions of the world. Because of their greater longevity, there are more women than men in Western Europe and North America. However, in countries such as China, India, Pakistan, and Bangladesh, there are fewer women in the population than men because of sex-selective abortion and the preferential treatment of boys over girls in nutrition and access to health care. The result is that there are

upward of 100 million women "missing" in the world (Sen 1999).

Gender inequalities are therefore a persistent feature of our world. Nonetheless, the status of women globally has improved measurably during the past half century. Some of this improvement can be attributed to women's rising levels of literacy, the spread of human rights and women's political participation, and access to contraception and reproductive technology. In this chapter we address the impacts of globalization on women's status and health.

Globalization has both positive and negative impacts on women's health, and these impacts are unequally distributed among different groups of women. For example, foreign direct investment has expanded women's employment opportunities and, hence, their economic autonomy. Globalization has also aided the international transfer of reproductive technologies, such as contraception. The closer integration of societies, particularly through telecommunications and the Internet, has mobilized the international women's movement. At the same time, many features of globalization pose a threat to women's health. For example, economic migration from developing countries to rich countries enhances women's earning power, but it also exposes them to the threat of exploitation and discrimination (Ehrenreich and Hochschild 2003). Some forms of reproductive technology, such as antenatal ultrasound, are prone to abuse, such as when they are used to assist sex-selective abortion.

Tracing out the consequences of globalization for women's health is a challenging task, not least because "gender is everywhere" one looks (Benería et al. 2000). That is, gender *cross-cuts* all other areas of globalization. Women are more vulnerable to, or disproportionately affected by, the global health threats described in the rest of this book. For example, poverty and gender inequality are the driving forces behind the "feminization" of the global HIV/AIDS pandemic. Seventy percent of the world's poor are women (UNDP 1995), and economic hardship in turn forces women and girls into commercial sex work or transactional sex (entering into relationships with older and wealthier men in exchange for money), putting them at risk of sexually transmitted diseases and HIV/AIDS (UNICEF 2005). The result is that nearly 60% of HIV-infected individuals in sub-Saharan Africa are women, and the proportion rises to 75% among young people 15–24 years of age in the region.

Women, particularly in developing countries, are vulnerable to targeting by the transnational tobacco industry (see chapter 3). Already in the West, cigarette smoking has become a "feminized" habit, and the rest of the world is surely not far behind. Women and children constitute 80% of the 50 million people affected by violent conflicts, civil wars, disasters, and displacement (Maclean and Sicchia 2004). Women and children also represent the majority of trafficked individuals in the world (see chapter 9).

For specific accounts of how women are disproportionately affected by the emerging global threats to health, readers are referred to the individual chapters in the rest of this book. In this chapter, we focus on how the processes of globalization operate through the gendered structures and institutions of the *economy* to influence the health and well-being of women. Economic policies related to global integration, trade, and financial liberalization have profound impacts on the lives and well-being of women and

their family members. Despite the profound relevance of gendered analysis, feminist critics have noted that the macroeconomic models underpinning globalization policies are frequently gender-blind (Elson 1995; UNRISD 2005). For example:

> While institutions such as the World Bank now concern themselves with gender inequalities in some institutional arenas—at the intra-household level in particular, as well as in the legal domain where traditions and customs have an important role to play—the attention to gender is selective and uneven. The silences and omissions in such frameworks are particularly revealing: significantly, markets and macroeconomic flows (trade, capital) are not subjected to the same gender analysis, the tacit assumption being that they are essentially benign and gender-neutral. (UNRISD 2005, p. 11)

The structural adjustment policies of the 1980s and 1990s are one prominent example of "globalized" economic policies[1] that had specific gender effects (Elson 2002; Jaggar 2002). Reflecting the rise of the "Washington Consensus" in the 1980s (see chapter 1), these policies emphasized government budget cuts and the commercialization of welfare services (through privatization and cost recovery, i.e., user charges on education and health care) (see chapter 13). The result was that the burden of adjustment was shifted onto women, who were forced to become "shock absorbers" of the economy and serve as care providers of the last resort within households on the edge of survival (UNRISD 2005).

Both the International Monetary Fund and World Bank have seemingly moved on from the rigid neo-liberal orthodoxy represented by the structural adjustment policies of the 1980s and 1990s. Nevertheless, the same questions remain—and continue to be debated—about the impacts of economic globalization on gender equality and women's well-being. For example, has trade liberalization promoted women's participation in paid employment, or improved their status and autonomy vis-à-vis men?

ECONOMIC GLOBALIZATION AND GENDER EQUALITY

The impoverishment of women throughout the world is determined by many factors, including their lack of access to education, constrained access to capital and land, disproportionate responsibilities for the provision of unpaid domestic and care work, discrimination in the labor market, and their subordinate status in society through systems of patriarchy.[2]

Does economic globalization and, in particular, trade liberalization promote women's autonomy? According to one view, trade liberalization promotes economic growth (see chapter 7), and in turn, higher incomes improve women's access to education. Therefore, trade liberalization increases gender equality and women's well-being. Others contend that economic growth alone does not automatically lead to a closing of gender gaps in income and well-being (Seguino 2000). We now turn to a closer examination of these contested claims.

Market Liberalization and Women's Labor Force Participation

In theory, trade liberalization in the developing world is expected to stimulate demand for labor-intensive manufactured goods in sectors such as textiles, apparel, electronics, and food processing. Women are an attractive source of labor for firms because of their lower wages (relative to men) (Elson and Pearson 1981). As Fontana et al. (1998) phrased it,

> Women's universally disadvantaged position in labor markets in developing countries—the wage and job discrimination they face—paradoxically redounds to their advantage under the competitive conditions brought in with trade liberalization, at least in those countries which have a comparative advantage in labor-intensively produced goods. (p. 49)

Trade liberalization should therefore lead to increased female employment (UNRISD 2005). Similarly, liberalization of foreign direct investment is theoretically linked to increased female employment, for example, through multinational enterprises operating in export processing zones and *maquiladoras* (see chapter 8). Thus, hypothetically, increased export volume due to liberalization should result in the following:

- Increased participation of women in paid employment, and therefore decreased gender gaps in labor force participation, as well as improved opportunities for women's economic, social, and political participation

- Decreased unemployment rates for women and therefore a reduced gender gap in unemployment

- Higher wages for female workers and therefore a decreased gender gap in earned income

Some empirical evidence suggests that women's labor market participation and share of employment have risen over the last two decades in developing countries as a result of liberalized trade and foreign direct investment (UNRISD 2005). In regions such as Southeast Asia and Latin America, increased trade (export expansion) resulted in increased female employment.

At the same time, the data also suggest that women's employment gains are often precarious. Trade increases women's access to labor markets, but they may find themselves locked in "dead-end" jobs with low pay, poor working conditions, and little opportunity for skill acquisition or advancement. Because of gender discrimination, women's jobs have been phased out in some cases as export production is diversified and manufacturing becomes more capital intensive (Joekes 1995; Fussel 2000). Furthermore, as developing countries "mature" industrially, they tend to lose labor-intensive manufacturing jobs to even lower wage countries. As these jobs are shed, women are usually the first to be laid off, and many find difficulty in finding reemployment in the more capital-intensive manufacturing sectors. In rapidly industrializing economies such as Taiwan, Korea, and Thailand, data suggest that there has been a net decline in women's share of employment in the manufacturing sector during 1991–2000 (Berik 2000; Jomo 2001). The share of women has fallen markedly in export-processing zones in Singapore and Mexico, prompting one interpretation of trade expansion as "offer[ing] women a once-off benefit in terms of improved access to the labor market, but with no sustained improvements in labor market status thereafter" (Fontana et al. 1998, p. 49).

In Bangladesh, jobs for women in the garment industry are projected to fall by up to 1 million with the phase-out of the Multi-Fibre Agreement in 2005.[3] Similar observations have been made in African countries (e.g., Zimbabwe, Tanzania, Nigeria, Kenya, Ghana, and South Africa) that lost export-oriented, labor-intensive (and female-dominated) jobs due to competition from cheaper Asian imports (Malhotra 2003). In these countries, local small-scale producers in the informal sector (most of whom are women) have also lost market share to cheaper imports. One example is female basket makers in Kenya, who lost their livelihood as local consumers began to import mass-produced cheaper substitutes from East Asia (Weston 1994).

When we turn to predominantly agriculture-based economies (e.g., in sub-Saharan Africa), evidence suggests that trade liberalization may have actually jeopardized women's livelihoods and well-being (Ça-ðatay and Ertürk 2004). In these countries, trade liberalization has stimulated the production of cash crops while simultaneously increasing import competition for food crops. Women have been adversely affected by these trends due to their concentration in small farms that produce food crops (see "Trade and Food Security," below).

Female employment has been disproportionately affected in industrialized countries (e.g., the United States) by liberalization of trade in textiles and apparel (Kucera and Milberg 2000). In summary, there is evidence for increased female employment parallel to increased international trade, although the quality of women's jobs tends to be less secure compared to traditionally male-dominated sectors.

Market Liberalization and Gender Equality

In theory, increased competition in the manufacturing sector should reduce discrimination against women in the long run, because discrimination is costly to employers who forgo profits in order to indulge their "taste for discrimination."[4] Indeed, there is some circumstantial evidence to bear this out. For example, in the Bangladeshi garment industry, female factory wages are reported to be two to three times higher than male agricultural workers' earnings (Fontana et al. 1998). In the United States, both the gender wage gap and the volume of imports as a share of gross domestic product remained fairly constant between 1960 and 1980, but during the most recent two decades (i.e., during the period of accelerated globalization), the female:male wage ratio increased dramatically in tandem with the rise in imports (Black and Brainerd 2002).

Economists Sandra Black and Elizabeth Brainerd (2002) compared the gender wage gap within the United States between 1976 and 1993 in industries

that formerly faced little competitive pressure to reduce gender discrimination (e.g., electronics) with competitive manufacturing industries (e.g., textiles). After controlling for gender differences in educational attainment and labor market experience, the authors found that increased competition through trade did appear to contribute to an improvement in female wages in concentrated relative to already competitive industries. In other words, although trade may raise wage inequality (particularly by reducing the relative wages of less skilled workers—see chapter 7), at the same time it appeared to benefit women by reducing the ability of firms to discriminate (Black and Brainerd 2002).

Not all empirical studies agree with the findings for the United States just described. An important question is the extent to which trends in the gender wage gap are attributable to trade liberalization, rather than to other factors such as a rise in female educational attainment relative to men. Improvements in women's labor market position are threatened by counteracting forces, such as the tendency to "crowd" women in labor-intensive sectors of the market, leading to an artificial oversupply of female labor (UNRISD 2005). In addition, the firms that hire women face constant pressure to keep costs low, and they can also relocate with relative ease. The result is that women's employment conditions make it structurally difficult to raise their wages and to close the gender wage gaps (UNRISD 2005). Indeed, some evidence suggests that trade liberalization has resulted in *downward* pressure on women's wages in some countries, for example, Taiwan, Hong Kong, and China (UNRISD 2005).

Although we have dwelt on the relationship between trade and the gender wage gap, we hasten to point out that the latter is only one indicator of gender inequality. The impact of trade on gender equality needs to be evaluated in a number of ways. Fontana et al. (1998), as well as researchers at nongovernmental organization Women in Development Europe (WIDE), recommend examining the effects of trade on gender equality at different levels: (a) individual socioeconomic effects (educational attainment, income, and livelihood), (b) effects at the meso level (labor markets), and (c) macroeconomic effects (economic growth, gender-equality policies).

In a detailed case study of trade liberalization between the European Union and Latin American countries (Argentina, Brazil, Chile, Mexico, Paraguay, Uruguay), researchers at WIDE focused on three sets of indicators describing the impacts on gender relations: situational indicators, indicators of political will, and dynamic indicators (WIDE 2001). *Situational* indicators provide an overview of gender inequality within the societies and economies of trading partners. The specific indicators within this domain describe the social and economic situation of women, including women's labor market position (female and male employment rates and unemployment rates), their relative earnings (the gender wage gap), share of export credit obtained by women, and access to education and credit. One macro-level indicator of gender equality within this domain is the UNDP's Gender-Related Development Index).[5] *Political will* indicators measure the consistency between trading partners' gender policies as they negotiate trade agreements. Specific indicators in this domain include the share of women in official trade delegations. Finally, *dynamic* indicators link situational indicators with trade variables over time, enabling an analysis of the effects of trade on gender equality, and vice versa. Data on trade includes trade tariff reductions, trading volumes, exports and imports (WIDE 2001).

In the WIDE analysis, dynamic indicators were calculated for the period 1995 to 1999/2000, during which trade between the European Union and Latin American countries increased by 23.4%. The analyses showed that there was no relationship between increased trade liberalization and macro-level measures of gender equality such as the Gender-Related Development Index, either in the European Union or in Mexico. Nor did the gender wage gap decrease with increased trade in either the European Union or in Argentina, Brazil or Mexico. In fact, in spite of the strong increase in European Union exports to Latin American countries, the gender unemployment gap in the European Union did not decrease. Among Latin American countries, Mexico experienced an explosive increase in trade with the European Union, but this did not translate into improved women's unemployment rates relative to men. On the contrary, the gender gap in unemployment rates appeared to increase considerably more than in other Latin American countries during the same period. The analyses also showed no relationship between increased trade and the gender composition of trade delegations that negotiated agreements between the European Union

and Latin American countries (WIDE 2001; Fontana and Wood 2000).

The WIDE analysts were careful to note the complexities of interpreting their findings. Because of the likely reciprocal relationships between trade and pre-existing gender inequalities in society, it can be difficult to tease out the direction of causality—that is, to what extent women gain or lose from increased trade, versus to what extent existing gender inequalities affect trade.

Two examples illustrate this complexity. Some countries in South Asia, such as Korea, Taiwan, and Singapore, have succeeded in increasing their exports as a result of increased international trade. These countries have been able to export industrial products at low prices, mainly by exploiting cheap labor, particularly of women, who earn substantially less than men. In these countries, preexisting gender inequalities (the high gender wage gap) spurred an increase in export trade.

By contrast, in sub-Saharan Africa, there is a strong gender division of labor in agriculture. Women grow food crops to feed the family, while men grow cash crops to earn income. Because of gender inequality in access to returns, women often refuse to labor in the cash crops of their husbands. At the same time, their food production is reduced due to the expansion of cash crops on available cultivable land. In this example, trade has resulted in a worsening of gender inequality in access to resources.

In summary, the effects of trade on gender equality are quite mixed. The reason is because any women's gains in employment through trade are *filtered* through structures of gendered occupational segregation, both in paid versus unpaid work and within paid work. Generating jobs for women is not a sufficient guarantee for closing the gender gaps in wages and working conditions, and a number of significant obstacles besides occupational segregation stand in the way of achieving gender equality, including women's overengagement in household tasks and childcare; women's lack of access to land, credit, transportation, and other resources; and the absence of women's voices in political and macroeconomic decision making. Needless to add, gender inequalities in the social, political, and economic spheres have been powerfully linked to women's longevity and well-being (Williamson and Boehmer 1997; Kawachi et al. 1999; Sen 2000).

Trade and Intrahousehold
Gender Relations

Ideally, increased female employment through trade should have a positive impact on women's autonomy, bargaining power within the household, and incentives for investing in their human capital. Nonetheless, the reality remains that, in spite of more women earning their own income than at any time during the history of the world, substantial inequalities remain in the division of household power and authority. Patriarchal cultures and norms throughout the world mean that men continue to have the dominant say over how incomes within households should be allocated. Economic progress does not necessarily change the social constraints on women's independence.

In many poor regions of the world, men solely decide how the household income is to be used regardless who earns it. Evidence from Bangladesh, Pakistan, India, and Sri Lanka suggests that one-third to one-half of women workers in agriculture and in industry hand over their wages to their husbands or other family members (Erfan 2004). A study in Thailand and the Philippines showed that a majority of women working in the export processing zones had to hand over their earnings to their natal households and even sometimes used them to support the education of their younger brothers (Sainsbury 1996). In rural areas of Indonesia and Tunisia, women workers are often recruited by male labor agents (e.g., their father or another male third-party), and wages are paid to the agents.[6]

On the other side of the balance sheet, however, it is important not to lose sight of the effects of employment and earnings on women's autonomy. There is no doubt that wage employment has resulted in women's increased self-esteem and expansion of life choices (e.g., leaving an unfavorable marriage), life satisfaction, and ability to delay marrying at a young age (Amin et al. 1998). A striking vignette of these benefits is provided by Jeffrey Sachs (2005), here describing the lives of young women working in the Bangladeshi garment factories:

> One by one, [the women] recounted the arduous hours, the lack of labor rights, and the harassment. . . . Nearly all of the women interviewed had grown up in the country-side, extraordinarily poor, illiterate, and unschooled, and vulnerable to chronic hunger and hardship in a domineering,

patriarchal society. Had they (and their forebears of the 1970s and 1980s) stayed in the villages, they would have been forced into a marriage arranged by their fathers, and by seventeen or eighteen, forced to conceive a child. Their trek to the cities to take jobs has given these young women a chance for personal liberation of unprecedented dimension and opportunity. . . .

> The Bangladeshi women told how they were able to save some small surplus from their meager pay, manage their own income, have their own rooms, choose when and whom to date and marry, choose to have their children when they felt ready, and use their savings to improve their literacy and job-market skills. (p. 12)

Increased earnings for women are also beneficial for their children's nutritional status because women tend to have a more family-oriented expenditure pattern than men. That is, women tend to spend a higher proportion of the income that they earn on health care, food, and the education of family members, whereas men tend to spend on items of personal consumption (Dwyer and Bruce 1988; Haddad et al. 1997). As women's incomes rises with trade-generated employment, one can expect improvements in child nutritional status and other human development indicators. Trade-related employment gains for women also set in train a wider change in gender relations. For example, demonstration of women's income-earning capability changes parental perceptions of girls away from being a liability toward seeing them as potential income earners and contributors to the household (Fontana et al. 1998). As a result, attitudes and incentives for investing in the human capital of girls are improved (Kabeer 1995).

GLOBALIZATION AND CAREGIVING

So far, we have discussed the impacts of economic globalization on women's paid employment and incomes. A less visible, and therefore often neglected, impact of globalization is on caring labor, that is, the unpaid work involved in providing care for children, the elderly, and the sick (UNDP 1999).[7] Throughout the world, women remain primarily responsible for caring labor. According to the UNDP (1995), women in developing countries spend two-thirds of their working hours on unpaid paid (compared to one-quarter for men), and most of these hours are for caring work. In Nepal, for example, women work 21 more hours each week than do men; in India, 12 hours more. In Kenya, 8- to 14-year-old girls spend 5 hours more on household chores than do boys (UNDP 1995).

How has globalization affected caregiving? The answer, in the words of the UNDP (1999), is that "globalization is putting a squeeze on care and caring labor" (p. 77). This is happening because the rise in women's paid work is not being offset by a proportionate expansion in state services (e.g., subsidized child care or community care) to support families. Nor have cultural norms kept pace with the rising labor market participation of women through increasing the role of men in caring labor. The result is that women increasingly labor under the "double burden" of paid and unpaid work responsibilities (Hochschild and Machung 1997; Fontana and Wood 2000).

The challenges of balancing work and family responsibilities have been documented by the Project on Global Working Families, led by Jody Heymann (Heymann et al. 2003). In thousands of interviews with working families in Mexico, Botswana, Vietnam, Honduras, Russia, and the United States, Heymann and colleagues document the ways in which poor working conditions combined with inadequate social supports threaten the health of women and children. Respondents in these surveys repeatedly cited how the absence of adequate maternity leave policies resulted in the premature cessation of breast-feeding or the inability to ensure that children receive their full set of immunizations. In the absence of affordable child care, working women throughout the developing world often have no choice but to leave their children alone at home, exposing them to increased risks of accidents and injuries. According to the Project on Global Working Families, more than one-third of parents in Mexico, Botswana, and Vietnam reported having to leave their children at home in the care of older siblings (often girls) without adult supervision (Heymann et al. 2003). Often, the children left in supervisory roles had to forgo schooling, resulting in lasting impacts on their future social mobility.[8] As noted by Heymann et al. (2003), "while child labor is a recognized problem affecting both boys and girls in the developing world, home-based work often remains unaddressed due to its informal nature" (p. 89).

Finally, global policies—exemplified by the structural adjustment programs imposed by the international financial institutions on debt-ridden countries during the 1980s and 1990s—have often exacerbated the burdens on working women. As described in chapter 13, these policies led to cutbacks in state-provided caring services, which effectively transferred the burden onto the shoulders of women.

In developed countries, the "care deficit" that has emerged as a result of more women entering paid employment is *pulling* migrants from the developing world to fill that vacuum (Ehrenreich and Hochschild 2002). The result is what Hochschild (2000) refers to as the "global care chain." For example, a family in a rich country (e.g., the United States) hires the caring labor of a immigrant woman from a poor country (e.g., the Philippines), who in turn has subcontracted the care of *her* children to a mother from a poorer (perhaps rural) family, who in turn has passed on the care of *her* children to her oldest daughter (Hochschild 2000). As asserted by Ehrenreich and Hochschild (2002), "The lifestyles of the First World are made possible by a global transfer of the services associated with a wife's traditional role—child care, home-making, and sex—from poor countries to rich ones" (p. 4).

The global care chain, in turn, is partly responsible for the feminization of migration, as millions of women from the poor countries in the world seek employment in the richer countries (see chapter 9).[9] During past episodes of globalization, males were predominant as economic migrants. Now more half of the world's 120 million legal and illegal migrants are believed to be women.

TRADE AND FOOD SECURITY

Women as Key Figures in Food Security

Many countries in Asia and Africa have more than two-thirds of their workforce engaged in agriculture and related activities. According to the Food and Agricultural Organization (FAO), low-income countries are primarily rural economies where women produce more than half of the food that is grown. Fifty percent of the developing world's female population is responsible for plowing and leveling land, while 70%

are involved in planting, tilling, and harvesting. In sub-Saharan Africa and the Caribbean, women produce up to 80% of basic foodstuffs. In Southeast Asia women account for between 50% and 90% of food production, while women in rural Africa produce, process, and store up to 80% of the food (FAO 1996). Thus, women play a major role in food security for their households and family members.

Yet access to productive resources, including land, credit, training, and technology, remains heavily biased in favor of men. In most rural households, men still control income from cash crop production, which is not necessarily used for household necessities or improvement of food security. Women's income on the other hand is used for food and other necessities within the household.

A major constraint on women is their lack of independent land rights to enable them to decide on the use of land. Women in many developing regions in the world have no inheritance rights for land, and when they marry, sole ownership of land usually passes to their husbands. Without formal ownership of land, women cannot obtain access to credit, creating a vicious cycle of poverty. In some countries, even when formal ownership of land by women is provided under the law, it may not be recognized in practice. In Gambia, it has been shown that even when women have formal land ownership rights, rice production was not under female management but under the control of the male head of household (Haddad et al. 1997).

Within this context, globalization and trade liberalization have promoted cash-crop farming, accompanied by a reduction in resources devoted to subsistence farming. Although total household income may be increased in households engaged in cash-crop farming, there is often a paradoxical adverse impact on food security (FAO 1996; Saito et al. 1994; Lado 1992).

Medium- and large-scale farms (most of which are run by men) have faced more favorable conditions for mechanization and integration into the world market. Furthermore, agro-processing multinationals often directly acquire land in many developing countries and then subcontract medium to large farmers to produce their crops. By contrast, small-scale farmers (many of whom are women) have been excluded from this process and have been forced to surrender their land for cash cropping. Women have been left to manage less valuable land. They are also slower to take advantage of new opportunities to upgrade their farming meth-

ods because of disadvantages in gaining access to credit, new technologies, and marketing networks (Çaðatay and Ertürk 2004).

Women in Uganda report that government incentives to produce beans for export have left them with no food crops for their families. In Kenya, women have been directed to plant tobacco but do not earn sufficient income to purchase food. Studies show that the nutritional status of women and children is worse among cash-crop farmers, particularly where the crops are tobacco, coffee, and cotton (McGow 1995).

HIV/AIDS and Food Security: A Looming Crisis

The HIV/AIDS epidemic has already had a substantial adverse impact on food security in sub-Saharan Africa. FAO estimates that 7 million agricultural workers have been killed by the pandemic, and 16 million more could die by 2020. In the nine most affected African countries, it has been projected that AIDS will reduce the agricultural workforce for the period 1985–2020 by the following proportions: Namibia, 26%; Botswana, 23%; Zimbabwe, 23%; Mozambique, 20%; South Africa, 20%; Kenya, 17%; Malawi, 14%; Uganda, 14%; and Tanzania, 13%.

The agricultural sector is also affected in other indirect ways related to HIV/AIDS. For example, households have been forced to sell their productive assets (land, livestock, tools, and machinery) to pay for medical and funeral bills; a greater number of dependents have been forced to rely on a smaller number of productive family members for income and food; farming knowledge and skills are lost before they can be passed on to the next generation. These factors combine to produce a poverty trap in sub-Saharan Africa that threatens human development in the region for generations to come.

Already in sub-Saharan Africa, the majority of HIV-infected individuals (60%) are women. This has led to a changing pattern of orphaning in the region, where it is estimated that 60% of AIDS orphans have lost their mothers, compared with 40% among orphaned children in Asia and Latin America. Recent household surveys indicate that maternal orphans are especially vulnerable to becoming "virtual" double orphans, because of the common pattern for the fathers to live elsewhere (UNICEF 2005). The HIV crisis in sub-Saharan Africa is further intensified by lack of well functioning health care systems in the region.

The World Trade Organization, the Agreement on Trade-Related Aspects of Intellectual Property Rights, and Food Security

The interests of developing countries and rich nations are frequently at odds when it comes to international trade regime. Agricultural subsidies in the north make it especially difficult for women farmers in the south (who are generally small-scale food producers) to remain competitive (Çağatay and Ertürk 2004). Trade agreements negotiated under the World Trade Organization (WTO), such as the Agreement on Trade-Related Aspects of Intellectual Property Rights (TRIPS)[10] also disadvantage the resource-poor south. In the area of agriculture, U.S. transnational firms have used TRIPS to insist on monopoly patents on seeds, a practice that has been vigorously opposed by people's organizations throughout the developing world.

TRIPS has also been invoked by transnational corporations (TNCs) to take out patents on indigenous medicines. Traditionally, women are the keepers and users of indigenous medicinal wisdom, and this knowledge is valuable to their families and communities. However, indigenous women have lacked the resources to market their knowledge to the rest of the world. TNCs are not required by TRIPS to compensate the communities from which they acquired their knowledge. Critics assert that TNCs have unfairly claimed intellectual property even when they have added little to existing indigenous knowledge.[11] By denying traditional healers the ability to put their indigenous knowledge to use, TRIPS policies potentially threaten the livelihoods of women healers in low income countries.

TOWARD GENDER-EQUITABLE GLOBALIZATION

Increasingly, the current patterns of globalization have been subjected to challenge and scrutiny, led by the efforts of feminist economists and civil society organizations (CSOs) throughout the globe. Following the framework developed by Çağatay and Ertürk (2004), the final section of this chapter describes the variety of initiatives that have emerged in recent years that have attempted to transform the processes of globalization toward the achievement of gender equity. These initiatives include the following:

- Attempts by CSOs to inject "gender-sensitive budgets" into national and international macro-economic frameworks
- Initiatives to incorporate a gender perspective into regional and multilateral trade agreements
- Initiatives to strengthen working standards for women, in both the formal and informal sectors of the economy, and to link labor standards to trade
- Initiatives to undertake "gender mainstreaming" in institutions of global governance (Çağatay and Ertürk 2004)

Gender-Sensitive Budgets

Since 1984, according to Çağatay and Ertürk (2004), more than 40 gender budget initiatives have been launched around the world.[12] They have been undertaken by both CSOs and governments and focus on the analysis of the differential impact of budgetary expenditures on women and men. Tools have been developed for undertaking this exercise (Elson 1998), and the different steps focus on such issues as gender-aware policy appraisals, beneficiary assessments, public expenditure incidence analysis, and gender-disaggregated analysis of the impact of budgets on time use. Although it is still early to determine the impacts of gender budgets on national priority setting and decision making, they have been endorsed by numerous international mandates, including the Beijing Platform for Action (United Nations 1995). In addition to gender budgets, the Economic Council for Africa has launched a new initiative, through its African Centre for Gender and Development, to develop new analytical tools to review macroeconomic policies from a gender and policy perspective (Çağatay and Ertürk 2004).

The Millennium Development Goals

The Millennium Development Goals (MDGs) have now become the central focus of development policy nationally and internationally (see chapters 16 and 17) and are regarded as a potentially powerful policy tool to further the agenda of gender equality and women's human rights. The MDGs have however been criticized for not complying with the broader Millennium Declaration (UNDP 2003; UNIFEM 2002; Sweetman 2005). The Millennium Declaration affirms the importance of gender equality and women's human rights, as well as the need to combat all forms of violence against women and to implement the Convention on the Elimination of All Forms of Discrimination against Women (CEDAW). Policy makers in many countries have been criticized for tending to focus exclusively on the target of achieving gender parity in primary and secondary education, while ignoring additional targets that relate to women's share of wage employment and the proportion of seats in national parliaments (Sweetman 2005). On the other hand, some countries have emphasized the importance of addressing the gendered patterns of violence in achieving the MDGs. Vietnam, for example, has targeted a reduction in the rate of violence against women as the basis for achieving goal 3 (promoting gender equality and empowering women).

In short, the MDGs are unlikely to be reached unless the concerns of gender inequality and discrimination against women are addressed by every aspect of the MDGs, not just goals 3 and 5 that mention women. The first goal on poverty reduction (goal 1) has been cited as a good example (see Sweetman 2005). The stated goal—eradication of extreme poverty and hunger—does not mention the gender dimensions of the phenomenon of poverty. Achieving the goal calls for a range of measures to tackle women's poverty, including the reform of laws and policies to secure women's equal access to economic resources, in particular, land and credit, and improvements in the measurement and monitoring of women's poverty and their access to information. At the country level, this means articulating and measuring the gender dimensions of each of the goals in national reports and ensuring, as a minimum requirement, that targets and indicators are compliant with CEDAW and other gender instruments. The 2005 review processes for both the MDGs and the Beijing Platform for Action are a good opportunity for women's organizations to remind their governments of the commitments they have each made and the actions needed to fulfill them (Sweetman 2005). Failure to address women's rights and gender inequality will ultimately doom the MDGs (World Bank 2001).

Gender Mainstreaming in the WTO

Among international financial institutions, the WTO has been singled out for criticism by feminist critics for being male dominated and ignoring women's views. At present, all seven members appointed to the dispute settlement body are male, and fewer than 10% of the 159 trade policy experts are women (Public Citizen Global Trade Watch 2003). In contrast to several international organizations—such as the United Nations Economic and Social Council, Asia-Pacific Economic Cooperation, and the World Bank—which have made attempts to mainstream a gender perspective in all their activities, the WTO has been particularly slow to incorporate a gender perspective into their policies.

Gender biases in international trade policies have been critiqued and brought to the attention of the world by a number of organizations, such as the Informal Working Group on Gender and Trade, a network of more than thirty CSOs. CSOs such as Development Alternatives with Women for a New Era (DAWN), International Gender and Trade Network, Alternative Women in Development (United States), WIDE, Women Working Worldwide (United Kingdom), and Women's Environment and Development Organization have advocated for the mainstreaming of gender in international trade agreements.

Women's Environment and Development Organization lists a number of recommended steps for mainstreaming trade agreements within the WTO, including mandating the inclusion of women in economic decision making and governance, resisting monopolization of food production and enacting policies that protect women's livelihoods in family- and community-based sustainable agriculture, preventing exploitation by TNCs of women's indigenous knowledge and plant genetic resources, and most important, mandating gender impact assessments of the effects of trade liberalization, highlighting harmful policies and building on areas where women have benefited from increased trade. (See the website of the Women's Environment and Development Organization, http://www.wedo.org.)

Enhancing Food Security

International organizations, such as the Technical Centre for Agricultural and Rural Cooperation[13] (http://www.cta.int), have identified a number of measures to promote food security. Many of these measures have the potential to strengthen women's position to ensure food security for all. These measures include improving women's access to productive resources such land, credit, and technology designed to increase production and consumption of food-producing crops; enhancing rural women's skills through training and networking; promoting and developing agricultural techniques that women can use for food production, harvest, and marketing; increasing women's access to and supply of clean water, thereby reducing the amount of time women spend searching for potable water; increasing access to and supply of domestic energy, to reduce amount of time women spend searching for wood fuel; establishing strategic monetary and grain reserves at the national, community, and village levels; expanding microcredit programs to women farmers and food traders; and lowering internal and external tariff barriers on food. In addition, women's land ownership rights and ownership of other assets should be strengthened throughout the developing world. Collective land purchases by local women's groups and other schemes that give women greater control over land should be encouraged by government policies. National policies in addition to the incorporation of gender equity oriented perspective into bilateral, regional, and multilateral trade agreements and policies related to agriculture may play a big role in enhancing household food security and nutrition.

Improving Labor Standards

As we have discussed above, there is no automatic link between trade liberalization and reduction in gender inequalities in paid or unpaid labor. Gender division between paid and unpaid work, gender segregation in labor markets, persistent gender wage gaps, gender discrimination, and gender inequalities in the quality of work continue to characterize work relations throughout the developed and developing worlds. As Çağatay and Ertürk (2004) noted, "it is important to eradicate such inequalities, not only because they constitute violation of women's human rights, but also because they are a fundamental cause of the reproduction of poverty" (p. 38).

The International Labour Office (ILO 2004) has championed the paradigm of "decent work" (see chapter 8), which emphasizes four strategic objectives: the promotion of employment, the promotion of rights at work, the expansion of social protection for workers, and social dialogue. Gender concerns cut across all four of these objectives. Thus, women workers' rights remain the most compromised because women are disproportionately engaged in sectors that

are difficult to organize, or they are underrepresented in unions, or they lack the time to organize due to their double burden of caring labor.

Within export processing zones, governments have often "relaxed" the application of their own labor laws with regard to minimum wages, as well as curtailed the ability of workers to bargain collectively for improved conditions of work (Çağatay and Ertürk 2004; see also chapter 8). Needless to add, women workers are disproportionately affected. Though many governments in the south claim that they cannot "afford" higher labor standards, globalization and assuring decent working conditions need not be zero-sum (Elliott and Freeman 2003).

When we turn to social protection for workers, women again end up holding the short end of the stick, because much for their work is unpaid and because the precarious nature of their employment means that they are less likely to be covered by social protection systems.

Despite the nearly universal recognition of the urgency of improving labor standards across the globe, the mechanisms for achieving that goal continue to be debated. For example, while activists and governments in the north have advocated linking labor standards to trade agreements, many in the south view this as a thinly disguised form of trade protectionism. However, as pointed out by Çağatay and Ertürk (2004), it is a mistake to view the improvement of labor standards as a north–south issue. To the extent that globalization forces developing economies to compete against each other, the attainment of decent work is also a south–south issue, and one that can be addressed only through global collective action. Within this context, the ILO (2003) has promulgated the establishment of a Global Social Trust that would be financed by a modest contribution from workers in Organization for Economic Cooperation countries. The ILO estimates that an average monthly contribution of 5 Euros from each worker in the north would suffice to launch a trust that would enable the poorest countries to establish a social floor for 80–100 million workers within the next two decades.

Improving labor standards in the informal sector will continue to pose a major challenge, but even here groups such as the Self-Employed Women's Association in India have demonstrated successful models of organizing women in the informal sector that could be scaled up elsewhere.

Strengthening Caregiver Support

Finally, improved working conditions for women need to go hand in hand with strengthening of social supports for working adults (Heymann et al. 2003). Adequate paid leave is needed to allow workers to take time to care for the health needs of children and elderly family members, as well as to attend to their own health. Despite numerous international agreements which have affirmed the right of workers to paid leave, substantial disparities persist in legislative provisions for paid leave (including maternity leave) between and within regions of the globe. Provisions for flexibility of work schedules similarly remain a priority for the formal work sector.

Outside of work, social supports, such as affordable child care, early childhood education, and elder care, are urgently needed to enhance the ability of working women and men to balance their work and family responsibilities (Heymann et al. 2003).

CONCLUSION

In conclusion, the effects of globalization on women's health defy simplistic characterizations. Slogans such as "globalization is the engine of women's employment" or "the benefits of trade trickle down to the poor" are insufficient to characterize the complex ways in which women's health and well-being (and that of their family members) have been affected by the closer integration of economies around the globe. What is abundantly clear is that the consequences of and benefits from globalization have been *gender-differentiated* because of the persistence of unequal opportunities faced by women and men throughout all societies, both in the north and the south. Within this context, the need for gender-equity–oriented macroeconomic, trade, and labor market policies remains an urgent priority for the future course of globalization. Gender "mainstreaming" means strengthening the capacity for analysis, action, monitoring, and evaluation across all activities of national governments and international institutions in the pursuit of human development.

Notes

1. Structural adjustment policies were "globalized" in the sense that they were imposed by the International Monetary Fund and the World Bank on many debt-ridden and crisis-prone countries throughout the world (see chapter 13).

2. For example, Nussbaum (1999) opens with a poignant vignette of a young widow in Rajasthan, India, who is forced to rely on the charity of her male relatives for survival. If she attempts to go outside her house, her in-laws will beat her.

3. The Multi-Fibre Agreement (Clean Clothes Campaign, 2001) was a quota system for textile imports to developed countries. With the phase-out of the agreement, low-cost manufacturers such as Bangladesh are expected to lose out to even lower-cost producers such as China.

4. A point made long ago by Becker (1957).

5. The Gender-Related Development Index (GDI) was introduced by the UNDP in 1995 as an extension of the Human Development Index (HDI) and accounts for inequalities in the achievements of women and men (UNDP 1995). The GDI is a composite, country-level index composed of measures of gender differences in school enrolment and literacy, life expectancy, and incomes. When there is gender equality across these domains, the GDI assumes the same value as the HDI. However, at present, the GDI is lower than the HDI for all countries, indicating that no country treats its women as well as its men.

6. At the same time, caution is warranted in interpreting these transfers. In many instances, women give part of their wages to parents not out of compulsion but voluntarily as a form of "parent repayment." Thus, according to Foo and Lim (1989), such transfers are "not viewed by women or their families as coercive or exploitative, rather it is voluntary, natural, logical, and a rational act of reciprocity" (p. 218).

7. Or what Nancy Folbre (2001) refers to as the "invisible heart" of the economy, to contrast with the "invisible hand" of markets.

8. Policy makers have begun to pay attention to preventing educational losses incurred as a result of children having to care for other children. For example, during the 1998 Asian financial crisis, efforts were made in Indonesia to keep poor children (especially girls) in schools through scholarships targeted to girls (see Aslanbegui and Summerfield 2000).

9. There is also significant south–south migration of women, as described by Ehrenreich and Hochschild (2002). One stream goes from Southeast Asia to the oil-rich Middle East and Far East—from Bangladesh, Indonesia, the Philippines, and Sri Lanka to Bahrain, Oman, Kuwait, Saudi Arabia, Hong Kong, Malaysia, and Singapore. Other streams go from the former Soviet bloc to Western Europe, as well as from Africa to various parts of Europe.

10. For a discussion of the implications of TRIPS for access to life-saving drugs, see chapter 15.

11. For example, a West African berry, *Pentadiplandra brazzeana*—which has a sweetness intensity that is 500 times greater than a 10% sucrose solution on a weight basis (Hellekant and Danilova 2005)—has been "patented" by scientists in the United States and Europe.

Similarly, more than 35 patents have been taken out on the neem plant in India, used as a pesticide and fungicide.

12. Also referred to as women's budgets, gender-sensitive budgets, or gender-responsive budgets.

13. The Technical Centre for Agricultural and Rural Cooperation was established in 1983 under the Lomé Convention between the ACP (African, Caribbean, and Pacific) Group of States and the European Union Member States.

References

Amin, S. Diamond, I., Neavel, R. T., & Newby, M. (1998). Transition to adulthood of female garment factory workers in Bangladesh. Studies in Family Planning 29(2):185–200.

Aslanbegui, N., & Summerfield G. (2000). The Asian crisis, gender and international financial architecture. Feminist Economics 6(3):83–103.

Becker, G. S. (1957). *The Economics of Discrimination.* Chicago: University of Chicago Press.

Benería, L., Floro, M., Grown, C., & MacDonald, M. (2000). Globalization and gender. Feminist Economics 6(3):7–18.

Berik, G. (2000). Mature export-led growth and gender wage inequality in Taiwan. Feminist Economics 6(3):1–26.

Black, S. E., & Brainerd, E. (2002). Importing equality? The impact of globalization on gender discrimination. National Bureau of Economic Research Working Paper 9110. Cambridge, MA: National Bureau of Economic Research. http://www.nber.org/papers/w9110.

Bonita, R., & Mathers C. D. (2003). Global health status at the beginning of the twenty-first century. Pp. 24–53 in *Global Public Health: A New Era,* edited by R. Beaglehole. Oxford: Oxford University Press.

Çağatay, N., & Ertürk, K. (2004). Gender and globalization: a macroeconomic perspective. World Commission on the Social Dimension of Globalization Working Paper No. 19. Geneva: International Labour Office.

Dwyer, D., & Bruce, J., eds. (1988). *A Home Divided: Women and Income in the Third World.* Palo Alto, CA: Stanford University Press.

Ehrenreich, B., & Hochschild A., eds. (2003). *Global woman: Nannies, maids, and sex workers in the new economy.* New York: Metropolitan Books.

Elliott, K. A., & Freeman, R. B. (2003). The role global labor standards could play in addressing basic needs. Pp. 299–327 in *Global Inequalities at Work,* edited by J. Heymann. New York: Oxford University Press.

Elson, D. (1995). Gender awareness in modeling structural adjustment. World Development 23(11): 1851–1868.

Elson, D. (1998). Integrating gender issues into national budgetary policies and procedures: some policy op-

tions. Journal of International Development 19(7): 929–941.

Elson, D. (2002). Gender justice, human rights, and neo-liberal economic policies. Pp. 78–114 in *Gender Justice, Development and Rights,* edited by M. Molyneux & S. Razavi. Oxford: Oxford University Press.

Elson, D. & Pearson, R. (1981). The subordination of women and the institutionalization of factory production. Pp. 59–80 in *Of Marriage and the Market: Women's Subordination in International Perspective,* edited by C. Young & R. McCullagh. London: Routledge.

Erfan, A. F., (2004). The rise of the Bangladesh garment industry: globalization, women workers, and voice. National Women's Studies Association Journal 16(2):34–45.

FAO (1996). *Rural Women and Food Security: Current Situation and Perspectives.* Rome: Food and Agriculture Organization.

Folbre, N. (2001). *The Invisible Heart: Economics and Family Values.* New York: New Press.

Fontana, M., Joekes, S., & Masika, R. (1998). Global trade expansion and liberalization: gender issues and impacts. Report No. 42, prepared for the Department for International Development (DFID). Brighton, UK: Institute of Development Studies. http://www.bridge.ids.ac.uk/reports/re42c.pdf.

Fontana, M., & Wood, A. (2000). Modeling the effects of trade on women at work and at home. World Development 28(7):1173–1190.

Foo, G., & Lim, L. (1989). Poverty, ideology, and women export factory workers in South-East Asia. Pp. 212–233 in *Women, Poverty and Ideology in Asia,* edited by H. Afshar & B. Agarwal. Basingstoke, UK: Macmillan.

Fussel, E. (2000). Making labor flexible: the recomposition of Tijuana's maquiladora female labor force. Feminist Economics 6(3):59–80.

Haddad, L., Hodinott, J., & Alderman, H., eds. (1997). *Intrahousehold Resource Allocation in Developing Countries. Methods, Models, and Policy.* Baltimore, MD: Johns Hopkins University Press.

Hellekant, D., & Danilova V. (2005). Brazzein—a small, sweet protein: discovery and physiological overview. Chemical Senses 30(suppl. 1):i88–i89.

Heymann, J., Fischer, A., & Engelman, M. (2003). Labor conditions and the health of children, elderly and disabled family members. Pp. 75–104 in *Global Inequalities at Work,* edited by J. Heymann. New York: Oxford University Press.

Hochschild, A. R. (2000). Global care chains and emotional surplus value. Pp. 130–146 in *Global Capitalism,* edited by W. Hutton & A. Giddens. New York: New Press.

Hochschild, A. R. & Machung, A. (1997). *The Second Shift: Working Parents and the Revolution at Home.* New York: Avon.

ILO (2003). Working out of Poverty. Report of the Director-General, International Labour Conference,

91st Session. Geneva: International Labour Office. http://www.ilo.org/public/english.standards/relm/ilc/ilc91/pdf/rep-i-a.pdf.

ILO (2004). *List of ILO Conventions and Recommendations.* Geneva: International Labour Office. http://www.ilo.org/public/english/protection/safework/standard.htm.

Jaggar, A. M. (2002). Vulnerable women and neo-liberal globalization: debt burdens undermine women's health in the global South. Theoretical Medicine 23:425–440.

Joekes, S. (1995). Trade-related employment for women in industry and services in developing countries. UNRISD Occasional Paper No. 5. Geneva: United Nations Research Institute for Social Development.

Jomo, K.S. (2001). Globalization, export-oriented industrialization, female employment, and equity in East Asia. UNRISD Programme Papers No. 34. Geneva: United Nations Research Institute for Social Development.

Kabeer, N. (1995). Necessary, sufficient, or irrelevant? Women, wages, and intra-household power relations in Bangladesh. IDS Working Paper No. 25. Brighton, UK: Institute of Development Studies, University of Sussex.

Kawachi, I., Kennedy, B. P., Gupta, V., & Prothrow-Stith, D. (1999). Women's status and the health of women and men: a view from the States. Soc Sci Med 48:21–32.

Kucera, D., & Milberg, W. (2000). Gender segregation and gender bias in manufacturing trade expansion: revisiting the "wood asymmetry." World Development 28(7):1191.

Lado, C. (1992). Female labor participation in agricultural production and the implications for nutrition and health in rural Africa. Social Science and Medicine, 34(7):789–807.

Maclean, H., & Sicchia, S. R., eds. (2004). Gender, globalization, and health. Paper presented at NIH Stone House Forum, April 27, 2004, Bethesda, MD.

Malhotra, K. (2003). *Making Global Trade Work for People.* London: Earthscan.

McGow, L. (1995). The Ignored Cost of Adjustment: Women under SAPs in Africa. The Development Gap. Discussion Paper presented at the Fourth World Conference on Women, Beijing, China, September 4–15, 1005.

Nussbaum, M. C. (1999). *Sex and Social Justice.* New York: Oxford University Press.

Public Citizen Global Trade Watch (2003). Unbalanced WTO dispute system—women need not apply: gender analysis of WTO dispute panelists. http://www.citizen.org/print_article.cfm?ID=5571

Sachs, J. D. (2005). *The End of Poverty. Economic Possibilities for Our Time.* New York: Penguin Press.

Sainsbury, D (1996). Gender, Equality and Welfare States. Cambridge: Cambridge University Press.

Saito, K., Mekonen, H., & Spurling, D., eds. (1994). *Raising the Productivity of Women Farmers in Sub-Saharan Africa.* Washington, DC: World Bank.

Seguino, S. (2000). Gender inequality and economic growth: a cross-country analysis. World Development 28(7):1211–1230.

Sen, A. (1999). *Development as Freedom.* New York: Alfred A. Knopf.

Sen, A. (2000). The population problem and gender inequality. Nation 271:24–31.

UNDP (1995). *Human Development Report 1995.* New York: Oxford University Press.

UNDP (1999). *Human Development Report 1999.* New York: Oxford University Press.

UNDP (2003). *Millennium Development Goals: National Reports, A Look through a Gender Lens.* New York: United Nations Development Program.

UNICEF (2005). *The State of the World's Children 2005.* New York: United Nation's Children's Fund.

UNIFEM (2002). *Progress of the World's Women: Gender Equality and the Millennium Development Goals.* New York: United Nations Development Fund for Women.

United Nations (1995). Beijing Declaration and Platform for Action. Adopted by the Fourth World Conference on Women: Action for Equality, Development and Peace, Beijing, September 15.

UNRISD. (2005). *Gender Equality: Striving for Justice in an Unequal World.* Policy Report on Gender and Development: 10 Years after Beijing. Geneva: United Nations Research Institute for Social Development.

Weston, A. (1994). The Uruguay Round: Unveiling the Implications for the Least-Developed and Low-Income Countries. Geneva: UNCTAD Secretariat.

WIDE (2001). *Instruments for Gender Equality in Trade Agreements: European Union—MERCOSUR—Mexico.* Brussels, Belgium: Women in Development Europe.

Williamson, J. B., & Boehmer, U. (1997). Female life expectancy, gender stratification, health status, and level of economic development: a cross-national study of less developed countries. Social Science Medicine 45:305–317.

World Bank (2001). *Engendering Development. Through Equality in Rights, Resources and Voice.* Washington, DC: World Bank.

Part II

Monitoring the Impact
of Globalization on Health

Chapter 11

Summary Measures of Population Health: Controversies and New Directions

Daniel D. Reidpath

That measurement is not a pure-hearted, rational endeavor sheltered from the vagaries of the human condition is not a new observation (Brown & Malone, 2004). When reflecting on the extension of that observation to the measurement of population health, very few would be surprised to learn that how health is measured is strongly grounded in a particular sociocultural context (Allotey & Reidpath, 2002; Porter, 1999) or that the process of measurement is intensely political (Hamlin, 1998).

The physicist Albert Einstein once famously observed that "not everything that can be counted counts and not everything that counts can be counted." The relevance of the adage to population health could be increased tenfold by adding that the meaning given to the counted varies according to rules of counting. The way that things are counted affects the interpretation of the results, and the choices that are made about how things should be counted are social and political.

The direction of health policy and allocation of health resources are directly affected by the estimated health of populations, particularly when the amount of health (or ill health) may be partitioned by condition or risk factor, including demographic characteristics. This means that changing the way one measures population health has the potential to affect policy and resource allocation profoundly. When the organizations involved in determining how population health should be measured are as significant as the World Bank and the World Health Organization (WHO), the sociopolitical context in which these events occur has global ramifications.

Notwithstanding this, when scientists working within large organizations are asked to speculate on appropriate measures of population health, it is easy for them to retreat into the specifics of the task, believing that their personal sense of objectivity will triumph over the weight of those external organizational or broader sociocultural forces that themselves pattern and influence thought.

The scientists' error is at once veiled by the dominance of the paradigm within which they work

(Kuhn, 1962) and, in the context of this chapter, significant because of the strategies that have been used to globalize and entrench those approaches to health measurement.

GLOBALIZATION

There is no single accepted definition of globalization. The International Monetary Fund has defined it in strictly economic terms as the "increasing integration of economies around the world, particularly through trade and financial flows around the flow of capital" (International Monetary Fund Staff, 2000). Its Bretton Woods twin,[1] the World Bank, described globalization more broadly in terms of "the global circulation of goods, services and capital, but also of information, ideas and people" (World Bank, 2000, p. 1).

As this book demonstrates, in considering the link between globalization and health, most researchers have thought about it in terms of the direct impact that globalization has on health and health service delivery (Navarro, 2002). Examples abound, including studies on the effect of globalization on the power of multinational pharmaceutical companies (Busfield, 2003), the impact of global capital systems on the environment and health (McMichael, 2000), and the global movement of health professionals—often to the detriment of developing countries (Marchal & Kegels, 2003).

Less obvious is the link between globalization and the issues surrounding the measurement of population health, and it is this link with which the present chapter is principally concerned. Attempts by the WHO and the World Bank to measure the global burden of disease provide one clear illustration of this link, and they highlight the social foundation of population health measurement and its global implications (Murray & Lopez, 1996; Ugalde & Jackson, 1995; World Bank, 1993). The example of the global burden of disease study is discussed in some detail below. It is worth bearing in mind, however, that the issues raised here are not exclusive to the present. For example, in the world of Edwin Chadwick, William Farr, and Louis-René Villermé, the nineteenth-century European champions of population health, health and measurement were interwoven with contemporary politics (Porter, 1999).

Now or then, a central issue would be the manner in which the claimed "objectivity" of measurement became a rhetorical device to support political and organizational ends (Porter, 1999). The starting point, therefore, is linguistic—the very definition of health—because controlling the language with which population health may be discussed is one way of trying to control the direction of future policy.

Before examining that, however, some background to the measures of population health under examination is needed.

MEASURES OF POPULATION HEALTH

A plethora of measures of population health exist. As technical instruments, these can be divided into two broad groups: measures related to health gaps and measures related to health expectancies (Murray et al., 2000).

The "health gap" refers to the difference between the actual and the ideal health of the population. In this case, the ideal is for each person in the population to live a full life in full health, where a full life is of some agreed length. Individuals experience premature mortality if they die before they have reached the age of the agreed full life. Premature morbidity refers to an individual's experience of a less than good health state before reaching the age of the agreed full life. Premature mortality or morbidity of any individual reduces the health of the population. By summing the number of healthy years of life lost (YLL) due to premature mortality or morbidity, one can estimate the burden of disease in a population.

The YLL due to mortality is straightforwardly calculated as the gap between the age of premature mortality and the idealized life expectancy. A discount rate is usually applied to YLL such that each future year accounts for slightly less value than the year before. Morbidity may be handled in much the same way except that only a part of a year is counted for each year lived in less than full health (years of life lost due to disability [YLD]), to reflect the "gap" between the disabled state and full health. A health state that is severely disabling is given a higher disability weight than a health state that is close to full health. This is to reflect the greater proportion of a full year of healthy life that is lost living in that health state for a year.

The health of the population is estimated as the sum of the YLLs and YLDs (for all individuals living or recently deceased in the population) over a year. Perhaps the best known of these measures is the disability-adjusted life year (DALY), which was developed initially for the World Bank/WHO global burden of disease studies (Murray, 1996; World Bank, 1993).

The population health measures based on "health expectancies" estimate a population's health as a function of average life expectancy at birth (Murray et al., 2000). In a fashion analogous to the DALY, life expectancy can be adjusted to take account of continued years of life in less than good health. The WHO developed a health expectancies measure, to complement the DALY, initially called the disability-adjusted life expectancy (Murray & Acharya, 1997) but later renamed healthy life expectancy (HALE).

The DALY and the HALE have contributed significantly to population health debates, particularly through the publication of the *World Health Reports*. Both measures have also been criticized on technical grounds (e.g., AbouZahr, 1999; Allotey et al., 2003; Anand & Hanson, 1997; Barker & Green, 1996; Reidpath & Allotey, 2003). The debates are not revisited here. Rather, the measures are sketched so that the discussion can progress about the social choices that have underpinned the globalization of population health measurement. These choices have included, among other things, quite specific decisions about how to define, operationalize, and write about health.

(RE-)DEFINING HEALTH

As the philosopher Ludwig Wittgenstein argued, definitions are tricky. Understanding conceptual categories such as a "game," for example, can frequently be achieved only with recourse to notions of resemblance within a family of "games," rather than to precise and well-bounded descriptions (Wittgenstein, 1953, 1969).[2] Health, in this regard, might be considered equally troublesome. Definitions of health are myriad, and the ways in which people conceptualize health probably conform better to a family resemblance rather than a single coherent idea.

Notwithstanding the linguistic and philosophical impediments, the WHO definition of health, which appeared in the preamble to the organization's 1948 constitution, remains one of the most widely acknowledged. Part of the appeal of the definition is its broad and generally inclusive nature, taking account

of physical, mental, and social states. Health is defined as "a state of complete physical, mental, and social well-being and not merely the absence of disease and infirmity."

For the purposes of measurement, an immediate difficulty arises. A necessary precursor to measurement is the development of a sound operational definition of the thing to be measured.[3] The operational definition needs to be a precisely measurable interpretation of the underlying concept. If the underlying concept is not a "thing" but a cluster of things brought together by a familial resemblance, then the mere act of operationalization may distort and corrupt the definition by focusing on some features of familial resemblance and ignoring others. The net result is an operational definition that no longer captures the essence of the underlying concept—a standard critique of positivist traditions in the social sciences.

The broad WHO constitutional definition of health does not in and of itself carry information about what of health is measurable. As it stands, therefore, it is unsuitable for tasks such as the measurement of population health. This does not make it an impossible starting point, but it adds to the complexity of the task. Notwithstanding this, the WHO's constitutional definition is said to provide the first building block in the development of an operational definition (Murray et al., 2002a, p. 732).

The reality, however, is that the WHO/World Bank discourse on the operational definition of health for their Global Burden of Disease studies often presents an inconsistent image seemingly detached from the constitutional roots of the WHO and often at odds with the broader health literature. The developers' arguments for the creation of their operational definition were predicated on a desire for an "objective" measure of health. Supporting arguments for their approach were based in part on "common sense," what was "natural," and "the intuitive societal notions of what constitutes health" (Murray et al., 2002a, p. 733).[4] Almost without exception, the definitions of health they chose to endorse supported the notion that health, universally, is intrinsic to the person, related to functional loss, and conceptually (and definitionally) separable from the social, cultural, and environmental context in which the life is lived (Reidpath et al., 2003). This position reflects some of the sociopolitical choices to be explored. Significantly, the notion of social well-being that appeared as a component of health in the constitutional definition (almost necessarily requiring the context of the lived experience to be taken into account) became ancillary.

The argument that locates health entirely within the person (Murray et al., 2002a) is widely applied within much of the health measurement literature (Murray et al., 2002b), although it is not consistent with the broader health literature that suggests a diversity of cultural views about the nature of health (Foucault, 1989/1963; Helman, 1994; Spector, 2000). For some groups, health represents internal balance between the humors or a balance between Yin and Yang, for other groups it represents a form of relational balance between the person and the environment, and for others, something different again. Even within a relatively homogeneous cultural group, substantial variations are identified in the manner in which health is conceived, often varying on age and gender lines (Blaxter, 1990). As Foucault observed in the opening of *The Birth of the Clinic*:

> For us, the human body defines, by natural right, the space of origin and of distribution of disease: a space whose lines, volumes, surfaces, and routes are laid down, in accordance with a now familiar geometry, by the anatomical atlas. But this order of the solid, visible body is only one way—in all likelihood neither the first, nor the most fundamental—in which one spatializes disease. (Foucault, 1989/1963, p. 1)

Although Foucault's focus was on disease, the point about the "natural right" is well made—there are multitudinous ways in which the intuitive and the commonsensical may be conceived. That one thinks in a particular way does not make it right, merely familiar.

Nonetheless, by narrowing and constraining the constitutional definition in the way it did, the WHO sought a definition of health that was institutionally palatable, globally applicable, and suitable for the task of measuring population health. The challenge was to operationalize this.

DEFINING HEALTH FOR THE GLOBAL BURDEN OF DISEASE STUDIES

Over the decade that the WHO/World Bank worked on estimating the global burden of disease, the operational definition of health evolved.

In 1993, the operational definition of health that was to inform a new globalized measure of population health focused on disability (World Bank, 1993). The definition continued the intent to project health as intrinsically related to the functioning of the body, thereby excluding relational considerations around the place of the person within a social, cultural, and environmental context (Musgrove, 2000; World Bank, 1993). Under this model, as disability increases (i.e., bodily functioning decreases), so health decreases—independent of any social or environmental externalities.

The next evolution in the following year (1994) saw disability again used for the operational definition of diminished health, but this time it was argued that disability was explicitly linked to the WHO's *International Classification of Impairments, Disabilities, and Handicaps* (ICIDH) definition of disability (Murray, 1994, p. 11; WHO, 1980). This shift does not seem to be a major one, except that it transpired that the operational definition was broader than intended and did not restrict the definition to intrinsic functional loss. Rather, the operational definition was "somewhere between disability and handicap" (Murray, 1996, p. 34). The distinction is important because the ICIDH definition of "disability" related exclusively to the functional loss, whereas "handicap" was used to characterize the relational aspect of disability within a social context. This definitional slippage between the intrinsic and the relational occurred unintentionally but unavoidably. It was ultimately meaningless to measure health in a context-free vacuum, and aspects of the interrelationship between the person (with the functional loss) and the context in which the person experienced the world had to be considered.

If a knee is damaged in some way, for instance, it may manifest itself as a limp, but a limp does not exist within the person—the limp is apparent only in the interaction between the person and the walking surface. The limp may be more pronounced and more deleterious when the person is traversing some surfaces than others.

By 1996, the WHO was confounded. Indeed, the arguments around the operational definition of health were contradictory. On the one hand, "one must focus on [functional loss] disability" (Murray, 1996, p. 33); on the other hand, the focus should be on a construct between disability and handicap, "best described as average level of handicap" (Murray, 1996, pp. 33–34).

By 1997, the position had settled to some degree. However, the inherent tension between health as a measurable performance loss directly associated with some functional or structural aspect intrinsic to the person, and health as a function of a relationship between body and context remained. Health was to be measured in terms of "functioning achievements (or lack of them) that can be specified due to illness" and that should be measured "by the degree of deprivation experienced by a person in being able to use one's own body" (Murray & Acharya, 1997, p. 724). This was to be done, however, by taking account of the relationship between the person with the functional loss and "the average social response or milieu for the world" (Murray & Acharya, 1997, p. 713). Thus, functional loss was circumscribed by the social and environmental context within which the body was to be used, while limiting the reach of context with an appeal to an average environment. The strategy was adopted to ensure that the loss attributable to a health state was counted the same across the globe—across the globally uniform environment. It was, to paraphrase Murray, to ensure that blindness in Bogota would be counted the same as blindness in New York.

Unfortunately, the logical problems with health measurement relying on functional loss in an "average environment" were significant. The difficulty was compounded when the data were to be disaggregated by population or geography because the arithmetic did not work (Reidpath et al., 2001, 2003), and this can be illustrated in the case of paraplegia.

The WHO argued that the health loss attributable to paraplegia could be calculated by examining the person (and their functional loss due to spinal cord injury) within an average social environment. The reality is, however, that, *ceteris paribus*, the health impact of paraplegia for a person living in Australia is quantitatively and qualitatively completely different from the health impact experienced by a person living in Cameroon (Allotey et al., 2003). There is no social milieu that is an average of a muddy rural village in the tropics and a city with well-developed physical infrastructure in temperate Australia. The consequence of this is that there is no coherent way of using an average context as the point of comparison of the health associated with paraplegia.

In 2002, the WHO tried again to create an operational definition of health that conformed to the organizational view that health was intrinsic to the

individual and separable from the context in which the life was lived. The new way to think about the measurement of the health of a person was in terms of their *capacity* in a "uniform environment," drawing on the new notion of capacity that had been introduced in the *International Classification of Functioning, Disability, and Health* (ICF; WHO, 2001):

> To assess the full ability of the individual, one would need to have a "standardized" environment to neutralize the varying impact of different environments on the ability of the individual. This standardized [uniform] environment may be: (a) an actual environment commonly used for capacity assessment in testing settings; or (b) in cases where this is not possible, an assumed environment which can be thought to have a uniform impact. . . . This adjustment has to be the same for all persons in all countries to allow for international comparisons. (p. 15)

Significantly, the paragraph in ICF continued, "The features of the uniform . . . environment can be coded using the [ICF] Environmental Factors classification" (p. 15), which include the "physical, social, and attitudinal environment in which people live and conduct their lives" (p. 171). This clearly acknowledges the relational nature of health, but by again fixing the social, cultural, and environmental context, they sought for the purposes of measurement to focus on the functional loss in isolation from the varied context in which life is lived. With respect to the operational definition of health "the ability to walk 100 metres on a level, well-lit, non-slippery surface" was provided as an example of capacity in the uniform environment (Murray et al., 2002a, p. 733). But the description is of a single, unrealistic, 100-meter journey that is divorced from the manner in which daily life is negotiated within a real, constrained physical and social infrastructure.

There should not be anything inherently special about the uniform environment used as an example in the ICF documentation. All that is required is that, for measurement purposes, the environment is the same everywhere. Consider instead an alternative "uniform environment." It is a village in a poor, tropical country in the rainy season. Roads and paths are reminiscent of rivers of mud. People with paraplegia are scorned, abused, and socially marginalized. If this uniform environment is used to measure the health of all the people in the world with paraplegia, then the wheelchairs (motorized or not) can be completely discounted, because they could not be moved through the mud. The relatively well-built environment of the socially conscious, modern city could also be ignored, as could a user-friendly public transport system or the provision of state assistance. The more congenial social relations of a less stigmatizing society could also be ignored.

It is certainly easy to appreciate the convenience that a uniform environment offers those who measure population health. The consequences, however, are that the health of the people with paraplegia who in reality live in the socially conscious, modern city would be underestimated (because the more congenial environmental factors were ignored). Under estimating health would indicate a more serious problem in those places than actually occurred. Conversely, if the uniform environment were based on that socially conscious, modern city, then the health of people with paraplegia in poor developing countries, with poor physical infrastructure, would be overestimated. Overestimating health would indicate a less serious problem in those places than actually occurred.

The situation becomes worse, however, when one considers the interrelationship between the myriad health states and the myriad environments one might select (Reidpath et al., 2003). It is quite conceivable that differently coded physical, social, and attitudinal "uniform environments" would see quite drastic global swings in the estimation of population health. Essentially, the criticisms that were made of average social milieu translate with almost no variation to the uniform environment (Reidpath et al., 2003).

The WHO/World Bank strategy to force one particular operational definition of health between 1993 and 2002 was in part linguistic. Where "disability" had failed, "average handicap" was introduced; where "average handicap" failed, "average social milieu" was introduced. With the failure of "average social milieu," the "uniform environment" was adopted. The linguistic shift was also often supported by changes in WHO classifications to notions of disability—again trying to constrain and separate the biomedical and the social, the structural, the functional, and the contextual. ICIDH (WHO, 1980), which the WHO/World Bank used in 1993 and 1994, gave way to ICIDH-2 (WHO, 1999), which was used to characterize the average social milieu. This in turn gave way to the ICF notion of capacity that utilizes the uniform environment (WHO, 2001).

The meanings of the words were also incredibly labile. In the 1980 parlance of ICIDH, "disability" was any restriction or lack of ability to perform an activity within the normal range due to a loss or abnormality of psychological, physiological, or anatomical structure or function (WHO, 1980, pp. 27–28). "Handicap" was a disadvantage from a disability explicable by contextual factors such as the social, cultural, and environmental setting (p. 29). By the time the ICF was published, however, this nomenclature had been twisted around completely, and disability was now an umbrella term that included body functions and structure interacting with the social, cultural, and physical environment (WHO, 2001, p. 8).

At each stage, the WHO/World Bank argument for the classification of functioning and disability and the argument for the measurement of population health were inextricably linked—a self-supporting infrastructure. Logically, however, the existence of one cannot be regarded as independent support for the correctness of the other.

When one juxtaposes the WHO constitutional definition of health with the conceptual writings about the nature of health, the best characterization for the continuous adjustments to the operational definition is "monster barring" (Lakatos, 1976).[5] Essentially, each time the WHO was alerted to a failure in its operational definition of health to restrict health to a functional loss intrinsic to the person, the definition was rewritten. In some circumstances the process of monster barring might be seen as a legitimate and useful mechanism for refining an operational definition of health, by excluding aberrant definitions. This would be particularly true if there was indeed strong evidence for a cross-cultural, "commonsense," "natural," and "intuitive" view of health. In the absence of that support, there are grounds for a reasonable suspicion that the barring of monsters from the operational definition was much more about the political economy of the WHO than it was about trying to capture a definition of health. In looking for support for the WHO position, the ICF and the work that led to its development warrant consideration. In the first instance, it warrants consideration because the ICF definitions of "capacity" and "handicap" were used in the operationalization of health, and in the second, because the development of ICF shared arguments about the universal nature of health with the Global Burden of Disease study measure of population health.

ICF

ICF is a part of a WHO "family" of international classificatory systems that codify information about health, using a "standardized common language" (WHO, 2001, p. 3). It was argued that it, in conjunction with *International Statistical Classification of Diseases and Health Related Problems* (ICD-10), which provides a primarily etiological framework for classifying disease (WHO, 1992), ICF "provides a valuable tool to describe and compare the health of populations in an international context" (WHO, 2001, p. 4). Using these classificatory systems, information on mortality (ICD-10) and morbidity (ICF) "may be combined in summary measures of population health for monitoring the health of populations and its distribution, and also for assessing the contributions of different causes of mortality and morbidity" (p. 4). This approach, it was further argued, moved ICF away from the *consequences* of health (which was the focus of the earlier ICIDH [WHO, 1980]) and focused on a component of health classificatory system. Three of the summary aims of the ICF were described as follows:

- To provide a scientific basis for understanding and studying health and health-related states, outcomes, and determinants
- To establish a common language for describing health and health related states
- To permit comparisons of data across countries, health care disciplines, services and time (WHO, 2001, p. 5)

The ICF, however, has not simply been claimed to be a "common" classificatory language for describing health states (Üstün et al., 2001a). It has been likened by the WHO to the Rosetta Stone, the Egyptian stone tablet that is synonymous with universal translation (Üstün, 2002, p. 348). Furthermore, the WHO has relied on the universal nature of the ICF (and of its older version, ICIDH-2) to support arguments about the universality of its approach to the measurement of population health (Murray, 1996; Murray & Acharya, 1997).

The discourse of universality raises an important question about what one might mean by a universal classificatory system and the extent to which the ICF (or measures of population health that rely on it) could reasonably be claimed to fulfill that role. To

answer the question requires a little background on the human process of classification and its application.

UNIVERSAL CLASSIFICATION

At its most basic, thinking involves classification (Körner, 1974), and humans by their nature classify (Bateson, 1988; Bowker & Star, 1999). It is in the identification of difference that we draw order out of chaos and make sense of relationships within and between objects and ideas (Slaughter, 1982). Whether we are "primitive" or "civilized," our systems of classification provide hierarchies of notions that permit us to develop an understanding of the surrounding world (Durkheim & Mauss, 1963, p. 81). Although the classificatory systems that evolve may vary radically between cultures, their role in connecting ideas and unifying knowledge within a culture is constant—even if the knowledge may itself be contested between cultures.

In the Western scientific tradition, classificatory systems abound, with plant taxonomies based on morphology illustrating one of the richest historical traditions (Slaughter, 1982). Given, however, that different and sometimes competing classificatory systems exist, how does one decide which system is fundamentally right—that is, actually captures some universal truth—and which systems have only local value? The problem in determining the universality of any particular classificatory system is, as Körner (1974, p. 16) so aptly observed, that people have a natural inclination to elevate the peculiarities of their own thought into universal characteristics of all thought. This, then, can lead to the assumption that the mere development of a classification system is in and of itself evidence of a universal truth. Borges (1964) eloquently parodied this position in his brief essay "The Analytical Language of John Wilkins." In it he describes the *Celestial Emporium of Benevolent Knowledge*, a fictional Chinese encyclopedia, which he claimed contained a taxonomy of animals that included such categories as mermaids, sucking pigs, those animals drawn with a very fine camel hair brush, and those that from a long way off look like flies (p. 103).

The classification of Pap smears for the identification of cervical cancer is a useful illustration of the difficulties in developing an objective classificatory system in health. Given the essential simplicity of the technology involved, a priori one might imagine the task to be clear cut, and yet as Clarke and Casper (1996) show in their critical analysis of the developments in smear classification (1917–1990), it was a very human undertaking. Historically, there have been four major systems for the cytological classification of vaginocervical smears: the eponymously named Pap[anicolaou] smear classification, the dysplasia/WHO system, the CIN system, and the Bethesda/SIL system (p. 607). The rise of each system reflected social, political, scientific, guild, and health demands, not simply the need for a universal system for cytological classification. Furthermore, if one system were to become universally adopted, it would, in all likelihood, more properly reflect hegemony than objectivity. Clarke and Casper wrote of the development of the cytological classification as revealing (a) the subjectivity of the systems that developed and changed over time, with various actors (individual and organizational) attempting to protect their own goals and advance their own interests, and (b) the subjectivity of the boundary between the normal and the pathological cell.

Moving from the (apparently) strictly biological to the more complex classification of "mental disorders," a second salient example is observed in the American Psychiatric Association's (1994) *Diagnostic and Statistical Manual of Mental Disorders: DSM-IV*. In this instance, culture becomes an even greater challenge to universality.

Acutely aware of the cultural aspects of many mental health conditions, both in terms of the manifestations and understanding of the conditions, the American Psychiatric Association sought explicitly to include considerations of culture throughout the manual (Mezzich et al., 1999). The inclusion of cultural considerations, however, fell well short of that recommended by the Group on Culture and Diagnosis, sponsored by the National Institute of Mental Health, and has profound implications for the disease taxa described in *DSM-IV* (Mezzich et al., 1999):

> The clinical experience encoded in the diagnostic criteria of DSM-III and subsequent revisions were largely based on relatively homogenous clinical populations of patients at university clinics, initially in the Midwest and East Coast of the U.S. There has been strikingly little effort to appraise the clinical and predictive utility of DSM cate-

gories, criteria, and axes on culturally diverse populations within the U.S. (p. 462)

Mezzich et al. (1999) also observed that future iterations needed further research on cultural frameworks for diagnosis and care.

In fairness, *DSM-IV* was principally designed for domestic U.S. consumption. Notwithstanding that, it has been far more widely adopted with a presumption that it encoded something quite universal about the nature of mental health. Furthermore, given the cultural diversity of the United States, the applicability of *DSM-IV* even to that single heterogeneous context invited (and has received) speculation.

Clearly, theories of health, and the classifications of disease that arise out of those theories, are not protected from the whimsy of impermanent subjectivity. Any hint of privileged objectivity is challenged by history—ancient and modern. The development of the ICF itself (WHO, 2001), out of the roots of ICIDH (WHO, 1980) and its staging point for change, ICIDH-2 (WHO, 1999), unavoidably throws the objectivity of ICF into doubt. A sense of progressive improvement must almost inevitably arise out of the planned changes and revision of ICIDH that led to ICF, heightening the belief that universality has been achieved or at least progressive improvement has been made. This simply recalls Körner's observation.

The foregoing, however, is speculative and is open to refutation. There is evidence to suggest that there are universal ways of understanding some things (Berlin, 1992), although the notion of "understanding" may need to be distinguished from the universality of a taxonomy. Wittgenstein suggested that it was impossible to specify linguistically exclusive, well-bounded categories in complex areas, and often the best one could hope to achieve was a statement of "family resemblance" (Wittgenstein, 1953, 1969). This is a far cry from a universal classificatory system but is nonetheless valuable.

Considerable effort was expended developing and testing the universal applicability of ICF (WHO, 2001). Some of this work has also been used to support the universality of measures of population health, such as the DALY and the HALE. Given the role that this work has come to play in the manner in which population health is envisaged, its empirical support justifies thoughtful consideration.

UNIVERSALS IN POPULATION HEALTH

In essence, the argument holds that if people from different settings agree with each other, then this is evidence of universality. If they agree about the value of health states, then this is evidence that the value of health states reflects a universal truth about the nature and classification of disability and notions of health.

The argument was explicitly made in the development of ICF, where WHO "engaged in a comprehensive exercise of developing instruments for the diagnosis and classification of alcohol, drug, and mental disorders that can be used cross-culturally and internationally" (Üstün et al., 2001b, p. 3). The argument was used with barely more circumspection in the development of the DALY as a global measure of population health (Murray, 1996; Murray & Acharya, 1997).

ADDRESSING UNIVERSALITY

To support the universal nature of the WHO's measures of health, data were sought that would demonstrate a cross-cultural sameness and the occurrence of context-insensitive "values" for different health states. If globally, everyone agreed about the value of a health state—paraplegia versus blindness versus deafness, and so forth—then an argument could be made for a uniform counting rule for each health state that ignored the context in which the health state occurred.

The value of a health state was referred to as a "disability weight" (Murray, 1996; Reidpath et al., 2003), and it was arrived at by panels of judges who were presented with pithy descriptions of twenty-two indicator health conditions. Using the person trade-off,[6] the value of these twenty-two less-than-perfect health states was determined.

Multiple panels had been convened in different countries, and the level of agreement (Spearman's rho) between panels about the various indicator conditions was high (Murray, 1996, pp. 38–40). The high levels of agreement were taken as evidence that each panel's judgments tapped into the latent, universal, value of the health states. The panel exercises, however, were by design better suited to the confirmation of a view than the testing of a view, and a plausible alternative explanation is that the level of agreement was an artifact of the methodology:

- The panels of judges all had health backgrounds, predisposing them to particular (common) views of health in virtue of their disciplinary training. Although they came from different places, ostensibly bringing together a diversity of views, in their discipline they had a highly prized and shared common culture.
- The panel exercise used a modified Delphi technique, which is renowned (indeed, designed) for achieving high levels of agreement within panels. Given (a) the disciplinary background of the panelists, and (b) the bias of the conveners of the panels, this would also increase the likelihood of between panel agreement.[7]
- The measure of agreement that was used (i.e., correlation) was flawed because of the heteroskedastic nature of the data and the fixed end points of full health and death—discussed below (figure 11.1).

Consider the judgments made by two hypothetical panels asked to value three health states: a "hangnail," that irritating and often painful sliver of loose skin occurring near the side of a finger nail; "coma"; and "deafness." In the exercise, "0" indicated a panel's indifference between the health state, and full health and "1" indicated indifference between the health state and death. Figure 11.1 shows the bivariate plot of the conditions based on the judgments of the two hypothetical panels. The hangnail is shown as very close in value to full health (0). Conversely, "coma" is shown with a very high value close to death. Deafness is shown with a range of possible values. The ellipse enclosing the points illustrates the heteroskedastic nature of the task, where conditions near either of the two end points are likely to elicit much higher levels of agreement between the panels than are health conditions that are more centrally located. The level of agreement was, in effect, anchored artificially high because of the "pull" exerted by the end points. A priori, one might expect that severely disabling conditions and marginally disabling conditions would elicit much higher levels of agreement between panels than conditions that would be more influenced by the context in which the life was lived (Reidpath et al., 2003).

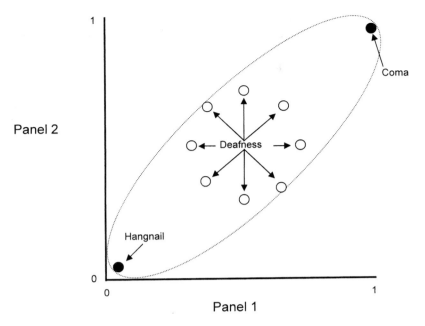

FIGURE 11.1. Heteroskedasticity in the bivariate distribution of panels' judgments about the value of health states

The combined effect of the disciplinary background of the panelists, the use of a group technique designed to elicit agreement, and the heteroskedastic nature of the data provide an inflated sense of agreement.

An adjunct approach used to support the development of the ICF was to elicit health state valuations from related country studies (Üstün et al., 1999, 2001a, 2002). In a series of fourteen small country studies, health professionals, policy makers, people with disabilities and their care providers (total $n = 241$) were required to rank order seventeen health state descriptions from the most to the least disabling (Üstün et al., 1999). High levels of agreement about the rank order of the health state were to be treated as evidence of universality. In one discussion of the results, the authors observed the following:

> The main result of this study is that the rankings of the disabling effect of health conditions were found to be relatively stable across countries, informant groups, and methods, although there is some variation. . . . Thus in the eyes of the respondents, the relative burden of different health conditions in terms of disability is fairly similar across the world. (Üstün et al., 2002, p. 589)

This all seems very positive and supports universality, except they go on to note that "the results also indicate that there are some quite pronounced differences between cultures and informant groups" (p. 589).

Three years earlier, the WHO had been somewhat more critical of the results, observing that "the differences [in ranks] are large enough to cast doubt on the assumption of universality of experts' judgments about disability weights" (Üstün et al., 1999, p. 111).[8] Interestingly, it was also noted that "the ranking of the conditions at both ends of the range showed less variability between informants than that for the intermediate conditions" (p. 113). This concise phrase elegantly captures the idea illustrated in figure 11.1 and directly supports the theoretical argument about the almost necessarily heteroskedastic nature of the bivariate relationships between informants' or panels' judgments.

Notwithstanding the doubt raised by the empirical data, when it comes to supporting universal measures of population health, the interpretation is barely qualified: "Fortunately, all empirical research suggests that the rank ordering of diseases . . . is rather invariant between populations and cultures" (van der Maas, 2002, p. 55).

The authorial technique adopted is reminiscent of the writings on "selective primary health care" (Rifkin

& Walt, 1986; Walsh & Warren, 1979; Werner & Sanders, 1997; Wisner, 1988). Control the language and create the field in which the work is to be judged. The WHO book intended to explore the issues of universality in ICIDH-2 using case studies from thirteen countries is a case in point (Üstün et al., 2001a). In the conclusion, there are no real surprises and a strong sense of the authors finding that which they had set out to find, including support for the universal nature of disability classification (Üstün et al., 2001c, p. 318). Cross-cultural difference is acknowledged only to the extent that it does not refute the theory.

Unfortunately, the conclusion does not sit well with the observation of the Nigerian team about disability in that country. "Policy-makers, professionals, persons with disabilities and their care-givers," wrote the team, "as well as the general populace would benefit from training sessions and public enlightenment campaigns to sensitize them to these concepts [of disability contained in ICIDH-2]" (Omigbodun et al., 2001, p. 192). Thus, rather than indicating agreement with a universal model, the Nigerian team appears to be suggesting that they could be educated to agree with that model. That is, the classification is not universal, but through the globalization of ideas, it could become universal. With this in mind, the conclusion of the Greek team appears too trite:

> An interesting finding from the pile sort study is that people in Greece and in all the other countries participating in the study share similar views and perceptions as regard the descriptions of disability and the relationships between concepts. This indicates that a universally applicable classification that is also culturally sensitive is possible. (Mavreas et al., 2001, p. 106)

CONCLUSION

The measurement of population health is a case study of globalization. Where the term "globalization" tends to stand as a marker of certain approaches to economic engagement and global trade, here it stands as a marker for the global management of an idea. The idea is that there exists a universally (i.e., cross-culturally) accepted notion of health as an attribute intrinsic to the individual based on loss of bodily function or structure that is unrelated to the social, cultural, or physical environment.

This idea may seem self-evident, and if it does, that probably reflects the globalization of the idea. The evidence supporting it is scant. It has, nonetheless, resulted in an intensive effort to develop measures of population health that are based on it, and to repudiate ideas that stand in opposition to it. Its power lies in the ready manner in which it coupled with the organizational requirements of multilateral agencies such as the World Bank and the WHO: health is individual, intrinsic, and an end in itself. It should also be recognized, however, that as this notion of health developed, so it also influenced the manner in which those organizations thought about health.

It is this latter observation that provides some promise for the future development of new, quite different, and more sophisticated measures of population health. Organizations can be influenced, and measures of population health need not be quite so arbitrary. The challenge is in the creation of the next generation of population health measures. It is in rethinking the operational definition of health that social, cultural, and environmental context can be taken into account, as can population well-being (Reidpath, 2005).

"Objectivity" had become a shibboleth in population health measurement where the measures actually relied on rhetorical style and the control of discourse as their pedestals. The naive realism that they embody will need to be traded in if population health measurement is going to serve the well-being of populations.

Notes

1. In 1944 a forty-five nation conference was held at Bretton Woods, New Hampshire. The purpose of the meeting was to discuss the postwar recovery of Europe and international monetary regulation. The Bretton Woods twins that emerged from that meeting were the International Bank for Reconstruction and Development (World Bank) and the International Monetary Fund.

2. Games are not all played with equipment; some are played alone, some with fixed numbers of players, some with any number. Some games are professional, some amateur. Some are physical, some purely mental. Nonetheless, people have a sense of what a game is.

3. The idea of an operational definition comes from the work of the 1946 Nobel Laureate in physics, P. W. Bridgman (1927), and specifies how an object or concept of interest is to be measured. In Bridgman's domain of physics, the operational definition of, say, temperature could relate to the observable property of mercury in a vacuum tube with the application of heat.

4. See, e.g., some of the arguments contained in Murray (1994, 1996).

5. The philosopher of science and mathematics Imre Lakatos introduced the notion of monster barring in his book *Proofs and Refutations* (Lakatos, 1976). In it he described a process in mathematics whereby an operational definition of polyhedra was specified as a function of vertices and edges. An example of a polyhedron would then be constructed that conformed to the definition but was, nonetheless, regarded as violating the quintessence of polyhedra. The aberrant polyhedron was then barred from membership of the class polyhedra as a "monster," and the operational definition reworked to create a consistent class of polyhedra that excluded the aberrant form.

6. The valuation exercise used a device known as the person tradeoff (PTO) (Murray, 1996; Nord, 1999). Erik Nord developed the PTO and describes a number of variants. The essential feature of the tradeoff, however, is that respondents are asked how many lives in one condition are "worth" how many lives in another. Arnesen and Nord (1999) give the following example:

> You are a decision maker who has enough money to buy only one of two mutually exclusive health interventions. If you purchase intervention A, you will extend the life of 1,000 healthy [nondisabled] individuals for exactly one year, at which point they will all die. If you do not purchase intervention A, they will all die today. The alternative use of your scarce resources is intervention B, with which you can extend the life of *n* individuals with a particular disabling condition for one year. If you do not buy intervention B they will all die today; if you do purchase intervention B, they will die at the end of exactly one year. (p. 1424)

7. Even supporters of the approach have in more conversational settings discussed the arduous and psychologically stressful nature of the exercise, including the requirement to conform. Others have been less kind (Bastian, 2000).

8. Oddly, in one discussion the WHO acknowledged that there was no reason to believe that disability is universal and that the experience of one disease in one setting may be quite different from the experience of the same disease in another setting (Üstün et al., 2002, p. 589).

References

AbouZahr, C. (1999). Disability adjusted life years (DALYs) and reproductive health: a critical analysis. *Reproductive Health Matters, 7*(14), 118–129.

Allotey, P. A., & Reidpath, D. D. (2002). Objectivity in priority setting tools in reproductive health: context and the DALY. *Reproductive Health Matters, 10*(20), 38–46.

Allotey, P., Reidpath, D., Kouame, A., & Cummins, R. (2003). The DALY, context and the determinants of the severity of disease: an exploratory comparison of paraplegia in Australia and Cameroon. *Social Science and Medicine, 57*(5), 949–958.

American Psychiatric Association. (1994). *Diagnostic and statistical manual of mental disorders: DSM-IV.* Washington, DC: American Psychiatric Association.

Anand, S., & Hanson, K. (1997). Disability-adjusted life years: a critical review. *Journal of Health Economics, 16*(6), 685–702.

Arnesen, T., & Nord, E. (1999). The value of DALY life: problems with ethics and validity of disability adjusted life years. *British Medical Journal, 319*(7222), 1423–1425.

Barker, C., & Green, A. (1996). Opening the debate on DALYs. *Health Policy and Planning, 11*(2), 179–183.

Bastian, H. (2000). A consumer trip into the world of the DALY calculations: an Alice-in-Wonderland experience. *Reproductive Health Matters, 8*(15), 113–115.

Bateson, G. (1988). *Mind and nature: A necessary unity.* New York: Bantam Books.

Berlin, B. (1992). *Ethnobiological classification: Principles of categorization of plants and animals in traditional societies.* Princeton, NJ: Princeton University Press.

Blaxter, M. (1990). *Health and lifestyles.* London: Tavistock.

Borges, J. L. (1964). The analytical language of John Wilkins (R. L. C. Simms, Trans.). In *Other inquisitions 1937–1952* (pp. 101–105). New York: Simon and Schuster.

Bowker, G. C., & Star, S. L. (1999). *Sorting things out: Classifications and its consequences.* Cambridge, MA: MIT Press.

Bridgman, P. W. (1927). *The logic of modern physics.* New York: Macmillan.

Brown, R. H., & Malone, E. L. (2004). Reason, politics, and the politics of truth: how science is both autonomous and dependent. *Sociological Theory, 22*(1), 106–122.

Busfield, J. (2003). Globalization and the pharmaceutical industry revisited. *International Journal of Health Services, 33*(3), 581–605.

Clarke, A. E., & Casper, M. J. (1996). From simple technology to complex arena: classification of Pap smears, 1917–90. *Medical Anthropology Quarterly, 10*(4), 601–623.

Durkheim, E., & Mauss, M. (1963). *Primitive classification* (R. Needham, Trans.). London: Cohen and West.

Foucault, M. (1989/1963). *The birth of the clinic: An archeology of medical perception.* London: Routledge.

Hamlin, C. (1998). *Public health and social justice in the age of chadwick: Britain, 1800–1854.* Cambridge: Cambridge University Press.

Helman, C. G. (1994). *Culture, health and illness* (3rd ed.). Oxford: Butterworth Heinman.

International Monetary Fund Staff. (2000). Globalization: threat or opportunity? *Issues Briefs,* April 12 (corrected January 2002). http://www.imf.org/exter nal/np/exr/ib/2000/041200.htm (accessed February 14, 2006).

Körner, S. (1974). *Categorical frameworks*. Oxford: Basil Blackwell.

Kuhn, T. (1962). *The structure of scientific revolutions*. Chicago: University of Chicago Press.

Lakatos, I. (1976). *Proofs and refutations: The logic of mathematical discovery*. Cambridge: Cambridge University Press.

Marchal, B., & Kegels, G. (2003). Health workforce imbalances in times of globalization: brain drain or professional mobility? *International Journal of Health Planning and Management, 18*(suppl. 1), S89–S101.

Mavreas, V. G., Kontea, M., Asimaki, M., Giouzelis, I., Katsikas, E., Kollias, K., et al. (2001). Greece. In T. B. Üstün, S. Chatterji, J. E. Bickenbach, R. T. Trotter, R. Room, J. Rehm, & S. Saxena (eds.), *Disability and culture: Universalism and diversity* (pp. 95–106). Seattle: Hogrefe and Huber.

McMichael, A. J. (2000). The urban environment and health in a world of increasing globalization: issues for developing countries. *Bulletin of the World Health Organization, 78*(9), 1117–1126.

Mezzich, J. E., Kirmayer, L., Kleinman, A., Fabrega, H., Parron, D. L., Good, B. J., et al. (1999). The place of culture in DSM-IV. *Journal of Nervous and Mental Disease, 187*(8), 457–464.

Murray, C. J. (1994). Quantifying the burden of disease: the technical basis for disability-adjusted life years. *Bulletin of the World Health Organization, 72*(3), 429–445.

Murray, C. J. L. (1996). Rethinking DALYs. In C. J. L. Murray & A. D. Lopez (eds.), *The global burden of disease: A comprehensive assessment of mortality and disability from diseases, injuries, and risk factors in 1990 and projected to 2020* (pp. 1–98). Cambridge, MA: Harvard School of Public Health.

Murray, C. J. L., & Acharya, A. K. (1997). Understanding DALYs. *Journal of Health Economics, 16*(6), 703–730.

Murray, C. J. L., & Lopez, A. D. (eds.). (1996). *The global burden of disease* (Vol. 1). Cambridge, MA: Harvard School of Public Health.

Murray, C. J. L., Salomon, J. A., & Mathers, C. (2000). A critical examination of summary measures of population health. *Bulletin of the World Health Organization, 78*(8), 981–994.

Murray, C. J. L., Salomon, J. A., Mathers, C., & Lopez, A. D. (2002a). Summary measures of population health: conclusions and recommendations. In C. J. L. Murray, J. A. Salomon, C. Mathers, & A. D. Lopez (eds.), *Summary measures of population health: Concepts, ethics, measurement and applications* (pp. 731–756). Geneva: World Health Organization.

Murray, C. J. L., Salomon, J. A., Mathers, C., & Lopez, A. D. (eds.). (2002b). *Summary measures of popula-*

tion *health: Concepts, ethics, measurement and applications*. Geneva: World Health Organization.

Musgrove, P. (2000). A critical review of "a critical review": the methodology of the 1993 world development report, "investing in health." *Health Policy and Planning, 15*(1), 110–115.

Navarro, V. (2002). Health and equity in the era of "globalization." In V. Navarro (ed.), *The political economy of social inequalities: consequences for health and quality of life* (pp. 109–119). Amityville, NY: Baywood.

Nord, E. (1999). *Cost-value analysis in health care: Making sense out of qalys*. Cambridge: Cambridge University Press.

Omigbodun, O., Odejide, O., & Morakinyo, J. (2001). Nigeria. In T. B. Üstün, S. Chatterji, J. E. Bickenbach, R. T. Trotter, R. Room, J. Rehm, & S. Saxena (eds.), *Disability and culture: Universalism and diversity* (pp. 185–194). Seattle: Hogrefe and Huber.

Porter, D. (1999). *Health, civilization and the state: A history of public health from ancient to modern times*. London: Routledge.

Reidpath, D. D. (2005). Population health: more than the sum of the parts? *Journal of Epidemiology and Community Health, 59*(10), 877–880.

Reidpath, D. D., & Allotey, P. (2003). Infant mortality rate as an indicator of population health. *Journal of Epidemiology and Community Health, 57*(5), 344–346.

Reidpath, D. D., Allotey, P. A., Kouame, A., & Cummins, R. A. (2001). *Social cultural and environmental contexts and the measurement of the burden of disease: An exploratory study in the developed and developing world*. Melbourne: Key Centre for Women's Health in Society, University of Melbourne.

Reidpath, D. D., Allotey, P. A., Kouame, A., & Cummins, R. A. (2003). Measuring health in a vacuum: examining the disability weight of the DALY. *Health Policy and Planning, 18*(4), 351–356.

Rifkin, S. B., & Walt, G. (1986). Why health improves: defining the issues concerning 'comprehensive primary health care' and 'selective primary health care.' *Social Science and Medicine, 23*(6), 559–566.

Slaughter, M. M. (1982). *Universal languages and scientific taxonomy in the seventeenth century*. Cambridge: Cambridge University Press.

Spector, R. E. (2000). *Cultural diversity in health and illness* (5th ed.). Upper Saddle River, NJ: Prentice Hall Health.

Ugalde, A., & Jackson, J. T. (1995). The World Bank and international health policy: a critical review. *Journal of International Development, 7*(3), 525–541.

Üstün, B. (2002). The international classification of functioning, disability, and health—a common framework for describing health states. In C. J. L. Murray, J. A. Salomon, C. Mathers, & A. D. Lopez (eds.), *Summary measures of population health: Concepts, ethics, measurement and applications* (pp. 343–348). Geneva: World Health Organization.

Üstün, T. B., Chatterji, S., Bickenbach, J. E., Trotter, R. T., Room, R., Rehm, J., et al. (eds.). (2001a). *Disability and culture: Universalism and diversity*. Seattle: Hogrefe and Huber.

Üstün, T. B., Chatterji, S., Bickenbach, J. E., Trotter, R. T., & Saxena, S. (2001b). Disability and cross cultural variation: the ICIDH-2 cross-cultural applicability research study. In T. B. Üstün, S. Chatterji, J. E. Bickenbach, R. T. Trotter, R. Room, J. Rehm, & S. Saxena (eds.), *Disability and culture: Universalism and diversity* (pp. 3–19). Seattle: Hogrefe and Huber.

Üstün, T. B., Chatterji, S., Bickenbach, J. E., Trotter, R. T., & Saxena, S. (2001c). Summary and conclusions. In T. B. Üstün, S. Chatterji, J. E. Bickenbach, R. T. Trotter, R. Room, J. Rehm, & S. Saxena (eds.), *Disability and culture: Universalism and diversity* (pp. 309–321). Seattle: Hogrefe and Huber.

Üstün, T. B., Rehm, J., & Chatterji, S. (2002). Are disability weights universal? Ranking of the disabling effects of different health conditions in 14 countries by different informants. In C. J. L. Murray, J. A. Salomon, C. Mathers, & A. D. Lopez (eds.), *Summary measures of population health: Concepts, ethics, measurement and applications* (pp. 581–592). Geneva: World Health Organization.

Üstün, T. B., Rehm, J., Chatterji, S., Saxena, S., Trotter, R., Room, R., et al. (1999). Multiple-informant ranking of the disabling effects of different health conditions in 14 countries. WHO/NIH Joint Project CAR Study Group [see comments]. *Lancet*, 354(9173), 111–115.

van der Maas, P. J. (2002). Application of summary measures of population health. In C. J. L. Murray, J. A. Salomon, C. Mathers, & A. D. Lopez (eds.), *Summary measures of population health: Concepts,*

ethics, measurement and applications (pp. 53–60). Geneva: World Health Organization.

Walsh, J. A., & Warren, K. S. (1979). Selective primary health care: an interim strategy for disease control in developing countries. *New England Journal of Medicine*, 301(18), 967–974.

Werner, D., & Sanders, D. (1997). *Questioning the solution: The politics of primary health care and child survival*. Palo Alto, CA: HealthWrights.

Wisner, B. (1988). Gobi versus PHC? Some dangers of selective primary health care. *Social Science and Medicine*, 26(9), 963–969.

Wittgenstein, L. (1953). *Philosophical investigations* (G. E. M. Anscombe, Trans.). Oxford: Basil Blackwell.

Wittgenstein, L. (1969). *Preliminary studies for the "philosophical investigations," generally known as the blue and brown books* (G. E. M. Anscombe, Trans. 2nd ed.). Oxford: Basil Blackwell.

World Bank. (1993). *World development report 1993: Investing in health*. New York: Oxford University Press.

World Bank. (2000). *Poverty in an age of globalization*. Washington, DC: World Bank.

WHO. (1980). *International classification of impairments, disabilities, and handicaps: A manual of classification relating to the consequences of disease*. Geneva: World Health Organization.

WHO. (1992). *International statistical classification of diseases and health related problems*. Geneva: World Health Organization.

WHO. (1999). *ICIDH-2: International classification of functioning and disability. Beta-2 draft, full version*. Geneva: World Health Organization.

WHO. (2001). *International classification of functioning, disability, and health*. Geneva: World Health Organization.

Chapter 12

Health Impact Assessment: Toward Globalization as If Human Rights Mattered

Eileen O'Keefe and Alex Scott-Samuel

Health impact assessment (HIA) is a set of tools, methods, and processes for policy making. It does this by examining potential consequences for health of policy options. Its objective is to improve policy. It aims to be systematic and rigorous. This chapter explores HIA as applied to globalization. We outline what HIA is, point to debate about its nature, and give an example of its use in the European Union. The European Union's use of HIA provides opportunities to examine consequences for less powerful players in global policy formation. Migrant communities in high-income regions such as the European Union can be key participants in HIAs relating to global policy.

Distinctive of our view of HIA is the link with human rights. The ability to assume minimal value agreement is crucial in policy analysis operating at a global level. Human rights is the prime candidate for a consensual base for fundamental values and rules for conducting essential common activities within and across all geographical, administrative, and cultural

boundaries. It is a discourse that enables us to make claims about impacts across these boundaries. Those at highest risk from damaging health impacts are often ambiguously located with respect to geographical, administrative, or cultural boundaries. This includes dissidents, displaced persons, legal and illegal diasporas (see also chapter 9), or poor people in low-, middle-, and high-income countries.

The link between human rights and HIA alerts us to the adverse (or positive) impacts of globalization that may be mitigated (or enhanced) by policies. The link is important for addressing the negative health impacts of globalization as well as enhancing positive impacts. This involves identifying structural and functional aspects of globalization such as its unevenness, regional structures, top-down forms of governance, and power brokerage, as well as its potential permeability to forces from "below." If, as we believe, opportunities to limit negative impacts involve targeting health-damaging concentrations of power, then identifying pressure points from which alternative power structures have a feasible chance of emerging is an important task. One of the important contributions that HIA can make at the global level is to reduce the likelihood that policy formation simply reflects dominant power relations. This has implications for the construction and use of HIAs. The agenda and methodology for HIAs should include issues of interest to, and promoted by, those who do not have a secure position of power within national boundaries or in the major regional constellations. The European Union offers some leverage in this regard (Deacon et al., 2003). Initially, globalization was treated by academics and international bodies and in popular culture as subject to economic determinism yielding little space for effective regulation or political contestation and as worthy of approval or disapproval. A more nuanced view, emphasizing the complexity and unevenness of globalization is emerging, indicating that economic constraints do not rule out contestation, political choice, and regulation and that globalization has both positive and negative tendencies. The view that globalization has dangerous impacts and that it cannot be abolished but can be reformed by addressing major macroeconomic issues is persuasive to us (Patomaki, 2001; Buse et al., 2002). If this is the case, HIA is exceptionally important to apply to policy operating at a global level.

HEALTH IMPACT ASSESSMENT

HIA is an increasingly popular approach to public decision making. It involves the systematic assessment of the effects on health of actions or interventions in the public sphere, such as policies, plans, programs, or projects. Ideally, HIA is prospective, involving the prediction of intended and unintended impacts of the policy under study (we refer throughout this chapter solely to HIA of policies). It is also possible to assess the health impacts of a policy currently in operation (concurrent HIA) or no longer operative (retrospective HIA). These latter forms involve different methods, being at least in part observational rather than predictive. Some prefer only to use the term "health impact assessment" in the prospective mode.

Although the need for HIA had been identified some time earlier, systematic methods were not developed until the early 1990s, when the (unpublished) HIA of the proposed second runway at Manchester airport was undertaken in 1993. Around the same time, the government of British Columbia

enacted legislation requiring prospective impact assessments (including HIA) of all new British Columbia government policy and published simple tools for undertaking this (Ministry of Health, 1994).

Prior to this, two parallel developments had set the scene for HIA (Scott-Samuel, 1996): the increasing importance of environmental and other forms of impact assessment, and the emergence of healthy public policy. Environmental impact assessment had been developing globally following its U.S. origins in the 1960s, culminating in the National Environmental Policy Act of 1969 (Vanclay and Bronstein, 1995). In the decades that followed, health began to be acknowledged within environmental impact assessments, but in a limited form that emphasized environmentally induced impacts on disease levels. Also of relevance was the development of social impact assessment, focusing on impacts on communities.

The notion of healthy public policy originated in the work of Nancy Milio (1981) and received international support—especially from the World Health Organization (WHO)—in the years following the 1986 Ottawa Charter for Health Promotion (WHO, Health and Welfare Canada, Canadian Public Health Association, 1986). The need for methods to assess the impacts on health of public policy was widely acknowledged within healthy public policy discourse.

The notion of a systematic methodological approach to HIA was developed at the Liverpool Public Health Observatory (Scott-Samuel et al., 2001; Fleeman and Scott-Samuel, 2000; Winters, 2001) and subsequently adopted by the WHO (Diwan et al., 2001; Ritsatakis et al., 2002). Methodology for HIA remains a contested territory. Here we outline our preferred approach and, in doing so, characterize the range of alternatives.

CHARACTERISTICS OF HIA

HIA is a tool that builds measurement of potential positive and negative consequences for health into policy-making procedures of all ministries and agencies. It can promote health awareness in policy making in ministries and agencies outside of the formal health care sphere, such as trade, leisure, environment, housing, agriculture, or transport. It has been influential in highlighting the impact of the determinants of health on inequalities in health status.

We locate HIA in the fields of politics, policy, and

decision making: an approach that lubricates the political and bureaucratic cogs of governance and citizenship by placing health considerations on public agendas. This requires that public health knowledge produced by epidemiologists be complemented and enriched by evidence from social sciences such as anthropology, sociology, and economics (Public Health Sciences Working Group, 2004). We acknowledge, however, that this view is not a universal one. The National Assembly for Wales (1999) talks of "broad" and "tight" perspectives on HIA: the former is more social scientific, democratic, and value-laden and incorporates both qualitative and quantitative methods, while the latter is more epidemiological, technocratic, value-neutral, and quantitative. These ideas are the subject of continuing debate (e.g., Douglas and Scott-Samuel, 2001; Parry and Stevens, 2001): while they represent ideal types, most approaches currently in use lean toward one or the other extreme.

HIA PROCEDURES AND METHODS

The elements of an HIA are summarized in boxes 12.1 and 12.2; many HIAs are rapid rather than comprehensive and may not include all of the stages we describe.

Debate: Effectiveness, Efficiency, and Public Health Values

The account of HIA presented above incorporates a social model of health, with emphasis on equity and participation. Debate about HIA includes concerns about effectiveness, efficiency, intrusion of public health values, and advocacy. These are interconnected. Kemm (2003) is concerned that effectiveness might be compromised by inadequate definitions and methods, the inappropriate intrusion of public health values and advocacy, and lack of support on the part of policy makers. Efficiency might be compromised if difficult to achieve aspects such as popular participation in HIA are required.

We agree that effectiveness is crucial and that thorough commitment to rigor should be employed. However, overreliance on a limited repertory of methods might confine HIA to entirely modest studies. HIA should engage with decisions that are most likely to have consequences for health and its distribution in populations. This is most apparent if HIA is to

come into play regarding transboundary threats to and opportunities for health characteristic of globalization.

Box 12.1 – The Elements of a Health Impact Assessment

- Apply a screening procedure to select policies for assessment
- Define the model of health impact to be employed
- Agree on the scope of the HIA in terms of depth, duration, spatial and temporal boundaries, methods, and outputs
- Conduct policy analysis
- Profile the areas and communities likely to be affected by the policy
- Collect qualitative and quantitative data from stakeholders and key informants on potential impacts and their distribution
- Evaluate the importance, scale, and likelihood (and if possible, cost) of potential impacts
- Search the evidence base to validate data
- Undertake option appraisal and developing recommendations for action
- Monitor and evaluate following implementation

Crucial to this is the distinction between HIA as a decision aid or as an algorithm. If it is a decision aid, as we believe, it should not be surprising that policy makers act only in part on the evidence regarding health. It is certainly true that, if decision makers do not make a commitment, a policy will not be implemented, and therefore, HIA practitioners should be very clear about what their task is. The HIA practitioner is not the decision maker. Politicians are on the front line of formal decision making. HIA is not designed to give a unique option providing a substitute for making policy choices. It may also be problematic due to multiple causality, long lead times, and inadequacy of data.

Furthermore, HIA cannot be evaluated solely in terms of impacts on health status in the short run since, again, it is a political matter what value health status is accorded by decision makers. Health cannot be presumed to be the highest or ultimate value from the point of view of decision makers. It is important for decision makers to know what the impact of options will be on health. But they will also have interests in knowing how proposals will affect the economy, their political prospects, and so on. Their decisions involve tradeoffs. Knowledge on its own does not carry the day with regard to policy implementation even when that policy has been endorsed by government. By the same token, the case for inclusion of a participatory approach to HIA needs to be considered on grounds other than its difficulty.

Box 12.2 – HIA Procedures and Methods

Screening

Often, an HIA of a specified policy will be commissioned. This will not always be the case—particularly when the HIA is being introduced in a new setting. In such circumstances, there will be a need to choose the policies on which HIA is to be undertaken. A screening procedure is a systematic way of doing this: in some senses, it is akin to a mini-HIA. Faced with a long list of policies (e.g., an agency's policy program for the coming year), there will clearly be a requirement to rapidly select the most important candidates for HIA. The screening procedure described in the Merseyside Guidelines for Health Impact Assessment (Scott-Samuel et al., 2001) employs the following criteria:

Economic Issues

- The size of the policy and of the population(s) affected
- The costs of the policy and their distribution

Outcome Issues

- The nature of potential health impacts of the policy (crudely estimated)
- The likely nature and extent of disruption caused to communities by the policy
- The existence of potentially cumulative impacts

Epidemiological Issues

- The degree of certainty (i.e., probability/risk) of health impacts
- The likely frequency (incidence/prevalence rates) of potential health impacts

- The likely severity of potential health impacts
- The size of any probable health care impacts
- The likely consistency of "expert" and "community" perceptions of probability, frequency, and severity of important impacts

Strategic Issues

- The need to give greater priority to policies than to programs, and to programs than to projects, all other things being equal (resulting from the broader scope—and hence potential impact—of policies as compared to programs and to projects)
- Timeliness—regarding ensuring that the HIA is prospective wherever possible and regarding planning regulations and other statutory frameworks
- Whether the policy requires an environmental impact assessment
- Relevance to local decision making

Model of Health

It is important to specify the model of health impact that will be used in the HIA. We favor a holistic, socioenvironmental model of health; using such a model implies the consideration of a potentially wide range of health impacts of any policy. Thus, the HIA of the European Employment Strategy (described later in this chapter) focuses broadly on social determinants of health, such as income or work/life balance, rather than narrowly on disease outcomes such as elevated levels of heart disease. Some others favor a "tight perspective" featuring a medical model focusing primarily on disease impacts.

Scoping

Large-scale HIAs are usually overseen by a steering group containing a range of relevant stakeholders such as representatives of the commissioning agency, the policy proponent, governmental or other public sector agencies involved with the policy, experts in the field covered by the policy, and representatives of population groups particularly affected. Those carrying out the HIA, once selected, will also be represented. The steering group will agree about the terms of reference of the HIA, including its scope and the model of health to be employed. Scoping covers a number of issues, including the following:

- The depth of the HIA—usually defined by the amount (if any) of fieldwork undertaken. The terms "rapid" and "comprehensive" are often used to refer to HIA depth
- The duration of the HIA—a rapidly undertaken HIA can obviously achieve greater depth by employing more staff
- The boundaries in space and time—in setting geographic and temporal limits the steering group needs to consider the potential spread of impacts (e.g., from airborne disease or cultural diffusion) and possible latent periods involved (some impacts may take months or years to become apparent)
- The methodology and methods to be employed
- The selection of practitioners to undertake the HIA
- The potential outputs and their dissemination—for example, technical and popular versions of any reports, media releases, journal papers, websites, videos
- Ownership, confidentiality, and copyright issues
- The budget and sources of funding for the HIA

Policy Analysis

Policy analysis in HIA is important insofar as it enhances understanding of potential impacts. It has tended to focus on a policy's content rather than on the policy process; both, however, are important determinants of the eventual health impacts.

Reviews of the policy context may include national and local reports, minutes of meetings, government, and other policies and may cover the public, private, and voluntary sectors. Detailed consideration may be required of the nature, origins, social, and political/economic significance of the policy.

The content of the policy is clearly important in terms of both direct and indirect, intended and unintended health impacts. The fixed or negotiable nature of the policy's detailed content may also be important. The dynamics of the policy's implementation require consideration: frequently, there will be a wide range of potential influences determining how the policy is (or is not) actually put into practice, resulting in an equally wide range of potential impacts on population health.

Profiling

Profiling highlights relevant health, social, demographic, and other recorded characteristics of those likely to be affected by the policy. It is important to include relevant population subgroups—especially vulnerable ones. Information reviewed should include not only routine data but also material available from research or previously collected for special purposes.

Impact Identification

Depending on the methodological approach adopted, a wide range of methods exists for identifying potential health impacts of a policy. Reviews of the relevant scientific, specialist, and everyday literature (including "gray" literature) take place in all but the briefest HIAs. The views of a wide range of stakeholders and key informants may also be obtained, using qualitative methods such as interviews, focus groups, or—less commonly—scenario exercises and Delphi studies. Quantitative methods may include surveys, mathematical or economic modeling, and specialist risk assessment methods.

When working with local people potentially affected by a policy, it is helpful for the interview or focus group schedule to include some reference to the model of health being employed, in order to ensure, for example, that the full range of health determinants that feature in a socioenvironmental model are considered by the respondents as potential health impacts of the policy.

Impact identification also includes wherever possible the characteristics of potential impacts, such as their importance, measurability and scale, severity, probability, and costs. In many situations, precise numerical data are unrealistic or do not exist. In order to avoid spurious attempts at quantification, the Merseyside Guidelines recommend simple characterizations of these parameters. For example, the measurability of a potential impact can be recorded as qualitative, estimable, or calculable; its probability of occurrence can similarly be described as definite, probable, possible, or speculative.

Recording these characteristics on a matrix can be helpful in considering the priority that should be given to them in the HIA's recommendations for modifying the policy. The inappropriateness of preferentially prioritizing quantifiable or probable impacts becomes apparent if one compares potential impacts such as "a definite increase of 0.05% in the prevalence of the common cold" and "the speculative possibility of a substantial increase in feelings of racism within a community."

Option Appraisal and Recommendations

Clearly, it cannot be assumed—even if there is total agreement about potential negative and positive health impacts of a developing policy—that the most health-enhancing option for modifying that policy will be adopted. A range of political, financial, and social considerations will mediate the outcome of any impact assessment. This in turn dictates that the results of an HIA will often be a series of options for policy change: which (if any) of these is adopted is frequently beyond the control of the Steering Group.

Monitoring and Evaluation

An HIA is not complete once its recommendations are delivered: although implementation lies beyond the scope of the HIA itself, it is important to evaluate the HIA and to monitor its effects. In brief, this can encompass the following:

- Process evaluation—the extent to which the HIA was undertaken in the manner intended
- Impact evaluation—whether the HIA was successful in modifying the policy it assessed
- Outcome evaluation—the benefits (or costs) to the affected populations resulting from the undertaking of the HIA

PUBLIC HEALTH VALUES AND HIA

Practical difficulties with community participation characterize critics' worries about efficiency and effectiveness. Parry and Wright (2003) assert that "HIA usually has to be done reasonably quickly, so as to operate within the policy-making timescale," resulting in the "radical solution" of "limiting involvement to a small group of experts" that "might be the most appropriate and efficient means to influence the policy-making process." If the objective is to "gain credibility with policy makers, it must fit policy makers' requirements" (p. 388). There are reasons for HIAs to include both equity and participation, distinct from the values held by the practitioner. We treat participation by those likely to be affected by a policy as essential. Where policy formation is a program rather than a one-off project, it is especially pressing. If there is focus on the long rather than short term, those policies may be given a

higher priority that are designed to equip people to be able to cooperate, understand, plan, and take responsibility for their lives. In such cases, involvement of those affected by an HIA is important. Participation can be built in at every level of impact assessment—local, national, and global. We should learn from the health care priorities debate, the key area where urgent attention has been given to evidence-based decision making and where attempts to implement expert systems come unstuck because of lack of legitimacy with politicians and/or the public. This led Klein (1998) to insist on the importance of consensus building among stakeholders in decision making, rather than just the expert marshaling of evidence. Consensus building was argued for, not as a value, but to achieve commitment so that policy that appears rational to epidemiologists carries weight with politicians.

This is also the case whenever the public themselves have to be part of the solution, a position that is increasingly relevant regarding personal lifestyle, or whenever the lay population are viewed as potential "expert patients" for whom self-care is part of the active management of chronic conditions. Wanless (2004) has argued that the population must be "fully engaged" if public health threats are to be countered and health improved in England. This applies also when it is recognized that the level of social capital affects health or that change in the behavior of a population is one of the variables. Dyson and Bhaskar (2003), in their contribution to a review on the tragedy of the commons, show the importance of popular participation in decision making with respect to resource management policy that misfired when the "problem of fuel wood scarcity, as perceived by government planners and donors, was quite different from the problems of primary concern to small farmers, who were trying to secure access to sustainable livelihood options" (p. 1915). Morgan (2003) asserts that there are major challenges regarding indirect impacts that "are especially associated with changes in the social, economic and cultural conditions in local populations likely to result from a given policy, plan or project" (p. 390). Aside from cases where the people's efforts are a necessary condition for achieving health improvement, the people may bear important costs that are a consequence of policy implementation. The interests of those on the receiving end of a policy who are worst off have a special moral claim when hard decisions are taken that will disproportionately affect them (Rawls, 1971).

HIA AND HUMAN RIGHTS

It would be a technical omission to carry out an assessment without looking at the distribution of potential health impacts within the population. Hence, at the very least an HIA should examine inequalities in health. The issue of equity is more complex. The notion of equity applies to those inequalities that are amenable to policy levers and are unjust (Whitehead, 1991). Kemm is correct to note the contestable nature of justice claims. Commitment to public health values, such as equity, is problematic in those cases when values are *only* subjective. But values are better founded when they have been subscribed to in international treaties. Human rights give us a way of identifying minimalist claims to which policy makers are bound. This is the case with respect to human rights instruments, such as the Convention on the Rights of the Child (United Nations, 1989), which has the widest acceptance globally. The reporting mechanisms used by the United Nations to assess a country's compliance with human rights treaties that they have signed can be used to provide evidence (O'Keefe and Hogg, 2000).

Globalization includes a process involving the emergence of cross-culturally foundational values. Hence HIA involves access to information and evidence-based policy making that is at the heart of human rights. Since 1946, the WHO has argued that health should be treated as a human right and subsequently that investment in health is necessary for development (WHO, 2002). The British Medical Association (2001) asserts "that the full range of human rights is essential and that different categories of rights are interdependent and indivisible" but that "industrialised countries frequently emphasise personal liberty and free markets but deny basic socioeconomic rights to underprivileged people" and concludes that "in many poor countries, attention must be given to the establishment of a healthy environment, including provision of food, water and sanitation, rather than prioritizing health care services" (p. 26). O'Keefe and Scott-Samuel (2002) argue that human rights discourse in the United States has been dominated by an atomistic individualist model that fails to accommodate social and economic rights. Dasgupta (1995) marshals wide-ranging empirical evidence from Africa, Asia, and Latin America indicating that the exercise of rights improves health status outcomes and that participation is instrumental to such outcomes. He argues further that redistributive strategies that promote the well-being of the aggregate can protect individuals. Braveman and Gruskin (2004) have shown that compliance with human rights standards can function as a global auditing tool; we believe that HIA should play an important part in this global audit effort.

Views taken on the effectiveness and efficiency of HIA have implications for questions about its applicability to large policy programs as compared with projects. The significance of power imbalances and the importance of maintaining a wide approach that engages with those imbalances are illustrated by the HIA of the largest World Bank–supported initiative in Africa. The bank instigated an environmental impact statement and HIA of an oil pipeline development involving a loan to the Chad Oil Export Consortium, including Exxon and the governments of Chad and Cameroon. Jobin (2003), a member of the assessment team, concluded that the decision makers addressed modest potentially damaging factors but did not engage with factors likely to be implicated in major impacts such as a rapid increase in HIV levels associated with specific, potentially modifiable transport arrangements that assessors had identified. Kemm (2003) suggests that the HIA of the Chad oil project was misguided in deviating from what the decision makers—the World Bank—wanted. Failure to implement its recommendations could be seen as an error in the original terms of reference of the HIA in which public health practitioners, driven by equity concerns, did not limit the study to what the partners would buy into in advance. We would disagree with this view.

If anything, globalization makes the use of public health values and advocacy in HIA in relation to big, unwieldy projects such as the Chad oil project urgent. Partnerships at the global level involving the commercial sector are characteristic of such planning (Buse and Walt, 2000) and the question is how far multilateral organizations such as the World Bank insert compliance with major findings into conditionality for agreeing to loans or, as in this instance, devolve implementation to partners without holding them to account. HIA faces threats similar to those besetting environmental impact assessment that is "usually funded and often commissioned by the developer, which may limit its independence" (Mindell and Joffe, 2003, p. 111).

What is odd about Kemm's (2003) position is the implication that an HIA must confine all options considered to ones that are known in advance to be within the policy makers' frame. An HIA is not impartial if it rules out questioning terms of reference, when the practitioner has reason to believe that avoidable negative health impacts at least partly within the policy competence of the decision makers are being excluded. The HIA task includes identifying the leverage available to policy makers to shift determinants of the relative distribution of health status among segments of the population.

Decision making at national level in low-income countries is constrained by multilateral funders such as the World Bank as well as through accreditation of countries for foreign direct investment. Multilateral actors shape the playing field and therefore should come within the purview of HIA. Since HIA draws on evidence, it should be as rigorous as the public health knowledge base and resources allow. The production of evidence about global impacts is problematic. We are heavily reliant on knowledge about health and health care produced by powerful stakeholders, such as the World Bank, which simultaneously make policy and provide us with the information to judge what the impacts of such policy might be. This is a problem because its policy framework is derived from a contestable macroeconomic paradigm. It is insufficient comfort for a population when the World Bank, evaluating the impact of its economic policy in a country, concludes that its approach was wrong and undertakes to do better in future (O'Keefe, 2003). There is an urgent need to widen capacity for producing knowledge that can inform HIA. Fortunately, as from 2005, the People's Health Movement, the Global Equity Gauge Alliance and Medact are planning a two-yearly report on global health issues that will examine the operation of organizations such as the World Bank (Katikireddi, 2004). It is essential to make use of materials produced in low and middle income regions such as the "framework for understanding globalization's impacts on health" devoted to examining how powerful global actors have shaped and are shaping prospects for health in Africa (Labonte et al., 2004, p. 5). HIA could and should be part of a knowledge producing process that includes an enterprise to "foster a public interest media that can truly accommodate global public debate" to inform much needed social change (Glasius et al., 2002, p. 8).

Demonstration of reduction in health inequalities in the short term is an unrealistic criterion of proof of effectiveness of HIA. HIA is an emerging tool for pol-

icy making. If we accept the logic of the difficulties, for example, that data are patchy, public health interventions have long lead-in times, public health problems are multicausal, and most important, power is unequal among stakeholders, it follows that an important potential outcome of the use of HIA is awareness raising within the policy-making community and the public at large of the concept of healthy public policy. This means that some of the changes we will be looking for are in slow, subtle shifts in the cultural environment surrounding health that are "determinants of determinants of health" and that are crucial to any enterprise in which people are expected to take responsibility for their health as the devotees of the concepts of social capital and active citizenship contend.

We would emphasize that these debates do not merely represent abstruse "paradigm wars" between epistemologists—in our view, failure to appreciate the ubiquitous nature of values and the scientific purpose of participation has important implications for both the validity and utility of HIAs. We would not accept that any activity can be described as value-neutral. Concepts from HIA practitioners, such as "the need policy-makers have for impartial advice may not fit in with the values of public health" (Kemm, 2003, p. 387) prevent our engaging with some health-damaging impacts of interest to less powerful groups. Similarly, proposals that "assessments almost certainly have to be predominantly 'top-down' professionally-led exercises" and that "limiting involvement to a small group of experts might be the most appropriate and efficient means to generate sufficient information to influence the policy-making process" (Parry and Wright, 2003, p. 388), restrict the use and utility of HIA when transboundary health threats are bound up with inequalities in power among stakeholders.

A CASE STUDY—HIA OF THE EUROPEAN EMPLOYMENT STRATEGY

The purpose of this brief case study is neither to focus on HIA methodology, which we have done in the preceding sections, nor to examine in great detail the health aspects of the policy under study—which may be of limited relevance to many reading this chapter. Rather, we use this case example to demonstrate the feasibility of HIA at the level of global public policy. This is necessary because of the very limited experience of applying HIA at this level: most HIAs undertaken have focused on neighborhood or regional projects rather than on national or international policies. Hirst and Thompson (1998) assert that the European Union is one of the three most powerful blocs in established global forums. They argue that the European Union countries' experience of the welfare state and regulation could be extended to the global level. This position is further developed in an analysis of the potential for a redistributionist global welfare policy (Deacon et al., 2003). Initiatives to develop HIA in the European Union may be particularly important, especially since the United States is the most powerful state-actor with respect to globalization but "exceptional" in its unwillingness to constrain its behavior in line with the developing international consensus regarding the control of negative global impacts.

The case study draws on reports from the Policy HIA for the European Union (Abrahams et al., 2004; Haigh and Mekel, 2004; Pennington, 2003). This thirty-month study was funded by DG Sanco, the health and consumer protection directorate of the European Commission (EC). The project partners were the International Health Impact Assessment Consortium at the University of Liverpool (IMPACT); Lögd, the Nord Rhein-Westphalia (NRW) Institute for Public Health in Bielefeld, Germany; the Institute for Public Health in Ireland, in Dublin and Belfast; and RIVM, the National Institute for Public Health and the Environment in Bilthoven, Netherlands.

The aim of the project was to synthesize and test a generic methodology for assessing the health impacts of European policies. In the first year of the project, literature reviews, selection tools, and in-depth discussions resulted in the development of a generic approach incorporating many of the principles, values, methods, and procedures described in preceding sections. In the second year, criteria were developed to select a policy on which to pilot the methodology. These criteria (box 12.3) do not constitute a generic HIA screening procedure, because they were developed for the purpose of selecting a policy that would fit within the parameters of the research project rather than being an optimal candidate for HIA. Nonetheless, these policy selection criteria may be of general interest.

Policies in the EC's work program for 2003 were screened using this procedure and the European Employment Strategy (EES) was selected for assessment.

HIAs were being undertaken in each member state and across Europe as a whole (Abrahams et al., 2004).

Box 12.3 – Policy Selection Criteria Used in the Policy Health Impact Assessment for the European Union Project

- The strength of the evidence base relating to potential health impacts of the policy
- The timing of the policy, in relation to the "window of opportunity" to undertake an HIA
- The degree of obligation on member states to implement policies of the type concerned
- The complexity of the policy
- The extent to which the policy is of general public interest
- The "health relevance" of the policy

The Policy

This case study provides a typical example of the European Union's use of HIA. The chief element of the EES is the employment guidelines, which are reviewed and modified at the annual European Council (of national ministers). The new guidelines are published in a package each April, together with specific recommendations for member states. The employment guidelines reflect common policy at the overarching European Union level. In addition, every member state draws up a national action plan (NAP) that describes how the previous year's employment guidelines have been put into practice. The NAP presents the progress achieved in the member state over the last 12 months, and the measures planned for the coming year. The EC and council together produce a joint employment report from the NAPs. This contains country-specific information as well as a comparison and synthesis of developments from a European perspective. The employment guidelines have three overall goals: full employment, quality and productivity at work, and cohesive and inclusive labor markets.

The European Council's 2000 Lisbon Agenda outlined Europe's "employment deficit" and proposed remedial labor market, fiscal, and structural policies. The features of the employment deficit identified by the council are as follows:

- A gender gap—only half of the women in the European Union are in work compared to two-thirds in the United States (though this statistic summarizes wide variations within Europe)
- A services gap—the European Union has relatively low levels of employment in the service sector
- Marked regional imbalances—European Union unemployment is concentrated in Germany, France, Italy, and Spain and is highest in the south, in outlying regions, and in declining industrial areas
- Long-term structural unemployment—half of those out of work have been unemployed for more than a year
- A skills gap—particularly in information technology, due to underinvestment in education and training
- An age gap—the employment rate in the 55–65 age group is too low

The proposed 2003 employment guidelines focused on 10 "priorities for action" (box 12.4).

THE HIA IN GERMANY

At the time of writing, the national HIAs within the four partner countries are almost completed. The German HIA will be used to exemplify the overall approach taken (Haigh and Mekel, 2004)—though detailed HIA procedures differed somewhat between countries.

A Steering Group was formed of stakeholders, key informants and experts. Previous reported HIAs and "snowballing" were helpful in identifying potential members. However, only one meeting of the Steering Group took place, because of the difficulty in achieving representative member participation. Attendance at this meeting, a participatory workshop, consisted of an expert in the implementation of the EES in Germany; an expert in the employment and health field; two employees of the Ministry for Environment, Conservation, Agriculture and Consumer Protection of the state of North Rhine-Westphalia; and an employee of the Federal Ministry of Health and Social Security.

The following were unable to attend: a representative of the Unemployment Association; an expert in European Union politics; and a representative from the Federal Ministry of Economics and Labour.

It was not possible to obtain the participation of other relevant stakeholders such as employer and employee unions.

Box 12.4 – Priorities of the 2003 Employment Guidelines

- Develop active and preventive measures for the unemployed and inactive
- Foster entrepreneurship and promote job creation
- Address change and promote adaptability in work
- Create more and better investment in human capital and strategies for lifelong learning
- Increase labor supply and promote active ageing
- Foster gender equality
- Promote the integration of and combat the discrimination against people at a disadvantage in the labor market
- Make work pay through incentives to enhance work attractiveness
- Transform undeclared work into regular employment
- Promote occupational and geographical mobility and improve job matching

---

Following introductions and presentations on HIA, the EES and the background to the project, draft terms of reference were discussed and agreed. There followed a facilitated workshop, at which a number of prepared questions and scenarios of "possible employment futures" were used to stimulate discussion. Introductions were first given on social determinants of health and evidence on the relationships between employment and health. The description of the EES had introduced the ten priorities and the five specific Recommendations for Germany—which relate to: helping the unemployed into jobs, promoting the adaptability of workers and companies, investing in human capital through lifelong learning, promoting gender equality in employment and pay and improving financial incentives to make work pay.

Pin boards were used to map the changing responses received as the prepared questions and scenarios were discussed in open forum. Participants confirmed the relevance of the five EC Recommendations for Germany. They also proposed that priority health impacts in the HIA should be pragmatically identified, based on the availability of evidence and the likely size, importance and interest of the impact.

Suggested priority areas for further examination included the health/employment implications of working conditions; job safety; low income; and social support.

Concentrating on one of the five EC Recommendations for Germany was also suggested. Appropriate examples could include an existing national program for countering unemployment; and changing work-life balances, such as to reduce the negative health impacts of compulsory flexibility.

On the basis of policy analysis of the EES in the German context and a literature review of the evidence linking work, employment policies and health, a model was devised to represent the causal linkages between these factors. The model was then applied to the EC's five recommended action areas for Germany in order to develop recommendations for enhancing the health impacts of the policy. While more than one area met prioritization criteria developed by the HIA team, it was agreed for the purposes of the pilot HIA to focus on health impacts relating to adaptability and flexibility of workers and companies.

There has been much research and much policy development within Germany in relation to adaptability and associated flexible forms of employment. Much of the research—and also many concerns expressed within the workshop in relation to flexibility—relate to precarious or marginal forms of employment. Examples include fixed term contracts, temporary work and part-time work. These are all characterized by job insecurity.

Impact identification included the development of three scenarios featuring differential shifts from permanent to fixed term contracts in the German labor force. The potential reductions in the health status of the population were predicted in relation to each scenario. Health-related absenteeism from work was used as an indicator of diminished health status.

At the time of writing, the recommendations of the HIA for enhancing the potential health impacts of flexible forms of employment were still in the process of development. Some of these, however, will be described here. We would also emphasize that alongside specific recommendations, the general conclusions of an HIA need equally to be considered. For example, one general conclusion of the HIA of the EES in Germany is that the overall aim of the EES—full

employment—is health promoting. In general, working is healthier than being unemployed. On the other hand, employment can also impact negatively on health. For example, the EES specifically encourages member states to balance flexibility with job security. It also emphasizes occupational health and safety, reducing discrimination, and gender equality.

The conclusions of the German HIA point out that flexible employment is likely to share some of the unfavorable characteristics of unemployment and may have similar negative effects on health—such as hazardous working conditions, job insecurity and dissatisfaction, lower levels of job control and less access to training and education opportunities. It points out that all these effects are potentially avoidable. There is, however, the risk of increased flexibility resulting in a split outcome whereby more adaptable 'winners' achieve career advancement and improved work-life balance while 'losers' suffer increased vulnerability, insecurity and ill health.

One recommendation of the HIA is to specifically encourage 'non-typical' people into flexible forms of employment in order to 'normalize flexibility.' Such mainstreaming of flexible work could result in some of the negative elements being reduced, such as through social benefit systems being adapted to fit in with these kinds of work.

Another recommendation of the HIA is to introduce a screening process at national level whereby employment-related policy is examined for possible discriminatory effects on flexible workers. Such effects might relate to having children, obtaining loans, retirement, or health insurance. The screening process should specifically consider population groups that are particularly vulnerable to the negative health effects of flexible forms of employment, such as women, older workers, disabled people, migrants and foreigners.

COMMENTARY

We have indicated throughout that HIA practitioners should carry out their work in the spirit of an independent ethical commitment to public health values that put the distribution and causes of inequalities of health status onto the agenda. This means for the European Union that HIA of employment should not be confined to citizens and legal migrants. The European Union experiences shortages of care workers needed by ageing populations and shortages of workers with specialist technical skills, alongside high unemployment amongst its citizens. Proposals to reduce welfare provision within the European Union are accompanied by racism orchestrated by populist media. Against a background of permeable borders and poverty on the E.U. periphery, in-migration of non-citizens presents an explosive mixture. The European Union has identified labor migration from countries on the border of countries joining the European Union, to be of particular interest in this regard (O'Keefe, 2003).

Diaspora communities could play a key role as stakeholders in HIA at the global level. The relative significance of their location in developed or developing countries has been blurred through processes of globalization (O'Keefe and Chinouya, 2004; see also chapter 9). Health policy in the wealthy countries is beset by shortages of essential workers. They are dependent on workers whom they recruit globally, often from countries where their skills are in even shorter supply (Stillwell et al., 2003). Countries losing skilled workers and those gaining them could examine the health impact of policies implicated in such flows. On the one hand, wealthier destination countries benefit from education and professional training of migrant staff subsidized by the source states. On the other, this can reduce the capacity of poorer countries to absorb the resource injections proposed by the Commission on Macroeconomics and Health (CMH) and other bodies. The extensive growth of global migrants as domestic workers in private homes in the European Union (Lutz, 2002) as well as in the workforce of commercial residential establishments in the wealthy countries, involves a global division of labor that has been characterized as an internationalized care chain (Hochshild, 2000). From the point of view of public health some of the most vulnerable residents in the European Union are likely to be undocumented workers in the informal economy (O'Keefe and Chinouya, 2004). These communities are of special significance in relation to health equity issues facing poor countries, most notably those in Africa, which have performed dismally economically following implementation of World Bank and IMF policy (Moyo and Kawewe, 2002; Mupedziswa and Gumbo, 2001). It is a matter of urgency for the European Union to widen HIA to examine the contradictory impact of global immigration governance on health. Employment studies should be widened to include

groups whose immigration and legal work status is compromised. This would strengthen the important recommendations regarding migration of health workers canvassed by international pressure groups (Swinson, 2001).

DISCUSSION: TAKING THE BROAD VIEW

The operation of HIA depends on positions taken on the conceptual, methodological and value issues addressed in this chapter. It is being used by individual countries such as the United Kingdom as well as by WHO and the World Bank. However, what it is, depends on essentially contestable notions of globalization itself. Stakeholder involvement may be required as sources of expertise or as buttresses to the legitimacy of the HIA. HIA can be pursued using a lens of increasing width that tracks the factors that impact on health. It requires a considerable widening to track the impact of global flows on the determinants of health and resources for health care. With the increased permeability of borders to the determinants of health, there is a pressing need to track impacts internationally to inform policy and practice across the full width of the lens. Individual countries, especially but not only poor ones, cannot insulate themselves against global threats to health.

Nevertheless, we need to consider potential limitations and drawbacks of HIA so that we do not raise expectations in an unrealistic manner. Ritsakakis (2004) notes that while HIA is important as a vehicle for promoting multisectoral planning, there is disagreement and confusion about the nature and methods of HIA and its relationship to other forms of impact assessment as well as questions about its effectiveness. She thinks that the private sector "mindful of their corporate image . . . could be encouraged to attempt HIA." Such a development raises the risk of capture by special interest groups that would not necessarily benefit population health. Commentators note that HIA might raise unrealistic expectations (Kemm and Parry, 2004). Finally, it is demanding to carry out assessments in light of the quality of evidence on which to draw to judge impact. The evidence base is often much less robust than the public supposes (Petticrew et al., 2004). There is also the potential risk that HIA promises too much, and disappoints various constituencies because policy-makers fail to act on the findings.

GLOBAL ECONOMIC POLICY
AS HEALTH POLICY

HIA should underpin measures needed to promote a health enhancing global economic, finance and trade regime. Equity in health is shaped by the operation of the economic and social forces that constrain the health choices of individuals, communities and states. The governance arrangements of agencies working at trans-national level warrant review. The World Bank warrants special attention in the light of the impact on health resulting from its policy of encouraging states to facilitate movement of their citizens into an international labor market (O'Keefe, 2000). Critics argue that the Bank's macroeconomic policy has worsened poverty and inequality in low-income countries (Werner and Sanders, 1997); that the IMF, World Bank, and WTO operate as a "parallel government" promoting austerity, privatization, and free trade (Chassudovsky, 1997); and that South Africa's home-grown economic strategy in line with this menu resulted in the imposition of cost-recovery programs on water and sanitation with negative consequences for public health (Bond, 1997; see also chapter 13). The wide lens, which has been in abeyance for several decades, is now re-emerging with the problems thrown up by globalization. It is acknowledged that "some of the most fundamental forces and processes determining the nature of life chances within and across political communities are now beyond the reach of nation-states. . . . If the most powerful geo-political forces are not to settle many pressing matters simply in terms of their own objectives and by virtue of their power, then the current institutions and mechanisms of accountability need to be reconsidered" (Held et al., 1999). The challenge is to reshape the "institutional arrangements for making accountable those sites and forms of power that presently operate beyond the scope of democratic control." This can be promoted by extending an explicit policy framework to the international level and applying the framework to the impact of the determinants of equity in health status between countries. Accountability for stewardship for health—which WHO applies to national govern-

ments (WHO, 2000)—needs to be extended to global players. This requires acknowledgement of and engagement with global power imbalances in the policy making process. The widest lens would require attention to the economic policy of major players such as the World Bank, not just its policies for health care. Stewardship can, arguably apply to impact on health including the distribution of health status within populations. Under Dr. Brundlandt's leadership, WHO widened the lens to encompass the impact of global factors on health, including global trade. The WHO established the CMH in 2000, to put flesh on the notion of investing in health. The Commission's task was to propose evidence-based health measures that would have as their consequence maximizing economic development while minimizing poverty. While we were told that the major thrust was to be the impact of health on "development and equity in developing countries," there was no indication that these might involve trade-offs. One component of CMH was a review of the evidence on the impact of structural adjustment programs on health (Breman and Shelton, 2001; see also chapter 15). This showed mixed outcomes with "an overwhelming majority [that] was negative about structural adjustment." Countries investigated showed declines in child mortality and maternal mortality and increased life expectancy, as well as increase in malnutrition. Most studies show decreases in health personnel per capita and severe deterioration in quality of care, and strengthening of the bias in favor of curative as against cost effective preventive care. The complexity of the picture disclosed in this review points to the possible complicity of the powerful players in globalization, in the plight of low-income countries and is at odds with the simple picture presented in the final CMH report. The picture is consistent with the detailed examples of structural adjustment programs analyzed by MacDonald (2001).

The more segregated the economic and social resources are in the wealthy world, the less does a commitment to equity get onto agendas and the less do determinants of equity get onto the agenda in global fora. This is apparent in policy formation that dominated the IMF and World Bank throughout the 1980s and particularly the 1990s with the focus on "poverty alleviating growth." This allows humanitarian concentration on the bottom rungs of social groups while leaving the rest of the society to widen inequalities due to the operation of market forces—clearly a prime candidate for HIA.

CONCLUSION: HIA IN ONE WORLD

The impact of global actors on the public and private sectors that shape the nature and distribution of health within and between nations needs to be made transparent. Wealthy countries have exercised more than their fair share of influence over the global trade and finance regimes. There is a need to build consensus based on the notion of one world committed to civil, political, economic and social rights, which engage with the global distribution of power in any decision-making that impacts on health. Low and middle income countries could use HIA nationally and within global fora when engaging in collective action on the determinants of health and health care. This applies as well to collective action with respect to the WTO, IMF, and G8, as well as regional groupings such as the Southern African Development Community, Caricom and the European Union. We see HIA making an important contribution to "globalization as if health—and human rights—mattered."

References

Abrahams D, den Broeder L, Doyle C, Fehr R, Haigh F, Mekel O, Metcalfe O, Pennington A, Scott-Samuel A (2004). *Policy Health Impact Assessment for the European Union: Final Project Report.* Liverpool: International Health Impact Assessment Consortium (IMPACT). http://www.ihia.org.uk/ephia/reports/finalprojectreport.pfd (accessed February 14, 2006).

Bond P (1997). Homegrown structural adjustment: implications for services delivery and public health. In: Jeebhay M, Hussey G, and Reynolds L, eds. *The New World Order: A Challenge to Health for All by the Year 2000.* Durban: Health Systems Trust, pp. 18–34.

Braveman P, and Gruskin S (2004). Health, equity and human rights: what is the connection? In: Fox D, and Scott-Samuel A, eds. *Human Rights, Equity and Health.* London: Nuffield Trust, pp. 9–17.

Breman A, and Shelton C (2001). Structural adjustment and health: literature review of the debate, its role-players and presented empirical evidence. CMH Working Paper Series No. WG6. Geneva: World Health Organization.

British Medical Association (2001). *The Medical Profession and Human Rights.* London: Zed Books.

Buse K, Drager N, Fustikian S, and Lee K (2002). Globalisation and health policy: trends and opportuni-

ties. In: Lee K, Buse K, and Fustakina S, eds. *Health Policy in a Globalising World.* Cambridge: Cambridge University Press, pp. 251–280.

Buse K, and Walt G (2000). Global public-private partnerships: part II—what are the health issues for global governance. *Bulletin of the World Health Organization*, 78(5): 699–709.

Chassudovsky M (1997). The globalization of poverty and ill-health: assessing the IMF-World Bank structural adjustment programme. In: Jeebhay M, Hussey G, and Reynolds L, eds. *The New World Order: A Challenge to Health for All by the Year 2000.* Durban: Health Systems Trust Durban, pp. 67–84.

Dasgupta P (1995). *An Inquiry into Well-being and Destitution.* Oxford: Oxford University Press.

Deacon B, Ottila E, Koivusalo M, and Stubbs P (2003). *Global Social Governance.* Helsinki: Ministry for Foreign Affairs of Finland.

Diwan V, Douglas M, Karlberg I, Lehto J, Magnusson G, and Ritsatakis A, eds. (2001). *Health Impact Assessment: From Theory to Practice. Report on the Leo Kaprio Workshop, Gothenburg, 28–30 October, 1999.* Gothenburg: Nordic School of Public Health.

Douglas M, and Scott-Samuel A (2001). Addressing health inequalities in health impact assessment. *Journal of Epidemiology and Community Health* 55: 450–451.

Dyson J, and Bhaskar V (2003). Managing tragedies: understanding conflict over common pool resources. *Science* 302: 1915–1916.

Fleeman N, and Scott-Samuel A (2000). A prospective health impact assessment of the Merseyside Integrated Transport Strategy (MerITS). *Journal of Public Health Medicine* 22: 268–274.

Glasius M, Kaldor M, and Anheier H, eds. (2002). *Global Civil Society 2002.* Oxford: Oxford University Press.

Haigh F, and Mekel O (2004). *Pilot HIA of the EES in Germany.* Bielefeld, Germany: Nord Rhein-Westphalia (NRW) Institute for Public Health (lögd).

Held D, McGrew A, Goldblatt D, and Perraton J (1999). *Global Transformations.* Oxford: Polity Press.

Hirst P, Thompson G. (1998). *Globalization in Question: The International Economy and the Possibilities of Governance.* Oxford: Polity Press.

Hochshild A (2000). Global care chains and emotional surplus value. In: Hutton W, and Giddens A, eds. *On the Edge: Living with Global Capitalism.* London: Jonathan Cape, pp. 130–146.

Jobin W (2003). Health and equity impacts of a large oil project in Africa. *Bulletin of the World Health Organization* 81: 420–426.

Katikireddi V (2004). New regular report will monitor global health issues. *British Medical Journal* 328: 778.

Kemm J (2003). Perspectives on health impact assessment. *Bulletin of the World Health Organization*

81: 387. http://www.who.int/bulletin/volumes/81/6/en/ (accessed April 11, 2004).

Kemm J, and Parry J (2004). The development of HIA. In: Kemm J, Parry J, and Palmer S, eds. *Health Impact Assessment*. Oxford: Oxford University Press, pp. 15–23.

Klein R (1998). Puzzling out priorities: why we must acknowledge that rationing is a political process. *British Medical Journal* 317:959.

Labonte R, Schrecker T, Sanders D, and Meeuss W (2004). *Fatal Indifference: The G8, Africa and Global Health*. Lansdowne: University of Cape Town Press.

Lutz H (2002). At your service madam! The globalization of domestic service. *Feminist Review* 70: 89–104.

MacDonald T (2001). *Third World Health Promotion and Its Dependence on First World Wealth*. Lampeter: Edwin Mellen Press.

Milio N (1981). *Promoting Health through Public Policy*. Philadelphia: FA Davis.

Mindell J, and Joffe M (2003). Health impact assessment in relation to other forms of impact assessment. *Journal of Public Health Medicine* 25 (2): 107–112.

Ministry of Health (1994). *Health Impact Assessment Tool Kit: A Resource for Government Analysts*. Victoria, BC: Population Health Resource Branch, British Columbia Ministry of Health and Ministry Responsible for Seniors.

Morgan R (2003) Health impact assessment: the wider context. *Bulletin of the World Health Organiation* 81 (6): 390.

Moyo O, and S Kawewe. (2002). Dynamics of a racialized, gendered, ethnicized, and economically stratified society. *Feminist Economics* 8(2):163–181.

Mupedziswa R, and Gumbo P. (2001). *Women Informal Traders and the Struggle for Survival in an Environment of Economic Reforms*. Uppsala: Nordiska Afrikaintsitut.

National Assembly for Wales (1999). *Developing Health Impact Assessment in Wales*. Cardiff: Health Promotion Division, National Assembly for Wales.

O'Keefe E (2000). Equity, democracy and globalization. *Critical Public Health* 10 (2): 166–177.

O'Keefe E (2003). Contested macroeconomic policy as health policy: the World Bank in Ukraine. In: T MacDonald, ed. *The Social Significance of Health Promotion*. London: Routledge, pp. 122–138.

O'Keefe E, and Chinouya M (2004). Global migrants, gendered tradition and human rights: black Africans and HIV in the United Kingdom. In: Tong R, Donchin A, and Dodds S, eds. *Linking Visions: Feminist Bioethics, Human Rights and the Developing World: Integrating Global and Local Perspectives*. Lanham: Rowman & Littlefield, pp. 217–234.

O'Keefe E, and Hogg C (2000). Social inequality, policy formation and children's mental well-being. In: Hosin A, ed. *Essays on Issues in Applied Develop-mental Psychology and Child Psychiatry*. Lampeter: Edwin Mellen, pp. 226–238.

O'Keefe E, and Scott-Samuel A (2002) Human rights and wrongs: could health impact assessment help? *Journal of Law, Medicine and Ethics* 30: 734–738.

Parry J, and Stevens A (2001). Prospective health impact assessment: pitfalls, problems, and possible ways forward. *British Medical Journal* 323: 1177–1182.

Parry J, and Wright J (2003). Community participation in health impact assessments: intuitively appealing but practically difficult. *Bulletin of the World Health Organization* 81: 388. http://www.who.int/bulletin/volumes/81/6/en/ (accessed April 22, 2004).

Patomaki H (2001). *Democratising Globalization: The Leverage of the Tobin Tax*. London: Zed.

Pennington A (2003). A *Brief Overview of the European Economic Strategy*. Liverpool: International Health Impact Assessment Consortium (IMPACT).

Petticrew M, Macintyre S, and Thomson H (2004). Evidence and HIA. In: Kemm J, Parry J, and Palmer A, eds. *Health Impact Assessment*. Oxford: Oxford University Press, pp. 71–80.

Public Health Sciences Working Group (2004). *Public Health Sciences: Challenges and Opportunities*. London: Wellcome Trust, p. 489.

Rawls J (1971). A *Theory of Justice*. Cambridge, MA: Harvard University Press.

Ritsakakis A (2004). HIA at the international policy-making level. In: Kemm J, Parry J, and Palmer S, eds. *Health Impact Assessment*. Oxford: Oxford University Press, pp. 153–164.

Ritsatakis A, Barnes R, Douglas M, and Scott-Samuel A (2002). Health impact assessment—an approach to promote intersectoral policies to reduce socioeconomic inequalities in health. In: Mackenbach J, and Bakker M, eds. *Reducing Inequalities in Health: A European Perspective*. London: Routledge, pp. 287–299.

Scott-Samuel A (1996). Health impact assessment: an idea whose time has come. *British Medical Journal* 313: 183–184.

Scott-Samuel A, Birley M, and Ardern K (2001). *The Merseyside Guidelines for Health Impact Assessment*. 2nd ed. Liverpool: International Health IMPACT Assessment Consortium, Department of Public Health, University of Liverpool. http://www.ihia.org.uk/document/merseyguide3.pdf (accessed April 22, 2004).

Stillwell B, Diallo K, Zurn P, Dal Poz M, Adams O, and Buchan J (2003). Developing evidence-based ethical policies on the migration of health workers: conceptual and practical challenges. *Human Resources for Health* 1: 8. http://www.human-resources-health.com/content/1/1/8 (accessed April 26, 2004).

Swinson C (2001). *Migration of Health Workers from Commonwealth Countries: Experiences and Recommendations for Action*. London: Commonwealth Secretariat.

United Nations. (1989). Convention on the Rights of the Child. UN Doc. AA/44/49. Geneva: United Nations.

Vanclay F, and Bronstein DA, eds. (1995). *Environmental and Social Impact Assessment.* Chichester: Wiley.

Wanless D (2004). *Securing Good Health for the Whole Population.* London: HM Treasury.

Werner D, and Sanders D (1997). *Questioning the Solution: The Politics of Primary Health Care and Child Survival.* Capetown: Healthrights.

Whitehead M (1991). The concepts and principles of equity and health. *Health Promotion International* 6 (3): 217–227.

WHO (2000). *World Health Report 2000 Health Systems: Improving Performance.* Geneva: World Health Organization.

WHO (2002). *25 Questions on Health and Human Rights.* Geneva: World Health Organization.

WHO, Health and Welfare Canada, Canadian Public Health Association (1986). *Ottawa Charter for Health Promotion.* Ottawa, Ontario: International Conference on Health Promotion.

Winters LY (2001). A prospective health impact assessment of the international astronomy and space exploration centre. *Journal of Epidemiology and Community Health* 55: 433–441.

Part III

The International Responses
to Globalization

Chapter 13

Structural Adjustment Programs and Health

Anna Breman and Carolyn Shelton

Do structural adjustment programs (SAPs) cause poor health outcomes? Are SAPs responsible for improved health indicators? Does reduced spending in the health sector have a direct impact on infant mortality? These and other questions surrounding the relationship between health and SAPs have been highly debated for more than ten years. In this chapter we identify the major players in the debate and their arguments and track changes in the debate over time.

A charged debate on the effects of structural adjustment on health was launched in the mid-1980s. The debate has focused on issues such as the impact of adjustment on government spending for health care services, the quality of care, and rates of child and infant mortality.

Structural adjustment refers to a set of policy advice given to developing countries by international agencies, mainly the World Bank and the International Monetary Fund (IMF), but also other donor agencies such as USAID (U.S. Agency for International Development). The objective of SAPs has been to enhance economic growth through macroeconomic stability and elimination of market distortions. These policies are controversial for several reasons. Developing countries have had to implement recommended policies in order to receive grants or loans from donor agencies (conditional lending). SAPs have also been criticized for having adverse effects on health outcomes, especially for the poor.

We undertook a desk review of literature gathered from sources relevant to structural adjustment and health. Articles presenting empirical evidence of effects of structural adjustment on health outcomes were of particular interest. An in-depth analysis of the empirical literature helps clarify key questions in the debate. Through extensive searches on economic and medical databases (Econlit, Jolis, First Search, Medline, PubMed), we identified seventy-six relevant articles for inclusion in the review. Among these articles, twenty-eight present empirical evidence on the impact of SAPs on health outcomes.

In this chapter we synthesize the findings from the literature review. First, we discuss the debate, the role-players, their main arguments, and trends in the debate. In the second section we present a framework illustrating the causal arguments for how structural adjustment may affect health outcomes and discuss methodological issues in empirical estimations of this relationship. In the third section we summarize and analyze the empirical evidence, and finally we draw conclusions from the review.

THE DEBATE

Time Frame: Why, When, and How the Debate Started

SAPs were first implemented in the early 1980s. The debate began with the concern that structural adjustment would have the strongest impact among the poorest and most vulnerable groups of the population. Health workers saw a tendency for public health improvements achieved over the past decades to be reversed. Since health is cumulative over the life cycle, setbacks in nutrition and health cannot be recovered later on in life when the economy recovers. Those who initiated the debate did not demand that structural adjustment should come to a halt, yet they contended that programs be implemented in such a way that the negative impacts on health and other social outcomes were mitigated. This debate has been ongoing since the early 1980s, and there are no signs that it may slow down as new empirical evidence continues to be presented.

In 1987, Cornia, Jolly, and Stewart published their often-cited two-volume book, *Adjustment with a Human Face*, and the debate took off. Volume 1, *Protecting the Vulnerable and Promoting Growth*, discusses the impacts of structural adjustment on social welfare, especially for children. Volume 2, *Country Case Studies*, presents empirical evidence from ten countries where adjustment programs have been implemented. The authors are not opponents of SAPs. The case studies show both positive and negative health outcomes from SAPs, and based on these observations, the book focuses on how to implement SAPs in order to protect vulnerable groups. The authors suggest, for example, that the poor and children should be exempted from user fees and that social protection programs should be implemented to mitigate the cost of increased unemployment.

Major Role-Players and Their Arguments

Major players in the debate include the World Bank and IMF, United Nations organizations (mainly UNICEF), representatives of academic institutions, and nongovernmental organizations. The various arguments represented in this literature review illustrate how the respective disciplines and motives of each player are reflected in their perspective on SAPs. Being responsible for the design and implementation of SAPs, the World Bank and IMF are key players in the debate. The World Bank and IMF first implemented SAPs in the early 1980s in response to the debt crisis in developing countries. Opponents of SAP policies contended that the World Bank and IMF ignored the establishment of social safety nets for the poorest groups. World Bank publications began to respond to this criticism as early as 1990.

An internal review of World Bank and IMF policies from 1980 through 1987 prompted the acknowledgment that SAPs must address negative social outcomes and identify ways for borrower countries to take the poor into account during adjustment periods (McCleary 1990). One article published by the World Bank (Pitt 1993) presented a theoretical framework for measuring health outcomes in the context of SAPs. The author concluded that a disregard for health outcomes could lead to a serious underestimation of positive returns for investing in health.

The United Nations Development Program (UNDP) published studies that were neither anti-SAP nor pro-SAP. Their argument was not whether a country should adjust, but how. One UNDP study found that productive feedback between macroeconomic policies and social outcomes was just beginning to emerge in the mid-1990s (Taylor and Pieper, 1996). The main argument was that significant positive and negative feedback between social indicators, economic growth, income, and consumption could lead to either vicious or virtuous circles.

Authors from academic and research institutions and nongovernmental organizations represented a wide variety of disciplines ranging from public health and nutrition, to economics, to gender studies. As a result, their arguments and opinions contributed to differing perspectives in the debate. For example, one article, published in a journal on human rights, examined the World Bank's approach to poverty reduction from the 1970s through the early 1990s (Amobi 1993). The article aimed to put structural adjustment policies in their political and historical context. The author concluded that although the World Bank's actions showed a strong commitment to poverty reduction, when SAPs were implemented in the 1980s, the policy focus shifted toward mitigating the economic crisis, and the poor were forgotten.

Another article was published in a book on women's issues and the economic crisis (Elson 1992). The author contended that the macroeconomists' failure to account for unpaid human labor as a variable for successful SAPs represented a male bias toward women's productive roles in society. The conclusion argued that a transformation of both public and private sectors in SAP countries should be responsive to women's ability to become successful producers of society.

The Range and Trends of the Debate over Time

There are three main trends in the debate: the opening discussion on adjustment with a human face, the harsh criticism toward structural adjustment that followed and the World Bank and IMF response, and third, the present debate, which is characterized by more empirical studies presenting new evidence of the effects of SAP on health outcomes. As already mentioned, the debate started with a number of articles supporting arguments in favor of "adjustment with a human face." Structural adjustment was regarded as necessary in order to come to terms with the difficult economic situation that many developing countries faced in the beginning of the 1980s. The articles were generally theoretical and offered suggestions on how to implement adjustment without creating adverse effects on health (see, e.g., Cornia et al. 1987, Hill and Pebley 1989, Amobi 1993).

At the beginning of the 1990s, articles defending World Bank and IMF strategies began to appear in academic journals and in World Bank publications. They generally acknowledged that structural adjustment may have had a negative impact on health (and education) and suggested how the problem should be dealt with. Several articles also made an effort to empirically

investigate the effects of structural adjustment (McCleary 1990, Suh and Yeon 1992, Pitt 1993, Serageldin et al. 1994). It is noteworthy, though, that relatively few articles are official World Bank/IMF documents. A considerable number of articles are authored by World Bank/IMF staff but published as independent articles.

At the same time, an increasing number of articles strongly opposed to structural adjustment were published. They were often more normative than theoretical and typically were based upon findings in other articles. Editorial notes in prestigious medical journals, such as *Lancet* and *Journal of the American Medical Association*, severely criticized structural adjustment (see, e.g., *Lancet* 1990, 1994, Logie and Woodroffe 1993).

The nature and progress of the debate seemed to influence the World Bank and IMF, and strong arguments for "adjustment with a human face" led to changed policies. Social funds were established to mitigate the negative impacts on health and education, while SAPs were adapted to be more responsive to the needs of the poor.

The debate changed focused in the late 1990s as the World Bank and the IMF adapted their policies. Currently, the World Bank supports the provision of basic health services to poor people for free or, where specific community conditions warrant, at lowest possible cost. In the case of certain interventions that have large benefits for the community and vulnerable groups, such as immunization and maternal and child health care, the World Bank discourages user fees. User fees remain controversial, but at present the World Bank is mainly criticized for rejecting health as a human need and a social right and for promoting private provision of health care (see, e.g., Sen and Koivusalo 1998, Laurell and Arellano 1996). One author goes as far as stating that World Bank policies lead to "hell for all" instead of "health for all" (Antia 1995).

PARTICIPATORY POVERTY REDUCTION STRATEGIES

In 1999, the World Bank and IMF sharpened their focus on reaching the needs of the poor with the introduction of participatory poverty reduction strategies, which were to provide the basis for all concessional lending and debt relief, under the Heavily Indebted Poor Country (HIPC) initiative.[1] The strategies are developed through Poverty Reduction Strategy Papers (PRSPs) by national authorities with the central purpose of defining economic and social policies to address poverty issues and to promote equitable growth (see also chapter 14). PRSPs aim to engage broad participation from civil society groups, specifically including the poor, in the design of such strategies. According to the World Bank, the five core principles of the development and implementation of PRSPs should be:

- Country-driven, with broad participation by civil society and the private sector
- Results-oriented, focusing on outcomes that would benefit the poor
- Comprehensive in recognizing the multidimensional nature of poverty
- Partnership-oriented, with coordinated participation of development partners (bilateral, multilateral, and nongovernmental)
- Based on a long-term perspective for poverty reduction

Since PRSPs are used to access concessional loans and recognize that the health of the population is key to ensuring economic growth, there is potential for increased funding in the health sectors of some of the poorest countries. A recent preliminary report of the World Health Organization (Dodd and Hinshelwood 2002) reviewed the health components of several PRSPs. The review found that although several PRSPs address national health strategies and the poorest groups, few countries have used the PRSP process as an opportunity to reexamine their national health plans from a poverty perspective, nor do they present current health strategies with a focus on poverty.

Thus far, many countries have focused on targets, such as the reduction of infant or maternal mortality, without much detail on how such issues affect the poorest. Given the current evidence from the World Bank and elsewhere that the Millennium Development Goals could be reached without significantly affecting the lives of the poorest, the same could be implied by many of the strategies outlined in the health components of the PRSPs. Despite the insufficient attention placed on the most vulnerable groups, many PRSPs include general statements such as improving access to health services in "remote areas." Based on the findings of this review, it is clear that the inclusion of health issues in the PRSPs has a long way to go in terms of reaching the poorest groups; how-

ever, it is a good starting point for investing in improving the health of the poor.

Due to the recent introduction of PRSPs, evidence of its long-term impact and implications for the health sector is limited. However, adjustment programs continue to be implemented and have been employed for a sufficiently long time to make it worth investigating their impact on health outcomes. Thus, articles presenting empirical evidence have become more frequent. It is evident that the literature has become less negative toward the impact of SAPs over time (see, e.g., Mwabu 1996, Bassett et al. 1997, Van der Gaag and Barham 1998, Garenne and Gakusi 2000). The empirical data show both positive and negative impacts on health. Health expenditures have not declined as much as was first assumed. It seems as if many countries have tried to protect expenditures on health and other social services at the expense of cutbacks in other sectors, such as infrastructure and defense (Van der Gaag and Barham 1998).

ANALYSIS OF LITERATURE ON SAPS

In order to reveal trends in the SAP debate, we classified the seventy-six articles included in this review into four categories according to their main findings: positive, negative, neutral, and both positive and negative. In this context, positive (negative) has a broad definition referring to the authors' opinions on structural adjustment. Furthermore, the articles were divided into three categories according to their nature: normative, theoretical, and empirical. Although some of the articles belong to one or more of these categories, the categorical selection was based on the main content. For example, articles that are mainly theoretical and present empirical evidence from other studies are classified as theoretical, while an editorial note will be classified as normative.

Among the seventy-six articles that we have identified, 45% are negative, 8% are positive, 20% are neutral, and 27% are both positive and negative. It is clear that opponents of structural adjustment who believe, or find, that adjustment will have negative outcomes on health tend to dominate the debate. An interesting pattern is revealed if we map the positive and negative aspects to the nature of these articles. All but one of the normative articles are negative. The theoretical ones are mainly neutral, discussing possible positive and negative impacts of adjustment but without taking "sides." The empirical articles are mixed with respect to positive and negative effects of adjustment on health outcomes. There is no category with a majority of positive articles. However, a closer examination of the positive articles reveals that they are all empirical studies.

Regional Differences

Fifty-seven of the seventy-six articles are related to a certain country or region. The articles can be divided into five groups according to the country/countries investigated: Africa, Asia, Latin America–Caribbean, Middle East–North Africa, and "global." Global refers to cross-country studies that comprise countries from at least two of these regions. Africa is heavily overrepresented. Nearly half (47%) of the country-specific or regional studies are from Africa, 16% are studies from Latin America, and 16% are from Asia; 4% are specific for the Middle East–North Africa region. The remaining 18% of the articles are global.

Jayarajah et al. (1996) find in their cross-country study of fifty-three adjusting countries that health expenditures and health outcomes have improved in Asia and Latin America and the Caribbean, while outcomes have deteriorated in Africa and the Middle East–North Africa region. Interestingly, our review of studies does not illustrate the same pattern. In Africa and Asia, the vast majority of the studies are negative. In Latin America and Middle East–North Africa, the outcomes are both positive and negative. These observations, however, comprise all types of articles, normative as well as theoretical and empirical. In Asia, it is clear that the negative articles are normative while the empirical ones are more often both positive and negative. We further discuss regional differences in the empirical sections of this chapter, where we also examine the variables used to determine health outcomes.

THEORETICAL FRAMEWORK
AND METHODOLOGY

Our objective in this section is to illustrate the breadth and variety of the theoretical frameworks employed in the literature on structural adjustment and health (see, e.g., Pitt 1993, Peabody 1996, Musgrove 1997, Sen and Koivusalo 1998). Our aim is also to show which elements of this framework have been put to empirical test and to discuss methodological is-

sues regarding the empirical assessment of the effects of structural adjustment on health.

Policy Mechanisms through Which
Structural Adjustment May
Affect Health Outcomes

Figure 13.1 depicts the possible relationships between adjustment policies and health outcomes. It illustrates which structural adjustment policies may affect health outcomes, various links between policies and health outcomes, and which measurable health outcomes have been studied in the empirical literature. The figure is organized around three main policies of structural adjustment: reduction in government expenditure, liberalized markets, and exchange rate devaluation.

Structural adjustment aims to improve macroeconomic performance and enhance economic growth. If a country is facing a budget deficit, it is likely that *reduction in government expenditure* will take place. If the cutbacks affect expenditures on health and infrastructure, the access to and the quality of health care might be affected. User fees are often introduced as a cost-recovery measure to compensate for cutbacks in health expenditures (Pitt 1993). *Liberalized markets* affect food subsidies and prices but also the price of other commodities that will affect household incomes and thus ability to pay for health services (Pitt 1993, Sen and Koivusalo 1998). *Exchange rate devaluation* will affect the prices of imported goods such as medicines and medical equipment. At the same time, exports will be facilitated, and, for example, export crop farmers are likely to see their income rise (Peabody 1996).

The variables in figure 13.1 denoted with an asterisk are the variables estimated in the empirical literature on structural adjustment and health. Several studies focus on changes in government expenditure on health and how such changes are related to the quality of care. Other articles show how exchange rate devaluation has increased food prices and thus nutritional status. Among the various measurable health outcomes, infant, child, and maternal mortality are common. Life expectancy at birth is also often used. Disease burden has been suggested as an important variable in the theoretical literature but has not yet been used, to our knowledge, in empirical studies. Finally, malnutrition is employed in diverse studies to assess child health under structural adjustment.

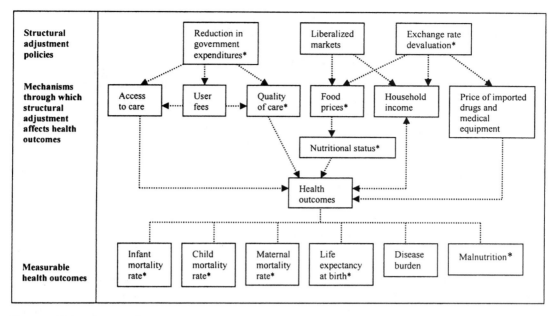

FIGURE 13.1. Theoretical Framework: Possible Relationships between Adjustment Policies and Health Outcomes. * Variables estimated in the empirical studies on structural adjustment and health. See text for further details and outcomes. *Sources:* Pitt (1993), Peabody (1996), Musgrove (1997), Sen and Koivusalo (1998).

Before summarizing the findings of the empirical literature, we first discuss various methodological issues that need to be addressed when empirically investigating these relationships.

Effects of Economic Recession versus Effects of Structural Adjustment

In discussing the results of structural adjustment, it is crucial to distinguish between the effects of economic recession and structural adjustment. Countries adopt SAPs in order to deal with economic crisis. It is not clear whether negative effects on health outcomes should be attributed to adjustment rather than to economic mismanagement, sheer bad luck, or other factors causing the crisis. Focusing on adjustment implies that the alternative would be not to adjust rather than how to adjust (Musgrove 1997). The relevant counterfactual question is therefore what would have happened if the reforms had not been implemented.

Various authors have dealt with this problem in different ways. Some simply state that it is impossible to distinguish between the effects of adjustment and the effects of economic crisis. Others ignore the problem, while a third group makes an attempt to separate

the impacts resulting from economic crisis and those of adjustment. The latter approach compares health outcomes before and after adjustment or compares adjusting to nonadjusting countries.

Serageldin et al. (1994) compare sixteen African countries before and after the introduction of SAPs in the 1980s. They find that per capita public health expenditure on health decreased while expenditures as a percentage of total government expenditures increased. At the same time, infant mortality as well as child mortality improved after the introduction of adjustment programs. The authors take this as evidence that the introduction of adjustment programs did not adversely affect health outcomes.

Thiesen (1994) and Van der Gaag and Barham (1998) compared adjusting to nonadjusting countries. Thiesen examined a set of twenty-nine African countries between 1970 and 1988. Expenditures and health were then compared between the nineteen adjusting and twelve nonadjusting countries. He showed that real absolute expenditure on health care decreased in both adjusting and nonadjusting countries. Moreover, the data showed that the rate of decline in infant mortality was slower in adjusting than in nonadjusting countries.

Van der Gaag and Barham (1998) took this method one step further. They performed a cross-country study where they divided a set of ninety-five countries into four groups: (1) early adjustment lending countries, (2) other adjustment lending countries, (3) nonadjustment lending countries with positive growth, and (4) nonadjustment lending countries with nonpositive growth. The last group was used as a control group, showing what happened to nonadjusting countries facing economic crisis, to be compared to the two groups of adjusting countries.

The major drawback of this type of study, as the authors point out themselves, is that the within-group variation is sometimes larger than the between-group variation. One way to deal with this problem would have been to try to use a matching methodology. Each country in a specific group could have been matched with a country in the control group that showed the same levels in key observable characteristics, such as gross domestic product (GDP) per capita, population size, real per capita health expenditures, and child mortality. To the extent that such country pairs were possible to identify, a difference-in-difference estimator could have been used to compare the expenditures on health and child mortality variables before and after adjustment occurred. The obvious difficulty with such a method is to identify countries that have sufficiently similar observable characteristics.

A second drawback with this type of study is the classification of countries. In the van der Gaag and Barham study, to be classified as an adjusting country, a country has to be engaged in a World Bank SAP. However, countries in the nonadjusting groups might have followed the same adjustment policies as the countries involved in World Bank adjustment programs. There is no discussion in the report on equivalent policies or any sensitivity analysis regarding the inclusion of countries.

Despite these drawbacks, the strength of the van der Gaag and Barham (1998) study is that it demonstrates that countries might do worse without adjustment. The nonadjusting countries performed worse in terms of real per capita spending on health care than did the adjusting countries. Case studies attempting to show a relationship between structural adjustment and health therefore need to carefully isolate the causal effect of the structural-adjustment–induced policy on the observed health outcome. A number of studies provide interesting methods to link these effects.

Linking a Specific Policy under Adjustment to Health Outcomes

To establish causality, researchers need to isolate the impact of specific adjustment policies on social outcomes. This is extremely difficult due to the multitude of intervening factors, which are difficult to control in a standard regression analysis. Moreover, the effects of adjustment policies often occur with a time lag and the lag itself will depend on the sequence of policy changes as well as institutional and structural features of the economy.

Handa and King (2003) investigate the exchange rate liberalization in Jamaica in 1991 and its effect on malnutrition. This structural adjustment induced a change in policy and led to a steep devaluation of the Jamaican currency. The authors argue that this event resembles a natural experiment. It occurred at a specific time with specific consequences that can be directly linked to food prices and hence to the availability of nutrients. The authors use synthetic cohort estimation techniques to decompose variations in children's weight into age effects, birth year effects, and time or year effects that capture common macroeconomic conditions. The study shows that the short-term nutritional status indicator of wasting (weight-for-height) declined significantly following the exchange rate liberalization. On the other hand, there was no significant effect on the long-term nutritional status indicator of stunting (height-for-age).

The success of this type of study depends on the authors' ability to link a specific policy under structural adjustment to a specific health outcome. It was possible in this study because Jamaica imports staple foods, and the increase in food prices could be directly linked to devaluation. Since the devaluation was sudden and unexpected, there were no possibilities for families to prepare beforehand for increased food prices. Moreover, it is noteworthy that the sharp devaluation was followed by currency appreciation and declining food prices. In subsequent periods, wasting decreased. The authors have thus succeeded in isolating one policy intervention and linked this policy to measurable health outcomes.

Kahn (1999) and Grootaert (1994) focused on the link between government expenditures on health and specific measurable health outcomes. As mentioned in the preceding section, SAPs are often accused of causing reduced levels of government spending on health. Government expenditure on health is also one of the most common variables in the empirical literature on structural adjustment and health. Kahn (1999) aimed to prove a direct link between expenditure and health outcomes, while Grootaert (1994) questioned any such direct relationship.

Kahn (1999) studied the affects of structural adjustment on health in Pakistan. The data suggested that health expenditures, as a percentage of GDP, have declined in Pakistan during the adjustment years. Due to economic growth, this percentage decline did not translate into a decline in absolute value. Real government expenditure on health increased over the adjustment period. At the same time, access to health personnel (as measured by population per doctor, dentist, and nurse) and facilities (as measured by population per hospital beds) increased. Health indicators such as life expectancy, infant mortality, and undernourishment improved.

One argument against the existence of a direct link between health expenditures and health outcomes is that government health expenditures are inefficient and subject to corruption. Household private expenditure on health should then have a more significant effect on health outcomes. To test these conflicting views, Kahn (1999) used a times series of average infant mortality rate in Pakistan spanning from 1972 to 1994. Infant mortality rate declined by 33% during this period. The independent variables used included government expenditure per capita, GDP per capita (as a proxy for private health expenditure), and remittances per capita (as an alternative measure of private health expenditures). Public health expenditure showed a positive and significant impact on infant mortality. GDP per capita was not significant, while remittances were positive and significant. Based on these findings, Kahn concluded that there is a direct relationship between government health expenditures and health outcomes.

The Kahn study, however, can be criticized in several ways. Among other things, there are problems of omitted variables and multicollinearity. It is a well-known fact that GDP per capita and government health expenditures are highly and positively correlated. Considering the shortcomings of the study, this can be considered only as weak evidence of a direct link between health expenditures and health outcomes.

In addition, Kahn's study is contradicted by the Grootaert (1994) study. Grootaert makes another significant contribution to the methodological aspect of evaluating the effects of SAPs on health outcomes. He argues that the focus should not be on aggregate social indicators, but on the distribution of the beneficiaries of social services. Is there an observable link between the aggregate levels of social spending and indicators of basic needs fulfillment?

The Grootaert (1994) study utilized data from the Côte d'Ivoire living standards survey, 1985–1988. In the mid-1980s, the economic crisis in Côte d'Ivoire quickly worsened due to a sudden appreciation of the real effective exchange rate. Despite economic difficulties, government expenditure on social welfare was protected during this time. The Grootaert study did not attempt to separate the effects of economic crisis and structural adjustment. The contribution of this report was in isolating the link between health expenditures and health outcomes among different socioeconomic groups. The poor do not comprise a homogeneous group, and the conditions of the poorest groups can evolve very differently from those of the poor as a whole. In order to separate socioeconomic groups, two poverty lines are used. The two lines distinguished between the bottom 30% (the poor) and 10% (the very poor) of the income distribution among the entire population.

Government spending in the social sectors was protected during the economic crisis. At the aggregate level, various health indicators remained at a constant level during these years. There was, however, little relation between the levels of government expenditures devoted to health and the service utilization indicators in health. Furthermore, countrywide data mask the vast differences in health outcomes between the poor and the nonpoor. For example, for the aggregate population, the percentage of ill people that consulted a doctor or a nurse remained relatively stable between 1985 (45.8%) and 1988 (41.3%), while the corresponding percentage among ill women in the poorest households decreased form 30.2% in 1985 to 16.2% in 1988.

This study highlights the fact that even though there is no detectable deterioration in aggregate health indicators, some groups, namely the poorest, have faced negative outcomes. Moreover, since health outcomes worsened for some groups while health expenditures remained constant, it can be very misleading to look at health expenditure as a determinant of positive or negative effects of SAPs.

Reverse Causality

Finally, Suh and Yeon (1992) introduce a diametrically opposed view to the rest of the empirical literature. In their report, the causal relationship between structural adjustment and health is reversed. Examining the Korean experience of structural adjustment and social welfare, they discuss the effects that social welfare might have on structural adjustment. The idea is that improvements in social welfare have a positive effect on worker productivity in the sense that workers will produce more efficiently under conditions of better health, nutrition, and general well-being. This in turn will have a positive effect on economic growth, which facilitates structural adjustment. In addition, social welfare can play a crucial role in promoting economic growth by easing social and political tensions. For a more detailed theoretical discussion, see McCleary (1990) and Taylor and Pieper (1996).

The Korean experience differs greatly from other countries' adjustment. The structural adjustment was not a result of severe economic crisis but a part of an economic development strategy where the government-led initiative to improve social welfare coincided closely with structural adjustment. Government expenditures on welfare showed a steadily increasing trend from the last half of the 1970s through 1986. Despite impressive economic and social progress, Korea faced an economic crisis in 1980. Compared to other countries, Korea quickly overcame the crisis. The authors argue that the investment in social welfare programs mitigated the economic crisis and reduced its duration. Unfortunately, they do not use their data to econometrically test the causal relationship.

The idea that social welfare and structural adjustment might be complementary is nevertheless highly interesting and deserves further investigation. To our knowledge, no such studies have been conducted. The fact that investment in health could be beneficial to structural adjustment is lacking in the debate. Considering the vast amount of literature on this topic, it is a misfortune that no attempts have been made to empirically establish such a reversed causal relationship.

A number of methodological issues regarding the relationship between structural adjustment and health have been raised. Only a handful of the twenty-eight empirical articles consider these issues, some of which are highlighted in this section. The following section summarizes the findings in the empirical literature.

EMPIRICAL EVIDENCE

This section includes a detailed analysis of the twenty-eight articles presenting empirical evidence of the correlation between structural adjustment and health (see Breman and Shelton (2001), appendix 1). The studies in this section differ substantially from each other and are therefore not directly comparable. Not only do they apply different methods and study different regions, but they also use a wide range of variables. We have therefore conducted a more in-depth survey of the empirical articles. In this section we aim first to compare the variables used in different studies. Which are the most common variables, and what do they tell us about the effects of structural adjustment on health? A discussion of comparable outcomes, trends, and differences between the articles with positive outcomes versus articles with negative outcomes follows. Finally, we examine outcomes by region and by author. Do outcomes depend on the person conducting the study?

Data and Methods

The twenty-eight empirical studies are well conducted with clearly defined data sources. Approximately one-third of our studies apply regression analysis to evaluate the correlation between variables that are specific for structural adjustment and health outcomes. Another third employ other statistical methods or a combination of several methods, and the last third present purely descriptive analysis of the data.

There are three main sources of data: government statistics from the countries investigated, for example, Vietnam living standard survey data; statistics from international organizations such as the World Bank, the IMF, and the United Nations; and data collected by the researchers. A surprisingly large number of studies (8 of 28) have collected their own data through focus group discussions or household surveys. The most common data sources are the international organizations, mainly the World Bank.

Variables

The two most common variables investigated are government health expenditures and child mortality.

Changes in the level of health expenditures may affect health outcomes if it affects access to health care and its quality. Child mortality, on the other hand, is a direct indicator of health status. Maternal mortality, life expectancy, and malnutrition are other measurements of health outcomes that have been investigated in several studies. Finally, a body of literature has tried to measure changes in the quality of health care under structural adjustment.

Health expenditures are likely to affect health outcomes, but it is not a direct measure of health status. Some authors have argued that health outcomes can be improved with a constant level of government expenditure on health through enhancing the effective use of existing funds (Serageldin et al. 1994). Restricting government expenditure would fuel the process toward better allocation of existing resources. Most authors, however, are of the opposite opinion. Health expenditures per capita are extremely low in developing countries, and to further restrict them would be devastating. As the preceding section shows, the empirical evidence of a direct link between health expenditures and health outcomes is weak.

Four different measurements of health expenditures are used (studies using this measurement):

- Per capita expenditure (Van der Hoeven and Stewart 1993, Serageldin et al. 1994, Van der Gaag and Barham 1998)
- Real total expenditure (Thiesen 1994, Sahn and Bernier 1995a, 1995b, Jayarajah et al. 1996)
- Percentage of GDP (Woodward 1992, Van der Hoeven and Stewart 1993, Serageldin et al. 1994)
- Percentage of total government expenditure (Suh and Yeon 1992, Van der Hoeven and Stewart 1993, Thiesen 1994, Jayarajah et al. 1996, El-Ghonemy 1998, Van der Gaag and Barham 1998)

There is evidence of both increasing and decreasing health expenditures. Authors investigating more than one country find evidence of both increases and decreases in health expenditures depending on the country and the time frame. There is no general conclusion to be drawn. Whether or not health expenditures have been protected seems to depend on the willingness of the government to prioritize the health sector, the depth of the economic crisis, and the success or failure of the SAP.

Child mortality can be divided into two subcategories (studies):

- Absolute decline (Suh and Yeon 1992, Van der Hoeven and Stewart 1993, Anderson and Witter 1994, Serageldin et al. 1994, El-Ghonemy 1998, Kahn 1999)
- Rate of decline (Hill and Pebley 1989, Woodward 1992, Thiesen 1994, Jayarajah et al. 1996, Mwabu 1996, Onyeiwu et al. 1997, El-Ghonemy 1998, Van der Gaag 1998, Garenne and Gakusi 2000)

Child mortality is a crucial indicator of health status. Health care for children is more price sensitive than is health care for adults, and child health is therefore likely to be an early indicator of deteriorating health status of a population. The empirical studies show that child mortality has declined in absolute terms in all investigated countries, although there are some countries where there are signs of increasing child mortality. However, there are not yet reliable data to support this (Cruickshank 2000). The rate of decline is much more disputed. Two studies indicate a slowdown in the rate of decline, two show an increase, and three find both. Two studies (Hill and Pebley 1989, Garenne and Gakusi 2000) conclude that there is no evidence that structural adjustment has either slowed or hastened the pace of decline in child mortality. These two cross-country studies focus solely on child mortality rates and use regression analysis to assess the effects of structural adjustment.

Maternal mortality and life expectancy at birth are more often measured in absolute terms than in rates of decline. The data show that maternal mortality (Suh and Yeon 1992, van der Hoeven and Stewart 1993, Kahn 1999) has declined and life expectancy increased (Anderson and Witter 2000, Mwabu 1996, Onyeiwu et al. 1997). Whether or not the rate of improvement has increased or slowed down is generally not known.

Malnutrition is the third most investigated variable. The outcomes are negative. Malnutrition appears to have increased under structural adjustment. Caloric intake has decreased in all studies involving malnutrition (see, e.g., Cornu 1995, Biljmakers et al. 1996, Onah 2000). Wasting (weight-for-height), which is considered as a measurement of short-term changes in nutritional status, has increased, while stunting (height-for-age), a long-term indicator, has improved (Cornu 1995, Biljmakers et al. 1996). The authors interpret this result as evidence of worsened nutritional status as a result of structural adjustment.

Several studies attempt to assess how structural

adjustment has affected the quality of health care. The method employed is to gather data through focus group discussions with health workers and patients. The overall pattern is a decline in the quality of care. One study from Pakistan finds that the number of people per doctor or nurse has decreased, which would imply better access to health personnel (Kahn 1999). However, seven other studies on this topic find a worsened situation with fewer health personnel per capita and severe deterioration in the quality of health care (see, e.g., Biljmakers et al. 1996, Lundy 1996, Onah 2000, Israr et al. 2000).

Furthermore, two studies examine how health expenditures are divided between preventive and curative care. In the past, most developing countries have had a strong bias toward curative care at the expense of more cost-effective preventive care. Both studies conclude that this bias has worsened rather than improved under structural adjustment (Sahn and Bernier 1993, 1995a, 1995b). In many instances, the lack of change that the authors could verify was matched by government pronouncements and plans suggesting that change was imminent.

POSITIVE VERSUS NEGATIVE STUDIES

We have reused the classifications from the preceding section for the outcomes of the twenty-eight empirical studies: positive, negative, both, and neutral. However, the definition of the categories is narrower in this section. Positive (negative) implies that the empirical evidence shows a positive (negative) effect of SAPs on health outcome. The authors' opinions are not relevant; the study must find evidence of negative outcomes to be categorized as a negative study. One empirical study was classified as neutral. The study examines fertility decline in Nigeria as a result of structural adjustment and economic recession (Onah 2000). The authors find a significant decline in fertility in Nigeria, but whether or not this fertility decline is a desirable outcome is not clear.

Upon examination of all seventy-six studies, an overwhelming majority was negative toward structural adjustment. As shown in table 13.1, a different pattern is revealed among the empirical studies. An almost equal number of studies show positive effects (29%), both positive and negative effects (32%), or negative effects (35%). It is not possible to conclude that the empirical evidence shows purely negative or

positive health outcomes resulting from structural adjustment. Furthermore, there is no evidence that more recent studies are more positive/negative than are previous ones. The outcomes seem to depend on the variables investigated, the country or region, and the method used.

Case Studies versus Cross-Country Studies

Fourteen studies are country-specific case studies, and fourteen are cross-country studies. The following ten countries are represented in the case studies (number of studies in parentheses if more than one): Brazil, Cameroon, Congo (2), Côte d'Ivoire, Jamaica (2), Nigeria, Pakistan, South Korea, Vietnam, and Zimbabwe (3).[2] A strong negative trend dominates the case studies; 50% find negative outcomes related to structural adjustment, and 21% show positive outcomes. Out of fourteen case studies, eight are from Africa. The African case studies mainly show negative effects (75%) of structural adjustment. The remaining 25% of case studies in Africa show both negative and positive effects.

The cross-country studies show a different pattern (see table 13.1). As a result of analyzing a larger number of countries, more studies are both negative and positive. The number of studies indicating positive outcomes (36%) is also considerable compared to the country-specific studies. It is interesting to examine more closely the method used in these cross-country studies. The positive studies investigate one single variable such as child health (Hill and Pebley 1989, Garenne and Gakusi 2000), compare adjusting countries to nonadjusting countries (Van der Gaag and Barham 1998), or conclude that health outcomes have improved in successful adjusters (Mwabu 1996). The negative cross-country studies compare outcomes in different countries, but in one region, Africa, in these cases.

Studies by Region

The overall literature review revealed a negative trend among Asian and African countries, while the articles from Latin America–Caribbean and Middle East–North Africa are generally both positive and negative. The objective of comparing different regions is to find out if the empirical evidence reinforces these trends.

Fifteen of the twenty-eight empirical studies were conducted in sub-Saharan Africa; 53% of these studies

TABLE 13.1. Nature of Study Related to Outcomes

Type of Study (Number of Studies)	Outcomes			
	Positive (%)	Negative (%)	Both Positive and Negative (%)	Neutral (%)
All studies (76)	8	45	27	20
Empirical studies (28)	29	35	32	4
Case studies (14)	21	50	21	8
Cross-country studies (14)	36	21	34	0

find negative effects of structural adjustment on health, and only 13% find positive outcomes. The empirical studies therefore reinforce the overall literature review in that they find mainly negative health outcomes in Africa during structural adjustment.

There are only three studies from Asia, and they are all case studies. It is therefore difficult to draw any conclusions on the effects of structural adjustment on health in Asia. The South Korean (Suh and Yeon 1992) and Pakistani (Kahn 1999) studies are positive, while the Vietnamese study (Gertler and Litvack 1998) is mainly negative.

Four studies are from the Latin America–Caribbean region. Two of them find both positive and negative health outcomes under structural adjustment. A study from Jamaica found strong negative effects of structural adjustment on the quality of health care (Lundy 1996), while the fourth study (Rios-Neto and De Carvalo 1997) found that health outcomes in Brazil have improved under structural adjustment.

Only one empirical study conducted in the Middle East–North Africa region was identified among those included in this literature review. This study (El-Ghonemy 1998) is a cross-country comparison of eight countries (Tunisia, Egypt, Morocco, Sudan, Turkey, Mauritania, Jordan, and Algeria). The results vary greatly between the different countries, showing both negative and positive outcomes.

Finally, five empirical studies cover countries from several continents. These studies are often designed to compare adjusting and nonadjusting countries. It is noteworthy that none of these studies is negative. Two studies found both negative and positive outcomes (Cornia and Stewart 1987, Jayarajah et al. 1996), and three studies are positive (Hill and Pebley 1989, Mwabu 1996, Van der Gaag and Barham 1998).

To conclude this section on regional differences, there are few discernable trends. Sub-Saharan Africa is the only region where there are a sufficiently large number of studies to identify a trend. Most of the evidence from the region shows negative health outcomes under structural adjustment. Too few studies in other regions made it difficult to draw any conclusions on any specific regional trends. The outcome depends on the variable used in the study, the method and whether or not it is a country-specific case study or cross-country study. Mwabu (1996) concluded in his cross-country study that structural adjustment has had a positive effect on health outcomes if the adjustment program has been successful. Zimbabwe and Jamaica are examples of countries where there is strong evidence of negative health outcomes that can be related to policies adapted as a part of SAPs. In contrast, South Korea and Brazil are examples of countries with successful adjustment programs, protecting social spending, and improving health outcomes.

THE AUTHORS

Having studied the variables used, methods, and regional differences, it is equally important to examine if the outcomes vary with the persons or institutions conducting the study. Who are the authors? Are they mainly from developed or developing countries? Are they economists or public health specialists? Is there a bias toward positive outcomes in the studies conducted by World Bank/IMF employees?

More than a third of the studies are conducted by university academics in developed countries. The majority of their studies found negative health outcomes in developing countries under SAPs. A small number of studies (5 of 28) were conducted by researchers in developing countries. They found positive outcomes as often as negative outcomes of structural adjustment. Another five studies were done in collaboration with researchers in developed and developing countries. Their results are both positive and negative.

A significant number of articles were published by employees of the World Bank (six) and United Nations (two). Only in a few cases were those articles written as official documents from these institutions. The authors are often both positive and negative toward structural adjustment. The assumption that World Bank employees would generally find a positive impact on health under structural adjustment cannot be justified in this study. Only one study found negative outcomes of structural adjustment (Grootaert 1994), and two found positive outcomes (Suh and Yeon 1992, Van der Gaag and Barham 1998); 50% of the studies conducted by World Bank or IMF employees found both positive and negative outcomes.

There is no category of authors that are overwhelmingly positive or negative. Therefore, we cannot conclude that the outcomes depend on the author. There is no evidence that researchers in developing countries should be more negative toward SAPs than are researchers in developed countries (it is rather the opposite), or that World Bank employees always conduct their studies in such a way that they find only positive outcomes of adjustment.

CONCLUSIONS

An analysis of the literature comparing empirical, theoretical, and normative articles on the relationship between SAPs and health outcomes has illustrated some interesting trends and changes in the debate over time. The most striking trend is that opponents of structural adjustment heavily dominate the debate despite the fact that empirical evidence shows positive outcomes of structural adjustment as often as negative. A considerable number of authors support adjustment on the condition that policies are implemented in such a way that they do not adversely affect health outcomes for the poor and most vulnerable groups. It is clear that the nature of the article is often correlated to the authors' opinions. Normative articles are generally negative while theoretical ones remain neutral. The empirical studies present both positive and negative outcomes of adjustment programs.

The regional distribution of the studies shows that sub-Saharan Africa is heavily represented both in the overall literature review and among the empirical articles. The majority of the studies in sub-Saharan Africa, whether theoretical or empirical, are negative toward structural adjustment and its effects on health outcomes. It is more difficult to find specific trends among other regions because they are underrepresented.

In order to assess health outcomes under adjustment, a wide range of variables have been used. Health expenditures and child mortality are the most common variables. It is important to note that the outcomes differ substantially: health expenditures have declined in some countries and increased in others. Child mortality has declined in absolute terms in all investigated countries, but in some countries there is evidence that the rate of decline has slowed significantly.

Furthermore, case studies, more often than cross-country studies, find negative outcomes as a result of adjustment policies. Case studies seem to be a useful tool to show adverse effects of adjustment, while cross-country studies find both positive and negative health outcomes depending on the country. Cross-country studies typically compare adjusting to nonadjusting countries and find that health outcomes and health expenditures have not deteriorated more in adjusting than in nonadjusting countries.

The debate on structural adjustment and health continues as various forms of SAPs remain in place. Although the debate is heavily concentrated with opponents of SAPs, the analysis of the literature presented in this chapter showed that positive or negative results of SAPs are not easily determined. Thus, a fairly large amount of research is being conducted on this subject, and new evidence is frequently presented. Although we cannot make definitive conclusions about the impact of structural adjustment on health, it is clear that this debate has helped to draw attention to how adjustment programs may be implemented without creating adverse effects for the poor.

Notes

1. The Heavily Indebted Poor Country initiative is an agreement among official creditors to provide debt relief to the most heavily indebted countries in Africa, Asia, Latin America, and the Middle East. The main objective is to reduce a country's debt burden to sustainable levels, while subject to satisfactory policy performance to ensure that adjustment and/or reform processes are not jeopardized by the burden of high debt levels.

2. All three studies on Zimbabwe were conducted by the same persons within a longer research project.

References

Amobi IC (1993). The World Bank approach to poverty reduction in debt and the human condition: structural adjustment and the right to development. *Studies in Human Rights*, No. 14. Westport, CT: Greenwood Press.

Anderson P, and Witter M (2000). Crisis, adjustment and social change: a case study of Jamaica. In: E Lefrank, ed. *Consequences of Structural Adjustment: A Review of the Jamaican Experience*. Jamaica: University of the West Indies, pp. 1–55.

Antia NH (1995). Structural adjustment and India's health. *National Medical Journal of India* 8(6): 277–278.

Bassett M, Bijlmakers L, and Sanders D (1997). Professionalism, patient satisfaction and quality of health care: experience during Zimbabwe's Structural Adjustment Programme. *Social Science and Medicine* 45(12): 1845–1852.

Biljmakers LA, Basset MT, and Sanders DM (1996). *Health and Structural Adjustment in Rural and Urban Zimbabwe*. Research Report No. 101. Uppsala, Sweden: Scandinavian Institute of African Studies.

Cornia GA, Jolly R, and Stewart F, eds. (1987). *Adjustment with a Human Face*. Vol. 1. *Protecting the Vulnerable and Promoting Growth*. Oxford: Clarendon Press.

Cornia GA, and Stewart F (1987). *Adjustment with a Human Face*. Vol. 2. *Country Case Studies*. Oxford: Clarendon Press.

Cornu A, et al. (1995). Nutritional change and economic crisis in an urban Congolese community. *International Journal of Epidemiology* 24(1): 155–164.

Cruickshank CJ (2000). Report from Nicaragua: midwifery and structural adjustment. *Journal of Midwifery & Women's Health* 45(5): 411–415.

Dodd R, and Hinshelwood E (2002). *Poverty Reduction Strategy Papers—Their Significance for Health*. Preliminary Report. Geneva: World Health Organization.

El-Ghonemy M (1998). *Affluence and Poverty in the Middle East*. London: Routledge.

Elson D (1992). From survival strategies to transformation strategies: women's needs and structural adjustment. In: L. Beneria and S. Feldman, eds. *Unequal Burden: Economic Crises, Persistent Poverty and Women's Work*. Boulder, CO: Westview Press, pp. 26–48.

Garenne M, and Gakusi E (2000). *Health effects of structural adjustment programs in sub-Saharan Africa*. Draft to be published as a CEPED working paper. Paris: French Center for Population and Development Studies.

Gertler P, and Litvack J (1998). Access to health care during transition: the role of the private sector in Vietnam. In: D Dollar, P Glewwe, and J Litrack, eds. *Household Welfare and Vietnam's Transition*. Washington, DC: World Bank.

Grootaert C (1994). Poverty and basic needs fulfillment in Africa during structural change: evidence from Côte d'Ivoire. *World Development* 22(10): 1521–1534.

Handa S, and King D (2003). Adjustment with a human face? Evidence from Jamaica. *World Development* 31(7): 1125–1145.

Hill K, and Pebley AR (1989). Child mortality in the developing world. *Population and Development Review* 15(4): 657–687.

Israr SM, et al. (2000). Coping strategies of health personnel during economic crisis: a case study from Cameroon. *Tropical Medicine and International Health* 5(4): 288–292.

Jayarajah C, Branson W, and Sen B (1996). *Social Dimensions of Adjustment, World Bank Experience, 1980–93*. Washington, DC: World Bank, Operations Evaluation Department.

Kahn S (1999). Structural adjustment and health. In: S R Kahn, ed. *Do World Bank and IMF Policies Work?* New York: St. Martin's Press.

Lancet (1990). Structural adjustment and health in Africa. Vol. 335: 885–886.

Lancet (1994). Structural adjustment too painful? Vol. 344: 1377–1378.

Laurell AC, and Arellano OL (1996). Market commodities and poor relief: the World Bank proposal for health. *International Journal of Health Services* 26(1): 1–18.

Logie DE, and Woodroffe J (1993). Structural adjustment: the wrong prescription for Africa. *British Medical Journal* 307: 41–44.

Lundy P (1996). Limitations of quantitative research in the study of structural adjustment. *Social Science and Medicine* 42(3): 313–324.

McCleary WA (1990). Policy implementation under adjustment lending. In: *The Path to Reform: Issues and Experiences*. Washington, DC: World Bank.

Musgrove P (1997). Economic crisis and health policy response. In: G Tapinos, A Mason, and J Bravo, eds. *Demographic Responses to Economic Adjustment in Latin America*. Oxford: Clarendon Press, pp. 37–53.

Mwabu G (1996). *Health Effects of Market-Based Reforms in Developing Countries*. UNU/WIDER Working Paper No. 120. Helsinki: UNU World Institute for Development Economic Research.

Onah HE (2000). Declining fetal growth standards in Enugu, Nigeria. *International Journal of Gynecology and Obstetrics* 68(3): 219–224.

Onyeiwu S, Shrestha H, and Botero C (1997). A welfare-based evaluability assessment of structural adjustment programs in Africa. *Canadian Journal of Development Studies* 28(special issue): 689–710.

Peabody JW (1996). Economic reform and health sector policy: lessons from structural adjustment programs. *Social Science and Medicine* 43(5): 823–835.

Pitt M (1993). Analyzing human resource effects: health. In: L. Demery, MA Ferroni, and C Grootaert, eds.

Understanding the Social Effects of Policy Reform. Washington, DC: World Bank.

Rios-Neto E, and De Carvalo J (1997). Demographic consequences of structural adjustment: the case of Brazil. In: G. Tapinos, A Mason, and J Bravo, eds. *Demographic Responses to Economic Adjustment in Latin America.* Oxford: Clarendon Press, pp. 37–53.

Sahn DE, and Bernier R (1993). *Evidence from Africa in the Intrasectoral Allocation of Social Sector Expenditures.* Cornell Food and Nutrition Policy Program, Working Paper 45. Cornell University, Ithaca, NY.

Sahn D, and Bernier R (1995a). Have structural adjustments led to health sector reform in Africa? *Health policy* 32: 193–214.

Sahn D, and Bernier R (1995b). Has structural adjustment led to health sector reform in Africa? In: P Berman, ed. *Health Sector Reform in Developing Countries— Making Health Development Sustainable.* Cambridge: Harvard University Press, pp. 247–275.

Sen K, and Koivusalo M (1998). Health care reforms and developing countries—a critical overview. *International Journal of Health Planning and Management* 13: 199–215.

Serageldin I, Elmendorf EA, and Eltigani EE (1994). Structural adjustment and health in Africa in the 1980s. *Research in Human Capital and Development.* Vol. 8. *Nutrition, Food Policy and Development*: pp. 131–195. JAI Press.

Suh S, and Yeon H (1992). Social welfare during the period of structural adjustment. In: V. Corbo and S-M Suh, eds. *Structural Adjustment in a Newly Industrialized Country: The Korean Experience.* Washington DC: World Bank, pp. 281–304.

Taylor L, and Pieper U (1996). *Reconciling Economic Reform and Sustainable Human Development: Social Consequences of Neo-Liberalism.* Discussion Paper, Series D-2. New York: UNDP.

Thiesen JK (1994). A study of the effects of structural adjustment on education and health in Africa. In: GW Shepard and KNM Sonoko, eds. *Economic Justice in Africa—Adjustment and Sustainable Development.* Studies in Human Rights No. 16. Westport, CT: Greenwood Press.

Van der Gaag J, and Barham T (1998). Health and health expenditures in adjusting and non-adjusting countries. *Social Science and Medicine* 46(8): 995–1009.

Van der Hoeven R, and Stewart F (1993). *Social Development during Periods of Structural Adjustment in Latin America.* Occasional Paper 18. Geneva: International Labour Office.

Woodward D (1992). *Debt, Adjustment, and Poverty in Developing Countries.* Vol. 2. *The Impact of Debt and Adjustment at the Household Level in Developing Countries.* New York: Save the Children, St. Martin's Press.

Chapter 14

Poverty Reduction Strategy Papers: Bold New Approach to Poverty Eradication or Old Wine in New Bottles?

Sarah Wamala, Ichiro Kawachi and Besinati Phiri Mpepo

Poverty reduction strategy papers (PRSPs) were introduced by the World Bank and International Monetary Fund (IMF) in September 1999 as a new requirement for countries to receive concessional funding and debt relief. PRSPs are national planning frameworks, and describe a country's macroeconomic, structural and social policies and programs to promote growth and reduce poverty, as well as associated external financing needs. The emergence of PRSPs reflects growing awareness on the part of the international financial institutions concerning the limited effectiveness of conditionalities imposed by traditional structural adjustment programs (SAPs) (see also chapter 13), as well as the disappointing poverty reduction performance in most highly indebted and aid-dependent countries during the past twenty years, despite substantial changes in policies and institutions (Booth 2001). Growing evidence has suggested that economic reforms are more likely to succeed when they are initiated and "owned" by the governments implementing them, as compared to being imposed by the IMF or World Bank (Fischer

2003). In principle, PRSPs give prominence to the national policy context for aid effectiveness, and the process for formulating them provides room for governments to garner public support for the programs.

PRSPs are the new basis for all foreign aid to poor countries. All heavily indebted poor countries (HIPCs) are now required to produce PRSPs as a basis for receiving loans and debt relief. In addition, the World Bank and IMF boards must approve a country's PRSP before a lending program is initiated (World Bank 2003). In accordance with the new regime, the IMF and World Bank have renamed their lending facilities for poor countries. The IMF has replaced its Enhanced Structural Adjustment Facility with the Poverty Reduction and Growth Facility (PRGF), while World Bank has established the Poverty Reduction Support Credit, a lending instrument designed to support the implementation of PRSPs and to complement traditional adjustment loans. Countries that previously received Enhanced Structural Adjustment loans from the IMF now receive PRGF loans. However, the interest rate and repayment conditions remain the same (Bretton Woods Project 2003). In addition, PRSPs largely extend the ideas previously developed by the World Bank's proposals to base its lending on a country-level Comprehensive Development Framework.

Five core principles underlie the development of poverty reduction strategies (World Bank 2003; Bretton Woods Project 2003):

- Country-driven: Unlike the SAPs, PRSPs are owned by respective governments, and it is emphasized that they should be prepared and written by countries themselves through a participatory process involving civil society and the private sector. In turn, broad public participation in the design of PRSPs is intended to achieve four goals (Sachs 2005): (i) better prioritization of investment plans, (ii) increased public awareness about poverty reduction programs, (iii) mobilization of nongovernmental organizations (NGOs) and community groups, and (iv) fostering more political awareness against corruption.
- Results-oriented: They focus on outcomes that are intended to benefit the poor, as opposed to being narrowly process oriented. In other words, PRSPs are supposed to start from the analysis and differential diagnosis of the causes of poverty and work backward to the design of appropriate policies. It was partly in response to the growing critique of SAPs (see chapter 13) that PRSPs were introduced to go beyond macroeconomic stabilization and liberalization and to begin to address the issues of poverty and equity in growth.
- Comprehensive: Recognizing the multidimensional nature of poverty and covering the different sectoral and cross-sectoral issues that affect the prospects for poverty reduction.
- Involving partnerships, including the coordinated participation of development partners (bilateral, multilateral, and nongovernmental), such that all funding sources are harmonized around a strategy developed under the leadership of the recipient government.
- Visualized as a medium- to long-term process, implying the need for long-term commitments by donors as well as careful consideration for timing and performance monitoring.

Whether PRSPs will actually lead to greater effectiveness and sustainability in antipoverty action remains a hypothesis (Booth 2001). Meanwhile, there is no boilerplate or blueprint for building a country's poverty reduction strategy. Rather, the process is supposed to reflect a country's individual circumstances and characteristics.

However, there are some core principles underlying the formulation of PRSPs, which include (i) a description of the participatory process—outlining the format, frequency, and location of consultations, as well as a summary of the main issues raised and the views of participants; (ii) an account of the impact of the consultations on the design of the strategy, as well as a description of the role of civil society in future monitoring and implementation; (iii) a comprehensive poverty diagnostics—describing the characteristics of poor people and their locations using existing data. At a minimum, PRSPs should have a description of appropriate targets, indicators, and systems for monitoring and evaluating progress—including the definition of medium- and long-term goals for poverty reduction outcomes (monetary and nonmonetary), the establishment of indicators of progress, and setting annual and medium-term targets. The indicators and targets must be easy to monitor and should be consistent with policy choices in the strategy.

THE PRSP CYCLE

The PRSP process involves three stages (Bretton Woods Project 2003):

- Completion of an interim PRSP (I-PRSP): As a way of enabling countries to qualify for debt relief while allowing time to develop a solid PRSP, countries have been permitted to develop I-PRSPs, which are required to diagnose poverty in the country and to outline a consultation process for drafting the final PRSP.
- Reaching a "decision point" upon presentation of the PRSP: This triggers partial debt relief (under the HIPC framework) or concessional loans. Importantly, the World Bank and IMF have argued that a recipient government can present whatever plan it wants (Bretton Woods Project 2003).[1] Upon being presented with a plan, World Bank and IMF staff then write a "joint staff assessment" (JSA) that highlights areas of disagreement and perceived weaknesses in the PRSP. In turn, the JSA indicates a "bottom-line" judgment as to whether the PRSP

presents a "credible" set of policies. Without a positive JSA, the government will not receive World Bank or IMF funding and will be unlikely to qualify for bilateral funding.

- Reaching a "completion point": After implementing a full PRSP for one year, the "decision point" is the date at which a heavily indebted country with an established track record of good performance under adjustment programs commits to undertake additional reforms. The completion point is the date at which the country successfully completes the key structural reforms agreed upon at the decision point. The country then receives the bulk of debt relief under the HIPC debt initiative without further policy conditions. The only exception is that governments should use the funds that would have been used to service the loan to increase public spending on education and health.

The successive steps (and various actors involved) in the PRSP cycle is illustrated in figure 14.1.

As of September 2004, forty-two countries have presented full PRSPs (table 14.1) (World Bank and IMF 2004).

In the following sections, we highlight two PRSPs—from Zambia and Uganda—to illustrate some successes and pitfalls in the process to date.

CASE STUDY: THE ZAMBIA PRSP

Zambia is one of the poorest countries in the world, with rural areas experiencing approximating 80% poverty levels. Similar to that of many other African countries, Zambia's poverty is higher in rural areas than in urban areas and higher among female-headed households than among male-headed households. Access to basic requirements such as water, sanitation, food, and shelter has been difficult for the majority of Zambians. Social services such as education and heath are out of reach of most people, especially in rural areas, while at the same time the quality of the existing services has been falling.

Women and children are the hardest hit by the poverty situation, and this has manifested in various ways. For instance, the under-five mortality rate is approximately 168 per 1,000 live births, the infant mortality rate is 95 per 1,000, the maternal mortality rate is 729 per 100,000 live births, and the HIV prevalence rate is approximately 16% among 15- to 49-

year-olds. Child poverty has been increasing due to the impacts of the HIV/AIDS pandemic. It is common to find child labor, street children, orphans, and child-headed households.

For a long time, the Zambian government has been exploring various ways of salvaging the national economy and has over the past decade and a half robustly implemented IMF/World Bank SAPs. The SAPs have been characterized by prescriptions such as privatization, trade liberalization, removal of subsidies, and a wage freeze for civil servants. For many Zambians, these prescriptions have meant job losses, low wages, high prices, and ultimately higher levels of poverty. The most recent IMF/World Bank prescription has been in the form of PRSPs, which are supposed to show a marked difference from SAPs in terms of their entry into the poverty debate and stakeholder participation in the program.

The preparation of a PRSP for Zambia was, as in many other countries, a precondition for the country to qualify and receive debt relief under the HIPC initiative. The preparation process began in 2000 and was spearheaded by the then Ministry of Finance and National Development.[2] The first step was the preparation of an I-PRSP, which, apart from providing a road map for preparing the final PRSP, was a precondition for Zambia to qualify for the HIPC decision point. Due to its linkage with HIPC and consequent time lines, the I-PRSP was prepared in a rushed manner with very little, if any, stakeholder involvement.

After successful approval of the I-PRSP, preparation of the full PRSP began. In line with two of the principles of the PRSP, that is, that the process must be "country driven" and "partnership oriented," the government set up multistakeholder working groups to dialogue and brainstorm on issues to be included in the PRSP. The working groups included representatives from government, civil society, the international community, and private sector. It should be noted that one critical stakeholder was left out of the formulation process—Members of Parliament (MPs). During the time that the PRSP was being formulated, politicians were in the throes of campaigning for 2001 presidential and parliamentary elections and had little time to engage with the PRSP. The few attempts that government made to bring MPs on board where futile.

Apart from the activities of the working groups, civil society came together to form a strong civil society network called the Civil Society for Poverty Reduction (CSPR), whose main objective was to ensure

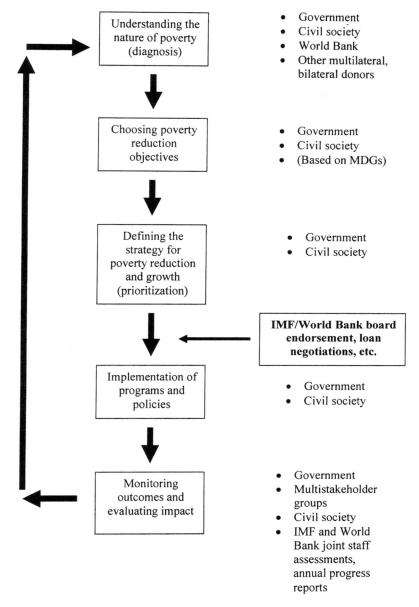

FIGURE 14.1. The PRSP Cycle: Successive Steps and Actors Involved.
Source: Adapted from Bretton Woods Project (2003).

meaningful civil society engagement in the PRSP process. CSPR conducted independent consultations in various provinces as well as provided a platform for civil society representatives working on poverty issues to contribute to the national document. The independent work of civil society resulted in a report entitled "A PRSP for Zambia—a Civil Society Perspective,"

(Mpepo 2002) the official civil society input to the PRSP submitted to the Ministry of Finance and National Planning.

In 2002, Zambia finalized the preparation of its PRSP, which reflected some good poverty-reducing plans. However, the primary tool for effecting PRSP expenditures, the budget, is yet to fully reflect the

TABLE 14.1. Countries with Full PRSPs by September 2004

Early PRSPs May 2000–June 2002	Later PRSPs July 2002–June 2003	Recent PRSPs July 2003–September 2004
Albania	Azerbaijan	Armenia
Bolivia (CP)	Benin (CP)	Bosnia and Herzegovina
Burkina Faso (CP)	Cambodia	Djibouti
Gambia (DP)	Cameroon (DP)	Kenya
Guinea (DP)	Chad (DP)	Lao PDR
Guyana (CP)	Ethiopia (CP)	Madagascar
Honduras (DP)	Georgia	Moldova
Malawi (DP)	Ghana (CP)	Mongolia
Mali (CP)	Kyrgyz Republic	Pakistan
Mauritania (CP)	Nepal	Serbia and Montenegro
Mozambique (CP)	Sri Lanka	
Nicaragua (CP)		
Niger (CP)		
Rwanda (DP)		
Senegal (CP)		
Tajikistan		
Tanzania (CP)		
Uganda (CP)		
Vietnam		
Yemen		
Zambia (DP)		

CP and DP indicate, respectively, that countries have reached the completion point and decision point under the HIPC initiative (see text for explanation).

Source: World Bank/IMF (2004).

importance of this plan. Further, the PRSP now sits at the center of a larger national plan—the Transitional National Development Plan—that, apart from centering largely on the PRSP, includes other issues such as national security.

Zambia's PRSP identifies the multidimensional characteristic of poverty and demands a multidimensional approach to tackling it. The main purpose of Zambia's PRSP is to promote sustainable economic growth (agriculture, tourism, industry, and mining), and to improve social services (health and education) and infrastructure (energy, transport and communications, water, and sanitation). The PRSP identifies HIV/AIDS, gender, and the environment as cross-cutting themes that affect all other sectors. The PRSP promotes good governance and appropriate macroeconomic policies, which will provide an enabling environment for implementation.

As with most PRSPs, concerns may be raised around how independent the preparation of the macroeconomic section was, given the interest of the IMF and World Bank in these issues. One could argue that it still emphasizes growth and stabilization in line with IMF/World Bank concerns and includes issues of privatization, a thorny issue in many poor economies.

Zambia's PRSP recognizes a two-way relationship between health and poverty. On the one hand, the PRSP points to poverty as being a source of ill health. It acknowledges that the poor in Zambia lack access to basic health services with qualified personal and essential drugs. Further, it acknowledges that the poor are unable to achieve good nutrition, which is essential for healthy and productive lives, and which has a direct bearing on the economic performance of a country. All in all, the poor suffer worse health outcomes and a heavier burden of disease.

At the same time, the PRSP views ill health as a cause of poverty and recognizes that health allows a poor person to work. It also recognizes that income is lost as a result of seeking care or caring for the sick. If health is an asset and ill health a liability, then protecting and promoting health care is central to the entire process of poverty reduction and human development. In recognizing the link between poverty and ill health, it is important to note that, for Zambia, ill health is more likely to lead to further impoverishment among the poor than among the wealthy. Meeting the health needs of the poor is important for preventing the increase in poverty.

In 1992, Zambia began a Health Reform Program. This program did not work because of insufficient resources to offer a decent health care package. The PRSP supports the Health Reform Program and commits to providing resources to it. The Health Reform Program sets up a basic health care package that is aimed at providing a decent level of health care to all Zambians. The PRSP commits to improved financial and human resource allocation to the health sector, better management of health services including improved drug supply, improvement of infrastructure, and access to health care in hard-to-reach and underserviced areas as well as vulnerable groups. Further, it commits to the replacement of obsolete equipment and provision of training staff.

Zambia's PRSP also lays out five key areas for public health: preventive programs and treatment for malaria; treatment and prevention of HIV/AIDS, tuberculosis, and other sexually transmitted diseases; an integrated approach to reproductive health, including family planning, pregnancy, delivery, postnatal care, teenage pregnancy, and other issues related to women's health; focusing on common childhood diseases that can be prevented or cured; and monitoring and controlling epidemic disease break outs. In addition to the above, the government will intensify interventions in nutrition by finalizing and implementing a National Food and Nutrition Policy, which will provide the National Food and Nutrition Commission with the mandate to coordinate and facilitate all nutrition activities in the country.

To expand on the HIV/AIDS intervention, first, the PRSP prioritizes the reduction of HIV/AIDS infections through behavioral change campaigns and condom distribution. Second, the PRSP aims to reduce the social and economic impact of HIV/AIDS by expanding access to quality voluntary counseling and testing, community home-based care, and antiretroviral treatment. Third, the PRSP proposes to improve the quality of lives of orphans and vulnerable children. Other interventions include improving the management of sexually transmitted infections, expansion of access to quality prevention of mother-to-child transmission of HIV, prophylaxis against tuberculosis, and drugs for opportunistic infections.

From the finalization of Zambia's PRSP in 2002, progress in implementation has been slow and characterized by low levels of disbursements.[3] The government has explained this in terms of unavailability of resources. In particular, some pledged funds from the international community have not been fulfilled, resulting in shortfalls in expected receipts. Further, Zambia continues to have a huge external and growing internal debt burden whose repayments have competed with resources for poverty reduction. However, the Zambian civil society feels that the perpetuation of poverty goes beyond resource availability to low government commitment, lack of priority setting, and low willingness to spend on PRSP programs. A study commissioned by CSPR reflects this by revealing how government releases more than approved allocations to some departments or ministries that have little to do with poverty reduction, for example, the cabinet office or state house, while at the same time spending less than allocated on poverty reduction programs.

To the dissatisfaction of civil society, it also appears that the government views the PRSP as more as a tool for international resource mobilization and as an HIPC trigger rather than a practical poverty-reducing plan. Thus, the PRSP does not appear to be exploited as an opportunity to begin addressing the plight of two-thirds of Zambians that live in unacceptable conditions. Once again, conditionalities appear to be the order of the day, as in the case with past SAPs.

On the positive side of the ledger, civil society, through the CSPR, has grown in strength, focus, and magnitude. There is a focus to monitor the implementation of the PRSP using budget tracking and participatory techniques.

In conclusion, the role for civil society and Zambian citizens in the process have been crucial in influencing the "contents" and "concepts" of PRSPs to the extent that these plans could actually bring about some tangible benefits for the poor. CSPR maintains that the PRSP should not be taken mainly as a tool to solicit funds and debt relief from the international community, but as a true tool for fighting the condition in which 80% of the Zambian population live today.

CASE STUDY: THE UGANDA PRSP

In April 1998, Uganda was the first country to benefit from debt relief under the HIPC initiative. In May 2000, it reached the completion point under the Enhanced HIPC Initiative.

Uganda's PRSP was developed through a participatory process and identified the following key goals: increasing the ability of the poor to raise their incomes, improving the quality of the life of the poor, creating an enabling environment for economic growth and structural transformation, and ensuring good governance and security. In November 2000, the World Bank's board approved a country assistance strategy for Uganda. According to this work plan for World Bank involvement in Uganda, the objective of the World Bank's strategy is to support Uganda's economic transformation and poverty reduction strategy as spelled out in the government's Poverty Eradication Action Plan (the formal title of Uganda's PRSP). While the work to maintain macroeconomic stability continues, the emphasis on assistance has shifted to the sector levels, for example, agriculture, health, education, water, and sanitation, and to cross-cutting public sector management issues.

Some positive impacts of the PRSP have been increased growth, as shown by growing gross domestic product (GDP) per capita of 4.9% in 2003 and 5.9% in 2004, and increased access to safe water from 58% in 2000 to 68% 2003. There is scarcity of data on how much of the Uganda's GDP is spent on school education. However, in spite of the initiatives to finance primary school education, 26% and 14% of young women and men (15–24 years old), respectively, cannot read or write. Yet even for those who get enrolled in primary school, only about 70% of males and 60% of females complete primary school. In addition, even when Uganda increased public health expenditure to 3.4% of GDP, 40% of children younger than one year of age still have no immunization coverage and 20% of children younger than five years suffer from malnutrition. Per capita income in 2004 is estimated to be about US$250. Life expectancy at birth remains low: forty-three years in 2002, compared to forty-seven years in 1990. It is yet to be seen how the PRSP will be beneficial to population health. Uganda's portfolio ratings were about as good as or better than the average ratings for Africa. Major challenges for the future are to reduce poverty disparities, promote rural development and service delivery, improve governance, and accelerate the development of infrastructure. In addition, a gender bias has been noted in Uganda's PRSP, in which most of the data are not sex disaggregated, rendering it difficult to monitor gender differences in poverty and health outcomes, and hence to develop gender-sensitive policies and strategies.

POVERTY–HEALTH LINKS IN PRSPS

There are high expectations that PRSPs will increase resources for health particularly for the poorest regions and most vulnerable groups. In 2002, the World Health Organization (WHO) developed a program of work to systematically monitor the place of health in PRSPs. The project analyzed the health component of the PRSP from a pro-poor perspective, and whether the overall PRSP document recognizes investments in health as important to poverty reduction. A desk review of a number of PRSPs was carried out using a standardized analytical framework, which was summarized in a report (WHO 2004; Dodd and Hinshelwood 2004).

According to the WHO review, all extant PRSPs at that time acknowledged the complexity of poverty stemming from its multidimensional nature. However, most of them lacked a comprehensive definition of poverty. In Sen's (1993) view, there are at least four dimensions of poverty: lack of opportunities (for employment and access to productive resources), lack of capabilities (access to public services, e.g., education and health), lack of security (vulnerability to economic risks and violence), and lack of empowerment (absence of voice, power, and participation) (Sen 1993). A comprehensive description of poverty needs to look beyond income and encompass these four dimensions. However, most of the poverty indicators used in the PRSPs focus on income poverty, using indicators such as the poverty line, consumption levels, and income distribution. There is no consensus on the definition and calculation of poverty, which varies across the range of PRSPs (Dodd and Hinshelwood 2004). There is often lack of clarity on the identification of poor groups as well as issues of vulnerability and social exclusion. The finance ministries seem to have had the dominant role and primary responsibility for the development of PRSPs in many countries, while health ministries, on the other hand, appear to have had a very limited role. Thus, it is not surprising that health issues are not well integrated in the macroeconomic targets or reflected within programs affecting other sectors such as trade, education, environment, or agriculture.

Although it is widely known and accepted that poor health and poverty are strongly linked, there is lack of clarity concerning the causal association between poverty and health in most PRSPs. Some PRSPs recognize poverty as a cause of poor health, while others view poor health as a cause of poverty. Economists have tended to emphasize the latter view and further argue that poor health dampens productivity, hampers economic growth and development, and limits international trade (Strauss 1998). Health does not enter as a basic human right in the design and implementation of the PRSPs, but rather as an engine for economic growth (Dodd and Hinshelwood 2004).

Many PRSPs include policies to benefit the poor such as plans to reallocate resources to poorer regions and to reduce the financial burden among the poor seeking health care. Individual PRSPs have sought to achieve this by improving the quality and availability of primary health care services to poor people in remote areas. At the same time, they rarely mention access to hospital care, thus failing to address the effects of impoverishment due to catastrophic illnesses. The private sector also plays a significant role in delivering health care services, but there is a lack of integration of private with government (public) sectors in making health care accessible to the poor and vulnerable groups.

PRSPS AND THE MILLENNIUM DEVELOPMENT GOALS

The Millennium Development Goals (MDGs) are long-term poverty reduction goals adopted by the United Nations as a result of the historic United Nations Millennium Assembly in September 2000 (Sachs 2005) (table 14.2). The eight goals and eighteen targets, to be achieved by 2015, focus on (1) the eradication of extreme poverty and hunger; (2) the achievement of universal primary education; (3) promoting gender equality and the empowerment of women; (4) reducing under-five child mortality; (5) improving maternal health; (6) combating HIV/AIDS, malaria, and other major diseases; (7) ensuring environmental sustainability; and (8) developing a global partnership for development (see also chapters 16 and 17, respectively, for further discussion of the roles of WHO and the G8 countries in meeting these goals).

It is noteworthy that three of the eight goals are directly concerned with public health improvements (reducing child mortality and maternal mortality and combating HIV/AIDS and malaria), while several others are strongly linked with health concerns (eradicating hunger and malnutrition, improving access to safe drinking water, and improving access to affordable essential drugs). In other words, the MDGs cannot be achieved without strong commitments to improving public health, and in turn, any poverty reduction strategy, if it is to succeed, needs to be specifically designed to meet the goals (Geithner and Nankani 2003).

Although there are no required set of indicators or goals that must be included in PRSPs, addressing the MDGs are essential for credible policies that can be financially supported. The earliest PRSPs were initiated prior to the establishment of the MDGs in September 2001; thus, it may be expected that they are less aligned with the MDGs than are the later ones. According to the review by Geithner and Nankani (2003), of the MDG targets (poverty head count, education, gender, health, environment, etc.), only poverty seems to have been fully addressed by most PRSPs. Health and education were monitored in about 70% of the PRSPs (Geithner and Nankani 2003). According to analyses carried out by Fetou et al. (2004), targets for reducing under-five child malnutrition have been more ambitious (relative to MDGs) in more recent PRSPs than in earlier ones. Other health-related targets, such as the proposed rate of reduction in maternal mortality rates, were less ambitious in the PRSPs than the in MDGs (Fetou et al. 2004).

Although most PRSPs recognize that health is a key ingredient for economic growth and include pro-poor strategies such as expanding primary health care, explicit linkages to health targets in PRSPs are patchy

TABLE 14.2. The United Nations MDGs

Goal	Targets
1. Eradicate extreme poverty and hunger	Halve, between 1990 and 2015, the proportion of people whose income is less than $1 a day
	Halve, between 1990 and 2015, the proportion of people who suffer from hunger
2. Achieve universal primary education	Ensure that by 2015 children everywhere, boys and girls alike, will be able to complete a full course of primary schooling
3. Promote gender equality and empower women	Eliminate gender disparity in primary and secondary education, preferably by 2005, and in all levels of education no later than 2015
4. Reduce child mortality	Reduce by two-thirds, between 1990 and 2015, the under-five mortality rate
5. Improve maternal health	Reduce by three-quarters, between 1990 and 2015, the maternal mortality rate
6. Combat HIV/AIDS, malaria, and other diseases	Have halved by 2015 and begun to reverse the spread of HIV/AIDS
	Have halved by 2015 and begun to reverse the incidence of malaria and other major diseases
7. Ensure environmental sustainability	Integrate the principles of sustainable development into country policies and programs and reverse the loss of environmental resources
	Halve by 2015 the proportion of people without sustainable access to safe drinking water and basic sanitation
	By 2020 to have achieved a significant improvement in lives of at least 100 million slum dwellers
8. Develop a global partnership for development	Develop further an open, rule-based, predictable, nondiscriminatory trading and financial system, including a commitment to good governance, development, and poverty reduction—both nationally and internationally
	Address the special needs of the least developed countries, including tariff- and quota-free access for least developed countries' exports, an enhanced program of debt relief for HIPC and cancellation of official bilateral debt, and more generous official development assistance for countries committed to poverty reduction
	Address the special needs of landlocked countries and small island developing states
	Deal comprehensively with the debt problems of developing countries through national and international measures in order to make debt sustainable in the long term
	In cooperation with developing countries, develop and implement strategies for decent and productive work for youth
	In cooperation with pharmaceutical companies, provide access to affordable, essential drugs in developing countries
	In cooperation with the private sector, make available the benefits of new technologies, especially information and communication

at best. For example, table 14.3 summarizes how specific indicators to meet MDG health targets were being monitored in eighteen early PRSPs completed prior to June 2002 (i.e., the countries listed in the left column of table 14.1). These data were based on information compiled by the World Bank (World Bank 2004).

Among health outcomes, most PRSPs target infant mortality ($n = 17$), maternal mortality (all), and access to improved sanitation ($n = 11$). However, most PRSPs did not include indicators that track how child and maternal mortality was being re-duced in each country. For example, only two out of eighteen PRSPs track immunization coverage, three out of eighteen track the proportion of pregnant women receiving prenatal care, and none of the PRSPs monitors prevalence of HIV/AIDS among younger pregnant women. In addition, only five of the eighteen PRSPs track access to health services (table 14.3). As Sachs (2005) has noted, often what PRSPs lack to date are practical linkages to meeting the MDGs, and all of the programs remain chronically underfunded (see also chapter 17 on this point).

TABLE 14.3. MDG Targets and Indicators (Related to Poverty and Health) That Countries Have Chosen to Monitor in Their PRSPs[a]

MDG	MDG Target	Indicator	No. of Countries
Extreme poverty and hunger	Poverty head count	Poverty line[b]	16
		<$1/day	2
		Poverty gap[c]	5
		Income distribution[d]	4
	Child malnutrition	<5 years old, underweight for age	5
		Children with low birth weight	3
	Malnutrition	Protein-energy malnutrition	1
		Vitamin A or/and iodine deficiency	3
		Food basket for vulnerable groups	0
Universal primary education	Enrollment	Net primary enrollment ratio	8
	Attendance	Rate of primary school attendance (%)	2
	Repeaters	No. of repeaters in primary school	8
	Dropouts	No. of dropouts in primary school	8
Literacy	Youth literacy rate (15–24 years)		0
	Adult literacy rate		7
Child mortality	Under-five mortality		11
	Infant mortality		17
	Immunization	% 1-year-old children immunized against measles	2
		Immunization rate for BCG (<1 year old)	2
		Immunization rate for DPT (<1 year old)	2
		Immunization coverage for children up to 2 years old	1 (Albania)
		% Immunized children under 6 years old	1 (Honduras)
Maternal health	% Maternal mortality		18 (all)
	Maternal care	Proportion of births attended by skilled health personnel	8
		% Pregnant women with adequate prenatal check-ups	3
		Contraceptive prevalence rate	2

(continued)

243

TABLE 14.3. (continued)

MDG	MDG Target	Indicator	No. of Countries
		Total fertility	5
HIV/AIDS, malaria	HIV/AIDS	Rate of anemia among pregnant women	1 (Zambia)
		HIV prevalence among pregnant women 15–24 years old	0
		Proportion of orphans to nonorphan 10–14 years old that are attending school	0
		HIV/AIDS prevalence rate	4
		% HIV/AIDS-infected people 15–19 years old	1 (Zambia)
		% HIV/AIDS-infected people 15–49 years old	1 (Zambia)
		Women infected with HIV	1 (Gambia)
		Rate of HIV prevalence among pregnant women	1 (Tanzania)
		Proportion of children infected by HIV/AIDS	1 (Vietnam)
Malaria		Prevalence and death rates related to malaria	0
		Malaria related mortality rate for children < 5 years old	2
		Households with mosquito nets (%)	1 (Mozambique)
Other		Prevalence and death rates related to tuberculosis	0
		% Children sickened by cholera, typhoid, hemorrhagic fever, plague, etc.	1 (Vietnam)
Environmental sustainability	Water	Proportion of population with sustainable access to improved sanitation (in both urban and rural areas)	11
		Rate of water pollution	2
		Rehabilitation or construction of new boreholes	1 (Malawi)
	Sanitation	Proportion of people with sustainable access to improved sanitation	12
Global partnership	Affordable drugs	Proportion of population with access to affordable, essential drugs on a sustainable basis	0
		Availability of essential, high-quality medicines at affordable prices	2
	Access to and use of health services	Population with access to health services (%)	5
		Households within 5 km of a health facility (%)	3

	Health facility utilization rate	2
	Consumer satisfaction index of health facilities	1 (Niger)
Noninfectious diseases	Incidence of diarrheal cases per 100,000	1 (Albania)
Population	Population growth rate	2
	Life expectancy at birth	5
	Crude death rate per 1 million people	1 (Guinea)
	Morbidity rate	1 (Yemen)

[a]Based on eighteen countries that completed PRSPs prior to June 2002 (Albania, Burkina Faso, Bolivia, Gambia, Guinea, Guyana, Honduras, Malawi, Mauritania, Mozambique, Nicaragua, Niger, Rwanda, Tanzania, Uganda, Vietnam, Yemen, Zambia). [b]Includes poverty line (national and international). [c]Includes both depth and severity of poverty. [d]Includes percent share of poorest quintile in national consumption and GINI coefficient.

Source: World Bank, Data and Statistics, http://www.worldbank.org/data/prsp/mdg.prsp.html.

GENDER IN THE PRSPS

Gender is a cross-cutting theme in all of the MDGs (see chapter 10 for further discussion). Given that women are overrepresented among the world's poor, PRSPs (whose primary objective is the alleviation of poverty) represent an important mechanism for improving the lives of women and for enhancing gender equity. However, since PRSPs were introduced in 1999, poor women in developing countries frequently have been ignored in the process. The poverty analyses in PRSPs have been criticized for their failure to reflect gendered aspects of poverty and the different ways in which men and women experience poverty (see Kabeer 2003; Whitehead 2003).

Gender cannot be isolated from major socioeconomic determinants of health, since gender interacts with all other social processes (Wamala and Lynch 2002). In fact, failure to plan for gender-sensitive poverty reduction strategies may well widen gender inequalities (Çağatay 2001). Bamberger et al. (2001) suggest three steps for integrating gender into country-specific poverty analyses: (a) addressing gender across the four dimensions of poverty (opportunities, capabilities, security, empowerment), (b) documenting the experiences of poverty in each of these dimensions, and (c) integrating the findings into the country's poverty diagnosis.

Civil society has often been critical of the neoliberal ideology that underpinned earlier SAPs and is now seemingly repeated in poverty reduction strategies. While PRSPs may represent an improvement over SAPs in terms of poverty diagnostics and the allocation of spending to pro-poor sectors, the core economic policies do not appear to have significantly departed from the Washington Consensus.[4] These policies (including privatization, market liberalization, and fiscal austerity) are often viewed as being detrimental to the lives of the poor, especially poor women (see also chapter 10). In many instances, the participatory processes in developing PRSPs have not included women activists or women's organizations, leading to the charge that resulting product is often gender-blind.

When it comes to monitoring the progress of PRSPs in improving the lives of poor women (or meeting the gender-specific MDGs), the lack of sex-disaggregated data is problematic. The situation is worsened by lack of understanding of gender issues by those in key positions of drafting the PRSPs, as well as lack of analytical capacity and expertise among women's groups in the civil society (Whitehead 2003).

Looking again at the eighteen early PRSPs that had reached either their decision point or completion point by 2004, we analyzed how gender targets had been set in each of them (table 14.4). Half of the PRSPs had set targets for primary school enrollment for girls in relation to boys. However, other targets related to gender equality, such as indices of gender development and empowerment, social and economic rights for women, income levels among poor women, and political participation and influence, were mentioned in only one or two countries.

In Rwanda's PRSP, for example, gender bias in education, health, law, and political participation were addressed, but the policy actions targeted only the gender gap in primary school education (Geithner and Nankani 2003). In most PRSPs where women's health was targeted, improving maternal health was listed as a priority, but they did not describe how this would be achieved.

The pattern demonstrated in table 14.4 is consistent with Whitehead's (2003) analyses that demonstrated that gender issues appeared in a fragmented and arbitrary way in the body of the PRSPs dealing with policy priorities and budget commitments. Some women's needs issues have been raised, especially in the sections on health and education, but gender has yet to be mainstreamed. Also, despite being recommended by the World Bank's PRSP Source Book (World Bank 2000), a separate chapter on gender was missing in half of the PRSPs reviewed.

CONCLUSION: AN ASSESSMENT OF PRSPS

Do PRSPs represent SAPs under another name? Are PRSPs merely window dressing for "business as usual" on the part of the international financial institutions? According to one view, PRSPs most of the time seem to be driven by recipient countries' expectations of what will be deemed acceptable and "sound policies" by the IMF and World Bank. Notwithstanding the core principle of "country ownership," there is an obvious tension between a country's poverty reduction goals, which may not be compatible with the conditionalities insisted upon by the Bretton Woods institutions. Loan negotiations still continue to be carried out behind closed doors within ministries of finance and central banks (Bretton Woods Project 2003).

According to another view, the PRSP process, especially as a means of achieving the MDGs, is currently

TABLE 14.4. Monitoring of Gender Inequality in Eighteen Early PRSPs[a]

Goal	Domain	Indicator	No. of Countries
Gender equality[b]	Education	Ratio of girls to boys in education[c]	9
		Literacy of under 40-year old women	1
	Employment (Share of women in nonagricultural sector)	Microenterprises and small businesses headed by women	2
		Women receiving technical training	0
		Proportion of all managerial/administrative positions held by women	2
		% Women among all members of professional organizations	1 (Zambia)
	Voices	No. women in elective bodies at provincial, district, and commune levels	1 (Vietnam)
		Participation of women in agencies and sectors at all levels (%)	1 (Vietnam)
		Proportion of women of all trade unions members	1 (Zambia)
Other non-MDG gender-related goals	Health	Women with access to basic health insurance (%)	1 (Bolivia)
	Gender inequality measures	Gender-Related Index (GDI)	3
		Gender Empowerment Measure (GEM)	2
		Work burden on women	1 (Niger)
		Gender-related violence (domestic)	1 (Niger)
		Level of gender disaggregation and analysis in reports, publications	3
	Social and economic rights	Women with identity card (%)	1 (Bolivia)
		Names of both husband and wife appearing on land-use right certificates (%)	1 (Vietnam)
		Proportion of land ownership transfers made to women (%)	1 (Zambia)
		Proportion women among all people accessing credit (%)	1 (Zambia)
	Income	Income levels of poor women	1 (Honduras)

[a]Based on eighteen countries with early PRSPs (see table 14-3 note). [b]Related to MDGs. [c]Education includes primary, secondary, and tertiary levels.

Source: World Bank, Data and Statistics, http://www.worldbank.org/data/prsp/mdg.prsp.html.

backward. As described by Jeffrey Sachs (2005), the IMF and World Bank begin by canvassing the international donor community to forecast the amount of aid that will be available in each year. They then instruct the recipient country to draw up "realistic" poverty reduction plans within the forecast budget. Thus:

> When it comes to real practice, where the rubber hits the road, in the poverty reduction plans, the Millennium Development Goals are expressed only as vague aspirations rather than operational targets. Countries are told to go about their business without any hope of meeting the MDGs. The

IMF and World Bank reveal split personalities, championing the MDGs in public speeches, approving programs that will not achieve them, and privately acknowledging, with business as usual, that they cannot be met! (Sachs 2005, p. 271)

The alternative approach would turn this process on its head, that is, raise donor funding *on the basis* of a country's requirements as set forth in its poverty reduction plans.

On the positive side, most observers agree with the assessment that the PRSP initiative has brought about a sharper focus on poverty reduction, as well as new opportunities for participation and inclusiveness. Here also there is room for improvement. Thus, broad-based participation in PRSPs so far seems to have been interpreted by most governments as seeking information or consultation on the extent and causes of poverty (i.e., the diagnostic step, illustrated in the first box in figure 14.1). So far there has been little encouragement for civil society to become engaged in detailed policy dialogue, including the content of macroeconomic policies. A priority is therefore to foster participation based upon standards such as inclusiveness (representing the poor, women's views, and other marginalized groups), and capacity to generate a higher quality of debate on technical issues as macroeconomic policies (CIDSE-Caritas Internationalis 2004).

The PRSP initiative is still new (entering its fifth year as of the time of writing), and international norms for design, implementation, and monitoring are still evolving. Key recommendations for the future point to the need for civil society groups and governments to invest strategically in developing analytical capacity. Many PRSPs have included detailed discussions in the areas of education, labor markets, and enterprise development. However, in many instances there have been limited discussions in topics such as land rights, rural development, environment and resource management, safety nets, and food security. Little discussion has been undertaken concerning structural adjustment measures, urban development, transport, or energy (Bamberger et al. 2001; Zuckerman and Garret 2003; Sanchez and Cash 2003). Civil society groups have an opportunity, within the PRSP framework, for holding their governments accountable through budget analysis, monitoring, and advocacy.

For governments, a priority is to institutionalize permanent and formal frameworks for the participatory process, one that fulfills more than a token information-gathering function. Toward that end, government budgets must become more transparent and accessible to civil society groups (CIDSE-Caritas Internationalis 2004). As the World Bank and IMF recently noted in a progress report, "the PRSP approach is still a work in progress" (World Bank/IMF 2004). It is still too early to tell if the PRSP approach will succeed in its stated aims. Simultaneously, they are seemingly at risk of being set up for failure unless there is radical change in the institutional behavior of the World Bank and IMF, that is, unless they start to act as if poverty reduction plans were truly owned and driven by the recipient countries.

Notes

1. The Bretton Woods Project was established by non-governmental organizations in 1995 with the aim to monitor the activities and initiatives of the World Bank and International Monetary Fund. It analyzes initiatives of the international financial institutions and disseminates information for advocacy.

2. New name is the Ministry of Finance and National Planning.

3. Disbursements have never matched budgetary allocations for the PRSP.

4. The Washington Consensus refers to the set of development policies advocated throughout the 1980s by an apparent consensus of the international financial institutions (the World Bank and IMF) and the U.S. Treasury Department. These policies included elements such as privatization of state enterprises, fiscal restraint, and trade liberalization.

References

Bamberger, M., Blackden, M., Fort, L., Manoukian, V. (2001). Gender. In: Review of PRSPs. Washington, DC: World Bank/IMF.

Booth, D. (2001). PRSP processes in 8 African countries. Paper presented to the WIDER Development Conference on Debt Relief, Helsinki, August 17–18, 2001. Accessed at: http://www.wider.unu.edu/conference/conference-2001-2/parallel%20papers/1_2_booth.pdf

Bretton Woods Project. (2003). Poverty reduction strategy papers (PRSPs): a rough guide. Accessed at: http://www.campaignforeducation.org/resources/Apr2002/prsp_roughguide.pdf

Çaðatay, N. (2001). Trade, gender and poverty. New York: United Nations Development Programme.

CIDSE (Cooperation Inernationale pour le Développement et la Solidarité)–Caritas Internationalis. (2004). PRSP: are the World Bank and IMF delivering on Promises? Background paper. Accessed at: http://www.globalpolicy.org/socecon/bwi-wto/wbank/2004/0428prsp.pdf

Dodd, R. and Hinshelwood, E. (2004). Poverty reduction strategy papers—their significance for health. Geneva: World Health Organization.

Dollar, D, Kraay, A. (2002). Growth is good for the poor. J Econ Growth 7(3):195–225.

Fetou, M, Harrison, M, Heyman, A, Hiraga, M, Swanson, E, Wang, V, Watanabe, N. (2004). Targets and indicators for MDGs and PRSPs: what countries have chosen to monitor. Washington, DC: World Bank.

Fischer, S. (2003). Globalization and its challenges. Richard T. Ely lecture. Am Econ Rev 93(2):1–30.

Geithner, TF, Nankani, G. (2003). Poverty reduction strategy papers—detailed analysis of progress in implementation. Washington, DC: International Monetary Fund and World Bank.

Kabeer, N. (2003). Gender mainstreaming in poverty eradication and the millennium development goals. A
handbook for policy-makers and other stakeholders.
Gatineau, Quebec: Commonwealth Secretariat/In-
ternational Development Research Center/Canadian
International Development Agency.

Mpepo, B. P. (2002). A poverty reduction strategy paper
(PSRP) for Zambia: a civil society perspective.
Paper presented at the Annual Poverty Review
Conference, Ministry of Finance and National
Planning, in conjunction with the Zambia Social
Investment Fund (ZAMSIF). Mulungushi Interna-
tional Conference Centre, Zambia.

Sachs, JD. (2005). The end of poverty: economic possibilities of our time. New York: Penguin Press.

Sanchez, D, Cash, K. (2003). PRSP. Partner perspectives
and positions. Diakonia: Church of Sweden, Save
the Children Sweden.

Sen, A. (1993). Capability and well-being. In: Nussbaum, M, Sen, A. (eds.). The quality of life. Oxford. Clarendon Press.

Strauss, T. (1998). Health, nutrition and economic development. J Econ Lit 36:776–817.

Wamala, SP, Lynch, J. (2002). Gender and social inequities in health—a public health issue. Lund:
Studentlitteratur.

Whitehead, A. (2003). Failing women, sustaining
poverty: gender in poverty reduction strategy papers. London: UK Gender and Development Network.

World Bank. (2000). Poverty reduction strategy papers.
Source Book. Washington, DC: World Bank.

World Bank. (2003). Overview of poverty reduction
strategies. Accessed at: http://www.worldbank.org/
poverty/strategies/overview.htm

World Bank. (2004). Development data and statistics.
Accessed at: http://www.worldbank.orgdata/prsp/
mdg-prsp.html

World Bank and International Monetary Fund. (2004).
Poverty reduction strategy papers—progress in implementation. Accessed at: http://siteresources.
worldbank.org/INTPRS1/Resources/prsp_progress_
2004.pdf

WHO. (2004). Poverty reduction strategy papers: their
significance for health: second synthesis report
(WHO/HDP/PRSP/04.1). Geneva: World Health
Organization

Zuckerman, E, Garret, A. (2003). Do poverty reduction
strategy papers address gender? A gender audit for
2002 PRSPs. A gender action publication. Accessed
at: http://www.sarpn.org.za/documents/d0000306/
index.php

Chapter 15

Health Policy and the World Trade Organization

M. Gregg Bloche and Elizabeth R. Jungman

Critics of international trade agreements often cast them as threats to human health, and they can point to some sobering warnings from world history. Infectious diseases have swept across political boundaries, carried by traders, colonists, and other agents of globalization. Transnational epidemics have laid economies low, undermining political stability. The spread of viruses and bacteria to peoples previously unexposed and therefore lacking immunity has decimated populations and changed the political course of continents. Trade, exploration, and warfare have repeatedly produced encounters between peoples at different levels of agricultural and technological development. Often, the results have been devastating for the disadvantaged group—economic marginalization, loss of sovereignty and culture, and collapse of public health. Yet the rise of civilization—plant and animal domestication, division of labor, technology, and resulting prosperity—was powered in large part by movement of products and knowledge along routes of trade and migration.[1] Peoples with poor access to these pathways, for geographic or other reasons, achieved neither the prosperity nor the health benefits associated with trade, migration, and ensuing development.

The World Trade Organization (WTO) will make the benefits of movement of goods, services, and knowledge available to an unprecedented degree. But concerns about the health impact of international trade, particularly in the poorest nations, have fed doubts about the value of globalization, especially for the world's worst off. Anxieties over food safety, environmental toxins, and access to life-saving medicines have fueled skepticism in many countries about the WTO and its associated agreements. This skepticism is compounded by perceptions that the WTO stands in opposition to national leaders' efforts to protect their citizens' lives and health. Rulings against national food safety regulations, mad cow disease and other transnational health scares, and, most visibly, the controversy over intellectual property protection for AIDS drugs have cast the WTO as a threat to health in the eyes of many. Within the WTO's dispute management scheme, these concerns have produced bitter conflicts.

On the political stump, in the press, and on the streets outside WTO meetings, the WTO's critics cast it in even harsher terms, as the enemy of the poor in general and people's health in particular. These critics' central claim has become familiar: the system the WTO superintends puts multinational corporations and rich countries' interests ahead of the lives and well-being of the world's poor. Goods, services, and money cross borders without regard for those without buying power, the story goes, and the WTO ensures the advantages enjoyed by the wealthy at others' expense. The consequences for people's health are catastrophic, the critics hold; they include lack of minimally adequate food and shelter, exposure to toxic substances and seductive tobacco advertising, and millions of avoidable deaths each year from AIDS and other infectious diseases.

Some of the leading advocacy groups working on behalf of the world's poor take a similarly dim view of the relationship between WTO governance and human health and well-being. Trade treaty language and the WTO's dispute settlement system, they hold, neglect health and human welfare.[2] The premise that WTO-related protections for intellectual property and limits on national regulatory authority leave little room for health is widespread among scholars who focus on public health and human development policy.[3] Some commentators on trade law have lent support to this premise by characterizing the WTO treaties as a self-contained legal scheme, to be construed without regard for international law bearing on human rights, the environment, and other matters.[4] The WTO agreements themselves make no reference to a role for non-WTO substantive law in the interpretation of trade treaty provisions.[5]

We contend in this chapter that portrayal of the WTO and its associated agreements as implacable threats to the health of people constitutes pessimism bordering on panic. Not only does this portrayal overlook potential synergies between trade and health; it all but ignores recent developments within the WTO that have affirmed member states' power to promote health. The WTO framers paid little heed to health policy. Over the past several years, however, politics and the AIDS pandemic have pushed health to center stage as a trade issue. The WTO has responded with heightened deference to national authority

when member states' health polices conflict with other values protected by trade agreements.

On their face, the principal WTO agreements bearing on health are frustratingly vague in their approach to the task of balancing protection for health against other trade-related concerns. Provisions in the General Agreement on Tariffs and Trade (GATT '94), the Agreement on Sanitary and Phytosanitary Measures (SPS), and the General Agreement on Trade in Services (GATS) allow, in general terms, for trade restrictions to reduce risks to health. But these treaties do not speak to such matters as the magnitude of risk needed to justify trade restrictions, standards of proof for assessments of risk, and methodology for weighing health dangers against the consequences of limits on trade. Likewise, the Agreement on Trade-Related Aspects of Intellectual Property Rights (TRIPS) contains language that can be read to allow poor countries to elide patents on lifesaving medicines. But TRIPS says little about the prerequisites or procedures for invoking its ambiguous exceptions to patent protection.

Despite this absence of clear direction, the WTO system, we contend below, has come to treat protection for health as a de facto interpretive principle when disputes arise over the meaning of trade agreements. To be sure, such a principle is nowhere stated in WTO associated treaties, declarations, or jurisprudence; nor is health even mentioned as a purpose in the preambles to the major WTO agreements.[6] Yet the special weight accorded to health in WTO decision making is evident across a broad range of trade issues.

The proposition that protection for health is an interpretive principle within the WTO system squares with broad recognition of a "right to health" outside the WTO framework. The notion of health as a human right has been affirmed in many international instruments, including the Universal Declaration of Human Rights[7] and the International Covenant on Economic, Social, and Cultural Rights.[8] Some have urged on this basis that a right to health be recognized as customary international law.[9]

The amorphous nature of this right—its ambiguity, its elasticity,[10] and the difficulty of translating it into enforceable legal standards[11]—has frustrated efforts to give it meaning in international or domestic law. But more modest efforts to make this and other similarly amorphous social and economic rights legally relevant show potential. The treatment of social and economic rights as "directive principles," nonjusticiable in themselves but important as guides to judicial construction of rights conferred by national constitutions,[12] is a promising model for the WTO system—and for the law of the global economy more generally. We conclude this chapter by contending that WTO law recognizes a right to health, in this modest form, in all but name. Those concerned with public health on a global scale should push the WTO's member states and governance organs to make this recognition explicit.

HEALTH, DEVELOPMENT, AND LIBERAL TRADE

Critics who cast the WTO as the foe of public health all but ignore the empirical evidence of a win–win relationship between health and economic development. It is well established that economic and social factors are more important contributors to the health status of populations than is medical care.[13] It is equally well established that, within nations, socioeconomic status (including income and education levels) correlates closely with measures of health status.[14] There is lively debate over whether economic inequality in itself, apart from people's wealth or poverty within a society, contributes to citizens' health status. Some read the data to support a correlation between the steepness of wealth gradients within societies and the health status of these societies,[15] while others admit only a correlation between people's health status and their levels of personal wealth.[16] There is near-consensus, though, that health is closely linked to personal wealth and therefore to levels of economic development. This connection, it is generally agreed, goes both ways: economic well-being fosters physical and mental health, and populationwide good health promotes development and wealth.[17]

The ways by which personal wealth promotes health are poorly understood. Hypotheses, not mutually exclusive, include superior nutrition, living arrangements that insulate people from environmental and psychological stresses, greater social connectedness, lower childbearing rates, and the propensity of people less preoccupied by immediate needs to take a longer view of life and to maintain healthier lifestyles. The role of economic development in this equation is even less well understood, beyond the obvious link between a society's level of development and per capita income and wealth. Societies with similar per capita gross

domestic product (GDP) vary widely in their performance on such common health indicators as life expectancy and infant mortality, though per capita income and health status correlate in a general way.[18] Hypothesized causal links between economic development and people's health include public spending on education, health, and other social programs;[19] sufficient earning power to avoid deprivation of food, nutrition, and shelter;[20] female literacy and the social status of women;[21] respect for political and civil rights; and social connectedness. All of these factors correlate in general with per capita income. But international comparisons have found that poor people's income and public spending on health explain much of the correlation between per capita GDP and life expectancy, to the point that when these variables are assessed separately, per capita GDP adds little or no explanatory power.[22]

Other evidence suggests that education spending, female literacy, political freedom, and social connectedness have independent explanatory power. Amartya Sen has observed that among countries with rapid economic growth—for example, the industrializing states of the Pacific Rim, Asia, and Latin America— better performance on health status indicators correlates with higher spending on education, health, and other social services.[23] Thus, for example, South Korea and Taiwan have for years spent more on basic education and health promotion than has Brazil, and they outperform Brazil on measures of health status. Among low-growth countries, a similar correlation obtains. Sen points to Costa Rica, Sri Lanka, and the Indian state of Kerala as examples of poor, low-growth societies that have made large investments (compared to other less-developed nations) in education and health programs and have much higher life expectancies than do their economic peers.[24]

Female literacy, in particular, correlates closely with reduced fertility and lower mortality rates for children younger than five years of age, even after researchers control for educational spending and income levels.[25] Sen ascribes this connection, which he treats as causal, to literacy's enhancement of women's command over their own lives.[26] He tells a similar story, albeit with less empirical support, about the import of political and civil rights. They empower people to come together to formulate their needs and to seek popular and government support for efforts to meet these needs.[27] Enhanced personal agency and greater public investment in social programs that foster populationwide health are the unsurprising results. Thus, all else equal, states that respect political and civil rights tend to perform better on measures of population health than those that do not. The most dramatic illustration of this is the virtual absence of famine in democracies, however poor.[28]

The common thread running through these putative economic, social, and political determinants of health is personal and community empowerment and capability. More research on the causal links between trade, economic development, personal wealth, people's capabilities, and population health is much needed. But the best available data support the following, admittedly oversimplified storyline: liberal trade (with judicious protection for intellectual property) can promote development, which can reduce poverty and bring about a broad-based increase in personal wealth. Amelioration of poverty and increases in personal wealth, in turn, empower people in both the private and public spheres, fostering personal choices and public policies that promote populationwide health and well-being.

This storyline is at odds with WTO naysayers' claims of irreconcilable conflict between liberalized trade and the health and welfare of the worst off. But there are important caveats. Trade that advantages only an elite few without contributing to a society's wider economic development, including reduction of poverty and raising of incomes, is unlikely to promote public health and well-being.[29] Trade agreements that limit national governments' ability to issue regulations reasonably calculated to promote public health do pose a threat to human well-being. Intellectual property protection that yields windfalls to firms for endeavors they would have engaged in anyway transfers wealth (often from the poor and working class to the rich) without fostering innovation. To the extent that this transfer reduces poor and working class people's purchasing power, it undermines capabilities that bear upon health. And to the extent that patent-protected prices put medical treatments out of people's reach, patent law subverts health visibly and poignantly. It would thus be Pollyanna-ish to expect WTO policies and jurisprudence to align perfectly with the goal of promoting health. On the other hand, as we argue presently, the WTO system has moved much further than many imagine toward recognition of health as a privileged value in the construction of trade law.

AN INTRODUCTION TO THE WTO

The WTO is composed of approximately 150 member states. It superintends the operation of a system of trade agreements governing the exchange of goods and services, the limits of national regulatory authority, protection for intellectual property, and other matters. Although leading industrial nations have a great deal of influence on WTO policies, the WTO governance scheme affords smaller and poorer countries considerable influence, including veto power over many matters. The veto threat and representation of smaller and poorer states on the bodies that oversee WTO trade agreements ensure at least a hearing for these states' concerns, especially when they band together.[30]

The WTO's Ministerial Council, comprised of cabinet-level representatives from every member state, oversees development of trade policy pursuant to all the WTO trade agreements but meets infrequently—typically every two years. WTO state parties provide ongoing supervision through the General Council, composed mostly of ambassadorial rank representatives, and specialized councils for each trade agreement. Three such councils oversee WTO agreements that bear on health policy—the Council for Trade in Goods (Goods Council), the TRIPS Council, and the Council for Trade in Services (Services Council). The Goods Council superintends the GATT and the Agreement on the Application of Sanitary and Phytosanitary Measures (SPS), which limit member states' authority to impose regulations that restrict trade in agricultural or industrial products on public health grounds. The TRIPS Council oversees TRIPS, which sets minimum safeguards for intellectual property (including patent-protected pharmaceuticals). The Services Council will superintend the GATS, which, when fully implemented, will limit national barriers to provision of services (including health care) by foreign firms and individuals.

The WTO system also includes a mechanism for resolving disputes between member states.[31] This mechanism begins with a "consultation" period for negotiation, but it includes a binding adjudication process, something rare in international law. This process incorporates both trial-type proceedings, conducted by panels of trade experts convened on a case-by-case basis, and the right to appeal panel findings to a permanent "appellate body" with review authority akin to that of a court of last resort in the

United States. The results of this process bind all parties to a dispute unless WTO member states (including the prevailing party) vote unanimously to overrule—a highly unlikely scenario.

HEALTH AND THE LAW
OF THE GATT

The GATT, which preceded the WTO's creation by almost a half century, has been the governing framework for international trade in agricultural and industrial products since 1947.[32] Article XX(b) of the GATT allows member states to take actions that restrict trade and that are otherwise proscribed by the GATT if they are "necessary to protect human . . . life or health."[33] Read in conjunction with the WTO standard for reviewing such actions—the requirement that dispute settlement panels "make an objective assessment" of relevant facts and law[34]—this provision appears to permit close scrutiny, by panels and the appellate body, of claims of health necessity made to support trade restrictions.

Outside the health context, the appellate body has invoked the "objective assessment" standard to support robust scrutiny of member states' trade remedies and restraints. Purported justifications for other trade-restricting measures, including antidumping laws,[35] countervailing duties,[36] and so-called "safeguards" for vulnerable industries,[37] are painstakingly parsed, weighed, and found wanting in appellate body opinions. Although the WTO agreement governing antidumping measures appears to give members broad discretion to ascertain dumping by exporters and to impose restrictive measures,[38] the appellate body has read much of this discretion out of the agreement.[39] And in a series of countervailing duty and safeguards cases, the "objective assessment" standard has been invoked to justify close review of national authorities' assessments of export subsidies and threats to domestic industries.[40] The WTO Agreement on Safeguards, for example, instructs a country contemplating action to protect a domestic industry to conduct a quantitative assessment of the threat posed to the industry by imports,[41] but the agreement says nothing about the standard for scrutiny of this assessment in the event of a trade dispute. The appellate body has filled in this gap, by advising panels to "critically examine" this assessment "in depth" and to reject it if an alternative assessment is merely "plausible."[42]

In sharp contrast, the appellate body has been highly deferential to member states' trade restrictions in the GATT Art. XX(b) context. Although it has construed the "objective assessment" standard to require that restrictions purportedly "necessary to protect human . . . life or health" be based on some scientific evidence of health risk,[43] it has held that such restrictions need not rest on "majority scientific opinion."[44] In its 2001 decision upholding a French import ban on asbestos-containing products, the appellate body stated that "a member may rely, in good faith, on scientific sources which . . . may represent a divergent, but qualified and respected, opinion."[45] Some have seen this deference to member states' discretion in the face of scientific uncertainty as a step toward WTO adoption of international environmental law's "precautionary principle."[46] Alternatively, this deference follows from treatment of protection for health as an interpretive principle, calling for less onerous standards of proof and review for trade restraints when health is at stake.

Indeed, the appellate body has gone further in the Article XX(b) context than the precautionary principle requires. In its 2001 *Asbestos* opinion, it announced that "WTO members have a right to determine the level of protection of health that they consider appropriate in a given situation."[47] France's decision to reduce the risk of new, asbestos-related health risks to zero by barring the manufacture, domestic sale, and import of asbestos-containing products was within this right, the tribunal held. National discretion to adopt zero risk policies is a matter beyond the reach of the precautionary principle, which addresses the separate question of how states (and transnational authorities) should treat scientific uncertainty about estimates of risk.

Assume, for example, that a regulatory agency has set a goal of one or fewer cases of cancer caused by "toxin T" per 100,000 exposed people. Assume, in addition, that state-of-the-art scientific understanding of the relationship between exposure level and incidence of cancer caused by toxin T is imprecise in the following sense: there is a two-orders-of-magnitude (10^2) range of uncertainty (based on conventional statistical methods) concerning the exposure level needed to induce cancer in one out of 100,000 people. The precautionary principle holds that the agency should designate the lowest exposure level in this range as the highest permissible exposure. The key point here is that the precautionary principle speaks to the setting of exposure limits once health policy goals (e.g., disease incidence targets) have been specified. The precautionary principle cannot, by itself, define these goals. Allowing national regulators to set a zero-risk goal and to bar imports accordingly constitutes exceptional deference to member states' health policies.

This deference is underscored by the appellate body's approach to the possibility of less restrictive alternate regulatory measures under Article XX(b)'s necessity test. In a pre-WTO decision criticized by public health activists, a GATT dispute settlement panel construed the necessity test to bar Thailand's discriminatory taxes on imported cigarettes, defended by that country on health grounds.[48] Thai authorities argued (with support from the World Health Organization) that enabling foreign tobacco firms to compete with domestic producers would boost the incidence of smoking—and thereby increase tobacco related morbidity and mortality—because foreign firms' marketing programs would overwhelm public health authorities' antismoking message. But the GATT panel concluded that the Article XX(b) necessity standard requires a finding that there is "no alternative measure consistent with [GATT], or less inconsistent with it," which the importing country could "reasonably be expected to employ to achieve its health policy objectives."[49] The panel declined to make this finding, concluding instead that nondiscriminatory taxes on both domestic and foreign cigarette producers could achieve Thailand's stated health goals in more GATT-friendly fashion.[50]

Whatever the merits of this controversial, pre-WTO ruling,[51] the appellate body signaled in its *Asbestos* opinion that member states now have wide latitude to specify health policies that rule out less restrictive alternatives. In response to the exporting country's claim that France could stop the spread of asbestos-related risks through a less restrictive policy of "controlled use" of asbestos-containing construction materials, rather than resorting to an outright ban, the appellate body said France's "chosen level of health protection"—no asbestos-related risk—precluded any alternative to an outright ban.[52] The countervailing health risks posed by substitute, nonasbestos building materials were of no moment, from this perspective, since France had specified its health policy more narrowly, as the elimination of asbestos-related risks.

From a rational risk regulation perspective, such deference to members' health policies is questionable, since it can lead to approval of regulations that

both restrict trade and (by disregarding the health dangers posed by substitute products) increase populationwide health risk. But if one assumes that national regulators are institutionally more competent than WTO panels (and the appellate body) to identify and weigh competing health risks and economic possibilities,[53] then deference to national health policy is the preferred means for promoting health. The *Asbestos* opinion's discussion of the Article XX(b) necessity test is striking for its emphasis on the high weight to be given to health in comparison with other goals. The more "vital or important" the ends at issue, "the easier it [is] to accept as 'necessary' measures designed to achieve those ends." And health, the opinion holds, is "both vital and important in the highest degree."[54]

HEALTH RISKS FROM FOOD: SPS

In 1998, the appellate body ruled that the European Community's (EC) import ban on beef from hormone-fed cattle violated the WTO agreement governing member states' food and agricultural safety regulations.[55] Supporters and critics of this decision agree on its landmark importance as a statement of WTO law governing regulation of food safety. Activists opposed to giving cows growth-promoting hormones condemned the ruling, as did many who worry about the ebb of national authority over food safety more generally. Street protests targeted the WTO's approach to food-borne health risks. A leading trade law scholar warned that the appellate body's treatment of food safety could gain the WTO "a reputation as a naysayer to health and biosafety regulation."[56] Yet the appellate body's reasoning in the *Hormones* case treats health as no less "vital and important" in the food safety context than in the GATT Article XX(b) setting. The outcome of the case was disappointing from a vantage point that sees subjective perceptions of health risk as sufficient justification for regulation that restricts trade. However, as we argue presently, the opinion displays the same deference to national health policy that is evident in the *Asbestos* ruling.

The EC lost the *Hormones* case on narrow grounds. Applying language in the relevant WTO treaty, SPS,[57] requiring regulators to act "based on" a risk assessment,[58] the appellate body found that the EC failed to conduct a risk assessment to evaluate its claim that poor control over hormone doses given to animals gives rise to health hazards for humans.[59] Had the EC done such a risk assessment and found dangers of this kind, it could have counted the risk of poor control over hormone administration, the appellate body said.[60] This risk, by itself, could have justified the EC's import ban.

Other language in the *Hormones* opinion strongly supports member states' discretion to regulate food and agriculture related health risks. Consistent with its tolerance for members' zero-risk policies in the GATT Article XX(b) context,[61] the appellate body rejected the proposition that the SPS risk assessment provision requires a showing of a threshold level of risk to justify trade-restricting regulation.[62] The appellate body also held that risk assessment can count concerns not reducible to "quantitative analysis" by "laboratory methods."[63] This allows national regulators to weigh subjective factors that influence both the perception and reality of risk. Beyond this, the appellate body read the precautionary principle into the SPS provision authorizing countries to regulate "where relevant scientific evidence is insufficient. . . ."[64] In addition, the opinion states that regulators need not show they in fact took into account the risk assessment data and conclusions presented to a WTO panel.[65] This enables member states to present state-of-the-art scientific data when defending their regulations in dispute resolution proceedings, and it eases the administrative (and financial) burden on governments concerned about crafting regulations to survive WTO scrutiny.

Moreover, the opinion treated the SPS mandate that regulation be "based on" a risk assessment as requiring only a "rational relationship" between the regulatory measure and the risk assessment.[66] As in the GATT Article XX(b) setting, the appellate body allowed for the possibility of "divergent" scientific opinion from "qualified and respected sources."[67] Such opinion, the appellate body said, could suffice to establish the requisite "rational relationship" between a risk assessment and a regulation. The appellate body put teeth in its rational relationship test by holding that a single dissenting scientist without supporting research data cannot constitute a "divergent" opinion.[68] But if the notion of divergent scientific opinion is to have any content—if it is to be more than euphemism for mere assertion that a regulation is rational—then some minimum threshold of empirical support and peer acceptance is appropriate.[69]

An emerging transatlantic conflict over European restrictions on the importation and use of genetically modified foods (GMFs) and seeds will require the WTO to revisit these issues, absent a negotiated settlement. In May 2003, the United States filed a complaint against the EC, alleging that European restrictions on GMFs are not scientifically justified and thus violate SPS.[70] A dispute resolution panel has been requested (indicating the failure of "consultation" efforts).[71] A negotiated settlement is still possible. Seeds genetically modified to yield pest-resistant crops are widely used in the United States[72] and accepted by most American consumers. In Europe, however, consumer anxiety about possible health hazards from GMFs is widespread,[73] and the EC has restricted GMF imports.[74] American food producers point to multimillion dollar annual losses from these restrictions, and they note the absence of scientific evidence, so far, documenting health risks from GMFs. European regulators counter that genetic engineering of food products is in its infancy and that its long-term health effects are unknown.[75]

The appellate body's insistence in its *Hormones* opinion that supporting research data is necessary to legitimate a "divergent" scientific opinion for SPS risk assessment purposes augers poorly for the EC in the GMF case, absent the emergence of scientific data showing danger to human health. On the other hand, the novelty of GMFs and the lack of empirical evidence bearing on long-term health risk support application of the precautionary principle, also endorsed in the *Hormones* opinion. The appellate body's characterization of SPS risk assessment as a matter of subjective judgment, not merely "quantitative analysis," also leaves some room for deference to Europe's treatment of GMFs. In our view, however, it would be an abuse of the precautionary principle— and the premise of deference to member states' subjective judgments about health risk—to permit prohibitions on GMFs to survive without any empirical support.

To sum up, although the *Hormones* decision went against EC regulators, the appellate body's opinion laid a foundation for future evolution of food and agricultural trade law in accordance with the principle of special deference to national authority to protect health. The *Hormones* decision requires that there be some empirical substance to claims of health risk if they are to pass muster in the dispute settlement process: subjective perceptions and popular fears are not by themselves enough. But once this low empirical barrier is crossed, emerging SPS jurisprudence protects health to a remarkable degree, through a policy of exceptional deference to member states' assessments of and responses to health risk.

INTELLECTUAL PROPERTY AND LIFESAVING MEDICINES

Nowhere have perceptions of conflict between the WTO system and protection for health been as strong as in the area of trade in lifesaving medications. The AIDS pandemic in sub-Saharan Africa has made WTO treatment of drug companies' intellectual property rights into one of the most visible and poignant international issues of our time. Of the 3 million worldwide deaths from AIDS in 2000, 2.4 million occurred in sub-Saharan Africa.[76] At least 12 million African children have been orphaned by AIDS, a number that could soar to 40 million by 2010 without more effective HIV control.[77] Of an estimated 36 million people now living with HIV worldwide, 95% live in developing countries. Twenty-five million—more than two-thirds—abide in Africa, and about 4 million of these suffer from advanced HIV-related illness.[78] Yet only a small fraction of infected Africans receive antiretroviral therapy, the state-of-the-art drug treatment that has transformed AIDS from a sure, short-term killer into a disease with which one can live indefinitely.[79]

High, patent-protected prices for antiretroviral agents are part of the story behind the minuscule proportions of HIV-infected Africans receiving treatment. Patent-protected prices also put some drugs for malaria, tuberculosis, and other endemic diseases out of reach for most Africans and others among the third-world poor.[80] It is widely held that TRIPS makes it more difficult for generic drug makers and "gray market" importers to undercut patent-protected prices by exploiting permissive intellectual property law in poor countries.[81] African and South American governments,[82] public health activists, and some scholars[83] have criticized TRIPS on this ground, for sacrificing the health of the world's poor to protect pharmaceutical firms' revenues. The pharmaceutical industry's standard response is that patent-protected monopoly pricing is necessary to promote research on breakthrough drugs of value to all, including the poor.[84] Foreign aid from wealthy nations, donations from pharmaceutical firms, and protection for international price discrimination against the threat of gray market arbitrage are among the industry's answers to the challenge of getting life-saving drugs to the world's poorest people.[85]

The appellate body has not yet opined on member states' flexibility, under TRIPS, to issue compulsory licenses, permit parallel importing, or import generic drugs manufactured elsewhere. Conflict over these issues has played out within the WTO's political organs. To a remarkable degree, this political process has responded to the desperate medical needs of sub-Saharan Africa and other impoverished regions. In the face of opposition from the pharmaceutical industry and industrialized nations,[86] the WTO's highest governing body, the Ministerial Conference, issued a pronouncement in November 2001 declaring that members have a "right to protect public health, . . . to promote access to medicines for all," and "to use, to the full, the provisions in TRIPS, which provide flexibility for this purpose."[87]

This ministerial pronouncement, generally referred to as the Doha Declaration, cleared a path for parallel importing—acquisition of patent-protected drugs at lower prices through arbitrage[88]—by construing TRIPS to allow members to make their own rules for exhaustion of patent rights.[89] It also construed the rather convoluted TRIPS provision on compulsory licensing, or "use without authorization of the right holder,"[90] to grant countries several, overlapping "right[s]": (i) the "right to determine what constitutes a national emergency or other circumstances of extreme urgency"[91] for the purpose of compulsory licensing without prior efforts to obtain "reasonable commercial terms"[92] from the patent holder, (ii) the more general "right to grant compulsory licenses,"[93] and (iii) the "freedom to determine the grounds upon which such licenses are granted."[94] Moreover, it pronounced that "public health crises, including those relating to HIV/AIDS, tuberculosis, malaria and other epidemics, can represent a national emergency or other circumstances of extreme urgency."[95] The Doha Declaration's use of rights language to construe the TRIPS provision on compulsory licensing contrasts with the provision itself, which is framed as a list of constraints on members' authority to issue compulsory licenses.[96]

The Doha Declaration also addressed a quandary confronted by poor nations without indigenous, generic pharmaceutical industries.[97] The TRIPS compulsory licensing provision mandates that use of patented subject matter without the right holder's authorization be "predominantly for the supply of the domestic market" of the country conferring a compulsory license. On its face, this rules out compulsory licensing and generic manufacture of patent protected medicine in one country, followed by export to impoverished consumer countries without generic drug manufacturers. And unless this pattern of manufacture and export is permitted, compulsory licensing can do little to address the drug access problems of the poor, since only a few of the world's developing nations have substantial drug manufacturing capacity and large domestic markets.[98]

The Doha Declaration instructed the Council for TRIPS (the TRIPS governing body) to "find an expeditious solution to this problem" by the end of 2002.[99] Within the council, U.S. negotiators insisted that compulsory licensing for export be permitted only for HIV/AIDS, malaria, tuberculosis, and other severe infectious illnesses.[100] Less developed countries sought the power to make it available for other health problems, and the TRIPS Council remained deadlocked over this issue as the Doha deadline passed.[101] Amidst mounting criticism of U.S. unilateralism[102] and the humanitarian consequences of failure to reach agreement, the Bush Administration relented, signing onto an August 2003 implementation agreement that authorizes individual member states to decide which health problems merit compulsory licenses for export.[103] Critics have expressed concern that the agreement's safeguards against illicit diversion of drugs produced under compulsory license could slow poor countries' efforts to make legitimate use of its provisions to save lives.[104] This risk bears close monitoring by member states and nongovernmental organizations. But the Doha Declaration and the 2003 implementation agreement are consistent with the principle of special deference, within the WTO scheme, to national authority to protect health.

The formal legal significance of the Doha Declaration and implementation agreement are uncertain. What the declaration clearly did not do is either amend TRIPS[105] or interpret the agreement in accordance with the procedure for interpretation established by multilateral treaty when the WTO was created.[106] As Steve Charnovitz has observed, language in the Marrakesh agreement establishing the WTO[107] permits the argument that the Doha pronouncements on TRIPS constitute "decisions" of the Ministerial Conference

on the WTO's behalf.[108] But the legal import of such "decisions," absent proceedings to amend or formally interpret TRIPS, is uncertain.

More plausibly, the Doha Declaration and implementation agreement have interpretive weight under the Vienna Convention on the Law of Treaties,[109] as either a "subsequent agreement between the parties regarding the interpretation"[110] of TRIPS or "subsequent practice in the application of the treaty which establishes the agreement of the parties regarding its interpretation."[111] Formally, this weight is limited: "subsequent agreement" and "subsequent practice" are to be "taken into account,"[112] the convention says, but the "ordinary meaning to be given to the terms"[113] of a treaty is paramount. As a practical matter, though, it is difficult to imagine that Doha will carry less than decisive weight in WTO dispute resolution proceedings and, more important, in the trade talks that settle most potential disputes between member states without resort to adjudication. Of even greater significance is Doha's reduction of TRIPS-related legal uncertainties that have inhibited public and private efforts to make lifesaving medicines affordable. Pharmaceutical manufacturers, importers, sellers, and medical clinics face diminished regulatory risk and are thus better able to invest in needed production capacity, distribution networks, and health care infrastructure.

The Doha Declaration and implementation agreement, in short, reduced the TRIPS threat to member states' health promotion efforts by construing ambiguous treaty terms in health-friendly fashion. There will be debate over Doha's legal authority, its implications for particular manufacturing and importing scenarios, and whether it should be seen as changing or merely clarifying WTO members' legal obligations.[114] But the declaration's broad affirmation of members' "right to protect public health" and to "use, to the full," TRIPS's "flexibility for this purpose" is consonant with the larger picture we have sketched in this chapter, of an emerging WTO norm that treats health as reason for special deference to national authority.

CONCLUSION: AS A HEALTH INTERPRETIVE PRINCIPLE

The principle that protection for health merits special regard as a basis for deference to member states' policies is a common strand running through WTO law.

This principle has emerged since the Marrakesh agreement creating the WTO. It appears nowhere in the Marrakesh treaty or the associated multilateral trade agreements, but it has animated the appellate body's approach to national health regulation under GATT and SPS, as well as the Ministerial Conference's treatment of TRIPS in the Doha Declaration.

This principle is the product of post-Marrakesh politics as much as law. It is also the product of flexible institutional design. To be sure, the advent of the appellate body, empowered to issue binding rulings,[115] moved the WTO from the more politicized model of GATT arbitration toward a "rule orientation" in trade disputes.[116] Yet creation of dispute settlement panels on a case-by-case basis, from a list of candidates formulated by the WTO Secretariat and made up largely of people with experience in government service,[117] ensures a process sensitive to political currents and cues. The appellate body's composition—seven members "broadly representative" of the WTO, appointed by the Dispute Settlement Body to staggered four-year terms—also assures a measure of responsiveness to international trade politics. Some have characterized the WTO's two-tiered litigation process—fact-finding and treaty application at the panel level, followed by appellate body review—as akin to the U.S. system of trial and appellate courts. But a closer analogy may be to a U.S. administrative agency that construes its enabling statute case by case, through adjudication and ensuing review by politically appointed board members or commissioners.[118] Such a scheme pursues a balance between "rule-orientation" and accommodation to concerns that find political expression. The Ministerial Conference, moreover, ensures wider institutional flexibility, as Doha illustrates, when the breadth and urgency of such concerns transcend the limits of case-by-case adjudication.

The influences that have pushed protection for health to a special place in post-Marrakesh WTO law are not difficult to discern, though precise causal relationships are impossible to prove. The power of developing nations and EC states within WTO institutions has mattered greatly. The United States, which has tended to resist heightened WTO deference to other nations' health policies, has proven strong but not dominant within the WTO scheme.[119] The influence of nongovernmental organizations, often acting in concert with developing nations, is part of the story, particularly in the TRIPS/HIV treatment context.

Press attention to the catastrophic human consequences of the AIDS pandemic, to more general concerns about the health and environmental consequences of globalization, and to the size (and aggressive tactics) of anti-WTO street protests has helped to put WTO-related health issues on the public agenda in developed countries. The growing realization that the AIDS pandemic and other health crises are threats to social and political stability—and thus to national security—has intensified wealthy countries' worries about the health of the third-world poor.[120] And, for some, the moral shame of millions of avoidable deaths per year, from AIDS and myriad other causes, has inspired a search for legal tools to save lives.

The special regard that the WTO accords to health has taken the form of heightened deference to national health policies rather than a WTO (or member state) duty to protect health. This reflects the WTO's role, as prescribed by its creators. Its institutions are reactive to health policies that restrict trade or intrude upon intellectual property protection. The WTO can say no to such policies, instruct offending countries to change them, and even authorize limited retaliation by states offended against. But the WTO can neither formulate its own health policies nor instruct members to do so.

This reactive role was hardly inevitable. The drafters of the Marrakesh agreement and its associated trade pacts were proactive in specifying detailed rules for liberal trade and protection for intellectual property. In theory, they could have been similarly proactive in setting out minimum health standards for production processes and exported goods, as well as criteria for compromise between intellectual property protection and medical need. That they were not might be ascribed to the power of interest groups concerned about the benefits of liberal trade and inattentive to people's health. But there is a case to be made for an interpretive principle of protection for health that takes the form of heightened deference to member states' health policies instead of an affirmative transnational duty.

This case rests on the intensely subjective, highly variable nature of people's beliefs about health danger. We appreciate and respond to health risks in ways shaped much less by statistical magnitudes than by the feelings these risks evoke[121] and by our sense of control over these risks. Our feelings about risk, in turn, are shaped by our character styles, values and culture, and personal and social experience. These influences tend to be local phenomena. They vary within small communities, more so among subnational regions, and even more so across international boundaries. Health policies that fail to take account of these influences risk departing too sharply from people's subjective needs. And public decision-making mechanisms that fail to offer opportunities for community control, or at least engagement, tend to raise people's anxieties about the risk–benefit judgments reached. Health politics is peculiarly local. Regional and national resource differences magnify this localism, by influencing judgments about regulatory and other public priorities. National, let alone transnational, efforts to systematize and rationalize health policies encounter skepticism and resistance.[122] Pushed too far, these efforts undermine the credibility, indeed the perceived legitimacy, of governments and multinational institutions.

One might object that parochial resistance to these rationalizing efforts should not be treated as a challenge to their desirability, since these efforts are our best chance to maximize the welfare of the whole.[123] But the more removed these efforts are from democratic oversight, the more tenuous are their claims to political legitimacy in both theory and practice.[124] The question of transnational health regulation's legitimacy in theory is beyond our scope in this chapter. We limit ourselves here to the point underscored by the caricatures of globalization often heard in political speeches and street protests—that distrust of transnational rationalizing efforts distorts many people's understanding of them. Keeping such distortion in check, even at the cost of a measure of worldwide consistency, is a central challenge for the governance of international trade. WTO deference to national health policy is responsive to this challenge. It serves as a steam valve for domestic anxieties about globalization while incorporating protection for health as an interpretive principle.

Protection of health as an interpretive principle, rather than an internationally justiciable right, allows room for national variations in resource availability, perceptions of risk, and balancing between health and other goals. The Indian experience with so-called "Directive Principles of State Policy," a separate category of constitutional norms that closely track international social and economic rights, suggests the potential for further development of this approach. The Indian Constitution states that Directive Principles "shall not be enforced by any court" but "are

nevertheless fundamental in the governance of the country. . . ."[125] Moreover, the constitution proclaims that "it shall be the duty of the State to apply these principles in making laws."[126] The Indian Supreme Court has read this language as authority to look to Directive Principles for interpretive guidance when construing other constitutional provisions. The Court's oft-cited 1985 decision in a case involving hundreds of thousands of Bombay squatters who claimed a right to stay based on their justiciable "right to life"[127] is illustrative. The squatters successfully argued that Directive Principles calling upon the state to secure "an adequate means of livelihood" and "the right to work" enlarged the content of the constitution's "right to life." The "right to life" barred the Bombay authorities from evicting the squatters, the Court held, because they needed to remain in their illicit abodes to be within commuting range of their jobs.[128]

Protection for health can play a similar "directive" role in shaping justiciable obligations within both domestic and international legal fora. Treatment of health as an interpretive norm, nonjusticiable in itself, sheds much of the problematic baggage of the right to health (and of social and economic rights generally). This baggage includes the line-drawing difficulties associated with agreeing on how much health is "attainable," as well as the power of adjudicative decision makers to command public resources in nondemocratic fashion and to displace political authority. In the international arena, special deference to domestic health policy, subject to rational relationship review, finesses the question of infringement on sovereignty that social and economic rights "enforcement" presents.

Heightened consciousness of health as a vital concern has already pushed WTO law in directions not envisioned by the framers at Marrakesh. The appellate body's near-total deference to national regulators' risk–benefit judgments and choices from among health policy objectives was not compelled by treaty language, but it is consistent with the legal premise that health is special. The Ministerial Conference's interpretive reinvention of TRIPS as a health-friendly agreement is the most striking example so far of health's elevated legal status. Upcoming negotiations over liberalization of trade in services offer an additional opportunity to define the place of protection for health within the WTO scheme.[129]

No WTO organ has explicitly embraced the premise of an international human right to health.[130] For some proponents of such a right, this has been disheartening. Yet the WTO's tacit endorsement of protection for health as an interpretive principle, effected through heightened deference to national health policies, has done as much to establish health as a value in international law as have actions by international bodies more directly focused on health. Indeed, the WTO has arguably done more. Its judicial and ministerial pronouncements have created state practice, through both their legal force and member countries' compliance with them. The WTO has thereby become a prime mover of customary as well as treaty-based international health law. It has recognized a soft, nonjusticiable right to health[131] in all but name. Member states, nongovernmental organizations, and others concerned about the place of health in transnational law should press WTO institutions to make this recognition explicit.

Notes

1. Jared Diamond, Guns, Germs, and Steel: The Fates of Human Societies (New York: W.W. Norton & Company, 1997).

2. E.g., John Hilary, The Wrong Model: GATS, Trade Liberalization and Children's Right to Health, Save the Children, 46 (October 2001) (stating that WTO dispute settlement panels that consider cases involving member states' health regulations "rule . . . on the basis of trade considerations, not public health concerns"). Save the Children contends generally in this report that the WTO dispute resolution process pays little more than lip service to language in the 1994 General Agreement on Tariffs and Trade (GATT '94) and other WTO-associated agreements permitting health-based exceptions to liberal trade rules.

3. Gilles de Wildt et al., "Which Comes First—Health or Wealth?" Lancet 357, 9262 (April 7, 2001): 1123–1124, at 1123 (discussing the UN Subcommission on Human Rights proclamation that the Agreement on Trade-Related Aspects of Intellectual Property Rights [TRIPS] "does not adequately reflect the fundamental nature and indivisibility of all human rights," including the right to health); David Price et al., "How the World Trade Organization Is Shaping Domestic Policies in Health Care," Lancet 354, 9193 (November 27, 1999): 1889–1892 (arguing that WTO policies conflict with the basic priorities undergirding many national health systems).

4. See Joost Pauwelyn, "The Role of Public International Law in the WTO: How Far Can We Go?" American Journal of International Law 95 (2001): 535–578, at 561 n. 175 (summarizing commentary taking the position that WTO law does not assimilate other international law, aside from rules of treaty interpretation).

5. A consensus of opinion holds that Art. 3.2 of the Understanding on Rules and Procedures Governing the Settlement of Disputes, known as the Dispute Settlement Understanding (DSU), I.L.M. 33 (1994): 112–135 (instructing dispute settlement panels and the DSU appellate body to "clarify" WTO treaty provisions "in accordance with customary rules of interpretation of public international law") incorporates the customary international law rules of treaty interpretation codified in Arts. 31–33 of the Vienna Convention on the Interpretation of Treaties. E.g., John. H. Jackson, The World Trading System: Law and Policy of International Economic Relations (Cambridge, MA: MIT Press, 1997): 120–121. But scholars and member states have differed over whether and to what degree substantive customary and conventional international law outside the trade realm—e.g., environmental and human rights law—is thereby brought within the WTO sphere for purposes of treaty interpretation. Although the appellate body has from time to time referenced international agreements outside the trade realm, it has not spoken clearly and generally to this question.

6. The preambles to the agreement establishing the WTO, GATT '94 (a revised version of GATT), the GATS, and TRIPS make reference to economic development and employment but not to public health. Only the Agreement on the Application of Sanitary and Phytosanitary Measures (SPS), devoted specifically to the application of GATT '94 to member states' public health regulations, affirms human health as an objective in its preamble.

7. See Art. 25(1) (declaring that everyone has "a right to a standard of living adequate for the health of himself and his family, including food, clothing, housing, and medical care").

8. See Art. 12(1) (declaring "the right of everyone to the enjoyment of the highest attainable standard of physical and mental health"). Other international law instruments that make reference to a right to health include the International Convention on the Elimination of All Forms of Racial Discrimination, Art. 5(e)(iv) open for signature, I.L.M. 3 (1966): 161–165, at 164; the Convention on the Elimination of All Forms of Discrimination against Women, Art. II (1)(f) and Art. 12 open for signature March 1, 1980, 1249 UNTS 13; and the Convention on the Rights of the Child, Art. 24 adopted by General Assembly, I.L.M. 28 (1989): 1448.

9. See Eleanor D. Kinney, "The International Human Right to Health: What Does This Mean for Our Nation and World?" Indiana Law Review 34 (2001): 1457–1475, at 1464 (discussing prospects for recognizing health as a right in customary international law).

10. Daniel Callahan, What Kind of Life? The Limits of Medical Progress (New York: Simon & Schuster, 1990): 31–68.

11. Cass Sunstein, "Against Positive Rights," Eastern European Journal of Constitutional Review 2 (1993): 35–38.

12. See, generally, Bertus De Villiers, "The Socioeconomic Consequences of Directive Principles of State Policy: Limitations on Fundamental Rights," South African Journal on Human Rights 8 (1992): 188–199.

13. James A. Auerbach and Barbara K. Krimgold, "Improving Health: It Doesn't Take a Revolution," in James A. Auerbach and Barbara K. Krimgold, eds., Income, Socioeconomic Status, and Health: Exploring the Relationship (Washington, DC: National Policy Institute, 2001): 1.

14. S. Leonard Syme, "Understanding the Relationship between Socioeconomic Status and Health: New Research Initiatives," in James A. Auerbach and Barbara K Krimgold, eds., Income, Socioeconomic Status, and Health: Exploring the Relationship (Washington, DC: National Policy Institute, 2001): 12. Syme observes:

> There is no more important environmental issue than socioeconomic status. The relationship between SES and health is well-known. It produces disease in all bodily systems—digestive genitourinary, respiratory, circulatory, nervous, blood, and endocrine. It also results in higher rates of mortality for most malignancies, congenital abnormalities, infections, parasitic diseases, accidents, poisoning, violence, perinatal mortality, diabetes, and musculoskeletal impairments. Id. at 14

15. E.g., Ichiro Kawachi and Tony A. Blakely, "When Economists and Epidemiologists Disagree," Journal of Health Politics, Policy, & Law 26, 3 (2001): 533–541; Richard D. Wilkinson, Unhealthy Societies: The Affliction of Inequality (London: Routledge, 1996). See Jennifer M. Mellor and Jeffrey Milyo, "Reexamining the Evidence of an Ecological Association between Income Inequality and Health," Journal of Health Politics, Policy, & Law 26, 2 (2001): 487–522 (disputing the validity of the statistical reasoning employed by those who contend that the steepness of wealth gradients in societies is a determinant of health, independent of levels of personal wealth).

16. James S. House, "Relating Social Inequalities in Health and Income," Journal of Health Politics, Policy, & Law 26 (2001): 523; A. Wagstaff and Evan Doorslaer, "Income Inequality and Health: What Does the Literature Tell Us?" Annual Review of Public Health 21 (2000): 543.

17. WHO Commission on Macroeconomics and Health, Macroeconomics and Health: Investing in Health for Economic Development (2001): 21–40; J. P. Smith, "Healthy Bodies and Thick Wallets: The Dual Relation between Health and Economic Status," Journal of Economic Perspectives 13 (1999): 145–166.

18. Amartya Sen, Development as Freedom (Oxford: Oxford University Press, 1999): 43–49.

19. Sudhir Anand and Martin Ravallion, "Human Development in Poor Countries: On the Role of Private Incomes and Public Services," Journal of Economic Perspectives 7 (1993): 133–150.

20. Id.

21. Martha Nussbaum, Women and Human Development (Cambridge, UK: Cambridge University Press, 2000): 294–295.

22. Anand and Ravallion, supra note 19.

23. Sen, supra note 18 at 45–47.

24. Id.; Jean Dreze and Amartya Sen, Hunger and Public Action (Oxford: Clarendon Press, 1989).

25. Sen, supra note 18 at 195–198.

26. Id. at 198–199.

27. Id. at 146–159.

28. See id. at 178–188 (arguing that political and civil rights empower people threatened by potential famine to mobilize the state to provide income support, employment, or other aid necessary to enable those in need to purchase food when they cannot grow or afford it themselves).

29. See generally Joseph E. Stiglitz, Globalization and Its Discontents (New York: W. W. Norton & Co., 2002).

30. At the Cancun Ministerial Conference in September 2003, e.g., a group of developing countries that became known as the "Group of 21," or "G-21," acted in concert to oppose the positions of the United States, Europe, and Japan in agriculture negotiations. See Ginger Thompson, "Protesters Swarm the Streets at WTO Forum in Cancun," New York Times, September 14, 2003, at A14.

31. The dispute settlement process is established by the Dispute Settlement Understanding, which was one of the Uruguay Round agreements that established the WTO. See Agreement Establishing the World Trade Organization, 1994, Annex 2: Dispute Settlement Understanding, available at http:// www.wto.org/english/docs_ e/legal_e/28-dsu.pdf (accessed October 19, 2003). For the WTO's official description of the dispute settlement process, see World Trade Organization, A Unique Contribution, at http:// www.wto.org/english/thewto_e/ whatis_e/tif_e/disp1_e.htm (accessed October 19, 2003).

32. The GATT was completed in 1947 and went into effect in 1948. It has since evolved through a series of multilateral negotiating "rounds," and in 1994 it was incorporated into the newly created WTO.

33. GATT 1994, Art. XX(b). This authorization is subject to the chapeau (introductory clause) to Art. XX, which requires that such measures not be applied in a manner that would constitute a means of arbitrary or unjustifiable discrimination between countries where the same conditions prevail or a disguised restriction on international trade.

34. Understanding on Rules and Procedures Governing the Settlement of Disputes, supra n. 5, Art. 11.

35. Dumping has been variously defined as the sale of goods abroad for a price below the price charged in the "home" (or exporting) market and as the sale of goods abroad for a price below their cost of production. Definition of dumping and consideration of policy responses to it is complicated by possibilities for expanding production at low marginal cost and for increasing profitable sales through price discrimination. Jackson, supra note 5, at 251–261.

36. Countervailing duties are assessed and collected by importing countries for the asserted purpose of neutralizing the market impact of exporting nations' subsidies. Id. at 281–283.

37. "Safeguards" are restrictive trade measures (typically temporary) in response to imports that purportedly pose a serious threat to a competing domestic industry, or to a country's economy in general, absent any recognized unfair trade practice. Id. at 175–181.

38. See Agreement on Implementation of Art. VI of GATT '94, Art. 17.6 (stating (i) that if national authorities' "establishment of the facts was proper and the evaluation was unbiased and objective, even though the [WTO dispute resolution] panel might have reached a different conclusion, the evaluation shall not be overturned," and (ii) that "[w]here the panel finds that a relevant provision of the [antidumping] Agreement admits of more than one permissible interpretation, the panel shall find the authorities' measure to be in conformity with the Agreement even if it rests upon one of those permissible interpretations"). To the extent that panels and the appellate body are willing to concede the possibility of multiple, permissible inferences from facts and treaty text, instead of imposing their preferred interpretations in formalistic fashion, Art. 17.6 gives member states discretion to take antidumping measures. Daniel Tarullo points to the parallel between Art. 17.6 and U.S. administrative agencies' discretion, under Chevron, USA v. National Resources Defense Council, 467 U.S. 837, 842–843 (1984), to adopt any "permissible construction" of an ambiguous statute. Daniel K. Tarullo, The Hidden Costs of International Dispute Settlement: WTO Review of Domestic Anti-dumping Decisions 5–6 (2002) (unpublished manuscript, on file with the author).

39. It has done so largely by purporting to ascertain single, correct interpretations of facts and law, thereby eliding treaty language, see Tarullo, supra note 38, that allows member states to choose from among multiple permissible interpretations. Id. at 8–24.

40. E.g., United States' Imposition of Countervailing Duties on Certain Hot-Rolled Lead and Bismuth Carbon Steel Products Originating in the United Kingdom, WT/DS138/AB/R (May 10, 2000); United States—Definitive Safeguard Measures on Imports of Circular Welded Carbon Quality Line Pipe From Korea, WT/DS202/AB/R (February 15, 2002); United States—Safeguard Measures on Imports of Fresh, Chilled or Frozen Lamb Meat from New Zealand and Australia, WT/DS177/AB/R (May 1, 2001).

41. See Agreement on Safeguards, Art. 4.2(a) (instructing national authorities to "evaluate all relevant factors of an objective and quantifiable nature having a bearing on the situation of that industry, in particular, the rate and amount of the increase in imports of the product concerned in absolute and relative terms, the share of the domestic market taken by increased imports, changes in the level of sales, production, productivity, capacity utilization, profits and losses, and employment").

42. U.S–Safeguard Measures on Imports of Fresh, Chilled, or Frozen Lamb Meat from New Zealand and Australia–AB-2001-1, WT/DS177,178/AB/R, para. 106 ("[p]anels must, therefore, review whether the competent authorities' explanation fully addresses the nature, and especially, the complexities, of the data, and responds to other plausible interpretations of that data. A panel must find, in particular, that an explanation is not reasoned, or is not adequate, if some alternative explanation of the facts is plausible, and if the competent authorities' explanation does not seem adequate in the light of that alternative explanation.").

43. European Communities—Measures Affecting Asbestos and Asbestos-Containing Products, WT/DS135/AB/R, para. 155 (April 5, 2001).

44. Id. at para. 178.

45. Id.

46. See Laurent Ruessman, "Putting the Precautionary Principle in Its Place: Parameters for the Proper Application of a Precautionary Approach and the Implications for Developing Countries in Light of the Doha WTO Ministerial," American University International Law Review 17 (2002): 905–949, at 926 (suggesting that EC-Asbestos (supra note 43) and an earlier decision, U.S.–Import Prohibition of CertainShrimp and ashrimp Products–AB-1998-4,WT/DS58/AB/R, "arguably afforded deference to a precautionary approach"); Sonia Boutillon, "The Precautionary Principle: Development of an International Standard," Michigan Journal of International Law 23 (2002): 429–469 at 457 (contending that "in Asbestos, the appellate body relied upon the precautionary principle as a standard in its analysis"). The "precautionary principle" holds, in general terms, that where scientific proof of a practice's adverse health and environmental impact is uncertain, policymakers should err on the safe side by curtailing the practice sufficiently to ensure that its health and environmental risks do not exceed accepted levels.

47. EC-Asbestos, supra note 43, at para. 168.

48. Thailand Restrictions on Importation of and Internal Taxes on Cigarettes, November 7, 1990, GATT B.I.S.D. (37th supp.) at 200 (1991).

49. Id. at para. 75.

50. Id. at para. 81.

51. It is defensible, in our view, without undercutting the importance of national public health aims. High-enough nondiscriminatory taxes would surely undermine cigarette-marketing efforts as effectively as would discriminatory taxes on imports. To be sure, nondiscriminatory taxes would be more politically difficult to enact because of opposition from domestic producers. But it is hardly clear that the power of domestic interest groups to push national policy in protectionist directions should count in favor of a finding that discriminatory treatment of foreign products is necessary to achieve national health goals.

52. EC-Asbestos, supra note 43, at paras. 173–174.

53. Institutional competence here might incorporate a variety of factors, including scientific and technical know-how, closeness to popular sentiments concerning health risks, respect for national sovereignty in health and safety matters, and the democratic legitimacy of national vs. transnational balancing among risks and benefits.

54. Id. at para. 172. The appellate body's treatment of health as a "vital and important" value is also evident in its decision to overturn the EC-Asbestos panel's ruling that similarly employed construction materials with and without asbestos are "like products" under GATT Art. 111(4), for purposes of GATT's "national treatment" requirements. In reversing the panel, which emphasized the shared end uses of these materials, the appellate body put primary emphasis on the different health risk profiles of materials that do and do not contain asbestos. Id. at paras. 125–141.

55. European Communities—Measures Concerning Meat and Meat Products (Hormones), AB Report, WT/DS26/AB/R, WT/DS48/AB/R (February 13, 1998).

56. Steve Charnovitz, "The Supervision of Health and Biosafety Regulation by World Trade Rules," Tulane Environmental Law Journal 13 (2000): 271–302, at 301.

57. Agreement on the Application of Sanitary and Phytosanitary Measures, decision date April 14, 1995 1867 U.N.T.S. 493.

58. Id. at Art. 5.1

59. EC-Hormones, supra note 55, at paras. 207–208.

60. See id. at paras. 205–206 (rejecting, as "fundamental legal error," the dispute resolution panel's view that risk resulting from poor administrative control cannot be counted in an SPS risk assessment).

61. See supra, text accompanying note 47.

62. EC-Hormones, supra note 55, at para. 186.

63. Id. at para. 187.

64. Id. at para. 124 (construing SPS Art. 5.7).

65. Id. at para. 188–189. The appellate body treated the SPS Art. 5.1 requirement that regulation be "based on" a risk assessment as a requirement that there be a logical ("objective") relationship between the risk assessment and the regulation at issue, not as a requirement that the risk assessment play a role in the regulatory decision-making process as a matter of historical fact. Id.

66. Id. at para. 193.

67. Id. at para. 194.

68. Id. at para. 198. Citing several scientific reports concluding that use of hormones to promote growth in cattle is safe, the appellate body declined to recognize, as a divergent scientific opinion, a single scientist's expressed view (not based on his own studies) that use of some of the hormones at issue posed a tiny but nonzero risk. Id. at paras. 196–198.

69. The content of such a threshold test is beyond our scope here, but one might imagine something similar to the approach taken to admissibility of scientific testimony in Daubert v. Merrill Dow Pharmaceuticals, 509 U.S. 579 (1993), relying on both empirical grounding and peer support for the scientific viewpoint at issue.

70. "U.S. to Push WTO Case Unless EU Biotech Moratorium Lifted," Inside U.S. Trade, May 16, 2003, at 5–6. The U.S. complaint also alleged violations of the Agreement on Technical Barriers to Trade, another component of the WTO scheme. Because it preceded the adoption of the European Union's final GMF regulations, the WTO complaint cites only the moratorium as its basis for action, not the new regulations. Id.

71. Washington Post, August 8, 2003, at E2.

72. Almost 40% of American grown corn is genetically modified. David Leonhardt, "Talks Collapse on U.S. Efforts to Open Europe to Biotech Food," New York Times, June 20, 2003, at A1. Because almost one-third of American crops are exported, the American Farm Bureau describes the European Union's moratorium on GMFs as a "nightmare." Elizabeth Becker and David Barboza, "Battle over Biotechnology Intensifies Trade War," New York Times, May 28, 2003, at C1.

73. Leonhardt, supra note 72.

74. From 1998 until 2003, the EC maintained an informal moratorium on GMF imports. Elizabeth Becker, "U.S. Contests Europe's Ban on Some Food," New York Times, May 14, 2003, at C1. In response to American objections, the EC implemented a new regulatory scheme in 2003 that in principal permits introduction of GMF products. "New EU Law on Biotech Food," Washington Post, July 3, 2003, at E2. But the Bush Administration says this scheme is unsatisfactory, since it mandates that GMFs be labeled and traceable, a requirement U.S. agricultural firms claim would be prohibitively expensive and virtually impossible to meet. See "U.S. Agriculture Groups Weigh WTO Case against New EU GMO Rules," Inside U.S. Trade, July 11, 2003, 4–5 (describing the details of the traceability and labeling rules and the U.S. position that the regulations are a "pyrrhic victory" because they are as restrictive as the moratorium).

Some EC member states have refused to allow even GMFs that comply with these regulations, and the EC has initiated enforcement action against these states. See European Union, Press Release, Genetically Modified Organisms: Commission Takes Court Action against Eleven Member States, July 15, 2003 (on file with author). In a 2003 case, the European Court of Justice considered whether member nations could take protective measures against foods containing transgenic proteins. Case C-236/01, Monsanto Agricoltura Italia SpA and Others v. Presidenza del Consiglio dei Ministri and Others, September 9, 2003. The Court held that protective measures were only justified if the "Member State has first carried out a risk assessment which is as complete as possible given the particular circumstances of the individual case, from which it is apparent that, in the light of the precautionary principle, the implementation of such measures is necessary in order to ensure that novel foods do not present danger for the consumer." Id. at paras. 84, 114. The court stated that the risk targeted by a nation's ban must not be based on a purely hypothetical approach to risk, founded on mere suppositions that are not yet scientifically verified. Id. at para. 106. To be valid, a ban on novel foods must be based on "detailed grounds" to suspect health risks, the court said. Id. at para. 108; Paul Meller, "Italy Loses Ruling on Modified Food," Washington Post, September 10, 2003, at W1.

75. Justin Gillis, "U.S. Attacks European Biotech Ban," Washington Post, May 14, 2003, at E1.

76. WHO Commission on Macroeconomics and Health, supra note 17, at 47.

77. Id.

78. Id. at 51.

79. Many of these can afford antiretroviral agents only sporadically and therefore receive ineffective treatment. Id.

80. Patent-protected prices are hardly the whole story behind large-scale failure to make treatment for AIDS and other life-threatening infectious diseases available to the third-world poor. As pharmaceutical industry representatives often point out, inadequate medical clinics and other public health infrastructure constitute enormous barriers to drug access in poor countries.

81. Harvey E. Balf, Jr., "Patent Protection and Pharmaceutical Innovation," New York University Journal International Law & Politics 29 (1997): 95–107. Robert Weissman, "A Long, Strange TRIPS: The Pharmaceutical Industry Drive to Harmonize Global Intellectual Property Rules, and the Remaining WTO Legal Alternatives Available to Third World Countries," University of Pennsylvania Journal of International Economic Law 17 (1996): 1069.

82. See Daniel Pruzin, "Intellectual Property: Call for Affordable Medicines to Be Put on Doha Ministerial Agenda," BNA International Trade Report 18 (2001): 737–738 (reporting on concerns expressed by African and South American trade officials).

83. E.g., Patrick L. Wojahn, "A Conflict of Rights: Intellectual Property under TRIPS, the Right to Health, and AIDS Drugs," UCLA Journal of International Law & Foreign Affairs 6 (2001): 463–497, at 476–480. Weissman, supra note 81, at 1100.

84. Henry Grabowski, "Patents, Innovation and Access to New Pharmaceuticals," Journal of International Economic Law 5 (2002): 849–860.

85. Consideration of these competing claims from the pharmaceutical industry and its critics is beyond our scope here. We confine ourselves here to the proposition that in the TRIPS context, as in the GATT and SPS settings, the WTO has come to treat health as a value with privileged status when interpretive questions arise.

86. Daniel Pruzin, "Intellectual Property: Rewriting TRIPS Could Hurt Research, Pharmaceutical Industry Strongly Warns WTO," BNA International Trade Report 18, September 27, 2000: 1507–1508. International pharmaceutical industry leaders warned that any perceived weakening of TRIPS patent protection would be "disastrous" for research investment. The United States, Switzerland, Canada, Japan, and Australia proposed that the November 2001 WTO Ministerial Conference issue a declaration stating, inter alia, that "strong, effective, and balanced protection for intellectual property is a necessary incentive for research and development of life-saving drugs...." Id. The declaration on TRIPS and public health eventually issued by the Ministerial Conference included no such statement.

87. Declaration on the TRIPS Agreement and Public Health, Ministerial Conference, 4th Session, Doha, November 9–14, 2001, WT/MIN(01)/DEC/2, para. 4 (November 20, 2001) [hereinafter Doha Declaration].

88. Arbitrage opportunities result from the different prices that pharmaceutical firms charge for the same patent-protected drugs in different countries. Such price discrimination enables firms to increase revenues and to expand access to drugs (through prices as low as marginal cost), but it creates opportunities for movement of drugs (parallel importing) from higher price to lower price countries.

89. See id. at para. 5(d) (stating that TRIPS provisions relevant to exhaustion of intellectual property rights "leave each Member free to establish its own regime for exhaustion . . . , subject to the most favored nation and national treatment provisions"). "Exhaustion" frees buyers of patent-protected intellectual property (from a patent holder or licensee) to resell this property to others. Once the patent holder (or licensee) has sold the property, it cannot claim intellectual property rights against subsequent buyers and sellers; hence, the rights are said to be exhausted. So-called national exhaustion regimes, preferred by the pharmaceutical industry, treat intellectual property rights as exhausted only within the country of initial sale: subsequent sellers and users must comply with the rights in every other country. Thus, national exhaustion, with robust enforcement, precludes parallel importing. "International" exhaustion schemes, by contrast, treat intellectual property rights as exhausted throughout the world after the initial sale. They thus permit parallel importing and are disfavored by drug patent holders. So-called regional exhaustion regimes represent a compromise, barring patent holders from claiming the rights against subsequent sellers and users within a group of nations but requiring subsequent sellers and users to comply with the rights in countries outside this group. The TRIPS agreement itself explicitly declines to speak to the question of exhaustion: Art. 6 states that "subject to the provisions of Arts. 3 and 4 [TRIPS' "National Treatment" and "Most-Favored Nation Treatment" clauses] nothing in this Agreement shall be used to address the issue of the exhaustion of intellectual property rights." Thus, the Doha Declaration went well beyond the TRIPS text in construing the agreement to leave member states free to choose their exhaustion regimes.

90. TRIPS, Art. 31.

91. Doha Declaration, supra note 87, para. 5(c).

92. TRIPS, Art. 31 (b). Absent (i), "national emergency or other circumstances of extreme urgency," or (ii), "public non-commercial use," Art. 31 (b) permits compulsory licensing only after "the proposed user has made efforts to obtain authorization from the right holder on reasonable commercial terms and conditions and such efforts have not been successful within a reasonable period of time."

93. Doha Declaration, supra note 87, para. 5(b).

94. Id.

95. Id. at para. 5(c).

96. TRIPS, Art. 31, opens as follows: "Where the law of a Member allows for other use of the subject matter of a patent without the authorization of the right holder . . . the following provisions shall be respected. . . ."

97. This issue is frequently referred to as the "paragraph 6" issue because it was raised and left unresolved by paragraph 6 of the Doha Declaration. See Doha Declaration, supra note 87, para. 6.

98. Brazil and India are the principal examples, and they are rare exceptions. No sub-Saharan African nation (except, to some degree, South Africa) has significant pharmaceutical manufacturing capacity.

99. Doha Declaration, supra note 87, para. 6. The declaration directed the TRIPS Council to report back to the WTO General Council with a solution. Id.

100. Elizabeth Becker, "Trade Talks Fail to Agree on Drugs for Poor Nations," New York Times, December 21, 2002, at C3.

101. Paul Blustein, "Talks on Low-Cost Drugs for Poor Nations Stall," Washington Post, December 21, 2002, at E1.

102. Elizabeth Becker, "U.S. Unilateralism Worries Trade Officials," New York Times, March 17, 2003, at A8.

103. WTO General Council, Implementation of Paragraph 6 of the Doha Declaration on the TRIPS Agreement and Public Health, WT/L/540 (August 30, 2003), available at http://www.wto.org/english/news_e/news03_e/trips_stat_28aug03_ e.htm ["Implementation Decision"] (accessed December 9, 2003). When, in 2003, U.S. pharmaceutical firms backed away from their previous insistence on limiting compulsory licensing for export to HIV/AIDS and other life-threatening infections, U.S. negotiators followed suit. They pressed instead for assurances that only countries that truly lack domestic capacity could exercise this option, as well as safeguards against illicit export of drugs produced under compulsory licenses. The industry and the G.W. Bush administration sought to include these assurances and safeguards in the implementation agreement so they would have more legal force, but they eventually agreed to accept a General Council chairman's statement outlining these conditions. "Zoellick Vows to Work for TRIPS Deal, Lays Out U.S. Conditions," Inside U.S. Trade (August 1, 2003): 7–8; see also General Council Chairperson Carlos Pèrez del Castillo, The General Council Chairperson's Statement (August 30, 2003), available at http:// www.wto.org/english/news_e/news03_e/trips_stat_28aug03_e.htm ["Chairperson's Statement"] (accessed November 12, 2003).

104. See, e.g., Flawed WTO Drugs Deal Will Do Little to Secure Future Access to Medicines in Developing Countries, Doctors Without Borders (August 20, 2003), at http://www.msf.org/content/page.cfm?articleid=C1540425-7F56-4D60- A6CB9D7ABA6D627F (accessed December 9, 2003); Tony Smith, "Mixed View of Pact for Generic Drugs," New York Times, August 29, 2003, at C3.

105. See Agreement Establishing the World Trade Organization, Art. X (setting out procedures for amendment of WTO multilateral agreements, including TRIPS).

106. Steve Charnovitz, "The Legal Status of the Doha Declaration," Journal of International Economic Law 5 (2002): 207–211; see also Agreement Establishing the World Trade Organization, Art. IX(2) (setting out procedure, not followed at Doha, for adoption of formal interpretations of a WTO multilateral agreement by a three-fourths vote, on the basis of a recommendation by the council overseeing the agreement).

107. Marrakesh Agreement Establishing the World Trade Organization, 1967 U.N.T.S. 14, 33 I.L.M. 1143 (1994).

108. Charnovitz, supra note 106. Art. IV(1) of the Marrakesh agreement states as follows: "The Ministerial Conference shall have the authority to take decisions on all matters under any of the Multilateral Trade Agreements, . . . in accordance with the specific requirements for decision-making in this Agreement and in the relevant Multilateral Trade Agreement." Art. III(2) states that the WTO provides "a framework for the implementation of the results" of multilateral trade negotiations "as may be decided by the Ministerial Conference." These ambiguous references to Ministerial Conference decisions leave open the question of whether the conference's decision-making authority concerning the meaning of TRIPS and other multilateral trade agreements extends beyond its power, under Art. X, to amend these agreements and its authority, under Art. IX(2), to formally interpret them.

109. The Vienna Convention on the Law of Treaties, with annex, UNGA UN Doc. A/Conf, 39/27, May 23, 1969.

110. Id. Art. 31(3)(a).

111. Id. Art. 31(3)(b).

112. Id. Art. 31(3).

113. Id. Art. 31 (1).

114. See generally Charnovitz, supra note 107.

115. This power, of course, is subject to the unlikely possibility of the appellate body's being overruled (or "not adopted") by consensus in the Dispute Settlement Body within 30 days of circulation of the appellate body report. Understanding on Rules and Procedures Governing the Settlement of Disputes, supra n. 5, Art. 17(14).

116. Jackson, supra note 5, at 124–127.

117. Understanding on Rules and Procedures Governing the Settlement of Disputes, supra n. 5, Art. 8.

118. A classic example is the National Labor Relations Board. This awkward mingling of rule orientation and responsiveness to political currents raises nettlesome legitimacy questions, beyond our scope here. These questions are even more difficult for the WTO than for domestic administrative agencies, owing to (i) the contractual nature of member states' commitments to the WTO and its associated treaties, and (ii) the absence of any international institutional or constitutional system, analogous to legislative oversight and presidential supervision of administrative agencies, by which WTO decision makers can be held to account for the balances they strike between trade concerns and other public values. For a discussion of these problems and some ideas about how to ameliorate them, see Robert L. Howse and Kalypso Nicolaidis, "Legitimacy and Global Governance: Why Constitutionalizing the WTO Is a Step Too Far," in

R. B. Porter et al. eds., Efficiency, Equity, and Legitimacy: The Multilateral Trading System at the Millennium (Washington, DC: Brooking Institution Press, 2001): 227–252.

119. The Declaration on the TRIPS Agreement and Public Health is illustrative. The Ministerial Conference reached agreement only after the United States dropped its efforts to obtain language portraying pharmaceutical firms' intellectual property rights more expansively. Gary G. Yerkev and Daniel Pruzin, "Agreement on TRIPS/Public Health Reached at WTO Ministerial in Doha," BNA International Trade Report 18 (November 15, 2001): 1817–1819. Some developing nations had threatened to hold up the issuance of another ministerial statement, launching a new Doha round of trade talks (a high priority for the United States and other industrialized countries), unless the United States compromised on TRIPS. Daniel Pruzin, "Global Drug Industry Association Blasts 'Nutty' WTO Text on TRIPS, Public Health," BNA International Trade Report 18 (November 8, 2001): 1782–1783; EC-Hormones, supra note 55, is also illustrative. Although the United States prevailed, it did so on narrow grounds, with the appellate body endorsing a more deferential approach to member states' health risk assessment under the SPS than the United States had urged. See supra, text accompanying notes 57–69.

120. See National Foreign Intelligence Board, Global Trends 2015: A Dialogue about the Future with Nongovernment Experts (Washington, DC: National Intelligence Council, 2000) (warning that AIDS and other health crises undermine development of effective economic and political institutions and aggravate domestic and international conflicts); Jordan S. Kassalow, Why Health Is Important to U.S. Foreign Policy (Washington, DC: Council on Foreign Relations & Milbank Memorial Fund, 2001) (urging that U.S. foreign policy work toward improving international health through a variety of economic and political means).

121. See George F. Loewenstein et al., "Risk as Feelings," Psychology Bulletin 127 (2001): 267–286 (arguing, based on review of empirical literature, that people's beliefs and decisions concerning risk often vary from those predicted by expected utility and rational choice theory); see also M. Gregg Bloche, "The Invention of Health Law," California Law Review 91 (2003) 247–322 (weighing legal and policy implications of subjectivity and variation in perceptions of health and medical risk).

122. See Bloche, supra note 120 (discussing obstacles to pursuit of systematic rationality in health policy).

123. See Stephen Breyer, Breaking the Vicious Circle: Toward Effective Risk Regulation (Cambridge, MA: Harvard University Press, 1993) (offering proposals for more expeditious pursuit of systemic rationality in U.S. risk regulation and arguing that visible striving toward this goal, by highly competent federal authorities, would enhance the actual and perceived legitimacy of regulatory governance).

124. There is an analogy here to the contention that international criminal tribunals for human rights abusers are problematic because their interpretations of law are not nested in a single, national legal and political culture, as are rulings by domestic criminal courts.

125. Indian Constitution of 1950, Art. 37.

126. Id.

127. Olga Tellis v. Bombay Municipal Corp., A.I.R. (Bom.) 1996.

128. Id. at paras. 32–33. The Court opined that "[T]he State may not, by affirmative action, be compellable to provide adequate means of livelihood or work to the citizens," but "any person, who is deprived of his right to livelihood except according to just and fair procedure established by law, can challenge the deprivation as offending the right to life. . . ." Id. at para. 33.

129. GATS Art. XIX calls for progressive rounds of negotiation over liberalization of trade in services. The Ministerial Conference in Doha set out a "Work Programme" calling for a round of such talks, leading to an exchange of trade liberalization commitments. Ministerial Declaration, Ministerial Conference, 4th Session, Doha November 9, 2001, WT/MIN(01)/DEC/1 para. 15 (November 20, 2001). Hospital management services, competition between the private and public sectors in health care, managed health care, and other medical insurance products are among the activities and ventures that fall within the GATS. See Debra J. Lipson, "The World Trade Organization's Health Agenda," British Medical Journal 323 (2001) 1139–1140, warning that liberalized trade in health services, pursuant to GATS, could reduce poor people's access to care.

130. Indeed, at Doha, the Ministerial Conference explicitly declined to recognize such a right. A draft ministerial declaration proposed by a group of developing countries called for the Conference to present its TRIPS pronouncements as, in part, a "discharging" of "the obligation to protect and promote the fundamental human rights to life and the enjoyment of the highest attainable standard of physical and mental health, including the prevention, treatment and control of epidemic, endemic, occupational and other diseases and the creation of conditions which would assure to all medical service and medical attention in the event of sickness, as affirmed in the International Covenant on Economic, Social and Cultural Rights." TRIPS: Proposal: Draft Ministerial Declaration: Proposal from a Group of Developing Countries, IP/C/W/312, WT/GC/W/450, October 4, 2001 (01–4803), http://www.wto.org/english/tratop_e/trips~_e/mindecdraft_ w312_e.htm (visited February 11, 2002). The Ministerial Conference did not include such a statement in its declaration on TRIPS.

131. For some, this idea is an oxymoron: many hold that there is no such thing as a right without a legal remedy. We are of the view that the idea of a nonjusticiable right can make pragmatic sense, but consideration of this complex jurisprudential question is beyond our scope here.

Chapter 16

Promoting Public Health in the Twenty-First Century: The Role of the World Health Organization

Ruth Bonita, Alec Irwin, and Robert Beaglehole

In memory of
Dr. Lee Jong-wook
April 12, 1945–May 22, 2006

The World Health Organization (WHO), a specialized agency of the United Nations, is the leading global health agency. WHO's constitution defines health as "a state of complete physical, mental and social well-being and not merely the absence of illness or infirmity," and it identifies WHO's objective as "the attainment by all peoples of the highest possible level of health" (WHO 1946). This broad concept of health and the vocation to serve all peoples equitably point to the challenges WHO confronts. Public health is increasingly shaped by global processes and international cooperation in health is more vital than ever before.

One of the paradoxes of globalization is that an increasingly interconnected and interdependent world is simultaneously marked by widening health gaps between privileged and less advantaged groups, both between and within countries (WHO 2003a). Ambitious development and health objectives, most prominently the Millennium Development Goals (MDGs), have been set by the global community

to promote a fairer distribution of the benefits of progress. But gains toward the targets are too slow, particularly in the countries with the greatest needs. "Old" diseases continue to inflict avoidable suffering and death, while the HIV/AIDS pandemic eludes control, and new health threats loom on the horizon. To assess WHO's capacity to lead in meeting these challenges, in this chapter we begin by recapping key stages of WHO's history. We then rapidly survey the current state of global public health. Finally, we explore strategic directions set by WHO's current leadership to respond and help shape a healthier, more equitable future for all. Globalization is an irreversible reality. But the character and consequences of that reality are not set in stone. The speed and distribution of health progress in the twenty-first century will be influenced by how effectively the international community uses institutions of democratic cooperation such as WHO. This in turn will influence the *kind* of globalized world future generations inhabit.

ORIGINS AND HISTORY

A historical perspective is helpful to understand both WHO's constraints and its unique strengths. The conceptual and institutional foundations of WHO were laid, along with those of other United Nations agencies, at the close of the Second World War. Like the United Nations itself, WHO is a product of the fact that globalization was underway long before the term was coined. Indeed, WHO's 1946 constitution was the culmination of more than a century of efforts to provide concerted action, for example, through the International Sanitary Conventions, against the spread of diseases associated with expanding international trade, colonization, and mobility of populations (Burci and Vignes 2004). To this was added in the late 1940s the moral aspirations of a world chastened by two catastrophic world wars and inspired by the conviction that equitable progress in health would help assure future peace (WHO 1997).

The WHO constitution, originally signed by 61 countries and now subscribed to by 192 member states, became the legal framework for the activities of WHO. The constitution's famous multidimensional definition of health and the universality of the stated mission served a twofold purpose: to establish the principle of a fundamental right to health services and to embed this right within a social agenda aimed at guaranteeing the necessary basic conditions for human flourishing (Burci and Vignes 2004).

Present in WHO's founding document are thus both an optimistic view of what health services can achieve and a recognition of the social and political dimensions of health. The constitution affirms that "Governments have a responsibility for the health of their peoples which can be fulfilled only by the provision of adequate health and social measures." It stipulates that WHO's core functions include supporting health-promoting actions in such social fields as "nutrition, housing, sanitation, recreation, economic or working conditions and other aspects of environmental hygiene" (WHO 1946). The interplay between the scientific and social-political dimensions of WHO's agenda, and the relative weight assigned to each at different periods, helped shape WHO's evolution.

The view that science and technology could solve the world's problems was prevalent in WHO's early years, a time that can be characterized as a strongly vocational phase (Sartorius N. Personal communication, 2004). The top priorities at the outset were malaria, maternal and child health, tuberculosis, venereal diseases, nutrition, and environmental sanitation (Burci and Vignes 2004). This period was followed by mass campaigns against tuberculosis, smallpox, malaria, and yaws, the so-called militaristic period.[1] With the successful eradication of yaws and smallpox in the 1970s, WHO's reputation reached its peak.

Concern with the social and economic context of health and health care reasserted itself in the Health for All movement, launched at the 1978 International Conference on Primary Health Care in Alma-Ata, Kazakhstan. The Declaration of Alma-Ata denounced health inequalities between and within countries, stressed that equitable health improvement would require "the action of many other social and economic sectors, in addition to the health sector," and argued for the strengthening of primary health care (PHC) as the key to reaching Health for All by the year 2000 (International Conference on Primary Health Care 1978).

The Declaration of Alma-Ata articulated a compelling vision, but in the 1980s and 1990s, despite important advances in some countries, action to achieve its bold objectives generally fell far short. The halting progress toward Health for All had much to do with global political and economic changes to which WHO was slow to respond convincingly. Most important was the rise of economic neo-liberalism, with its emphasis on privatization, deregulation, shrinking the public sector, and freeing markets. Government involvement in many fields, including health, was to be reduced, in favor of the private sector and the efficiencies ostensibly generated by the free play of market forces. Neo-liberal theory presented this as the best path to economic growth, poverty reduction, and health improvement (Hofrichter 2003; Kim et al. 2000; Navarro 2004).

Throughout the 1980s and early 1990s, international financial institutions espousing neo-liberal principles, most prominently the World Bank and International Monetary Fund, encouraged numerous developing countries to undertake structural adjustment programs, often involving drastic cuts in public sector spending, including for health. The neo-liberal economic paradigm and related health sector reform processes drove a far-reaching reconfiguration of the health sector in many countries. WHO's leadership struggled to find its bearings in this new context, and WHO's credibility suffered. By the mid 1990s, despite innovative work by groups such as the WHO-sponsored Task Force on Health in Development,

WHO appeared disengaged and relatively powerless to influence global processes affecting health. With the publication of the World Bank's landmark *World Development Report 1993: Investing in Health*, global leadership in health policy seemed to have passed from WHO to institutions such as the World Bank (1993).

With the arrival of Gro Harlam Brundtland as Director-General in 1998, a period of strategic thinking and reform took place, which helped to restore WHO's credibility. During Brundtland's five-year term, the evidence base for public health actions was strengthened, health attained new prominence in international development agendas, linkages between health and human rights were clarified, and gender and human rights perspectives were firmly integrated into WHO strategies for country support. Intensified partnership-building efforts initiated or strengthened collaborative relations with a variety of global health actors (box 16.1). Broad strategic directions were established for the General Programme of Work (box 16.2). Of particular significance, WHO established itself at the forefront of international tobacco control efforts by confronting the tobacco industry. The stage was set for the first public health treaty developed by WHO, the Framework Convention on Tobacco Control (see chapter 3).

Box 16.1 – WHO and Other Global Health Actors

No institution can hope to resolve global health problems single-handedly. In a complex landscape, WHO's effectiveness depends increasingly on WHO's ability to build strong partnerships. While the number and prominence of partnerships have increased dramatically in the last decade, cooperation with other actors has been important throughout WHO's history.

Most fundamental is WHO's relationship to the United Nations. WHO is a specialized technical agency of the United Nations system. The United Nations Secretary-General is the formal depositary of the WHO constitution, which is similar in most respects to the constitutions of other United Nations bodies, with its commitment to the fundamental principle of "one member state, one vote." However, WHO also maintains considerable autonomy vis-à-vis the United Nations. A country can belong to WHO without being a United Nations member, as Switzerland did from 1947 to 2002 (Burci and Vignes 2004).

WHO collaborates closely with other United Nations agencies, such as the United Nations Development Programme and the United Nations Children's Fund (UNICEF), on policy issues and specific health-related projects, for example, vaccination programs. Historically, WHO's relationship with UNICEF has been particularly close, given the latter's concern with the health of children and mothers. WHO and UNICEF cosponsored the landmark 1978 International Conference on Primary Health Care at Alma-Ata. WHO, other United Nations organizations and the World Bank are cosponsors of the United Nations Joint Programme on HIV/AIDS (UNAIDS). Within UNAIDS, WHO is responsible for leading the health sector response to the pandemic.

WHO's regional structure is unique among United Nations agencies. Important regional health organizations predated WHO's creation and were incorporated into the new body, while maintaining some of their specificities. The most important case is that of the Pan American Health Organization. Created as the Pan American Sanitary Organization in 1902, this body began to serve as the WHO Regional Office for the Americas in 1949 but has continued to exercise a high degree of autonomy (Burci and Vignes 2004).

While differences between WHO's positions and those advocated by the World Bank have been apparent on a number of health and development issues, the two agencies have also shown the ability to work together, for example, within the framework of the Special Programme for Research and Training in Tropical Diseases and the Global Alliance for Vaccines and Immunization (GAVI), of which both are cosponsors, or in the coordination of efforts to fight HIV, involving cooperation between WHO's 3-by-5 campaign and the World Bank's Multi-country AIDS Programme. Currently, the two agencies are working with other partners to coordinate global support for the health-related MDGs through the High Level Forum.

WHO also works with the World Trade Organization (WTO) in areas where trade policies may influence health, for example, intellectual property rights and access to medicines and the health implications of the General Agreement on Trade in Services (see WHO/WTO 2002). How far consensus and collaboration between the organizations can extend remains to be seen; however, the 2001 Doha Declaration on the Agreement on Trade-Related Aspects of Intellectual Property Rights and Public Health created an important foundation by reaffirming the priority of public health concerns in the formulation and application of trade policy.

Among WHO's other important relationships are those with civil society organizations and with the private sector. The late 1990s and early years of the subsequent decade saw WHO involved in a proliferation of public–private partnerships in health, including GAVI and the Medicines for Malaria Venture.

Box 16.2 – Four Basic Strategic Directions for WHO

- Reducing excess mortality, morbidity, and disability, especially in poor and marginalized populations
- Promoting healthy lifestyles and reducing risk factors for human health that arise from environmental, economic, social, and behavioral causes
- Developing health systems that equitably improve health outcomes, respond to people's legitimate demands, and are financially fair
- Framing an enabling policy and creating an institutional environment for the health sector and promoting an effective health dimension to social, economic, environmental, and development policy

Source: WHO (1999).

A key element in Brundtland's effort to reposition WHO was the Commission on Macroeconomics and Health (CMH). In its December 2001 report, the CMH calculated the global economic costs of ill health in developing countries and argued for increased investment in health as a key development input (WHO 2001). The CMH showed that health improvements in poor countries and communities, in addition to their intrinsic value, would accelerate economic growth and generate significant gains for the global economy. By quantifying the importance of health for global economic performance, the CMH helped reposition health as a decisive development issue and restored WHO's credibility as an actor in the new global economic and political environment. However, critical voices strongly challenged the emphasis on health as a means to the end of economic development, rather than an end in itself (Banerji 2002; Waitzkin 2003).

The latest WHO administration, led by Jong-Wook Lee, took office in July 2003. Lee has strongly reasserted the connection between health, equity, and social justice as fundamental for WHO (Lee 2004). The new administration seeks to build on the improved policy credibility achieved during the Brundtland years, while firmly reorienting WHO to the moral compass of the constitution and the vision of health and social justice affirmed at Alma-Ata. Thus, the emphasis is on country-level outcomes, accountability to member states, equitable health progress as a prerequisite for collective "peace and security," and a balance between strengthening health care services and working with partners to address the broader social and political dimensions of health. The overarching ambition is to intensify WHO's work on health inequities and strengthen health systems to deliver essential and effective interventions, especially to poor and marginalized populations (Lancet 2004) at the same time as fulfilling the core functions for WHO (box 16.3).

Box 16.3 – Six Core Functions for WHO

- Articulating consistent, ethical, and evidence-based policy and advocacy positions
- Managing information by assessing trends and comparing performance, setting the agenda for and stimulating research and development
- Catalyzing change through technical and policy support in ways that stimulate cooperation and action to help build sustainable national and inter-country capacity
- Negotiating and sustaining national and global partnerships
- Setting, validating, monitoring, and pursuing the proper implementation of norms and standards
- Stimulating the development and testing of new technologies, tools, and guidelines for disease control, risk reduction, health care management, and service delivery

---

In the remainder of this chapter, we explore today's major health challenges and consider whether the new approach to WHO's work can influence the global public health agenda and improve health, especially for the most vulnerable.

THE STATE OF GLOBAL
PUBLIC HEALTH

While aggregate global health indicators have improved substantially since the middle of the last century, the gross health inequalities highlighted in 1978 by the Declaration of Alma-Ata persist. Indeed, the gaps are widening between the world's poorest people and those better placed to benefit from economic development and public health progress. Over the last 50 years, average life expectancy at birth has increased globally by almost 20 years, from 46.5 years in 1950–1955 to 65.2 years in 2002. The large life expectancy gap between developed and developing countries in the 1950s has changed to a gap between the very poorest developing countries and all other countries. Thus, life expectancy at birth in 2004 ranged from 86 years for women in developed countries to less than 37 years for men in sub-Saharan Africa, a more than two-fold difference in total life expectancy. By contrast, the life expectancy of the Chinese population increased to 71 years in 2002, and this largely contributed to the overall outstanding performance of the low mortality in developing countries.

Of the 59 million deaths in 2005, 10.5 million were among children younger than five years of age, and more than 98% of these were in developing countries. Globally, considerable progress has been made since 1970, when over 17 million child deaths occurred. In 14 African countries, however, current levels of child mortality are higher than they were in 1990. Overall, 35% of Africa's children are at higher risk of death today than they were 10 years ago. Across the world, children are at higher risk of dying if they are poor and malnourished, and the gaps in child mortality between the haves and the have-nots are widening in many regions. Despite the progress in improving child survival, available interventions, if applied equitably, have the potential to dramatically reduce the number of childhood deaths to about 1 million. The continuing inability of national and global health agencies to ensure that these interventions reach the children in the poorest countries indicates the need for WHO and its partners to work more vigorously in this area.

Closely related to the challenge of reducing child survival is the continuing problem of unacceptably high maternal mortality rates in many poor countries. Although responsible for only about 1% of global mortality, almost all of the 500,000 deaths that occur each year could be readily prevented if all women of the world had access to basic maternal services that are taken for granted in most middle- and high-income countries. Of course, maternal mortality is also closely entwined with the more fundamental issues of female literacy and human rights more generally.

An overview of the state of adult health at the beginning of the twenty-first century is characterized by two major trends: slowing of gains and widening health gaps and the increasing complexity of the burden of disease. The most disturbing sign of deteriorating adult health is that adult mortality in Africa has reversed so drastically that, in parts of sub-Saharan Africa, current adult mortality rates today exceed those of thirty years ago. The most important immediate cause of the reversal is the HIV/AIDS pandemic. Worldwide in 2002, despite trends of overall declining communicable disease burden among adults, HIV/AIDS was the leading cause of mortality and the single most important contributor to the burden of disease among adults 15–59 years of age. In many countries in sub-Saharan Africa, the effects of HIV/AIDS are overwhelming already weakened health systems and threatening the very survival of some societies.

Although minor from the perspectives of mortality or burden, the outbreak of SARS in early 2003 reminded the world of the shared vulnerability to new infections (WHO 2003a; Lancet 2003). It also highlighted the weakened state of essential public health services, not only in Asia but also in several wealthy countries such as Canada. In addition to approximately 8,000 cases and more than 900 deaths, SARS caused serious economic damage.[2] Such effects show the importance that a severe new disease can assume in a closely interdependent and highly mobile world. While SARS was the first major lethal infection to emerge in the twenty-first century, it will not be the last, as witnessed by the concern over avian influenza in 2005–2006.

Alongside the threat of new infections, the growing burden of chronic noncommunicable diseases (NCDs) in developing countries looms as a major health challenge. Even very poor countries will increasingly have to grapple with the "double burden" of NCDs on top of persistent infectious epidemics. Already, almost 50% of the adult disease burden in the highest mortality regions of the world is attributable to NCDs. Twice as many deaths from cardiovascular disease (CVD) now occur in developing countries as in developed countries. Overall, in developing countries, injuries, neuropsychiatric disorders, and CVD are the top three contributors to overall disease burden (WHO 2003a).

AREAS FOR URGENT ACTION

Faced with this array of challenges, WHO has targeted several areas for urgent action—judging that the consequences of delay in these fields would be especially destructive. Accelerating a comprehensive global response to HIV/AIDS is one objective and includes rapid scale-up of antiretroviral HIV/AIDS treatment in developing countries. Another priority is spurring progress toward the health-related MDGs. It is also likely that WHO will intensify its attention to the chronic NCD agenda, in recognition of the global burden of these conditions.

The millions of deaths caused by HIV/AIDS in the last decades of the twentieth century could be dwarfed by the pandemic's toll in the twenty-first— unless bold action is taken to halt the spread of the virus and prolong the lives of those already infected. A comprehensive attack on HIV/AIDS involves multiple dimensions, including prevention, treatment, care, and support for people living with HIV/AIDS, their families, and communities. These dimensions are interrelated and mutually supporting. In developing countries, for many years treatment was the most seriously neglected component of the comprehensive strategy. By mid 2003, of the estimated 6 million people in urgent need of antiretroviral treatment for HIV/AIDS in developing countries, only 400,000, or about 7%, had access to it (WHO 2004a). In September 2003, to focus attention on this situation and spur action, WHO, UNAIDS, and the Global Fund to Fight AIDS, Tuberculosis, and Malaria joined forces to declare lack of access to antiretroviral HIV/AIDS therapy in developing countries a global health emergency. WHO and its partners committed themselves to the "3 by 5" target: providing 3 million people in developing regions with antiretroviral treatment by the end of 2005. Although this target was not reached, it generated considerable momentum. The goal now is universal access to anti-retroviral drugs.

WHO's approach to expanding HIV/AIDS treatment embodies a major shift in its way of working. The changes have reached far beyond the 3 by 5 target. They mark a reaffirmation of core WHO values and a commitment to intensified action to confront the most urgent health challenges of poor and vulnerable communities. Fundamentally, WHO has embraced AIDS treatment scale-up as a question of justice. Millions of people in the developing world face death from an illness that is routinely and effectively treated in high-income countries. The moral case is clear: we cannot accept the idea that these people are "too poor to treat" (Castro and Farmer 2003). Committing to a highly ambitious, time-bound target (3 by 5) was seen to be the best way to focus the international spotlight on the AIDS treatment gap, energize the communities already working on this issue, and mobilize new partners and fresh resources.

HIV/AIDS has so far inflicted its greatest toll on some of the world's poorest and most fragile countries and communities, particularly in sub-Saharan Africa. By weakening and then killing prime-age adults— women and men in the midst of their active years of work and parenting—the pandemic has a devastating effect on economic productivity, family structures, educational opportunities for younger generations, and the transmission of knowledge and skills. Studies have shown the crippling impact of HIV/AIDS on knowledge transmission and human capital formation in key sectors such as agriculture (De Waal and Whiteside 2003). Drawing on these insights, recent analyses have suggested that earlier calculations seriously underestimated the long-term economic and social damage of HIV/AIDS on high-burden countries. Emergency action to tackle the pandemic including the rapid scale-up of antiretroviral treatment is vital to save some of the world's poorest and most vulnerable countries and communities from economic implosion and social collapse (Bell et al. 2003)

WHO's commitment to a stronger leadership role in HIV/AIDS reflects its responsibility to provide balanced guidance on health sector investment and priority setting. To be credible, WHO has to be engaged and technically strong in those sectors to which the global community is in fact channeling health investment. By far the greatest share of new resources flowing into global health at the time 3 by 5 was launched were being committed to HIV/AIDS work. WHO has a responsibility to ensure that countries have the normative and technical support they need to get the best use out of these new resources (World Health Bulletin 2004).

Most important, it is vital that investment in AIDS treatment scale-up support the broader strengthening of national health systems, for example, through innovative action to address critical human resource shortages (Kober and Van Damme 2004). WHO's commitment is to help countries respond to the HIV/AIDS emergency in a manner which will not deprive other health programs of essential resources and energy, but instead enable a long-term strengthening of health infrastructure. Rolling out antiretroviral treatment presents a tremendous challenge to the health systems of countries heavily burdened by HIV/AIDS; in many countries, systems are drastically underfunded, poorly run, and barely functional. Some critics object that attempting a comprehensive response to HIV/AIDS in these settings will divert resources and weaken systems further. However, scaling up antiretroviral therapy has the potential to strengthen key components of the health system in low-income countries by increasing investment in physical infrastructure, reinforcing drug procurement and distribution systems, catalyzing the recruitment and training of new health workers, improving compensation and motivation among the health work force, and creating capacities for the delivery of chronic care which may then be applied to other disease challenges. Examples from Thailand and Haiti show how HIV/AIDS treatment scale-up can combine with and support the strengthening of PHC (WHO 2004a; World Health Bulletin 2004). In any case, in the hardest hit countries, the assault of HIV/AIDS has already pushed health systems to the edge of disintegration. A comprehensive response to the disease is vital if these systems are to be saved from collapse.

The HIV/AIDS fight is a test for new work patterns at WHO and new forms of cooperation across the global health community. There is a sense of urgency, clear goal setting, and intensified cooperation with countries. Resources have been channeled away from headquarters and into on-the-ground action in regions and countries. Early 2004 saw large numbers of HIV department staff members based at WHO's Geneva headquarters redeployed to country level to engage with national health officials and partners and accelerate the response to country needs. Deployed WHO staff worked with national partners in preparing applications to the Global Fund, addressing technical issues in drug procurement and management, designing national antiretroviral therapy scale-up plans, and other key activities.

Partnership has been key to progress in expanding a comprehensive response to HIV/AIDS. To drive rapid scale-up of antiretroviral therapy in the hardest

hit areas, WHO's HIV department constituted a partners group with membership from governments, international organizations, donors, the private sector, the academic community, nongovernmental organizations (NGOs), and community-based organizations, centrally including groups of people living with HIV/AIDS. The partners group's input has been decisive in orienting WHO's HIV/AIDS strategy. In relation to other international and bilateral agencies, efforts have been made to move beyond familiar tensions over turf toward real openness and a shared pragmatic focus on results. The effects of this new approach will remain as a legacy beyond December 2005. Creative international collaboration will continue to be vital in addressing such issues as the health workforce crisis, cited by many sub-Saharan African countries as their greatest obstacle in tackling HIV/AIDS (Kober and Van Damme 2004).

MULTISECTORAL ACTION FOR HEALTH AND DEVELOPMENT: THE MDGS

Success in comprehensive HIV/AIDS control, including access to treatment, will bring benefits across many sectors of health and development. In countries with high HIV burdens, many of them in sub-Saharan Africa, HIV/AIDS is currently blocking progress not only on goal 6 (combating the major infectious diseases) but also on many of the other MDGs (box 16.4). Thus, AIDS treatment scale-up is closely joined to another prime objective for WHO: cooperation with countries to achieve the health-related MDGs.

The eight MDGs are linked to quantitative targets to be reached by 2015. Many of the MDG objectives were first set out by international conferences and summits held in the 1990s. They were later compiled and became known as the International Development Goals. In September 2000, United Nations member states unanimously adopted the Millennium Declaration. Following consultations among international agencies, including the World Bank, the International Monetary Fund, the Organization for Economic Cooperation and Development, and the specialized agencies of the United Nations, the United Nations General Assembly recognized the MDGs as part of the road map for implementing the Millennium Declaration.

Box 16.4 – The Impact of HIV/AIDS on the MDGs

HIV/AIDS epidemics undermine poverty reduction efforts by sapping economic growth, thus hampering efforts to reach goal 1, eradicating extreme poverty and hunger. HIV/AIDS has cut annual growth rates by 2–4% per year in some high-burden countries in Africa. The pandemic has decimated the agricultural workforce in some areas and interrupted the transmission of vital agricultural skills, thus entwining with the effects of drought to increase vulnerability to hunger in parts of sub-Saharan Africa (De Waal and Whiteside 2003). HIV/AIDS cuts family incomes and forces people to spend money on medical care and funerals, thus reducing educational opportunities and the chances of reaching goal 2, universal primary education. In Zambia, the number of teachers killed by AIDS in 1998 was equivalent to two-thirds of the number of teachers trained in the same year (United Nations Children's Fund 2000). Millions of orphans created by HIV/AIDS have even fewer educational opportunities. Goal 3, gender equity and women's empowerment, is undermined because HIV/AIDS disproportionately adds to the caregiving burdens of women and girls, reducing their chances of pursuing education and paid work. HIV-positive women face many forms of discrimination and psychological and physical abuse. Goal 4, to reduce child mortality, and goal 5, to reduce maternal mortality, are both under threat, particularly in the seven African countries with the highest adult HIV prevalence, where AIDS has resulted in a 36% rise in under-five mortality. In Uganda, maternal mortality was five times higher among HIV-positive women than among HIV-negative women (Sewankambo et al. 2000). The pandemic also adversely affects the chances of contending with malaria and tuberculosis as part of goal 6, to combat HIV/AIDS, malaria, and other diseases. People living with HIV/AIDS are seven times more likely to develop tuberculosis than are those who are not infected with the virus HIV infection (Glynn et al. 1997). There is some evidence that HIV-infected women are more likely to develop malaria during pregnancy than are HIV-negative women, and mother-to-child HIV transmission rates were more than twice as high among women with placental malaria compared with women without malaria (Brahmbhatta et al. 2003). Goal 7, ensuring environmental stability, includes the target to have achieved "a significant improvement in the lives of at least 100 million slum dwellers" by 2020. As HIV/AIDS spreads suffering and death in some slum areas, it further weakens already fragile local economies, social capital, and educational opportunities, making this target more remote. All goals depend on goal 8, developing an equitable global partnership for development. HIV/AIDS constrains development progress in hard-hit countries, for example, through its decimation of countries' skilled workforces. Meanwhile, wealthy countries' slowness to respond seriously questions the credibility of their commitment to a new development compact.

Source: WHO (2004a).

The force of the MDGs stems from their multisectoral breadth. The eight goals embrace: poverty and hunger, education, gender inequality, child mortality, maternal mortality, HIV/AIDS and other major infectious diseases, environmental sustainability, and the need for global partnership in development. While three goals are explicitly health focused, all have strong links to health. Accordingly, WHO has embraced the MDGs as a main direction of WHO's work through 2015. The MDGs offer a chance to underscore the close linkages between health and other development priorities and to address health and development through coordinated multisectoral action.

The MDGs emphasize reciprocal obligations between high-income and developing countries. In return for developing countries' adopting the MDGs as priorities in their domestic agenda, goal 8 encourages wealthy countries to support developing countries by respecting the rules of fair trade and by providing development assistance, debt relief, access to essential medicines, and technology transfer. In this sense the MDGs are a mutually reinforcing framework contributing interactively to human development (Haines and Cassels 2004). They hold to account the authorities responsible for providing health services, and they help define the role of health in development. At the same time, the MDGs provide a focus for governments planning poverty reduction strategies and the budgets required to achieve these. By setting quantitative targets and encouraging steady monitoring of progress, the MDGs maintain awareness of the urgent need for action.

Major changes are needed if the MDGs are to be achieved. The most stubborn problem remains the shortfall in financial resources (Lee et al. 2004). Halfway between the baseline year (1990) and the outcome year (2015), many countries are already falling behind the required performance levels, particularly in lowering child and maternal mortality. In developing countries the average annual reduction rate of under-five mortality was only 2.4% during the 1990s, well short of the MDG target of 4.2% (World Bank/WHO 2004); in many countries, this rate improved little after 2000. Indeed, in sixteen countries in Africa, mortality rates for children under five years have been *rising*, not falling (WHO 2003b). One estimate suggests that, if current patterns continue, sub-Saharan Africa will not reach the poverty MDG until 2047, nor the target for child mortality until 2165 (UNDP 2003). The creation of an international finance facility has recently been proposed, which would provide a framework to increase aid from US$50 billion in 2001 to US$100 billion annually in the years until 2015. This would significantly accelerate gains toward the MDGs (Lee et al. 2004).

One of the challenges raised by the MDGs is measuring progress. Sound information is essential for tracking progress, evaluating impact, and attributing changes to different interventions, as well as for guiding decisions on program scope and focus (Haines and Cassels 2004). WHO has a key role in coordinating health information systems at country level. However, the task is often complicated by the presence of a plethora of development partners, many of whom impose their own monitoring systems on countries, duplicating work and stretching scarce human and financial resources.

Although the MDGs are assuming increasing importance for many international organizations, development agencies, and governments, there are some criticisms that the health MDGs are at once too narrow and too broad. On the narrow side, the MDGs ignore chronic NCDs. On the side of excessive breadth, many MDG targets are formulated in terms of averages across the total population. Thus, analysts have been able to show that it would be mathematically possible for countries to achieve key MDGs by making improvements primarily for the wealthiest population quintiles, leaving the needs of the poorest unaddressed (Gwatkin 2002). WHO aims to support countries in fulfilling the spirit as well as the letter of the MDG commitment—this means ensuring poor and vulnerable social groups do not lose out. In general, WHO sees the MDG process as a chance to reaffirm WHO's fundamental commitment to measurable health improvements in countries, including for

NCDs, based on objectives member states themselves endorse and own. With WHO's resources increasingly shifting from Geneva to regional and country offices, WHO is positioned to support countries' efforts toward the MDG targets and a wider set of country-relevant health goals. At the same time, through country cooperation strategies with an explicit equity component, WHO aims for deprived groups to share fully in the progress achieved.

THE GLOBAL BURDEN OF CHRONIC NCDS

The lack of attention to chronic NCDs in the MDG framework is out of step with key health trends. These diseases now represent the largest share of the total disease burden in all regions except sub-Saharan Africa (table 16.1). Unfortunately, the growing burden of chronic, NCDs has been relatively neglected by global policy makers, international health donors, national governments, nongovernmental agencies, academics, and civil society. Almost 50% of the adult disease burden in the high-mortality regions of the world is now attributable to chronic diseases; the majority of this burden is preventable on the basis of existing knowledge, with a few common risk factors explaining a large proportion of new chronic disease events (WHO 2002a). The challenge is to convert this knowledge into effective national prevention policies and program (WHO 2005).

Despite evidence of the magnitude of this burden, the preventability of its causes, and the threat it poses to already strained health care systems, national and global responses remain inadequate. Even within WHO, surveillance, prevention, and management of chronic diseases receive only a tiny proportion of WHO's total budget, although these conditions account for 60% of all deaths and 47% of the burden of disease (WHO 2005). The leading chronic diseases are CVD, especially coronary heart disease and stroke (17 million deaths); cancer (8 million deaths); chronic respiratory disease (3.5 million deaths); and diabetes (almost 1 million deaths). Mental health problems are leading contributors to the burden of disease in many countries and contribute significantly to the incidence and severity of many chronic diseases, including CVD and cancer.

Regional estimates indicate that only in Africa are communicable diseases more frequent as causes of

TABLE 16.1. Ten Leading Causes of Deaths, Globally and in Developed and Developing Countries: Estimates for 2002

Rank	Disease	% Total Deaths
World		
1	Ischemic heart disease	12.6
2	Cerebrovascular disease	9.7
3	Lower respiratory infections	6.6
4	HIV/AIDS	4.9
5	Chronic obstructive pulmonary disease	4.8
6	Perinatal conditions	4.3
7	Diarrheal diseases	3.2
8	Tuberculosis	2.7
9	Malaria	2.2
10	Trachea, bronchus, lung cancers	2.2
Developed Countries[a]		
1	*Ischemic heart disease*	*22.9*
2	*Cerebrovascular disease*	*13.3*
3	*Trachea, bronchus, lung cancers*	*4.5*
4	*Lower respiratory infections*	*3.4*
5	*Chronic obstructive pulmonary disease*	*3.1*
6	*Colon and rectum cancers*	*2.6*
7	*Diabetes mellitus*	*1.8*
8	*Stomach cancer*	*1.7*
9	*Other self-inflicted injuries*	*1.7*
10	*Breast cancer*	*1.7*
Developing Countries		
1	*Ischemic heart disease*	*9.5*
2	*Cerebrovascular disease*	*8.5*
3	*Lower respiratory infections*	*7.9*
4	*HIV/AIDS*	*6.3*
5	*Perinatal conditions*	*5.5*
6	*Chronic obstructive pulmonary disease*	*5.3*
7	*Diarrheal diseases*	*4.1*
8	*Tuberculosis*	*3.4*
9	*Malaria*	*2.9*
10	Road traffic accidents	*2.3*

[a]Developed countries are European countries, former Soviet countries, Canada, United States, Japan, Australia, and New Zealand.

Source: World Health Organization, internal data

death than are chronic diseases, with 2.8 million CVD deaths in China and 2.6 million in India occurring each year. Chronic diseases also contribute significantly to adult mortality in central and eastern European countries.

Chronic diseases are an important contributor to health inequalities within and between countries and generally predominate among poor populations largely because of inequalities in the distribution of major chronic disease risk factors (Mackenbach et al. 2000; Leon and Walt 2001). It has been estimated that by 2030, heart attacks, stroke, and diabetes will together account for four in ten deaths among adult labor force (35–64 years) in low and middle income countries compared with one in eight deaths in the same age group in the United States and other wealthy countries (Leeder and Raymond 2004). This reinforces the need for a realignment of global public health programs, which have until now focused almost exclusively on longstanding campaigns to vaccinate children, improve child and maternal health, and staunch the toll of infectious diseases.

There are positive signs of attention to chronic disease, exemplified by the Framework Convention on Tobacco Control, which was adopted in 2003 by the World Health Assembly, signed by 168 countries and ratified by 120 countries. It was put into force on February 18, 2006, and, when implemented, will help to save millions of lives (see chapter 3).

Another facet of WHO's role in promoting the global public health agenda is illustrated by the development of the Global Strategy on Diet, Physical Activity and Health. This strategy was endorsed by the World Health Assembly in May 2004 after considerable international debate (WHO 2004b). The development of the strategy broadened the debate in the complex area of public health, nutrition, and food policy. The strategy aims to achieve optimal diets and increased physical activity for entire populations; this will involve broad-based partnerships and alliances as well as the use of incentives, in contrast to the binding international legislative approach required to achieve successful control of tobacco (Yach et al. 2004b). While there are a few areas of easy agreement such as promotion of consumption of fruits and vegetables and promotion of physical activity, major shifts in food production and marketing processes will also be needed. In particular, reduction of salt, sugar, and saturated fat levels in processed foods and changes in marketing strategies for cheap energy-dense, nutrition-poor foods may be more difficult to achieve and will require the active participation of the food industry (see also chapter 4).

The Global Strategy provides member states with a comprehensive range of policy options from which to choose and emphasizes that reducing the burden of disease requires partnership across sectors. The strategy suggests recommendations for action by all stakeholders—member states, United Nations agencies, NGOs, and the private sector. Key principles are proposed to guide the development of policies and strategies to address unhealthy diets and physical inactivity using the best available scientific evidence combined with comprehensive, multidisciplinary approaches.

The strategy sees governments assuming a steering role in changing the environment to improve the nutritional and physical activity patterns of their populations. It stresses the importance of building on existing structures and national mechanisms rather than creating new ones. It suggests that national legislation and appropriate infrastructure are critical in introducing effective policies. The main policy recommendations of the strategy are for countries to develop national dietary and physical activity guidelines; provide accurate and balanced information to consumers, in particular with regard to nutrition labeling and nutrition and health claims; and address issues related to marketing of foods, especially to children. The strategy recommends that countries review and evaluate their food and agriculture policies to be consistent with a healthy and adequate diet. The resources to implement this strategy have yet to be committed. A number of strategies are required to elevate chronic diseases on the international health agenda, including a recognition that the influence of global economic factors impedes progress, better data and better evidence of the impact of risk factor control, and a shift of orientation around health systems—from a focus on acute problems to one oriented toward managing chronic diseases (Yach et al. 2004a; WHO 2002b).

STRENGTHENING HEALTH SYSTEMS

Most countries will make only limited advances in population health in the years ahead without significant strengthening of their health care systems (WHO 2000a). Current health challenges mean that systems need to be able to integrate health promotion and disease prevention while providing treatment for acute and chronic illness. It is clear that in many low- and middle-income countries, the health-related MDG targets will not be attained, let alone sustained, in the absence of significant strengthening of health systems (Freedman et al. 2004). WHO's work toward specific targets such as the MDGs and 3 by 5 is being organized so as to drive a broad buildup of health care system capacities largely through the PHC approach.

To improve health care access and outcomes while narrowing equity gaps, health care systems based on the principles of PHC are again being emphasized, while taking into account the profound changes in the global health landscape since Alma-Ata (WHO 1998a, WHO 2003c). Enduring fundamental principles include a needs-based approach, community participation, recognition that intersectoral action is crucial to achieving substantial health gains among the most vulnerable populations, and prevention and treatment as complementary activities. WHO's cooperation with countries to strengthen health care systems is part of a broad strategic reconfiguration of WHO's work in measurement, evidence, and health systems analysis.

Health care systems in low- and middle-income countries face a wide array of challenges: the global health workforce crisis, the need for improved health information, sustainable financing, and the stewardship challenge of implementing pro-equity health policies in a complex and pluralistic environment (WHO 2003a). The health workforce crisis is an especially urgent concern, particularly in sub-Saharan Africa. The shortage of qualified personnel slows progress toward health targets and contributes directly to the HIV/AIDS treatment gap. In some instances, workforce constraints threaten to undermine the benefits of new financial resources and technologies being made available to the health sector (Kober and Van Damme 2004). While new workers must be trained in large numbers, it may also be possible to reactivate already trained health professionals who have left the field. For example, a WHO mission to Kenya in September 2003 found that around 4,000 nurses, 1,000 clinical officers, 2,000 laboratory staff, and 160 pharmacists or pharmacy technicians were unemployed in the country at that time. HIV/AIDS treatment scale-up and other health objectives can advance in the short term by enabling and encouraging such qualified people to reenter health work, even as longer term solutions are sought to address the wider structural issues underlying the workforce crisis (WHO 2003a).

Fundamental requirements for health care systems guided by PHC principles also include pro-equity financing and stewardship mechanisms that can ensure that quality health care services are accessible for the whole population, including poor and marginalized groups. National and local health care delivery needs are far more complex than at the time of Alma-Ata 25 years ago. But pro-equity, PHC-driven health systems development strategies offer hope for the future. The success of such strategies will be measured by results in countries. This is the fundamental indicator which will tell us that WHO is "getting it right."

GLOBAL HEALTH PARTNERSHIP

While WHO can play a key leadership role in promoting public health in the twenty-first century, WHO has no pretension of being able to achieve progress by acting alone. Processes such as expanding comprehensive action against HIV/AIDS have shown that collaboration among a broad range of partners will be necessary to meet the health objectives of the new century. On the other hand, simply forming a partnership is no guarantee that a given problem will be solved—especially when the partners include disparate actors (international organizations, national governments, civil society groups, and for-profit corporations) whose long-term interests and fundamental values may diverge. To be effective, partnership must rest on a precise delineation of respective roles and responsibilities and on a clear understanding of where commonalities among the actors begin and end.

At this time, there is an unprecedented opportunity for WHO and its partners to act together to achieve rapid and demonstrable progress. WHO's advocacy around the importance of health in development and the need for greater investment in global health has begun to bear fruit. Commitments in selected areas have drawn substantial new funding into the global health field: a planned US$15 billion over five years from the U.S. president's Emergency Plan for AIDS Relief; commitments of US$2 billion through mid-2004 to the Global Fund to Fight AIDS, Tuberculosis and Malaria; and US$1.4 billion from the Bill and Melinda Gates Foundation for global health programs, augmented by a further US$900

million for tuberculosis in 2006. These resources can "jump start" aggressive action in key health areas.

Still, current commitments in the health sector should be relativized against the US$1 trillion poured annually into global military budgets and the US$300 billion that rich countries pay each year in agricultural subsidies, to the detriment of developing nations. Development aid from almost all high-income countries remains far from the target of 0.7% of gross domestic product agreed at the Monterrey Summit in 2002, while combined health investment by most low-income countries and donors lags well below the levels the CMH calculated would be necessary for universal provision of a basic package of health care services (United Nations 2002; Lee 2004). WHO, with an annual budget of US$1.2 billion, struggles to fulfill its global health mandate and to meet the requests of member states and other partners for normative guidance and technical support. This means that WHO must continue and intensify its global advocacy role, emphasizing health strategically as a crucial development input and—most important—as one of the human ends toward which economic development itself is a means.

WHO's success in serving member states depends increasingly on collaboration with numerous national and international partners. However, WHO's participation in such processes must also be grounded in a clear set of values—those described in WHO's constitution and reaffirmed in documents such as the Declaration of Alma-Ata and the World Health Declaration signed by WHO's member states in 1998 (WHO 1998). The power of WHO's technical and scientific leadership is indissolubly linked to its moral credibility, which must be vigilantly maintained (Navarro 2004). This is a key part of WHO's "value added" in any partnership.

In particular, WHO must be both visionary and pragmatic in its commitment to "the ethical concepts of equity, solidarity and social justice" (WHO 1998). Addressing health equity means that WHO will have to be increasingly concerned with the way health systems can function as *redistributive* mechanisms, understanding "redistribution" broadly to mean "all social processes that create increasingly inclusive or egalitarian access to resources" (Mackintosh and Tibandebage 2004, cited in Freedman et al. 2004).

From a practical political standpoint, WHO will have to make the case convincingly that social justice, health equity, and increased inclusiveness will ultimately bring benefits *for all*, and not only for se-lected target populations (the poor, indigenous com-munities, HIV-positive Africans) who may be the first to gain from some redistributive processes. The WHO constitution warns that failure to respect some people's right to health may put the security of all at risk. "The health of all peoples is fundamental to the attainment of peace and security," whereas "[u]nequal develop-ment in different countries in the promotion of health and the control of disease . . . is a common danger" for humanity as a whole (WHO 1946). The connections between health and security, often separated in na-tional and international debates in the last decades of the twentieth century, are increasingly being recon-nected. This connection should further elevate health in the global development agenda.[3] The founding doc-uments of WHO and the United Nations provide guid-ance by underscoring that lasting security depends upon justice in the distribution of the goods and oppor-tunities people need to live a dignified life (Lee 2003).

Political implementation of redistributive reforms remains the defining challenge (Freedman et al. 2004). How can equity-oriented redistributive pro-cesses in health be achieved in a global context where market forces dominate and power is unequally shared among stakeholders (governments, multinational cor-porations, international organizations, donors, civil society)? National policy makers may have the best of intentions, but the real autonomy of political leaders and officials in developing countries is often severely constrained by resource shortfalls, debt loads, global economic patterns beyond the control of national pol-icy, and pressures from powerful international finan-cial institutions, donors, and the business sector. On the other hand, national elites in developing states can often position themselves to benefit from eco-nomic processes (e.g., privatization) that may nega-tively affect health and well-being for the majority of a country's population.

To fulfill its mission, WHO must be able to support countries in identifying, implementing, and sustain-ing policies to improve health and health equity in this complex political and economic environment. WHO has shown its commitment to grapple with these challenges through processes such as the Frame-work Convention on Tobacco Control; the ongoing work of numerous technical units, including those fo-cused on globalization and trade, poverty, health sys-tems, and the MDGs; and special instruments such as global commissions.

A commission on the social determinants of health, launched in 2005, constitutes one of WHO's important efforts in this direction. The commission is assembling and analyzing evidence on how factors such as social position, early-life conditions, housing, and working conditions affect people's health. Even more important, the commission will spearhead a po-litical process to drive change. It will identify policies that have successfully improved health and health eq-uity through action on the social determinants of health, particularly in developing countries, and it will work with decision makers and stakeholders in countries and the wider global health community to promote uptake of these successful models. The com-mission will spur WHO itself further in the integra-tion of priority-targeted programs (e.g., HIV/AIDS treatment scale-up), health systems strengthening, and action on the social determinants of health. Inte-grated action embracing all three dimensions will be needed to meet global health objectives in the years ahead.

CONCLUSION

Shaping a better future for the global community re-quires closing health gaps between the privileged and the excluded. To achieve progress in health equity, strong scientific, and ethical leadership are needed in the international health field. WHO is the only agency with responsibility for improving the health of all populations. At its best, WHO unites on-the-ground efficacy at country level with the exercise of global authority and coordination functions. It bonds the most advanced science to a normative commit-ment to justice and human rights.

Various views have been expressed as to how WHO should best address the challenges of the twenty-first century. One extreme is the essentialist approach in which the appropriate focus for WHO is seen to be only on health issues that concern the global community as a whole, meaning that WHO should only undertake those responsibilities that af-fect many or all countries simultaneously, such as transborder disease control and coordination of a global health information system (Frenk et al. 1997). Another view assumes greater responsibility for reinte-grating health policies with development strategies, a "social justice view." This approach, strongly backed by the current WHO leadership, requires a more interventionist role: mobilization and reallocation of health sector aid, advocacy of principles of social justice, provision of scientific and technical support to countries, the targeting of vulnerable groups (women, migrants, indigenous peoples, ethnic minorities, etc.), and monitoring the practices of big business and government (Lucas et al. 1997; Lee 1998).

As an intergovernmental organization accountable to 192 member states, WHO faces unique difficulties in achieving its broad goal. Tensions emerge between WHO's need to be responsive to the agendas of member states and its mandate to provide leadership based on scientific evidence. Likewise, the interests of different countries clash, as can those of NGOs and representatives of the for-profit sector, when they seek to collaborate within the public–private partnerships so important to many aspects of WHO's global health work today. When such difficulties arise within WHO, they must be resolved through painstaking compromise, rather than by unilateral executive decision. Unwieldy as they may be, however, democratic processes remain preferable to any known alternative, especially in the promotion of such fundamental public goods as health. It is within a democratic forum that the voices and health needs of vulnerable groups stand the best chance of being heard.

The global community must confront today's emergencies while laying sustainable foundations for a healthier future. This means synergizing targets such as 3 by 5 with the broad scale-up of equitable, integrated health systems that can meet the needs of communities and make quality health services available to everyone. Neither WHO nor indeed any single institution can accomplish such a task. But, working closely with countries and partners, WHO can lead the way. It remains to be seen whether the global community will muster sufficient political commitment to shape a healthier future for all people, especially the most disadvantaged. Enormous technical and political challenges stand in the way. Democratic, inclusive institutions such as WHO must be used to their full potential if progress toward health equity is to be a reality. The law of the market will not suffice.

Notes

1. Although smallpox and yaws were brought under control, resources were never sufficient to tackle tuberculosis and malaria on an adequate scale, and 50 years later, both remain, together with HIV/AIDS, the focus of

efforts by international partnerships, including WHO. Indeed, with the exception of venereal diseases, all of the original priorities continue to pose major challenges.

2. International travel to affected areas fell by 50–70%. Businesses, particularly in tourism-related areas, failed, while some large production facilities were forced to suspend operations when cases appeared among workers. The Asian Development Bank (2003) estimated the total cost of the epidemic to Asian economies at US$60 billion.

3. The United Nations Security Council and national bodies acknowledge the growing security impact of HIV/AIDS (National Intelligence Council 2002). The threat of new infections, arising naturally or as a result of human action, demands new forms of cooperation between security and public health.

References

Asian Development Bank. (2003). Assessing the impact and costs of SARS in developing Asia. Asian development outlook update 2003. http://www.adb.org/Documents/Books/ADO/2003/update/sars.pdf.

Banerji D. (2002). Report of the WHO Commission on Macroeconomics and Health: a critique. Int J Health Serv 32: 733–754.

Bell C, Devarajan S, Gersbach H. (2003). The long-run economic costs of AIDS: theory and application to South Africa. Washington, DC: World Bank.

Brahmbhatta H, Kigozi G, Wabwire-Mangen F, Serwadda D, Sewankambo N, Lutalo T, et al. (2003). The effects of placental malaria on mother-to-child HIV transmission in Rakai, Uganda. AIDS 17: 2539–2541.

Burci GL, Vignes C-H. (2004). World Health Organization. Kluwer Law International.

Castro A, Farmer P. (2003). Infectious disease in Haiti: HIV/AIDS, tuberculosis and social inequalities. Eur Mol Biol Organ Rep, no. 4, pp. 520–523. http://www.medanthro.net/docs/Castro&Farmer%20embor844.pdf.

De Waal A, Whiteside A. (2003). New variant famine: AIDS and food crisis in southern Africa. Lancet 362: 1234–1237.

Freedman L, Wirth M, Waldman R, et al. (2004). Millennium Project Task Force 4, Child health and maternal health. Interim report. New York: United Nations Millennium Project. http://www.unmillenniumproject.org/documents/tf4interim.pdf

Frenk J, Sepulveda J, Gomez-Dantes O, McGuiness MJ, Knaul F. (1997). The future of world health: the new world order and international health. Br Med J 314: 1304–1307.

Glynn JR, Warndorff DK, Fine PEM, Msika GK, Munthali MM, Ponnighaus JM. (1997). The impact of HIV on morbidity and mortality from tuberculosis in sub-Saharan Africa: a study in rural Malawi and review of the literature. Health Trans Rev 7(suppl. 2):75–87.

Gwatkin D. (2002). Who would gain most from efforts to reach the MDGs for health? An enquiry into the possibility of progress that fails to reach the poor. Washington, DC: World Bank.

Haines A, Cassels A. (2004). Can the Millenium Development Goals be attained? Br Med J 329: 394–397

Hofrichter R, ed. (2003). Health and social justice. San Francisco: Jossey Bass.

International Conference on Primary Health Care. (1978). Declaration of Alma-Ata, September 1978. http://www.who.int/hpr/archive/docs/almaata .html. Kim J, Miller J, Irwin A, Gershman J. (2000). Dying for growth: global inequality and the health of the poor. Monroe, ME: Common Courage Press.

Kober K, Van Damme W. (2004). Scaling up access to antiretroviral treatment in southern Africa: who will do the job? Lancet 364: 103–107.

Lancet. (2003). Will SARS hurt the world's poor? [editorial]. 361: 1485.

Lancet. (2004). Kick starting the revolution in health systems research [editorial]. 363: 1745.

Lee JW. (2003). Global health improvement and WHO: shaping the future. Lancet 362: 2083–2088.

Lee JW. (2004) Address to the 57th World Health Assembly. Geneva, 17 May 2004. http://www.who.int/dg/ lee/speeches/2004/wha57/en/.

Lee K. (1998). Shaping the future of global health cooperation: where can we go from here? Lancet 351: 899–902

Lee K, Walt G, Haines A. (2004). The challenge to improve global health: financing the Millennium Development Goals. JAMA 291: 2636–2637.

Leeder S, Raymond S. (2004). Race against time: the challenge of cardiovascular diseases in developing economies. New York: Columbia University. http://www.earthinstitute.columbia.edu//news/news /2004/images/raceagainsttime_FINAL-0410404.pdf

Leon DA, Walt G. (2001). Poverty, inequality and health: an international perspective. Oxford: Oxford University Press.

Lucas A A, Morgedal S, Walt G, et al. (1997). Cooperation for health development: the World Health Organization's support to programmes at country level. London: Governments of Australia, Canada, Italy, Norway, Sweden, and United Kingdom.

Mackenbach JP, Cavelaars AEJM, Kunst AE, et al. (2000). Socioeconomic inequalities in cardiovascular disease mortality. An international study. European Heart J 21: 1141–1151.

National Intelligence Council. (2002). The Next Wave of HIV/AIDS: Nigeria, Ethiopia, Russia, India and China. Washington, DC: National Intelligence Council.

Navarro V. (2004). The world situation and WHO. Lancet 363: 1321–1323.

Sewankambo NK, Gray RH, Ahmad S, Serwadda D, Wabwire-Mangen F, Nalugoda F, et al. (2000). Mortality associated with HIV infection in rural Rakai district, Uganda. AIDS, 14: 2391–2400.

UNDP. (2003). Human development report 2003. The Millennium Development Goals: a compact among nations to end human poverty. New York: United Nations Development Programme/Oxford University Press.

United Nations. (2002). Report of the International Conference on Financing for Development, Monterrey, Mexico, 18–22 March 2002. New York: United Nations.

United Nations Children's Fund. (2000). Progress of Nations 2000 (background paper). New York: United Nations Children's Fund.

Waitzkin H. (2003). Report of the WHO commission on macroeconomics and health: summary and critique. Lancet 361: 523–526.

WHO. (1946). Constitution of the World Health Organization. New York: World Health Organization.

WHO. (1997). Health: the courage to care. Geneva: World Health Organization.

WHO. (1998a). Health for all in the twenty-first century. Geneva: World Health Organization, p. 6.

WHO. (1998b). World health declaration. Annex to World Health Assembly Resolution WHA51.7. Geneva: World Health Organization.

WHO. (1999). Executive board paper EB 105/3, December. Geneva: World Health Organization.

WHO. (2000a). World health report 2000. Health systems. Improving performance. Geneva: World Health Organization. http://www.who.int/whr/2001

WHO. (2000b). Design and implementation of health information systems. Geneva: World Health Organization.

WHO. (2001). Macroeconomics and health: investing in health for economic development. Geneva: World Health Organization.

WHO. (2002a). World health report, 2002. Reducing risks, promoting health. Geneva: World Health Organization. http://www.who.int/whr/2002

WHO. (2002b). Innovative care for chronic conditions: building blocks for action. Geneva: World Health Organization.

WHO. (2003a). World health report 2003: shaping the future. Geneva: World Health Organization. http:// www.who.int/whr/2003

WHO. (2003b). WHO 3 × 5 Initiative assessment mission to Kenya, 6–11 October [unpublished report]. Geneva: World Health Organization.

WHO. (2003c). Primary health care: a framework for future strategic directions. Geneva: World Health Organization.

WHO. (2004a). World health report 2004: changing history. Geneva: World Health Organization. http:// www.who.int/whr/2004

WHO. (2004b). WHO global strategy on diet, physical activity and health. Geneva: World Health Organization. http://www.who.int/gb/ebwha/pdf_files/ WHA57/A57_R17-en.pdf

WHO. (2005). Preventing chronic diseases: a vital investment. Geneva: World Health Organization. http://www.who.int/chp/chronic_disease_report/en

WHO/WTO. (2002). WTO agreements and public health: a joint study by the WHO and WTO secretariat. Geneva: World Health Organization/World Trade Organization.

World Bank. (1993). World development report 1993: investing in health. Washington, DC: World Bank.

World Bank/WHO. (2004). Overview of progress toward meeting the health MDGs. Issue paper 1 for the High Level Forum on the Health MDGs. Geneva, January 8–9, 2004. http://unstats.un.org /unsd/mi

World Health Bulletin. (2004). WHO's HIV/AIDS strategy under the spotlight. World Health Bull 82(6): 474–476.

Yach D, Hawkes C, Epping-Jordan JE, Galbraith S. (2004a). The World Health Organization's Framework Convention on Tobacco Control: implications for global epidemics of food-related deaths and disease. J Public Health Policy 24: 274–250.

Yach D, Hawkes C, Gould CL, Hofman K. (2004b). The global burden of chronic diseases: overcoming impediments to prevention and control. JAMA 291: 2616–2622.

Chapter 17

What's Politics Got to Do with It? Health, the G8, and the Global Economy

Ted Schrecker and Ronald Labonte

The HIV/AIDS pandemic made the concept of "global health" intelligible to people outside a narrow circle of activists and visionary professionals. It also demonstrated the need for a frame of reference, in research and policy, that transcends both biomedical perspectives and epidemiological categories to focus on the complicated and multistage causal relations that lead from the international political economy to create fatal vulnerabilities at the household and community level (see, generally, Kalipeni et al., 2004). In this vein, medical anthropologist Brooke Grundfest Schoepf has pointed out that as long ago as 1988, people in Zaire (now the Democratic Republic of the Congo) "had another name for AIDS (SIDA in French) that encapsulated their understanding of its social epidemiology," which included rapid social change, endemic economic insecurity, and the subordination of women: *Salaire Insuffisant Depuis des Années* (Schoepf, 1998: 110; see also Schoepf, 2002). Schoepf's work is especially valuable because she

consistently foregrounds the relations between micro-level outcomes and such macro-level factors as falling commodity prices, domestic austerity policies that involved cuts in public sector employment and in subsidized access to health care, and migration driven by economic desperation (Schoepf, 1988, 2002, 2004; Schoepf et al., 2000).

A recent review (Bates et al., 2004a, 2004b) of research on HIV/AIDS, tuberculosis, and malaria—the priority diseases of the Global Fund for AIDS, Tuberculosis, and Malaria established in 2002—concludes that vulnerability to all three diseases is closely linked; that poverty, gender inequality, development policy, and health sector "reforms" that involve user fees and reduced access to care are important determinants of vulnerability; and that "[c]omplicated interactions between these factors, many of which lie outside the health sector, make unravelling of their individual roles and therefore appropriate targeting of interventions difficult" (Bates et al., 2004a: 268). These are not the only obstacles to effective interventions. Both malaria and tuberculosis are recognized as diseases of poverty, so investments in research on treatment are unlikely to be attractive on commercial grounds, and investments in prevention and control can be expected to yield limited health and economic benefits outside the affected regions or classes.

People outside the industrialized world are increasingly affected by a "double burden" of disease, as vulnerabilities to communicable disease that were (erroneously) supposed to be taken care of by economic growth coexist with exposure to industrial pollution and to risk factors for noncommunicable diseases such as cardiovascular disease and diabetes, which arise from rapid growth-related transition to patterns of production and consumption more typical of the industrialized world (WHO, 2003). Injury is another term in the equation. Road traffic accidents, or "road violence" (Chen and Berlinguer, 2001: 37), in developing countries kill more than a million people each year, most of whom never had the chance to own a vehicle, and injure many times that number (WHO, 2003: 95–100; see also Nantulya et al., 2003, and chapter 6). The toll of death and injury is augmented by workplace accidents (see chapter 8), by crime, and by the direct health damage and social and economic dislocation that occur in zones of war and intrastate conflict (Levy and Sidel, 1997; Stewart, 2003; see also chapter 9). Thus, recent literature (Lozano et al., 2001; Bradshaw et al., 2003) refers to triple burdens of disease, because of distinctive challenges presented by rapid increases in injuries, or even quadruple burdens, because of the special challenge presented by HIV both for health systems and social policy.

So, what's politics got to do with it? In this chapter, we describe a limited number of links between "globalization" and health determinants and outcomes, as identified by other authors (e.g., Cornia, 1987; Woodward et al., 2001) and synthesized for the World Health Organization (WHO) (Labonte and Torgerson, 2005). Globalization, more accurately described as "a *process* of greater integration within the world economy through movements of goods and services, capital, technology and (to a lesser extent) labor, which lead increasingly to economic decisions being influenced by global conditions" (Jenkins, 2004: 1, emphasis original), did not just happen.[1] It is best understood as the dynamic outcome of the inter-

actions of technological advance (itself driven, in part, by the imperatives of economic and geopolitical competition) and policy choices by the governments of the world's richest countries (Marchak, 1991; Gershman and Irwin, 2000). These policy choices have included aggressive promotion of trade liberalization and deregulation of national financial markets, which has facilitated rapid transnational movements of capital. In the global labor market that has begun to emerge as a result (World Bank, 1995), investors and corporate managers can engage in worldwide comparison shopping for the optimal combination of labor costs, labor productivity, regulatory regimes, and transportation costs (see chapter 8). This trend is sector specific and (so far) incomplete. Nevertheless, North American readers, in particular, should browse a local Wal-Mart (now the largest private employer in both the United States and Mexico and widely credited with transforming the retail sector), check out the national origin of the products on sale, and ask why so few familiar brands are manufactured in the industrial heartlands of a generation ago.

We concentrate on policy positions of the G7/G8 group of nations,[2] which together account for 46.6% of global gross domestic product and 46.8% of global exports—roughly half the planet's economic activity (IMF, 2003b: table A). Voting weighted by the size of national financial contributions gives G8 governments close to an absolute majority in the decisions of the World Bank and International Monetary Fund (IMF) (table 17.1)—institutions that have been crucial in promoting and, some would say, enforcing integration into the global economy. The same governments wield disproportionate power in the nominally more egalitarian World Trade Organization (WTO), where the size of their markets and the access to specialized expertise provided by ample central government budgets confer formidable bargaining advantages with respect to countries of the developing world (Jawara and Kwa, 2003), and the policies of all three institutions are converging around a common, market-oriented policy agenda (Brock and McGee, 2004). Thus, if a blueprint for managing the global economy can be said to exist, one of the best places to look for it is in the official statements that emanate from the annual G8 summits—the starting point for our earlier research (Labonte et al., 2004; Labonte and Schrecker, 2004)—and in the policies pursued by G8 national governments.

TABLE 17.1. G8 Voting Strength on World Bank and IMF Boards

	World Bank (IDA)	World Bank (IBRD)	IMF
Canada	4.24[a]	3.85[a]	2.94[b]
France	4.34	4.31	4.95
Germany	7.02	4.49	6.00
Italy	3.66[a]	3.51[a]	3.26[b]
Japan	10.92	7.87	6.14
Russia	0.28	2.79	2.75
United Kingdom	5.00	4.31	4.95
United States	13.91	16.41	17.11
Total G8	49.37	47.54	48.10

The IDA (Internal Development Association) is the arm of the World Bank that provides grants and "concessional" (below-market) loans to countries that could not easily borrow on commercial markets. The IBRD (International Bank for Reconstruction and Development, also part of the World Bank, provides financing at commercial rates, mainly to middle-income countries.

[a] Figure somewhat overstates country voting strength, because the director casts votes of other (smaller) countries, as well, and individual country voting strength figures are not provided.

[b] The director casts votes of other (smaller) countries, as well, but the figure represents actual country voting strength.

Source: World Bank (2003b) and IMF (2003a)

MEETING (OR NOT MEETING) BASIC NEEDS: AID

It is axiomatic in the study of population health that health care is only one determinant of health among many, and often not the most important (Evans and Stoddart, 1990). Much of the burden of disease outside the industrialized world is inextricably connected with poverty and economic insecurity; as just one example, WHO attributes 15.8% of the global burden of disease, almost all of that outside the industrialized world, to childhood and maternal undernutrition (WHO, 2002b: 52–56)—an underestimate of the full significance of nutritional factors, since it does not take into account such factors as the relation between adult nonmaternal undernutrition and infectious disease. Depending on the basis for estimation, 1.1–1.2 billion people around the world are living on less than $1/day, and 2.7–2.8 billion, almost half the world's population, on less than $2/day (World Bank, 2001a: 36–38; Chen and Ravallion, 2004).[3] The most recent estimates show that, on either measure, the number of people living in poverty in sub-Saharan Africa roughly doubled between 1981 and 2001 (Chen and Ravallion, 2004; see also chapter 7).

Against this background, the Millennium Development Goals (MDGs) (see chapter 16) have become a useful benchmark for assessing global progress toward meeting basic needs. The MDGs are derived from the Millennium Resolution (Resolution 55/2, § 19) adopted by the United Nations General Assembly in the year 2000. No binding commitment to implementing the goals exists, but they represent "the best summary of the efforts undertaken by the international community over the past 40 years to find a path for sustainable development for all members of the global community" (Global Forum for Health Research, 2004: 12) and have become the focus of an unprecedented effort on the part of the World Bank and a variety of agencies within the United Nations system to measure development progress in a systematic way and to advocate for additional resources for development with a special emphasis on meeting basic needs (De Silva and Tropp, 2003; United Nations Development Programme, 2003; United Nations System Standing Committee on Nutrition, 2004; World Bank, 2004). Three of the eight MDGs are directly concerned with health; they address child mortality, maternal health, and the spread of infectious diseases such as AIDS and malaria.

Several others address crucial determinants of health—notably, those dealing with "extreme poverty and hunger," access to safe drinking water and basic sanitation, educational opportunities, and improving the lives of slum dwellers.

G8 nations, as parties to the Millennium Resolution, have committed themselves to the MDGs and their associated targets, and have reiterated this commitment at recent summits; for example, "[W]e commit ourselves to the agreed international development goals including the overarching objective of reducing the share of the world's population living in extreme poverty to half its 1990 level by 2015" (G8, 2000, § 13), and, "We will work with developing countries to meet the International Development Goals [which are now, with some modifications, the MDGs]" (G8, 2001, § 14).[4] Without neglecting the responsibility of governments of poorer nations to mobilize what resources they can, it is not unreasonable to hold the G8 (or, more accurately in this instance, the G7) accountable for poorer countries' MDG successes or failures, particularly when the latter are due largely to a lack of resources rather than a lack of political will.

It should trouble G7 leaders, then, that numerous recent assessments are pessimistic about prospects for achieving the MDGs. After years of slow improvements in nutritional status, the number of undernourished people worldwide was almost unchanged during the 1990s, actually increasing in sub-Saharan Africa (UNFAO, 2005). This pattern refers only to chronically insufficient caloric intake, while micronutrient deficiencies affect much larger numbers of people (ACC/SCN, 2000: 23–32; UNFAO, 2003: 13–15, 19–21). World Bank data and forecasts indicate that an overall economic growth rate in the developing world twice as high as the rate during the 1990s will be required to meet the MDG for poverty reduction on a worldwide basis, and even if such a growth rate were to be achieved, a substantial number of countries—especially in southern Africa—would miss the goal (World Bank, 2001b; Arulpragasam and Prennushi, 2002). More recently, a World Bank assessment concluded: "Even if economic growth accelerates . . . and even if progress toward the gender and water goals were to be substantially accelerated, the developing world will wake up on the morning of January 1, 2016, some way from the health targets—sub-Saharan Africa a long way" (Wagstaff et al., 2003: 2.12).

Levels of spending on official development assistance (ODA, foreign aid) instantiate failure on the part of the industrialized world, and the G8 in particular, to take seriously the imperative of achieving the MDGs. The value of ODA expressed as a percentage of the total gross national income (GNI) of members of the Organization for Economic Cooperation and Development (OECD) Development Assistance Committee (DAC), which includes most of the world's substantial donors, slowly declined starting in the mid-1980s, although this trend has now started to reverse (OECD DAC, 2005). The decline in ODA provided by the G7, as compared to the strong performance of some other DAC members (figure 17.1), was much more pronounced, despite the occasional explicit summit commitment to increase assistance levels. In 1999, for example, the G7 promised "to strive gradually to increase the volume of official development assistance" (G8 1999, § 29), although subsequent commitments stressed only "strengthening the effectiveness" of such aid (G8, 2000, § 20). G7 and other donor country commitments made before, during, and after the United Nations' 2002 Monterrey Conference on Financing for Development will raise the inflation-adjusted value of development assistance from $58.2 billion in 2002 to $76.8 billion by 2006, if all these commitments are fulfilled (OECD DAC, 2004: 62). By comparison, one World Bank estimate is that achieving the first seven MDGs (i.e., all of them apart from the eighth and nebulous "global partnership for development") would require an additional $40–$70 billion per year in ODA (Devarajan et al., 2001). A 2003 briefing note for the World Bank board estimated the costs of meeting the "service delivery" MDGs (education, health, water supply, and sanitation, but not reducing hunger or poverty except to the extent that these benefits are associated with meeting other goals) as "in the range of at least an *additional* $35–65 billion per year" for low- and lower middle-income countries, and the authors warn that the figures represent "*significant underestimates* of the total amount of resources that will be required to meet all the MDGs" (World Bank, 2003a: 4). All such estimates rely on "heroic assumptions" (Hanlon, 2000: 890; Devarajan et al., 2001: 30) about a number of variables, but they are nevertheless useful as indications of the gap between needs and available resources. They are also consistent with estimates published in 2005 by the UN Millennium Project (2005) and the Commission for Africa (2005), which

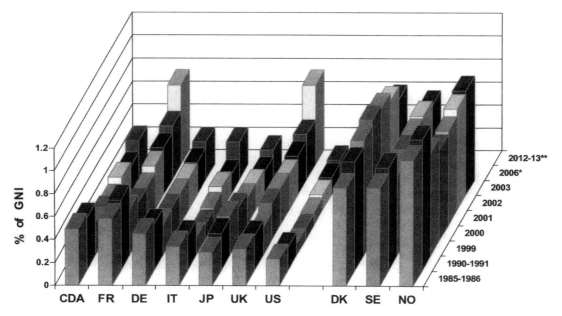

FIGURE 17.1. Trends in Development Assistance Flows, G7 and Selected Comparison Countries. CDA, Canada; FR, France; DE, Germany; IT, Italy; JP, Japan; UK, United Kingdom; USA, United States of America; DK, Denmark; NL, Netherlands; NO, Norway; SE, Sweden. * OECD estimates, assuming all commitments made at Monterrey in 2002 are fulfilled. ** Promised as of early 2005. *Source:* OECD Development Assistance Committee (2005 and earlier years); Chirac (2003); MacAskill (2004).

was established in the run-up to the 2005 G8 summit at Gleneagles as part of the United Kingdom's initiative to place African development high on the summit agenda.

Increasing ODA spending to 0.7% of the industrialized countries' GNI is a long-standing goal expressed over the years in various nonbinding United Nations documents, including the 1992 report of the Rio "Earth Summit" (United Nations, 1992) and, more recently, the Monterrey Conference (United Nations, 2002a). The key outcome of the 2005 G8 summit was a commitment to increase development assistance to Africa by US$25 billion by 2010, a commitment driven primarily by pre-summit announcements by France, Britain, and the European Union (EU) that they would raise their aid spending to the 0.7% target. (Canada, the United States, and Japan were conspicuous in their refusal to state timetables for reaching the target.) This commitment appeared to respond directly to the reports of the Millennium Project and the Commission for Africa, each of which recommended an approximate doubling of the current value of development assistance. However,

some civil society organizations, notably Jubilee Research (2005), were strongly critical of the commitment on the basis that much of it involved not genuinely "new" money, but rather recycled announcements made in advance of the Summit. This is perhaps a less serious limitation than at least two others. First, no specific financing mechanisms were described, leaving open the prospect that domestic resistance could compromise the commitments—even though increasing development-assistance spending to the 0.7% target in 2003 would have cost G7 countries only the price of 0.6–1.5 Big Macs per week for each of their residents (table 17.2). Second, some of the new spending could come in the form of debt relief or could simply offset substantial revenue losses from import liberalization by developing countries, for instance, as part of the Economic Partnership Agreements (EPAs) now being negotiated between the EU and Africa, Caribbean, and Pacific countries (Stevens and Kennan, 2005).

This is not to imply that aid is a panacea (Labonte et al., 2004: 123–132). Historically, aid has often served the political/strategic interests of donor nations

TABLE 17.2. G7 Aid Commitments, 2003

Country	Canada	France	Germany	Italy	Japan	United Kingdom	United States	Total
Value of ODA, 2003, $ million	2,031	7,253	6,784	2,433	8,880	6,282	16,254	42,555
ODA as percentage of GNI, 2003	0.24	0.41	0.28	0.17	0.20	0.34	0.15	
Additional resources that would be made available by meeting the 0.7% target, $ million	3,893	5,130	10,176	7,585	22,220	6,652	59,598	105,934
Population, million	31.40	59.50	82.50	57.70	127.20	59.20	288.40	
Value per capita of additional resources needed to meet the 0.7% target, $	124	86	123	131	175	112	207	
Cost of a Big Mac, 2003, $	2.17	2.89	2.89	2.89	2.18	3.08	2.71	
Additional annual cost of meeting the 0.7% target, in Big Macs per capita	57	30	43	45	80	36	76	

Source: OECD DAC (2005, tables 4 and 38), except Big Macs/capita calculation (based on national Big Mac cost figures from the Economist [2003]).

289

and major commercial interests within their borders. For example, the U.S. commitment at Monterrey to increase its annual aid spending to $15 billion by 2006, by way of the Millennium Challenge Account, indicated that new funds would be conditional on "sound economic policies that foster enterprise and entrepreneurship, including more open markets and sustainable budget policies" (United Nations, 2002b: § 8–9). This can be read as code for increasing marketing investment opportunities for U.S. firms. Much aid also serves domestic commercial clienteles by being "tied" to purchases of goods or services (in the form of "technical cooperation") from the donor country. Aid has often financed large-scale, environmentally destructive projects with limited relevance to basic needs (Rich, 1994; Bosshard et al., 2003). Further problems involve corruption in the use of aid funds (LaFraniere, 2004; Vasagar, 2004) or, less dramatically, the coexistence of cuts in public spending on basic needs with lavish spending on salaries and perquisites for the political elite (for African examples, see van de Walle, 2001: 101–109) or with high volumes of capital flight (Ndikumana and Boyce, 2003). All these issues demonstrate the urgent need for careful financial management and transparent mechanisms for ensuring accountability in the use of aid funds, not least in order to counteract the "donor fatigue" that set in during the 1990s. However, they should not distract attention from the fact that aid *can* work, and that—as pointed out by the Commission for Africa and the Millennium Project—much larger aid flows can and should be put to productive use with appropriate administrative safeguards in place. In other words, major increases in ODA flows are probably not a sufficient condition for faster progress toward the MDGs; they are a necessary condition. As shown in the next section, this is especially true for countries dealing with high levels of external debt.

MEETING (OR NOT MEETING) BASIC NEEDS: DEBT SERVICE AND DEBT RELIEF

Foreign debt represents a form of "bondage that ensnares hundreds of millions of the world's poorest people. . . . As though bound to feudal lords, their lives and labor have been mortgaged to rich country banks and governments, often by leaders they did not choose, to finance projects that did not benefit them"

(Ramphal, 1999). In 2000, developing countries received $46.6 billion in ODA, while paying out $330.4 billion to service their external debt. Outflows of funds for debt service dwarfed ODA receipts in every region except sub-Saharan Africa, where the two were roughly in balance (Pettifor and Greenhill, 2002; figure 17.2).[5] In many countries, a large proportion of the ODA received in any year is immediately committed to debt servicing (Hanlon, 2000; Utting et al., 2000: 27). Country-level comparisons of debt service payments and spending on basic needs are even more disturbing, for example, in 2001–2002, government expenditure on health services in Bangladesh was $492 million, while expenditure on external debt service was $1.08 billion. In Kenya, the figure for health spending was $189 million, and for debt repayment, $580 million (Rowson and Verheul, 2004: 8).

The specific causes of "debt crises" vary from country to country and over time (George, 1988; Strange, 1998; Hanlon, 2000), but it is widely agreed that major contributors include the oil price shocks of 1973 and 1979–1980; the rapid increase in inflation-adjusted interest rates during the early 1980s, resulting from the monetarist policies of the United States; falling world prices for the primary commodities that are the key exports (and foreign exchange earners) of many developing economies; increases in debt service payments and import prices resulting from devaluation of local currency against the U.S. dollar in which the debt is denominated, which is often a condition of structural adjustment lending; and "capital flight" as foreign investors and domestic elites shift their assets abroad, reducing the ability of governments to meet revenue requirements through taxation.[6] Ironically, the lowering of tariffs that was an element of many structural adjustment programs, and was subsequently entrenched in the Uruguay Round of trade negotiations that established the WTO, had a similar impact on government revenues: partly because they are relatively easy to collect, and collecting other forms of tax revenue may be beyond the capacity of the state in many developing countries, tariffs account for a far larger proportion of the revenues of many developing country governments than is the case in the industrialized world (World Bank, 2002: 252–255).

The destructive effect of debt service obligations on the ability of many developing economies to meet basic needs was identified at least as early as 1987 by the World Commission on Environment

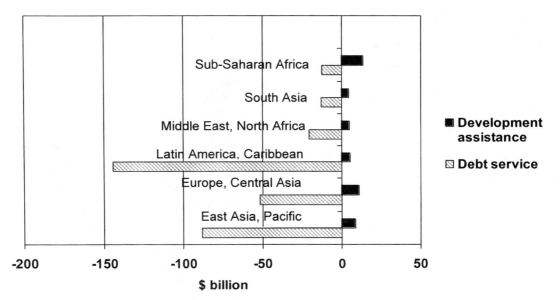

FIGURE 17.2. Development Assistance and Debt Service Flows Compared by Region, 2000. *Source:* Data in Pettifor and Greenhill (2002).

and Development (1987). In the same year, a UNICEF-sponsored study (Cornia et al., 1987) demonstrated that domestic austerity measures, adopted by recipient governments as the price of "structural adjustment" loans from the World Bank and the IMF (box 17.1), often resulted in deterioration of basic indicators of child welfare such as nutrition, immunization levels, and education (see also chapter 13). Despite this body of evidence and much subsequent research on the destructive human consequences of debt crises and structural adjustment, which are now recognized in some quarters as a human rights issue (Cheru, 1999, 2001), response on the part of the industrialized world was desultory at best until 1996, when the World Bank and IMF announced the Heavily Indebted Poor Country (HIPC) initiative. HIPC subsequently became the centerpiece of G7 debt reduction initiatives and was expanded in 1999 as Enhanced HIPC.

Box 17.1 – "Structural Adjustment," Past and Present

"Structural adjustment" entered the development policy lexicon in 1980, when the World Bank initiated structural adjustment loans to help developing coun-

tries respond to the impact of the 1979–1980 recession on their ability to service external debt. After 1982, when Mexico threatened default on billions of dollars in loans made by major U.S. banks, structural adjustment became more important as the industrialized countries agreed to provide new financing for debt rescheduling through the World Bank and the IMF. The new loans (and they were loans, not grants) came with "conditionalities": agreement to a relatively standard package of macroeconomic policies, including reduced subsidies for basic items of consumption; the removal of barriers to imports and foreign direct investment; and rapid privatization of state owned enterprises on the presumption that private service provision is inherently more efficient and that proceeds from privatization could be used to ensure debt repayment (Dixon et al., 1995; Milward, 2000; Sparr, 2000). The 1980s saw the IMF and World Bank transformed into "watchdog[s] for developing countries, to keep them on a policy track that would help them repay most of their debts and to open their markets for international investors" (Junne, 2001: 206). Early evidence of the negative impact of structural adjustment programs on the ability of many economies to meet basic needs (Cornia et al., 1987) did not prevent a "veritable explosion in the use of policy conditionality during the 1980s and into the 1990s" by the World Bank and the IMF (Killick, 2004: 12;

for documentation, see IMF, 2001). Admittedly, the impact of this "explosion" was probably mitigated by the fact that many conditions were only partly implemented or complied with, yet the World Bank and IMF seldom cut off subsequent lending (for African examples, see van de Walle, 2001: 67–85).

With a recent emphasis on poverty reduction, structural adjustment is no longer part of the official vocabulary of the World Bank and the IMF. However, the change may be cosmetic; the IMF's Poverty Reduction and Growth Facility is, in fact, "the reformed and renamed Enhanced Structural Adjustment Facility" (World Bank, 2001c: 201). Poverty reduction strategy papers (PRSPs), and periodic progress reports on their implementation, are now required of countries receiving concessional (below-market) loans from the World Bank or debt relief under the HIPC initiative and must be approved by the boards of the World Bank and IMF (see also chapter 14). Direct parallels exist between the process of qualifying for debt relief through the preparation of a PRSP and earlier forms of conditionality (Cheru, 2001; IMF, 2001: 50–52), and the macroeconomic policy elements often replicate those that were demanded as part of structural adjustment (Focus on the Global South, 2003; Labonte et al., 2004: 26–29). A recent study notes that World Bank and IMF requirements attached to funding that supports PRSPs "include trade-related conditions that are more stringent, in terms of requiring more, or faster, or deeper liberalization, than WTO provisions to which the respective country has agreed" (Brock and McGee, 2004: 20). For these and other reasons, many civil society organizations now argue strongly that PRSPs, whatever their potential merits, should not be tied to eligibility for debt relief and development assistance.

The initiative offered partial debt relief to forty-two of the world's poorest countries and has resulted in substantial increases in public spending on such basic needs as health and education in some recipient countries (Gupta et al., 2002). However, Oxfam International (2001: figure 1) has calculated that in fourteen of the eligible countries, annual debt servicing costs will exceed combined public spending on health and primary education even *after* the maximum debt relief available under the pre-2005 initiative is obtained. At this point, roughly half the HIPC countries' external debt would remain unpaid and uncanceled (Martin, 2004: 12), because for purposes

of HIPC a country's debt load is considered "sustainable" if its net present value[7] is less than 150% of annual export revenues. This criterion, based "on how much money could be squeezed out of a poor country" (Hanlon, 2000: 886), was adopted at the insistence of the G7, "balancing the need to include strategic G7 allies and the desire to help keep costs down" (Martin, 2004: 17–18). Thus, some of the poorest countries in the world are expected to rescue themselves from poverty by rapidly increasing the value of their exports in an increasingly competitive global marketplace ("trade not aid").

Patricia Goldstone (2001: 50) has described this approach to development policy as "internationalized workfare," invoking an analogy with U.S. welfare "reforms" that forced mothers into low-wage work on almost any terms, usually without eligibility for health insurance. In addition, one recent analysis indicates that even the relatively modest resources made available through HIPC may have come at the expense of ODA flows of other kinds, rather than representing an addition to them (Killick, 2004).[8] A more appropriate process for deciding on levels of debt relief would start by giving priority to a country's ability to meet such objectives as the MDGs and then determine how much was left over for debt repayment (Greenhill, 2002; Greenhill and Sisti, 2003).

Even complete cancellation of the external debt of countries eligible for HIPC would make only $3.2 billion per year available for other budgetary purposes (Martin, 2004: 28). A background document for the United Nations Development Program's 2003 Human Development Report (Pettifor and Greenhill, 2002) argues that cancellation of *all* external debts of the HIPC countries, along with at least $16.5 billion per year in additional ODA, will be necessary if those countries are to meet the MDGs. In a larger scale exercise based on estimates of the social spending that would be required to meet a list of targets comparable to those associated with the MDGs in ninety-three countries, economist Joseph Hanlon concluded that giving priority to those targets would require canceling all the external debt of thirty-four countries, including some HIPCs and others such as Bangladesh that are not eligible for the HIPC initiative, as well as providing $15 billion per year in new ODA flows to those countries (Hanlon, 2000). Partial debt cancellation would be required for another thirty-seven countries, including, for example, debt cancellation worth $24 billion for now-beleaguered Argentina, $116 billion for Indonesia, and $98 billion for India—each a country that cannot qualify for HIPC despite the prevalence of poverty within its borders. Using 1998 as the base year, Hanlon estimates that these seventy-one countries would need an additional $85 billion per year in a combination of increased aid flows and reduced debt service to meet their development goals and targets. No such estimate is ever more than an approximation, but Hanlon's figures, like the World Bank cost estimates cited above, are on the same order of magnitude as the amount of new money that would be made available by bringing G7 ODA spending (including spending for debt relief) up to the target of 0.7% of GNI.[9]

After the 2005 summit, these obstacles appeared to have been overcome with the commitment to an additional US$40–$60 billion in cancellation of debts owed by HIPCs to the World Bank, the IMF, and the concessional arm of the African Development Bank, and with a separate partial debt cancellation deal for Nigeria (which is not a HIPC) worth US$31 billion (Elliott and Wintour, 2005). However, the commitment may not be entirely reliable, since as of early 2005, US$12.3 billion of commitments under the existing, enhanced HIPC initiative have remained unfunded (United Nations, 2005: 146). The Gleneagles response also may be inadequate because it fails to address the debts owed by low-income non-HIPCs (other than Nigeria), including debts owed to private creditors (Commission for Africa, 2005: 328). Recipients of additional debt relief will apparently have development assistance reduced by some portion of the amount (Joint World Bank/IMF Development Committee, 2005), repeating a pattern in which development assistance declined substantially during the late 1990s following the start of the HIPC initiative (Killick, 2004: 6–7). Finally, concerns persist about the conditions that are likely to be attached to debt cancellation—as indicated, for example, by post-summit World Bank warnings that the G8 debt cancellation announcement "offered no mechanism for suspending debt relief if a debtor country deviated from economic and social reforms" prescribed by the Bank and the IMF (Wroughton, 2005).

Late in 2004, proposals to increase the value of debt relief provided by the industrialized countries were under active consideration by G7 finance ministers, providing both tantalizing glimpses of what might be possible and insights into the hard politics of selling global obligations to domestic audiences (box 17.2).

Box 17.2 – The Current Politics and Future Possibilities of Debt Relief

In advance of the G7 finance ministers' meeting in October 2004, at least two proposals for expanded debt relief for low-income countries were being actively promoted. The United States was proposing that the World Bank and IMF cancel an additional $70 billion in debt owed by the world's poorest nations, as part of a package that included canceling a comparable amount of external debt owed by Iraq. (A strong argument can be made that debts incurred by the regime of Saddam Hussein should be regarded as odious, and therefore uncollectible; see note 9.) Britain advanced a twofold proposal, offering to pay an additional £100 million per year of the debts owed by all the HIPC-eligible countries and some others, as part of its increased commitment to ODA, and proposing that further debt relief be financed by revaluing and selling some of the IMF's gold reserves, currently carried on its books at artificially low values (Bright and Keegan, 2004; U.K. Department for International Development, 2004).

The G7 finance ministers failed to agree on either proposal (Bright and Keegan, 2004), with Canada expressing particular concern that the sale of IMF gold reserves might depress the revenues of its gold mining industry (McKenna, 2004)—a minor industry in national terms, but one that is locally important in a country where many regional economies remain tied to resource industries. The Canadian objection illustrates the difficulties that even well-intentioned political leaders face when development policies offer positive effects on the determinants of health but also involve costs that must be borne within their own borders. This problem looms even larger with respect to the imperative of improving market access for the products of developing economies.

BASIC NEEDS, MARKET ACCESS, AND HEALTH: DO AS WE SAY NOT AS WE DID?

In *The Lexus and the Olive Tree*, Thomas Friedman described a visit to Hanoi, where "every inch of sidewalk seems to be covered by someone selling something off a mat, out of a trunk or from the shelves of a storefront." One of those people was a woman crouched on the sidewalk with a bathroom scale, and every morning, he would pay to have himself weighed as his "contribution to the globalization of Vietnam. To me," he wrote, "her unspoken motto was: 'Whatever you've got, no matter how big or small—sell it, trade it, barter it, leverage it, rent it, but do something with it to turn a profit, improve your standard of living and get into the game'" (Friedman, 2000: 348–349). In a similar vein, former Mexican president Ernesto Zedillo and former Canadian finance minister (then prime minister) Paul Martin, who cochaired a United Nations commission on the role of the private sector in development, appealed to the latent "entrepreneurial energy" of the developing world: "Visit the tiniest town in the poorest country on market day and you will see this incipient private sector in action" (Martin and Zedillo, 2003).

This almost magical view of the capabilities of markets, which underscores the value of the "internationalized workfare" analogy, pervades contemporary development policy. It is exemplified by the statement issued by the G8 in 2001 that "[w]e are determined to make globalization work for all our citizens and especially the world's poor. Drawing the poorest countries into the global economy is the surest way to address their fundamental aspirations" (G8, 2001, § 3). More recently, by the G8 Action Plan on Applying the Power of Entrepreneurship to the Eradication of Poverty, released at the 2004 G8 Summit, enthusiastically embraced the approach of Martin and Zedillo. For many observers, a key question remains on whose terms developing countries are to be drawn into the global economy. To whose advantage, and with what social consequences (Chang, 2002)? For example, in Vietnam, in many respects a poster child for the supposed benefits of economic integration (in addition to Friedman, see Hiebert, 1996), "[o]ut-of-pocket payments for health care pushed 2.6m Vietnamese into poverty in 1998" (Wagstaff and Yazbeck, 2004). Although more research is needed on the health consequences of local and regional situations in which domestic producers are decimated by import competition, as in the case of the Zambian textile industry and corn production in southern Mexico[10] (Anon, 2002; Jeter, 2002), dismissing "the losers of free trade and investment" as "a variety of stakeholders related to inefficient incumbents facing increased foreign competition" (Rugman and Verbeke, 2003: 96) is an inadequate response to the potential health consequences of such transitions. Furthermore, only a few countries "grew out of poverty" since the end of the Second World War, and many analysts believe this is

attributable to a development path that included strategic tariff and nontariff barriers to imports (rather than import liberalization) with support for key export industries, rigorous controls on foreign capital flows, and various degrees of *dirigisme* [state direction] in industrial policy (Amsden, 1994; Hertzman and Siddiqui, 2000; Rodrik, 2001; Chang, 2002).[11]

Development policy specialists who disagree about much else agree on the importance of income growth for the determinants of health, *if* the benefits of growth are widely shared. This is a crucial point: historical evidence indicates that *even if* integration into the global economy represents a path to riches for the developing world, specific policy interventions will be needed in order to ensure that benefits are shared in ways that lead to improvements in population health (Szreter, 1999, 2003). With this condition in mind, if improved market access for the products of the world's poorest countries would result in substantial increases in income, then such improvements could represent an important route toward improved population health. Taking up this theme, Oxfam has developed a "double standards index" (DSI) that compares the European Union, Canada, United States, and Japan on a number of dimensions of free trade rhetoric versus protectionist practice (Watkins and Fowler, 2002: 97–121). "Taken individually, each of the trade restrictions considered in the DSI is deeply damaging to developing countries. Considered collectively, they help to explain why developing countries have been unable to increase their share of world trade, and why the links between international trade and poverty reduction are so weak" (Watkins and Fowler, 2002: 100).

The World Bank has similarly noted that, while agricultural exports can reduce rural poverty and exports of textiles, clothing, and other labor-intensive manufactures can reduce urban poverty, "the world's poor face tariffs that are, on average, roughly twice as high as those imposed on the non-poor" (World Bank, 2001b: 37). The effect may be to create a substantial impediment to the upgrading of primary production within global commodity chains (Gibbon, 2001) that many economists envision as a most promising pathway for growth for low-income economies. Because many low-income economies rely on exports of agricultural commodities, subsidies and other barriers to market access represent a special problem. It has been estimated that total support to agriculture in OECD countries in 2000 amounted to US$327 billion—several times the value of industrial countries' annual ODA budgets (World Bank, 2001b: 47). Such subsidies not only limit developing countries' market access, as industrialized country producers can offer artificially low prices in their domestic markets, but also offer domestic producers an incentive to generate surpluses that are dumped on international markets, as in the case of sugar from the United States and wheat from the European Union (Watkins, 2003).

On the other hand, some development policy activists claim that both Oxfam and the World Bank have excessive faith in the potential of export-oriented development strategies, especially in the agricultural sector (Bello, 2002; Shiva, 2002). They argue that diversion of resources from domestic to export production might actually worsen the situation of smallholders and subsistence producers, undermining food security and placing greater stresses on the environment. Conversely, "agroindustralization" may mean that economic benefits flow to large-scale commercial producers within developing countries and to "upstream" actors such as the processors, distributors, and supermarkets that are increasingly important in global agricultural commodity chains (McMichael, 1993; Raynolds et al., 1993; Raikes and Gibbon, 2000; Reardon and Barrett, 2000; Lang, 2003).[12]

Considerable anticipation existed that a new round of trade talks begun at Doha, Qatar, in November 2001 would constitute a true "development round" in which the trade policy priorities of developing countries, including expanded market access, would be taken seriously. At the last summit (2001) before terrorism concerns came to dominate the G8 agenda, the G8 "agreed . . . to support the launch of an ambitious new round of global trade negotiations with a balanced agenda" (G8, 2001, § 10). The Doha process itself dampened that optimism somewhat (Third World Network, 2001), largely because of industrialized countries' intransigence on agricultural subsidies (Watkins, 2003); follow-up talks in Mexico ended in acrimony in September 2003 as it became apparent that the developed countries, notably several members of the G8 (the European Union, United States, and Japan) were unwilling to concede much in the area of market access, even while demanding expanded investment opportunities for their own firms (Denny et al., 2003; Denny and Elliott, 2003). Three years later, a similar failure at the Hong Kong ministerial meeting was narrowly averted by

agreement on both an end-date of 2013 for agricultural export subsidies and eventual reduction of domestic subsidies, albeit more slowly than developing countries had urged. Export subsidies for cotton—the bane of West African cotton producers who have already won two WTO disputes against the United States on this issue—must end by 2006. But this agreement actually means little: domestic subsidies, which account for 80% to 90% of U.S. support to cotton producers, will not be reduced until and unless agreement on an overall package of reductions in domestic agricultural subsidies is reached (International Centre for Trade and Sustainable Development, 2005; Third World Network, 2005).

Trade policy can affect not only the economic determinants of health but also the operation of health systems. By the end of the 1990s, it had become apparent that harmonization of patent law regimes under the 1995 Agreement on Trade-Related Intellectual Property Rights (TRIPS) would result in prohibitively high prices for the antiretroviral medications that are now a standard therapy for HIV/AIDS in the industrialized world. Prolonged campaigns by some developing country governments and civil society organizations resulted in the November 2001 Declaration on TRIPS and Public Health (WTO, 2001) and a subsequent interpretation by the WTO General Council in August 2003 (WTO, 2003; for overviews of these events, see 't Hoen, 2002; Sell, 2003: 146–162, 2004; Brysk, 2004). Despite resistance on the part of some industrialized countries, especially the United States, the declaration and its interpretation established that, within the provisions of TRIPS, medical necessity can justify both compulsory licensing (enabling production of lower cost generic versions of patented drugs) and production of generics for export to countries that lack domestic production capacity ("parallel imports," in WTO-speak). It remains to be seen how effectively the declaration will be used to increase access to essential medicines, especially for conditions other than HIV/AIDS, which is unlike other communicable diseases that affect large numbers of people in the developing world (e.g., tuberculosis, malaria, schistosomiasis, trypanosomiasis) in that it affects substantial numbers of people in the industrialized world with private assets, third-party (public or private) health insurance, and political clout.[13] Canada was the first G7 country to amend its patent legislation to permit domestic firms to produce generic drugs for export in accordance with the declaration (Orbinski, 2004), but the Canadian legislation is compromised in several respects: most notably, the schedule accompanying the legislation lists only a limited number of drugs, with others to be added only by cabinet approval—an approach that invites lobbying by pharmaceutical firms whose profits might be threatened (Elliot, 2004).

More basic limits on governments' health policy flexibility may result from the outcome of negotiations now under way on the General Agreement on Trade in Services (GATS) under the auspices of the WTO (Pollock and Price, 2003; Woodward, 2003). Governments can "reserve" particular services—that is, take them off the table—for purposes of these negotiations, but strong pressures exist not to do so, especially for countries concerned about market access for their own products or services. Once a particular service (e.g., part or all of the health sector) has been opened to foreign investment under GATS, privatization is essentially "locked in": if a foreign firm (e.g., a private insurer or a hospital management corporation) lost markets as a result of a subsequent effort to limit commercial activity, WTO dispute settlement procedures might come into play and expose a country wishing to curtail commercial health care provision or financing to demands for compensation in other areas of trade. U.S. managed care firms have already expanded into the Latin American market, predictably leaving the highest cost, lowest income patients for public health care systems (Stocker et al., 1999; Iriart et al., 2001), and GATS is being actively promoted, especially by the United States and the European Union, as a way of opening up markets for their service providers. The prospect of increased disparities in access to health care as a result of locked-in privatization is therefore not far-fetched.

HEALTH SYSTEMS

Health care matters, and the controversy over antiretrovirals is just one instance among many in which lack of access to interventions that would be taken for granted in the industrialized world is a matter of life and death outside it (Farmer, 1999, 2003). Money matters, too, and the single most important fact about health care outside the industrialized world is the desperate scarcity of money. Despite rhetorical acknowledgment of the importance of "[s]trong national health systems" (G8, 2001, § 17), the G8 have consistently avoided

concrete summit commitments to increase funding. In 2001, the WHO Commission on Macroeconomics and Health estimated the cost of a package of basic, relatively well-understood low-cost and low-tech interventions (Jha et al., 2002; see also Spinaci and Heymann, 2001) at $34 per person per year. Making these interventions widely available could save "at least 8 million lives *each year* by the end of this decade, extending the life spans, productivity and economic well-being of the poor" (Commission on Macroeconomics and Health, 2001: 11, emphasis original). The commission warned that its cost figures were "on the low end of the range of [cost] estimates," and that "[n]ot a lot of quality health services can be purchased at $30 to $45 per person. . . . Our estimates refer to a rather minimal health system, one that can attend to the major communicable diseases and maternal and perinatal conditions that account for a significant proportion of the avoidable deaths in the low-income countries" (Commission on Macroeconomics and Health, 2001: 55–56). Annual health budgets of $30–45 per person would nevertheless represent a dramatic improvement over the $14 per person that is available to provide health care for 1.1 billion people whose countries spend the least on health.[14]

The Commission estimated that scaling up provision of those essential interventions for 2.5 billion people, in sub-Saharan Africa and in countries outside that region with per capita gross national product of less than $1,200, would require $22.1 billion in new development assistance financing in 2007, rising to $30.7 billion in 2015 (Commission on Macroeconomics and Health, 2001: table A2.6, all figures in constant 2002 dollars). The Commission argued as well for rapidly expanded health surveillance and research on diseases of the poor, bringing its total estimate of the needed new money to $27 billion in 2007, rising to $38 billion in 2015. Its report assumed that universal access to basic health interventions in middle-income countries could be provided through the reallocation of resources already available from domestic sources—an assumption that may be arithmetically valid but ignores obvious political constraints. Emphasis was also placed on the need for "complementary investments" in health-related areas such as education, water and sanitation, and agricultural improvement but did not provide cost estimates (Commission on Macroeconomics and Health, 2001: 25). Such multiple downward biases in the Commission's estimates of the overall need for new money mean that it is even more disturbing to compare them with the value of total ODA for health. Although the amount has been increasing in recent years, with about half the new G7 aid commitments for Africa targeting health, total ODA for health (the amount given by all donors to *all* recipient nations) was still just $8.1 billion in 2002, the most recent year for which reliable figures are available (Michaud, 2003). This is about the same amount that people in the United States spend each year on bathroom renovations (Scott, 2002).

The international community may actually have contributed to health resource scarcities, in particular as they affect the poorest and most vulnerable, through promotion of a market-oriented concept of health sector reform (HSR) that strongly favors private provision and financing (Mackintosh, 2003; Petchesky, 2003: chapter 4; Koivusalo and Mackintosh, 2004). Multilateral institutions such as the World Bank have been especially important in this respect (see, e.g., Kim et al., 2000; Iriart et al., 2001); so pervasive is the influence of these agencies that HSR was once defined explicitly as "those activities undertaken cooperatively between the international development banks and a national government to alter in fundamental ways the nation's health financing and health provision policies" (Glassman et al., 1999: 115). The multilateral institutions are important not only because of their leverage as lenders,[15] but also, and more broadly, as knowledge producers (Mehta, 2001; Wade, 2002) and as nodes in a transnational network of professionals characterized by common assumptions, training experiences, and career paths (Lee and Goodman, 2002).

In 1987, the World Bank endorsed a set of policy prescriptions including partial cost recovery through user charges, expansion of insurance as a financing mechanism, strengthening "nongovernment provision of health services for which households are willing to pay," and decentralizing the delivery of health services (Akin et al., 1987: 25). In its widely cited 1993 World Development Report on Investing in Health, the World Bank was even clearer about its preference for markets as mechanisms for resource allocation: "There must be a basis for believing that the government can achieve a better outcome than private markets can" in providing and financing health services, and the cost-effectiveness of publicly financed health interventions ("value for money") must be determined by comparison "with the situation created by privately financed health interventions" (World Bank, 1993: 65). The World Bank often does not speak with a single

voice and may have moderated its enthusiasm for markets in recent years as part of a rediscovered interest in poverty reduction. On the other hand, marketization of the health sector is entirely congruent with the World Bank's position on the design of labor market institutions, pension funds, and social assistance as stated in its Social Protection Sector Strategy in 2000: "In an ideal world with perfectly symmetrical information and complete, well-functioning markets, all risk management arrangements can and should be market-based (except for the incapacitated)" (Holzmann and Jörgensen, 2001: 16). Social policies to help the nonincapacitated poor can be justified only because of market failures resulting from the fact that the poor "are more vulnerable than other population groups because they are typically more exposed to risk and have little access to appropriate risk management instruments" (Holzmann and Jörgensen, 2001: 10). More concretely, retrenchment in public sector health spending and the imposition of user fees and other cost recovery measures have often been mandated as part of structural adjustment conditionalities determined jointly by the World Bank and the IMF (Loewenson, 1993; Lundy, 1996; Schoepf et al., 2000; Yong Kim et al., 2000; Bassett et al., 2000; see also chapter 13). Although it is theoretically attractive to provide fee exemptions for the poorest users of health care (Gilson and Mills, 1995; Nolan and Turbat, 1995: 43–51; Gilson, 1997; Mills, 1998), in practice these have proved difficult to implement and are often ignored (Gilson et al., 2001: 60–63), at least partly because of "the conflict between financial sustainability and protection of the poor" (Gilson et al., 2001: 54; see also Nolan and Turbat, 1995: 26–28, 36–37). On equity grounds, the best that can be said for official user charges is that they may replace informal and even more inequitable patterns of side payments demanded by care providers or suppliers of medicines (Killingsworth et al., 1999; Ensor and Witter, 2001; Akashi et al., 2004).

The concept of HSR described here has proved remarkably resilient in the face of evidence that its effectiveness in generating revenue is limited and that it often leads to deterioration in access to health care for the poor and otherwise vulnerable.[16] That deterioration occurs because very large numbers of people in the developing world simply cannot afford necessary health care (Narayan et al., 2000; Whitehead et al., 2001). For example, national survey data in Mexico indicate that 51.8% of people who did not seek medical care for severe illness gave cost, or their own lack of money, as a reason (Leyva-Flores et al., 2001: 19). A smaller scale study of patterns of health service utilization in Lusaka, Zambia, found that costs were the most commonly given reason for choosing self-medication as a first resort in case of illness and also the most common reason for noncompliance with treatment regimes following a visit to the centralized university teaching hospital (Atkinson et al., 1999). Ethnographic research and the experiences of front-line care providers (Farmer, 1999, 2003; Mill and Anarfi, 2002) support the conclusion that the issue is often not one of unwillingness to pay, but rather of inability to pay, and understandable reluctance to sell off assets that may be critical to the household's economic survival (Russell, 1996; Narayan et al., 2000). In 1999, a Ghanaian columnist described the choices facing the poor in that country's increasingly marketized health care system as "pay cash or carry death" (quoted in Mill and Anarfi, 2002: 331).

On a global scale, a vision of health care that places primary reliance on markets is problematic in another way, as well. Because the private pharmaceutical industry now accounts for 41.5% of all health research spending (Global Forum for Health Research, 2004: 112), research directions are shaped by anticipation of commercial returns. Of 1,393 new drugs marketed between 1975 and 1999, only 16 were for tropical diseases and tuberculosis (Trouiller et al., 2002). "Apparently it is more profitable to develop and market Viagra than to research a new drug to treat patients with visceral leishmaniasis, a fatal disease if left untreated. Such a drug is more likely to be developed through veterinary research if it has economic potential on the pet market" (Veeken and Pécoul, 2000: 309; see also Picard, 2000; Reich, 2000). The result is the so-called "10/90 gap": roughly 10% of health research spending addresses conditions that account for 90% of the global burden of disease, overwhelmingly outside the industrialized world, reflecting the more general axiom that "money talks louder than need" in setting priorities for scientific research (United Nations Development Programme, 1999: 68–76).

CONCLUSION: THE POLITICS AND ETHICS OF HEALTH EQUITY

For Calabresi and Bobbitt (1978), tragic choices in health care and policy are exemplified by decisions that must be made when the number of candidates for organ transplants far exceeds the scarcity of donor organs. This is close to a situation in which scarcity is absolute, within constraints defined by today's natural and technological capabilities. Far more common are situations in which "scarcity is not the result of any absolute lack of a resource but rather of the decision by society that it is not prepared to forgo other goods and benefits in a number sufficient to remove the scarcity" (Calabresi and Bobbitt, 1978: 22). In other words, "scarcity cannot simply be assumed as a given" (Calabresi and Bobbitt, 1978: 151) but must be understood as the result of political and economic decisions that affect health and the determinants of health—for example, about how much to spend on ODA, or whether to give basic needs in developing countries priority over the balance sheets of creditor institutions in the industrialized world. Jeffrey Sachs, who chaired the Commission on Macroeconomics and Health, forcefully notes that "in a world of trillions of dollars of income every year, the amount of money that you need to address the health crises is easily available in the world" (Sachs, 2003: 3). This is the first, and most basic, answer to the question of what politics has to do with health and the global economy.

The question of how best to "pitch" advocacy in support of policies that improve the determinants of health, especially across national borders, is a matter not only of tactics but also of social science and, ultimately, of ethics. Certain interventions, including infection control and some forms of environmental protection, may represent genuine "public goods" that the rich world cannot feasibly purchase for itself while excluding others (Chen et al., 1999). On this line of reasoning, taken to its extreme in the claim that "better health for anyone, anywhere on earth, benefits everyone else" (Global Forum for Health Research, 2002: 35), global health is an investment in global security, and the economic costs associated with the recent outbreak of SARS show the value of infection control as a public good.

A more expansive economic argument was made by the Commission on Macroeconomics and Health, for which "investment in health" represented an investment in future development, because it can initiate virtuous cycles of human capital formation and growth. Conversely, failure to invest in health can result in a vicious downward spiral as households sell off assets necessary to their survival, falling into a "medical poverty trap" from which escape is extremely difficult (Whitehead et al., 2001; see also Narayan et al., 2000). This trap can ensnare not only households but also communities, regional economies, and ultimately entire nations, like many countries in sub-Saharan Africa that are hardest hit by HIV/AIDS (Brown, 2004).

Using the term "public good" in its technical economic sense, there may not be very many global public goods for health: eradication of diseases like smallpox and polio; control of HIV infection, because of the ease of cross-border transmission, and of epidemic influenza—which, curiously, is hardly ever mentioned in the global health literature; and control of antimicrobial resistance. Control of tuberculosis may also qualify, because multidrug-resistant tuberculosis presents a threat even to certain populations within the industrialized world. With these exceptions, control of communicable diseases that contribute most to the global burden of disease is at best a regional public good—and within the affected regions, protection from diseases such as malaria and tuberculosis is much more readily available to the rich than to the poor (Farmer, 2000; Woodward and Smith, 2003; Smith et al., 2004). For women, gender and class or social subordination often interact to magnify the dangers of HIV infection (see Schoepf, 1998, 2004, on southern Africa; see Epele, 2002, on the United States), emphasizing the extent to which HIV infection is now, like tuberculosis, primarily a problem of the powerless rather than the powerful. Benefits from control of injuries and noncommunicable diseases are inherently more place specific and often more closely related to economic situation and social position.

The body of evidence for the prevalence of "medical poverty traps" means that the Commission on Macroeconomics and Health discourse of investment in health, subsequently embraced by WHO (WHO, 2002a), has a stronger empirical foundation than a strategy of improving health equity by way of supplying public goods. At the same time, investing in health as an organizing principle for public policy arguably invites a form of economic triage that is inimical to health equity concerns: countries, regions, and populations at the front of the queue for investments in health may be those that offer the greatest promise of economic returns, for example, because of the availability of expanding consumer markets or the availability of healthy and relatively skilled yet low-cost labor. "Health redlining"[17] is a useful way of thinking about triages that direct resources away from populations that cannot be expected to generate adequate returns on investment; Bond (2001: 179–182) suggests that such a process underlies the South African government's reluctance to mobilize resources for treatment of HIV/AIDS, which "is killing workers and low-income consumers"—in other words, members of a population that are expendable for purposes of macroeconomic policy—"at a time when South African elites in any case are adopting capital-intensive, export-oriented accumulation strategies."

An emerging literature on health equity (Evans et al., 2001; Braveman, 2003; Braveman and Gruskin, 2003a, 2003b; McCoy et al., 2003) "reflects a concern to reduce unequal opportunities to be healthy associated with membership in less privileged social groups, such as poor people; disenfranchised racial, ethnic or religious groups; women; and rural residents. In operational terms, pursuing equity in health means eliminating health disparities that are systematically associated with underlying social disadvantage or marginalization" (Braveman and Gruskin, 2003b: 540). In a related vein, drawing on commitments made in the 1948 Universal Declaration of Human Rights and subsequent elaborations, some scholars and legal practitioners now put forward instead the concept of health as a human right in the global frame of reference (Attaran, 1999; Austin, 2001; Chapman, 2002; Hunt, 2003). The attractiveness of the argument is that if health (or, more precisely, access to opportunities to lead and protect a healthy life) is a right, then some claims on resources necessary to realize that right do not require vindication with reference to an external criterion such as current purchasing power or future earning power (the unspoken basis for triage in the discourse of investment in health). The rights-based position is also more in keeping with health equity as "a values-based commitment to tackle poverty and health, with or without conclusive evidence of aggregate utilitarian gains" (Braveman and Gruskin, 2003b: 540). The appointment of a United Nations Special Rapporteur on the right to health in 2002, the renewal of his appointment in 2005, and his willingness to define his mandate as including (for instance) the impact of trade agreements on the right to health (Hunt, 2004b), suggest that the rights-based approach may slowly be moving into the development and health policy mainstream (see Hunt, 2003; Hunt 2004a; Hunt, 2005).

Intellectual and institutional challenges facing proponents of this position are formidable: they need not only to establish a credible basis for obligations across national borders, when the primary focus of human rights law and policy has been the obligations of governments to those living under their jurisdiction, but also to establish foundations for articulating those obligations in the relevant political and legal forums. Adding to the difficulties is a political environment that, especially in the Anglo-American world, is generally hostile to redistributive policies even within national borders. Encouragingly, researchers in many fields related to international health are now refusing to accept "resource scarcity" as a fact of life (Berer, 2002; Petchesky, 2003; Narasimhan and Attaran, 2003; Sachs, 2003; Labonte et al., 2004). Arguably, a more appropriate strategy for research and advocacy is to investigate distributions of economic and political power that make resources scarce for some purposes, such as meeting basic health-related needs, but virtually limitless for private discretionary consumption (by the few) and public military adventures.

Our own experience as researchers investigating the links between G8 policies and health in the developing world indicates that pursuing this strategy requires alliances and collaborations that cross disciplinary, institutional, and sectoral boundaries, as well as national borders. These are difficult to establish under the best of circumstances, and especially so when they involve researchers and civil society organizations in developing countries that lack the resources (computers, reliable high-speed Internet service, rapid access to electronic journals through university libraries) that many researchers in the industrialized world take for granted.

The special importance of transdisciplinarity is evident from the range of literature canvassed for this chapter. Research into the pathways by which contemporary globalization affects health differently for winners and losers, within and between countries, is needed in order to continue developing an evidence base against which to evaluate market-driven development policies. Agencies that support research in the areas of international health and development policy must take into account the special requirements of such collaborations. At the same time, considerable evidence already exists that the fundamental health challenge presented by contemporary globalization is the necessity of a market-correcting system of wealth redistribution within and between nations. As Nancy Birdsall, president of the Washington-based Center for Global Development, has stated the issue:

> [G]lobalization, as we know it today, is fundamentally asymmetric. In its benefits and its risks, it works less well for the currently poor countries and for poor households within developing countries. Because markets at the national level are asymmetric, modern capitalist economies have social contracts, progressive tax systems, and laws and regulations to manage asymmetries and market failures. At the global level, there is no real equivalent to national governments to manage global markets, though they are bigger and deeper, and if anything more asymmetric. They work better for the rich; and their risks and failures hurt the poor. (Birdsall, 2002: 67–68)

Some vehicles for this redistribution are identified or suggested in this chapter. They include increases in development assistance; expanded debt cancellation, and debt relief calculated on the basis of the domestic expenditures necessary to meet basic human needs; trade agreements that allow low- and middle-income nations to achieve a level of domestic economic development that can make global market competition less unequal; and subordination of trade policy imperatives to human rights norms (i.e., the right to health) or attainment of the MDGs. Others include some form of tax on financial transactions to curb "hot money" speculation, perhaps supplemented by a carbon tax to reduce the profligate use of fossil fuels by high-income nations (notably several G8 countries), as the beginning of a rudimentary global taxation system that could be used for development/redistributive purposes.

These are not necessarily new ideas, but they challenge contemporary orthodoxies and entail a change in the present global distribution of wealth and power. History suggests that such changes often demand radical forms of political mobilization and action, although history has not yet encountered such a demand on a global scale. No simple precedents exist, but several forms of mobilization are already being pursued. These include, in no particular order of importance:

- The increasing prominence of human rights discourse in national and global frames of reference
- The simultaneous rise of a global civil society movement pressing for political actions to shift

the rules of contemporary globalization (see, e.g., People's Health Movement et al., 2005)

- Direct actions by local, national, and regional groupings of actors, attempting to hold their governments and multinational enterprises accountable for the impacts of their policies and practices on health and human development
- A growing web of linkages among labor, women's, environmental, and other groups, both within and across borders, that may prevent elites whose interests are threatened by economic and social justice or environmental sustainability from engaging in divide-and-conquer tactics

Whether or not the G8, and its annual summits, represents an appropriate target for such mobilization continues to be debated. Remaining silent on the links between G8 policies and health, however, is not an option (Labonte and Schrecker, 2006).

Notes

1. Not all globalization scholars, not even all those examining health impacts (e.g., Lee, 2001), would confine their analysis to economic dimensions. Nor are other approaches to the theorization of globalization, e.g., those emphasizing changed real and perceived dimensions of space (shrinking), time (speeding up), environment (stressed/depleted), and culture (blending/diffusing, or alternatively clashing), necessarily inaccurate or unhelpful.

2. The G8 (Group of 8 Nations) was formed in 1975 as the G6 in response to the challenges of economic management created by the first "oil crisis" (Webb, 2000). The six countries originally included were France, the United States, Britain, Germany, Italy, and Japan. Canada joined the club in 1976; Russia achieved partial membership in the group in 1998 and full membership as of 2003. However, in some circumstances it makes more sense to refer to the G7 than to the G8 — e.g., Russia is now in no position to provide development assistance. Our usage in the text reflects this economic disparity between Russia and other G8 members.

3. This calculation has been criticized for underestimating the true extent of poverty, notably because of shortcomings in the way "purchasing power parities" are calculated and the fact that neither $1 nor $2 per day reflects actual minimum costs of basic needs that are of primary concern to the poor (Reddy and Pogge, 2003; Satterthwaite, 2003; Wade, 2004).

4. All official documents from G8 summits and ministerial meetings cited here are available from the G8 Research Group (2006).

5. Individual countries vary widely in the proportion of their debt owed to private banks, national governments' export credit agencies (which are agencies that offer loans at below-market interest rates to purchasers of their country's exports), and multilateral institutions such as the World Bank and IMF.

6. Economic historian Thomas Naylor stated in 1987, "There would be no 'debt crisis' without large-scale capital flight" (Naylor, 1987: 1370). More recently, Ndikumana and Boyce (2003: 122) found that, "[d]uring 1970–96, roughly 80 cents on every dollar that flowed into [sub-Saharan Africa] from foreign loans flowed back out as capital flight in the same year," and the author who coined the phrase the "Washington Consensus" to describe the market-oriented axioms that guided development policy in the 1980s has warned that the possibilities for progressive taxation to finance social spending in Latin America are limited "because too many of the Latin rich have the option of placing too many of their assets in Miami" (Williamson, 2004: 13). For more extensive discussion of capital flight and its implications for fiscal capacity, see Helleiner (2001) and Labonte et al. (2004: 14–16, 32–34).

7. That is, the value of the debt (principal and interest) in today's dollars, after discounting for future inflation to reflect the fact that it need only be repaid in the future.

8. Debt cancellation costs are routinely included as part of a donor country's ODA budget. Thus, the $825 million that African countries owe to Export Development Canada (an export credit agency) and the Canadian Wheat Board (a marketing agency that guarantees minimum producer prices for wheat exports) will, as these debts are canceled over the next few years, be reckoned as part of almost 20% of Canada's staged increase in development assistance for African countries (Canadian Council for International Cooperation Africa-Canada Forum, 2002).

9. For reasons of space, we leave aside the important questions of whether taxpayers in the industrialized world should bear the costs of losses incurred by private lenders, and of whether some debts incurred by developing country governments — e.g., those incurred to finance domestic repression or foreign military ventures — are "odious debts" and therefore should be regarded as uncollectable as a matter of ethics and perhaps of international law (Kremer and Jayachandran, 2002).

10. In the Mexican case, the impact of low-cost imports was magnified, and in fact preceded, by domestic policies of restructuring agriculture to favor large-scale commercial farming and "dismantling of official assistance to small-scale producers of basic crops" (Preibisch et al., 2002: 68).

11. Such a development path is not necessarily benign in terms of its domestic social consequences: consider the high level of political repression in predemocratization South Korea (Cumings, 1989) as an instance of the axiom that "[t]he discipline of labor by the state lies at the heart of all late industrialization" (Amsden, 1990: 10).

12. This controversy is one of several illustrating (a) that policy analysis using a determinants-of-health approach in the international context, especially if it is

intended to be prescriptive, is difficult to disentangle from much broader debates about appropriate development strategies, and (b) that considerable caution is in order when generalizing about such appropriate strategies and their potential health implications.

13. This fact arguably explains the existence of anti-retrovirals in the first place: a critical mass of victims in the rich countries created financial and political incentives for their commercialization. As pointed out in the conclusion of this chapter, a resource allocation problem that logically precedes issues of licensing and intellectual property involves finding necessary financing for scientific research that could lead to new treatments for diseases of the poor.

14. Population-weighted average health expenditure from all sources (public and private), calculated for all countries where health expenditure is ≤$21/capita from data tables 2.1 and 2.15, World Bank Health, nutrition and population data series.

15. The World Bank, e.g., is "now the single largest external source of HNP [Health, Nutrition, and Population] financing in low- and middle-income countries" (Preker et al., 2000: ix).

16. Space does not permit even a summary of the evidence here (for key reviews and case studies, see Creese, 1991; Laurell, 1991; McPake et al., 1993; Gilson, 1997; Creese and Kutzin, 1997; Bloom, 1998; Barrientos and Lloyd-Sherlock, 2000; Yong Kim et al., 2000; Gilson et al., 2001; Liu et al., 2001; Hung et al., 2001; Laurell, 2001; Liu, 2002; Bloom et al., 2002; Wadee et al., 2003; Lister, 2005).

17. The term "redlining" derives from the practice of mortgage lending agencies financed by the U.S. federal government of drawing red lines on local maps around "neighborhoods that were dense, [racially] mixed, or aging." They would refuse to lend for home purchases within those areas, thereby accelerating their decline and undermining the quality of life of people not rich enough to move out (Jackson, 1985: 197–218).

References

ACC/SCN (2000). *Fourth Report on the World Nutrition Situation: Nutrition throughout the Life Cycle.* Geneva: United Nations Administrative Committee on Coordination Sub-committee on Nutrition, in collaboration with the International Food Policy Research Institute. Available: http://www.unsystem .org/scn/Publications/4RWNS/4rwns.pdf.

Akashi H, Yamada T, Huot E, Kanal K, and Sugimoto T (2004). User fees at a public hospital in Cambodia: effects on hospital performance and provider attitudes. *Social Science and Medicine* 58: 553–564.

Akin J, Birdsall N, and de Ferranti D (1987). *Financing Health Services in Developing Countries: An Agenda for Reform.* Washington, DC: World Bank.

Amsden A (1990). Third world industrialization: "global Fordism" or a new model. *New Left Review* 1820: 5–31.

Amsden A (1994). Why isn't the whole world experimenting with the East Asian model to develop? *World Development* 22: 627–633.

Anon (2002). Mexico's farmers: floundering in a tariff-free landscape. *The Economist,* November 30, 31–32.

Arulpragasam J, and Prennushi G (2002). *Poverty Reduction and the World Bank: Progress in Operationalizing the WDR 2000/2001.* Washington, DC: World Bank. Available: http://www.worldbank.org/poverty/ library/progr/2000-01/report.pdf.

Atkinson S, Ngwengwe A, Macwan'gi M, Ngulube TJ, Harpham T, and O'Connell A (1999). The referral process and urban health care in sub-Saharan Africa: the case of Lusaka, Zambia. *Social Science and Medicine* 49: 27–38.

Attaran A (1999). Human rights and biomedical research funding for the developing world: discovering state obligations under the right to health. *Health and Human Rights* 4(1): 26–58.

Austin W (2001). Using the human rights paradigm in health ethics: the problems and the possibilities. *Nursing Ethics* 8: 183–195.

Barrientos A, and Lloyd-Sherlock P (2000). Reforming health insurance in Argentina and Chile. *Health Policy and Planning* 15: 417–423.

Bassett MT, Bijlmakers LA, and Sanders D (2000). Experiencing Structural Adjustment in Urban and Rural Households of Zimbabwe. In: Turshen M, ed., *African Women's Health.* Trenton, NJ: Africa World Press, pp. 167–191.

Bates I, Fenton C, Gruber J, Lalloo D, Medina Lara A, Squire SB, et al. (2004a). Vulnerability to malaria, tuberculosis, and HIV/AIDS infection and disease. Part 1: determinants operating at individual and household level. *Lancet Infectious Diseases* 4: 267–277.

Bates I, Fenton C, Gruber J, Lalloo D, Medina Lara A, Squire SB, et al. (2004b). Vulnerability to malaria, tuberculosis, and HIV/AIDS infection and disease. Part II: determinants operating at environmental and institutional level. *Lancet Infectious Diseases* 4: 368–375.

Bello W (2002). What's Wrong with the Oxfam Trade Campaign. Focus on the Global South (online). Available: http://www.globalpolicy.org/socecon/ bwi-wto/wto/2002/04260xfam2.htm.

Berer M (2002). Health sector reforms: implications for sexual and reproductive health services. *Reproductive Health Matters* 10: 6–15.

Birdsall N (2002). A stormy day on an open field: asymmetry and convergence in the global economy. In: Gruen D, O'Brien T, Lawson J, eds., *Globalisation, Living Standards and Inequality: Recent Progress and Continuing Challenges,* Proceedings of a Conference held in Sydney, May 27–28, 2002. Canberra: Reserve Bank of Australia, pp. 66–87. Available: http://www.rba.gov.au/PublicationsAnd Research/Conferences/2002/.

Bloom G (1998). Primary health care meets the market in China and Vietnam. *Health Policy* 44: 233–252.

Bloom G, Lu Y, and Chen J (2002). *Financing Health Care in China's Cities: Balancing Needs and Entitlements during Rapid Change*. IDS Working Paper 176. Brighton, UK: Institute of Development Studies. Available: http://www.ids.ac.uk/ids/bookshop/wp/wp176.pdf.

Bond P (2001). *Against Global Apartheid: South Africa Meets the World Bank, IMF and International Finance*. Cape Town: University of Cape Town Press.

Bosshard P, Bruil J, Horta K, Lawrence S, and Welch C (2003). *Gambling with People's Lives: What the World Bank's New "High-Risk/High-Reward" Strategy Means for the Poor and the Environment*. Washington, DC: Environmental Defense. Available: http://www.foe.org/camps/intl/worldbank/gambling/Gambling.pdf.

Bradshaw D, Groenewald P, Laubscher R, Nannan N, Nojilana R, Pieterse D, et al. (2003). Initial burden of disease estimates for South Africa 2000. *South African Medical Journal* 93: 682–688.

Braveman P (2003). Monitoring equity in health and healthcare: a conceptual framework. *Journal of Health Population and Nutrition* 21: 181–192.

Braveman P, and Gruskin S (2003a). Defining equity in health. *Journal of Epidemiology and Community Health* 57: 254–258.

Braveman P, and Gruskin S (2003b). Poverty, equity, human rights and health. *Bulletin of the World Health Organization* 81: 539–545.

Bright M, and Keegan W (2004). G7 torpedoes Brown's debt write-off push. [London] *Observer*, October 3.

Brock K, and McGee R (2004). *Mapping Trade Policy: Understanding the Challenges of Civil Society Participation*. IDS Working Paper 225. Brighton, UK: Institute of Development Studies.

Brown LR (2004). Economic growth rates in africa: the potential impact of HIV/AIDS. In: Kalipeni E, Craddock S, Oppong JR, and Ghosh J, eds., *HIV and AIDS in Africa: Beyond Epidemiology*. Oxford: Blackwell, pp. 291–303.

Brysk A (2004). Human rights and private wrongs: constructing norms in global civil society. Presented to International Studies Association annual conference, Montreal, March 17–20. Available: http://archive.allacademic.com/publication/index.php?PHPSESSID=798ee11e8649a600de7ce22588ddf11e.

Calabresi G, and Bobbitt P (1978). *Tragic Choices*. New York: W.W. Norton.

Canadian Council for International Cooperation Africa-Canada Forum (2002). *Canadian Economic Relations with Sub-Saharan Africa: Recent Trends*. Ottawa: Canadian Council for International Cooperation. Available: www.ccic.ca/e/docs/003_acf_revised_sept_can_economic_relation_africa.pdf.

Chang H-J (2002). *Kicking Away the Ladder: Development Strategy in Historical Perspective*. London: Anthem Press.

Chapman AR (2002). Core obligations related to the right to health. In: Chapman A, and Russell S, eds., *Core Obligations: Building a Framework for Economic, Social and Cultural Rights*. Antwerp: Intersentia, pp. 185–215.

Chen L, and Berlinguer G (2001). Health equity in a globalizing world. In: Evans T, Whitehead M, Diderichsen F, Bhuiya A, and Wirth M, eds., *Challenging Inequities in Health: From Ethics to Action*. New York: Oxford University Press, pp. 34–44.

Chen L, Evans T, and Cash R (1999). Health as a global public good. In: *Global Public Goods: International Cooperation in the 21st Century*. New York: Oxford University Press (for United Nations Development Programme), pp. 184–204.

Chen S, and Ravallion M (2004). *How Have the World's Poorest Fared since the Early 1980s?* Policy Research Working Paper 3341. Washington, DC: Development Research Group, World Bank. Available: http://www.worldbank.org/research/povmonitor/MartinPapers/How_have_the_poorest_fared_since_the_early_1980s.pdf.

Cheru F (1999). *Economic, Social and Cultural Rights: Effects of Structural Adjustment Policies on the Full Enjoyment of Human Rights*. E/CN.4/1999/50. Geneva: Office of the United Nations High Commissioner for Human Rights. Available: http://www.unhchr.ch/Huridocda/Huridoca.nsf/TestFrame/f991c6c62457a2858025675100348aef?Opendocument.

Cheru F (2001). *Economic, Social and Cultural Rights: The Highly Indebted Poor Countries (HIPC) Initiative—a Human Rights Assessment of the Poverty Reduction Strategy Papers (PRSP)*. E/CN.4/2001/56. Geneva: Office of the United Nations High Commissioner for Human Rights. Available: http://www.unhchr.ch/Huridocda/Huridoca.nsf/0/d3b348546ad5fb91c1256a110056aca4/$FILE/G0110184.pdf.

Chirac J (2003). Speech to the Opening Meeting of the 58th Session of the United Nations General Assembly, September 2003. New York: Permanent Mission of France to the United States. Available: http://www.un.int/france/documents_anglais/030923_mae_charac_ag

Commission for Africa (2005). *Our Common Interest: Report of the Commission for Africa*. London: Commission for Africa. Available: http://www.commissionforafrica.org/english/report/thereport/english/11-03-05_cr_report.pdf

Commission on Macroeconomics and Health (2001). *Macroeconomics and Health: Investing in Health for Economic Development*. Geneva: World Health Organization. Available: http://www.cid.harvard.edu/cidcmh/CMHReport.pdf.

Cornia GA (1987). Economic decline and human welfare in the first half of the 1980s. In: Cornia GA, Jolly R, and Stewart F, eds., *Adjustment with a Human Face, Vol. 1: Protecting the Vulnerable and Promoting Growth*. Oxford: Clarendon Press, pp. 11–47.

Cornia GA, Jolly R, and Stewart F, eds. (1987). *Adjustment with a Human Face, Vol. 1: Protecting the*

Vulnerable and Promoting Growth. Oxford: Clarendon Press.

Creese A, and Kutzin J (1997). Lessons from cost recovery in health. In: Colclough C, ed., *Marketizing Education and Health in Developing Countries: Miracle or Mirage.* Oxford: Oxford University Press, pp. 37–62.

Creese AL (1991). User charges for health care: a review of recent experience. *Health Policy and Planning* 6: 309–319.

Cumings B (1989). The abortive abertura: South Korea in the light of Latin American experience. *New Left Review,* no. 173, pp. 5–33.

Denny C, and Elliott L (2003). G21 alliance of the poor fights subsidies deal. *Guardian,* September 15. Available: http://www.guardian.co.uk/Archive/0,4271,,00.html

Denny C, Elliott L, and Vidal J (2003). Alliance of the poor unites against west. *Guardian,* September 15. Available: http://www.guardian.co.uk/Archive/0,4271,,00.html

De Silva L, and Tropp S, eds. (2003). The Millennium Development Goals. *Development Policy Journal* 3, April (entire issue). Available: http://www.undp.org/dpa/publications/DPJ3Final1.pdf

Devarajan S, Miller MJ, and Swanson EV (2001). *Goals for Development: History, Prospects and Costs.* Washington, DC: World Bank. Available: http://econ.worldbank.org/files/13269_wps2819.pdf.

Dixon C, Simon D, and Närman A (1995). Introduction: the nature of structural adjustment. In: Simon D, van Spengen W, Dixon C, and Närman A., eds., *Structurally Adjusted Africa.* London: Pluto Press, pp. 1–14.

Economist (2003). McCurrencies. *Economist,* April 23 (online). Available: http://www.licenseenews.com/news/news188.html

Elliott L (2004). Deal on global trade holds out hope for poor nations. *Guardian,* August 2. Available: http://www.guardian.co.uk/Archive/0,4271,,00.html

Elliott L, Wintour P (2005). Biggest African debt rescue saves Nigeria £17.3 bn. *Guardian,* July 1.

Elliot R (2004). Canada's New Patent Bill Provides a Basis for Improvement. *Bridges Monthly Review* 8(5): 19–20. Available: http://www.ictsd.org/monthly/bridges/BRIDGES8-5.pdf.

Ensor T, and Witter S (2001). Health economics in low income countries: adapting to the reality of the unofficial economy. *Health Policy* 57: 1–13.

Epele ME (2002). Gender, violence and HIV: women's survival in the streets. *Culture, Medicine and Psychiatry* 26: 33–54.

Evans RG, and Stoddart GL (1990). Producing health, consuming health care. *Social Science and Medicine* 31: 1347–1363.

Evans T, Whitehead M, Diderichsen F, Bhuiya A, and Wirth M, eds. (2001). *Challenging Inequities in Health: From Ethics to Action.* New York: Oxford University Press.

Farmer P (1999). *Infections and Inequalities: The Modern Plagues.* Berkeley: University of California Press.

Farmer P (2000). The consumption of the poor: tuberculosis in the 21st century. *Ethnography* 1: 183–216.

Farmer P (2003). *Pathologies of Power: Health, Human Rights, and the New War on the Poor.* Berkeley: University of California Press.

Focus on the Global South (2003). *Anti Poverty or Anti Poor? The Millennium Development Goals and the Eradication of Extreme Poverty and Hunger.* Bangkok: Focus on the Global South. Available: http://www.dev-zone.org/cgi-bin/links/jump.cgi?ID=7135.

Friedman T (2000). *The Lexus and the Olive Tree.* New York: Anchor.

G8 (1999). G8 Communiqué Köln 1999. Köln: G8 Summit Secretariat. Available: http://www.g8.utoronto.ca/summit/1999koln/finalcom.htm

G8 (2000). G8 Okinawa Communiqué. Okinawa: G8 Summit Secretariat. Available: http://www.g8.utoronto.ca/summit/2000okinawa/finalcom.htm

G8 (2001). Final Communiqué. Genoa: G8 Summit Secretariat. Available: http://www.g8.utoronto.ca/summit/2001genoa/finalcommunique.htm

G8 Development Ministers (2003). Meeting of the G8 Development Ministers—Press Briefing from Mr Pierre-André Wiltzer (online). Available: http://www.g8.fr/evian/english/navigation/news/previous_news/ministerial_meetings_communiques/meeting_of_the_g8_development_ministers_press_briefing_from_mr_pierre-andre_wiltzer.html12003.

G8 Research Group (2006). G8 Information Centre. Toronto: University of Toronto. Available: http://www.g8.utoronto.ca/

George S (1988). *A Fate Worse Than Debt.* London: Penguin.

Gershman J, and Irwin A (2000). Getting a grip on the global economy. In: Kim JY, Millen JV, Irwin A, and Gershman J, eds., *Dying for Growth: Global Inequality and the Health of the Poor.* Monroe, ME: Common Courage Press, pp. 11–43.

Gibbon P (2001). Upgrading primary production: a global commodity chain approach. *World Development* 29: 345–363.

Gilson L (1997). The lessons of user fee experience in Africa. *Health Policy and Planning* 12: 273–285.

Gilson L, and Mills A (1995). Health sector reforms in sub-Saharan Africa: lessons of the last 10 years. *Health Policy* 32: 215–243.

Gilson L, Kalyalya D, Kuchler F, Lake S, Oranga H, and Ouendo M (2001). Strategies for promoting equity: experience with community financing in three African countries. *Health Policy* 58: 37–67.

Glassman A, Reich MR, Laserson K, and Rojas F (1999). Political analysis of health reform in the Dominican Republic. *Health Policy and Planning* 14: 115–126.

Global Forum for Health Research (2002). *The 10/90 Report on Health Research 2001–2002.* Geneva: World Health Organization. Available: http://www.globalforumhealth.org/pages/index.asp.

Global Forum for Health Research (2004). *The 10/90 Report on Health Research, 2003–2004*. Geneva: Global Forum for Health Research. Available: http://www.globalforumhealth.org/pages/index.asp.

Goldstone P (2001). *Making the World Safe for Tourism*. New Haven, CT: Yale University Press.

Greenhill R (2002). *The Unbreakable Link—Debt Relief and the Millennium Development Goals*. London: Jubilee Research. Available: http://www.jubilee2000uk.org/media/unbreakable_link.pdf.

Greenhill R, and Sisti E (2003). *Real Progress Report on HIPC*. London: Jubilee Research at the New Economics Foundation. Available: http://www.jubilee2000uk.org/analysis/reports/realprogressHIPC.pdf.

Gupta S, Clements B, Guin-Siu MT, and Leruth L (2002). Debt relief and public health spending in heavily indebted poor countries. *Bulletin of the World Health Organization* 80: 151–157.

Hanlon J (2000). How much debt must be cancelled? *Journal of International Development* 12: 877–901.

Helleiner E (2001). Regulating capital flight. *Challenge* 44(1): 19–34.

Hertzman C, and Siddiqui A (2000). Health and rapid economic change in the late twentieth century. *Social Science and Medicine* 51: 809–819.

Hiebert M (1996). *Chasing the Tigers: A Portrait of the New Vietnam*. New York: Kodansha International.

Holzmann R, and Jörgensen S (2001). *Social Protection Sector Strategy: From Safety Net to Springboard*. Washington, DC: World Bank. Available: http://wbln0018.worldbank.org/HDNet/hddocs.nsf/2d51 35ecbf351de6852566a90069b8b6/1628e080eb459 3a78525681c0070a518/$FILE/complete.pdf.

Hung P, Dzung T, Dahlgren G, and Truan T (2001). Vietnam: efficient, equity-oriented financial strategies for health. In: Evans T, Whitehead M, Diderichsen F, Bhuiya A, and Wirth M, eds., *Challenging Inequities in Health: From Ethics to Action*. New York: Oxford University Press, pp. 296–306.

Hunt P (2003). *The Right of everyone to the enjoyment of the highest attainable standard of physical and Mental Health*, A/58/427. New York: United Nations. Available: http://www.unhchr.ch/Huridocda/ Huridoca.nsf/0/306eaaf7b4938ba9c1256dd700514 35d/$FILE/N0356469.pdf

Hunt P (2004a). *The Right of Everyone to the Enjoyment of the Highest Attainable Standard of Physical and Mental Health*, A/59/422. New York: United Nations. Available: http://daccess-ods.un.org/access.nsf/ Get?Open&DS=A/59/422&Lang=E

Hunt P (2004b). *Economic, Social, and Cultural Rights: The Right of Everyone to the Enjoyment of the Highest Attainable Standard of Physical and Mental Health—Addendum: Mission to the World Trade Organization*, E/CN.4/2004/49/Add.1. Geneva: United Nations Economic and Social Council Commission on Human Rights. Available: http://www.unhchr.ch/Huridocda/Huridoca.nsf/e06a5300f90fa02 38025669700518ca4/5860d7d63239d82c1256e660 056432a/$FILE/G0411390.pdf

Hunt P (2005). *The Right of Everyone to the Enjoyment of the Highest Attainable Standard of Physical and Mental Health*, A/60/348. New York: United Nations. Available: http://daccessdds.un.org/doc/ UNDOC/GEN/N05/486/77/PDF/N0548677.pdf? OpenElement

IMF (2001). *Structural Conditionality in Fund-Supported Programs*. Washington, DC: International Monetary Fund. Available: http://www.imf.org/ External/NP/prspgen/review/2002/031502a.pdf.

IMF (2003a). *Annual Report 2003: Making the Global Economy Work for All*. Washington, DC: International Monetary Fund.

IMF (2003b). *World Economic Outlook September 2003: Public Debt in Emerging Markets*. Washington, DC: International Monetary Fund. Available: http://www.imf.org/external/pubs/ft/weo/2003/02/.

International Centre for Trade and Sustainable Development (2005). *Low Ambitions Met: Members Adopt Declaration*. Geneva: ICTSD. Available: http:// www.ictsd.org/ministerial/hongkong/wto_daily/19% 20December/en051219.pdf

Iriart C, Merhy EE, and Waitzkin H (2001). Managed care in Latin America: the new common sense in health policy reform. *Social Science and Medicine* 52: 1243–1253.

Jackson KT (1985). *Crabgrass Frontier: The Suburbanization of the United States*. New York: Oxford University Press.

Jawara F, and Kwa E (2003). *Behind the Scenes at the WTO: The Real World of International Trade Negotiations*. London: Zed Books.

Jenkins R (2004). Globalization, production, employment and poverty: debates and evidence. *Journal of International Development* 16: 1–12.

Jeter J (2002). The dumping ground: as Zambia courts western markets, used goods arrive at a heavy price. *Washington Post*, April 22, A01.

Jha P, Mills A, Hanson K, Kumaranayake L, Conteh L, Kurowski C, et al. (2002). Improving the health of the global poor. *Science* 295: 2036–2039.

Joint World Bank/IMF Development Committee (2005). *Development Committee Communiqué*, September 25. Washington, DC: International Monetary Fund. Available: http://www.imf.org/external/ np/cm/2005/0925905.htm

Jubilee Research (2005). *The G8 2005: What Are the Lessons?* August 11. London: Jubilee Research. Available: http://www.jubileeresearch.org/latest/ g8110705.htm

Junne GCA (2001). International organizations in a period of globalization: new (problems of) legitimacy. In: Coicaud J-M, and Heiskanen V, eds., *The Legitimacy of International Organizations*. Tokyo: United Nations University Press, pp. 189–220.

Kalipeni E, Craddock S, Oppong JR, and Ghosh J, eds. (2004). *HIV and AIDS in Africa: Beyond Epidemiology*. Oxford: Blackwell.

Killick T (2004). Politics, evidence and the new aid agenda. *Development Policy Review* 22: 5–29.

Killingsworth J, Hossain N, Hedrick-Wong Y, Thomas S, Rahman A, and Begum T (1999). Unofficial fees in Bangladesh: price, equity and institutional issues. *Health Policy and Planning* 14: 152–163.

Kim JY, Shakow A, Bayona J, Rhatigan J, and Rubin de Celis EL (2000). Sickness amidst recovery: public debt and private suffering in Peru. In: Kim JY, Millen JV, Irwin A, and Gershman J (eds.), *Dying for Growth: Global Inequality and the Health of the Poor*. Monroe, ME: Common Courage Press, pp. 127–154.

Koivusalo M, and Mackintosh M (2004). *Health Systems and Commercialisation: In Search of Good Sense*., Prepared for the UNRISD international conference on Commercialization of Health Care: Global and Local Dynamics and Policy Responses. Geneva: United Nations Research Institute for Social Development (UNRISD). Available: http://www.unrisd.org/80256B3C005BCCF9/httpNetITFramePDF?ReadForm&parentunid=32A160C292F57BBEC1256ED10049F965&parentdoctype=paper&netitpath=80256B3C005BCCF9/(httpAuxPages)/32A160C292F57BBEC1256ED10049F965/$file/koivmack.pdf.

Kremer M, and Jayachandran S (2002). *Odious Debt*. Washington, DC: Brookings Institution. Available: http://www.brookings.edu/views/papers/kremer/200204.htm.

Labonte R, and Schrecker T (2004). Committed to health for all? How the G7/G8 rate. *Social Science and Medicine* 59: 1661–1676.

Labonte R, and Schrecker T (2006). The G8 and global health: What now? What next? *Canadian Journal of Public Health* 97: 35–38.

Labonte R, Schrecker T, Sanders D, and Meeus W (2004). *Fatal Indifference: The G8, Africa and Global Health*. Cape Town: University of Cape Town Press.

Labonte R, and Torgerson R (2005). Interrogating globalization, health, and development: Toward a comprehensive framework for research, policy, and political action. *Critical Public Health* 15: 157–179.

LaFraniere S (2004). Donor mistrust worsens AIDS in Zimbabwe. *New York Times*, August 12. Available: http://query.nytimes.com/gst/fullpage.html?sec+health&res=9F0CE1D9163FF931A2575BC0A9629C8B63

Lang T (2003). Food industrialisation and food power: implications for food governance. *Development Policy Review* 21: 555–568.

Laurell AC (1991). Crisis, neoliberal health policy, and political processes in Mexico. *International Journal of Health Services* 21: 457–470.

Laurell AC (2001). Health reform in Mexico: the promotion of inequality. *International Journal of Health Services* 31: 291–321.

Lee K (2001). Globalization: a new agenda for health? In: McKee M, Garner P, and Scott R, eds., *International Co-operation in Health*. Oxford: Oxford University Press, pp. 13–30.

Lee K, and Goodman H (2002). Global policy networks: the propogation of health care financing reform since the 1980's. In: Lee K, Buse K, and Fustukian S, eds., *Health Policy in a Globalising World*. Cambridge: Cambridge University Press, pp. 97–119.

Levy BS, and Sidel VW, eds. (1997). *War and Public Health*. New York: Oxford University Press.

Leyva-Flores R, Kageyama ML, and Erviti-Erice J (2001). How people respond to illness in Mexico: self-care or medical care? *Health Policy* 57: 15–26.

Lister J (2005). *Driving the Wrong Way? A Critical Guide to the Global 'Health Reform' Industry*. London: Middlesex University Press.

Liu Y (2002). Reforming China's urban health insurance system. *Health Policy* 60: 133–150.

Liu Y, Rao K, Evans T, Chen Y, and Hsiao W (2001). China: increasing health gaps in a transitional economy. In: Evans T, Whitehead M, Diderichsen F, Bhuiya A, and Wirth M, eds., *Challenging Inequities in Health: From Ethics to Action*. New York: Oxford University Press, pp. 76–89.

Loewenson R (1993). Structural adjustment and health policy in Africa. *International Journal of Health Services* 17: 717–730.

Lozano R, Zurita B, Franco F, Ramirez T, Hernandez P, and Torres J (2001). Mexico: marginality, need, and resource allocation at the county level. In: Evans T, Whitehead M, Diderichsen F, Bhuiya A, and Wirth M, eds., *Challenging Inequities in Health: From Ethics to Action*. New York: Oxford University Press, pp. 276–295.

Lundy P (1996). Limitations of quantitative research in the study of structural adjustment. *Social Science and Medicine* 42: 313–324.

MacAskill E (2004). Aim is to meet UN target by 2013. *Guardian*, July 13. Available: http://www.guardian.co.uk/Archive/0,4271,,00.html

Mackintosh M (2003). *Health Care Commercialisation and the Embedding of Inequality*. RUIG/UNRISD Health Project synthesis paper. Geneva: United Nations Research Institute for Social Development. Available: http://www.unrisd.org/unrisd/website/document.nsf/d2a23ad2d50cb2a280256eb300385855/4023556aa730f778c1256de500649e48/$FILE/mackinto.pdf.

Marchak P (1991). *The Integrated Circus: The New Right and the Restructuring of Global Markets*. Montreal: McGill-Queen's University Press.

Martin M (2004). Assessing the HIPC initiative: the key policy debates. In: Teunissen J, and Akkerman A, eds., *HIPC Debt Relief: Myths and Realities*. The Hague: Forum on Debt and Development, pp. 11–47. Available: http://www.fondad.org/publications/hipc/BookComplete.htm.

Martin P, and Zedillo E (2003). Private investment must be the main source of income growth and job creation in poor countries—just as it is in industrialized nations. [Toronto] *Globe and Mail*, August 1, p. A15.

McCoy D, Bambas A, Acurio D, Baya B, Bhuiya A, Mushtaque A, et al. (2003). Global equity gauge alliance: reflections on early experiences. *Journal of Health Population and Nutrition* 21: 273–287.

McKenna B (2004). Canada resists British plan to revalue IMF gold reserves. [Toronto] *Globe and Mail*, October 4, pp. B1, B6.

McMichael P (1993). World food system restructuring under a GATT regime. *Political Geography* 12: 198–214.

McPake B, Hanson K, and Mills A (1993). Community financing of health care in Africa: an evaluation of the Bamako initiative. *Social Science and Medicine* 36: 1383–1395.

Mehta L (2001). Commentary: the World Bank and its emerging knowledge empire. *Human Organization* 60: 189–196.

Michaud C (2003). *Development Assistance for Health (DAH): Recent Trends and Resource Allocation, prepared for Second Consultation, Commission on Macroeconomics and Health, October 29–30, 2003.* Geneva: World Health Organization. Available: www.who.int/entity/macrohealth/events/health_for_poor/en/dah_trends_nov10.pdf.

Mill JE, and Anarfi JK (2002). HIV risk environment for Ghanaian women: challenges to prevention. *Social Science and Medicine* 54: 325–337.

Mills A (1998). To contract or not to contract? Issues for low and middle income countries. *Health Policy and Planning* 13: 32–40.

Milward B (2000). What is structural adjustment? In: Mohan G, Brown E, Milward B, and Zack-Williams AB, eds., *Structural Adjustment: Theory, Practice and Impacts*. London: Routledge, pp. 24–38.

Nantulya VM, Sleet DA, Reich MR, Rosenberg M, Peden M, and Waxweiler R, eds. (2003). Road traffic injuries and health equity. *Injury Control and Safety Promotion* 10(1–2) (entire issue).

Narasimhan V, and Attaran A (2003). Roll back malaria? The scarcity of international aid for malaria control. *Malaria Journal* 2: 1–8.

Narayan D, Chambers R, Shah MK, and Petesch P (2000). *Voices of the Poor: Crying Out for Change*. Oxford: Oxford University Press for the World Bank.

Naylor RT (1987). *Hot Money: Peekaboo Finance and the Politics of Debt*. Toronto: McClelland & Stewart.

Ndikumana L, and Boyce JK (2003). Public debts and private assets: explaining capital flight from sub-Saharan African countries. *World Development* 31: 107–130.

Nolan B, and Turbat V (1995). *Cost Recovery in Public Health Services in Sub-Saharan Africa*. Washington, DC: World Bank.

OECD DAC [Development Assistance Committee] (2004). Development co-operation 2003 report. *DAC Journal* 5(1) (entire issue).

OECD DAC [Development Assistance Committee] (2005). Development co-operation 2004 report. *DAC Journal* 6(1) (entire issue).

Orbinski J (2004). Access to medicines and global health: will Canada lead or flounder? *Canadian Medical Association Journal* 170: 224–226.

Oxfam International (2001). *G8: Failing the World's Children*. Washington, DC: Oxfam International. Available: www.oxfam.org/eng/pdfs/pp0107_G8_Failing_the_Worlds_Children.pdf

People's Health Movement, Global Equity Gauge Alliance, Medact (2005). Global *Health Watch 2005–2006*. London: Zed Books. Available: http://www.ghwatch.org/2005_report.php

Petchesky RP (2003). *Global Prescriptions: Gendering Health and Human Rights*. London: Zed Books.

Pettifor A, and Greenhill R (2002). *Debt Relief and the Millennium Development Goals*. New York: United Nations Development Programme. Available: hdr.undp.org/docs/publications/background_papers/2003/HDR2003_Pettifor_Greenhill.pdf.

Picard A (2000). A legendary killer allowed to get away. [Toronto] *Globe and Mail*, September 23. Available: http://www.andrepicard.com/sleepingsickness.html

Pollock AM, and Price D (2003). The public health implications of world trade negotiations on the General Agreement on Trade in Services and public services. *Lancet* 362: 1072–1075.

Preibisch KL, Rivera Herrejon G, and Wiggins SL (2002). Defending food security in a free-market economy: the gendered dimensions of restructuring in rural Mexico. *Human Organization* 61: 68–79.

Preker AS, Feachem RGA, and de Ferranti D (2000). *Health, Nutrition, and Population Sector Strategy Paper*. Washington, DC: World Bank. Available: http://www.worldbank.org/html/extdr/hnp/sector_strategy/hnp.pdf.

Raikes P, and Gibbon P (2000). "Globalisation" and African export crop agriculture. *Journal of Peasant Studies* 27: 50–93.

Ramphal S (1999). Debt has a child's face. In: UNICEF, ed., *The Progress of Nations 1999*. New York: UNICEF, pp. 26–29.

Raynolds L, Myrhe D, McMichael P, Carro-Figueroa V, and Buttel FH (1993). The "new" internationalization of agriculture: a reformulation. *World Development* 21: 1101–1121.

Reardon T, and Barrett CB (2000). Agroindustrialization, globalization, and international development: an overview of issues, patterns, and determinants. *Agricultural Economics* 23: 195–205.

Reddy SG, and Pogge TW (2003). *How Not to Count the Poor*, version 4.5. New York: Columbia University. Available: http://www.columbia.edu/~sr793/count.pdf.

Reich M (2000). The global drug gap. *Science* 287: 1979–1981.

Rich B (1994). *Mortgaging the Earth: The World Bank, Environmental Impoverishment and the Crisis of Development*. Boston: Beacon Press, 1994.

Rodrik D (2001). *The Global Governance of Trade as if Development Really Mattered*. New York: United Nations Development Programme. Available:

http://www.undp.org/mainundp/propoor/docs/pov_globalgovernancetrade_pub.pdf.

Rowson M, and Verheul E (2004). *Pushing the Boundaries: Health and the Next Round of PRSPs.* Amsterdam: WEMOS Foundation. Available: http://www.wemos.nl/en-GB/Content.aspx?type=PublicatieItem&id=1720

Rugman AM, and Verbeke A (2003). The World Trade Organization, multinational enterprise, and civil society. In: Fratianni M, Savona P, and Kirton J, eds., *Sustaining Global Growth and Development: G7 and IMF Governance.* Aldershot, UK: Ashgate, pp. 81–97.

Russell S (1996). Ability to pay for health care: concepts and evidence. *Health Policy and Planning* 11: 219–237.

Sachs J (2003). *Achieving the Millennium Development Goals: Health in the Developing World, Speech at the Second Global Consultation of the Commission on Macroeconomics and Health.* Geneva: World Health Organization. Available: http://www.earthinstitute.columbia.edu/about/director/pubs/CMHSpeech102903.pdf.

Satterthwaite D (1993). The Millennium Development Goals and urban poverty reduction: great expectations and nonsense statistics. *Environment and Urbanization* 15: 181–190.

Schoepf BG (1988). Women, AIDS, and economic crisis in Central Africa. *Canadian Journal of African Studies* 22: 625–644.

Schoepf BG (1998). Inscribing the body politic: AIDS in Africa. In: Lock M, and Kaufert P, eds., *Pragmatic Women and Body Politics.* Cambridge: Cambridge University Press, pp. 98–126.

Schoepf BG (2002). "Mobutu's disease": a social history of AIDS in Kinshasa. *Review of African Political Economy*, no. 93/94, pp. 561–573.

Schoepf BG (2004). AIDS in Africa: structure, agency, and risk. In: Kalipeni E, Craddock S, Oppong JR, and Ghosh J, eds., *HIV and AIDS in Africa: Beyond Epidemiology.* Oxford: Blackwell, pp. 121–132.

Schoepf BG, Schoepf C, and Millen JV (2000). Theoretical therapies, remote remedies: SAPs and the political ecology of poverty and health in Africa. In: Kim JY, Millen JV, Irwin A, and Gershman J, eds., *Dying for Growth: Global Inequality and the Health of the Poor.* Monroe, ME: Common Courage Press, pp. 91–126.

Scott A (2002). Interior Life. *New York Times Magazine*, December 1, pp. 19–20.

Sell SK (2003). *Private Power, Public Law: The Globalization of Intellectual Property Rights.* Cambridge: Cambridge University Press.

Sell SK (2004). The quest for global governance in intellectual property and public health: Structural, discursive, and institutional dimensions. *Temple Law Review* 77: 363–399.

Shiva V (2002). Export at any cost: Oxfam's free trade recipe for the third world. Dev-Zone (online).

Available: http://www.dev-zone.org/kcdocs/3120VandanaOxfam.html.

Smith R, Woodward D, Acharya A, Beaglehole R, and Drager N (2004). Communicable disease control: a "global public good" perspective. *Health Policy and Planning* 19: 271–278.

Sparr P (2000). What is structural adjustment? In: Sparr P, ed., *Mortgaging Women's Lives: Feminist Critiques of Structural Adjustment.* London: Zed Books, pp. 1–12.

Spinaci S, and Heymann D (2001). Communicable disease and disability of the poor. *Development* 44: 66–72.

Stevens C, and Kennan J (2005). *EU–ACP Economic Partnership Agreements: The Effects of Reciprocity.* Brighton, UK: Institute of Development Studies. Available: http://dfid.gov.uk/aboutdfid/organisation/epas-effects-reciprocity.pdf

Stewart F (2003). Conflict and the Millennium Development Goals. *Journal of Human Development* 4: 325–351.

Stocker K, Waitzkin H, and Iriart C (1999). The exportation of managed care to Latin America. *New England Journal of Medicine* 340: 1131–1136.

Strange S (1998). The new world of debt. *New Left Review*, no. 230, pp. 91–114.

Szreter S (1999). Rapid economic growth and "the four Ds" of disruption, deprivation, disease and death: public health lessons from nineteenth-century Britain for twenty-first-century China? *Tropical Medicine and International Health* 4: 146–152.

Szreter S (2003). The population health approach in historical perspective. *American Journal of Public Health* 93: 421–431.

Third World Network (2001). Everything but development: the Doha WTO outcome and process. *Third World Resurgence*, no. 135–136 (entire issue). Available: http://www.twnside.org.sg/title/focus27.htm.

Third World Network (2005). *Little to Celebrate in Hong Kong Outcome.* Penang: TWN. Available http://www.twnside.org.sg/statements/Final_TWN_Statement_end_of_WTO_MC_6.doc

't Hoen E (2002). TRIPS, pharmaceutical patents and access to essential medicines: a long way from Seattle to Doha. *Chicago Journal of International Law* 3: 27–46. Available: http://www.accessmed-msf.org/upload/PressClips/24620021440503/ChicagolawjournalTRIPS.pdf.

Trouiller P, Olliaro P, Torreele E, Orbinski J, Laing R, and Ford N (2002). Drug development for neglected diseases: a deficient market and a public-health policy failure. *Lancet* 359: 2188–2194.

U.K. Department for International Development (2004). UK to provide deeper debt relief (press release), September 26. London: Department for International Development. Available: http://www.dfid.gov.uk/news/files/pressreleases/deeperdebt.asp

UNFAO (2003). *The State of Food Insecurity in the World 2003.* Rome: United Nations Food and

Agriculture Organization. Available: ftp://ftp.fao.org/docrep/fao/006/j0083e/j0083e00.pdf

UNFAO (2005). *The State of Food Insecurity in the World 2005: Eradicating World Hunger—Key to Achieving the Millennium Development Goals.* Rome: United Nations Food and Agriculture Organization. Available: ftp://ftp.fao.org/docrep/fao/008/a0200e/a0200e.pdf

United Nations (1992). *Agenda 21.* New York: United Nations Division for Sustainable Development. Available: http://www.un.org/esa/sustdev/documents/agenda21/english/agenda21toc.htm.

United Nations (2002a). *Report of the International Conference on Financing for Development.* A/CONF.198/11. New York: United Nations Publications. Available: http://ods-dds-ny.un.org/doc/UNDOC/GEN/N02/392/67/PDF/N0239267.pdf?OpenElement.

United Nations (2002b). *Follow-up Efforts to the International Conference on Financing for Development.* Report by the Secretary-General, A/57/319. New York: United Nations Publications, August. Available: www.un.org/esa/ffd/a57-319-ffd-followup.pdf.

United Nations (2005). *World Economic and Social Survey 2005: Financing for Development,* E/2005/51/Rev.1, ST/ESA/298. New York: United Nations Department of Economic and Social Affairs. Available: http://www.un.org/esa/policy/wess/wess2005 files/wess2005web.pdf

United Nations Development Programme (1999). *Human Development Report 1999: Globalization with a Human Face.* New York: Oxford University Press.

United Nations Development Programme (2003). *Human Development Report 2003: Millennium Development Goals: A Compact among Nations to End Human Poverty.* New York: Oxford University Press.

United Nations Millennium Project (2005). *Investing in Development: A Practical Plan to Achieve the Millennium Development Goals.* London: Earthscan. Available: http://www.unmillenniumproject.org/documents/MainReport/Complete-lowres.pdf

United Nations System Standing Committee on Nutrition (2004). *Fifth Report on the World Nutrition Situation: Nutrition for Improved Development Outcomes.* Geneva: United Nations. Available: http://www.unsystem.org/scn/Publications/AnnualMeeting/SCN31/SCN5Report.pdf.

Utting P, Hewitt de Alcántara C, Bangura Y, Mkandawire T, Razavi S, Westendorff D, and Freedman J. (2000). *Visible Hands: Taking Responsibility for Social Development, an UNRISD Report for Geneva 2000.* Geneva: United Nations Research Institute for Social Development. Available: http://www.unrisd.org/unrisd/website/document.nsf/0/FE9C9439D82B525480256B670065EFA1?OpenDocument.

van de Walle N (2001). *African Economies and the Politics of Permanent Crisis, 1979–1999.* Cambridge: Cambridge University Press.

Vasagar J (2004). EU freezes £83m aid to "corrupt" Kenya. *Guardian,* July 22. Available: http://www.guardian.co.uk/eu/story/0,,1266206,00.html

Veeken H, and Pécoul B (2000). Drugs for "neglected diseases": a bitter pill. *Tropical Medicine and International Health* 5: 309–311.

Wade RH (2002). US hegemony and the World Bank: the fight over people and ideas. *Review of International Political Economy* 9: 201–229.

Wade RH (2004). Is globalization reducing poverty and inequality? *World Development* 32: 567–589.

Wadee H, Gilson L, Thiede M, Okorafor O, and McIntyre D (2003). *Health Care Inequity in South Africa and the Public/Private Mix.* Geneva: University of Geneva (UNIGE). Available: www.unige.ch/iued/new/recherche/ruig-dsd/docs/SAN-SA-01.pdf.

Wagstaff A, Claeson M, et al. (2003). *The Millennium Development Goals for Health: Rising to the Challenges.* Washington, DC: World Bank. Available: http://www1.worldbank.org/hnp/MDG/MDGESW.pdf.

Wagstaff A, and Yazbeck A (2004). *Measuring Inequalities in Health.* Presentation to World Bank Workshop on Reaching the Poor. Washington, DC: World Bank. Available: http://info.worldbank.org/etools/docs/library/1145271/RTPmaterials/Workshoppapers/adam%20for%20workshop%20session2.ppt

Watkins K (2003). *Northern Agricultural Policies and World Poverty: Will the Doha "Development Round" Make a Difference?* Paper presented at the annual Bank Conference of Development Economics, Paris, May 15–16, 2003. Washington, DC: World Bank. Available: http://wbln0018.worldbank.org/eurvp/web.nsf/Pages/Paper+by+Watkins/$File/WATKINS.PDF.

Watkins K, and Fowler P (2002). *Rigged Rules and Double Standards.* Washington, DC: Oxfam International. Available: http://www.maketradefair.org/assets/english/report_english.pdf.

Webb M (2000). The Group of Seven and political management of the global economy. In: Stubbs R, and Underhill G, eds., *Political Economy and the Changing Global Order,* 2nd ed. Don Mills, Ontario: Oxford University Press Canada, pp. 141–151.

Whitehead M, Dahlgren G, and Evans T (2001). Equity and health sector reforms: can low-income countries escape the medical poverty trap? *Lancet* 358: 833–836.

WHO (2002a). *Investing in Health, the New Dimension in Development Policy: Why and How to Do It.* Media Advisory No. 4. Geneva: World Health Organization. Available: http://www.who.int/inf/en/MA-2002-07.html.

WHO (2002b). *World Health Report 2002: Reducing Risks, Promoting Healthy Life.* Geneva: World Health Organization. Available: http://www.who.int/whr/2002/download/en/.

WHO (2003). *World Health Report 2003: Shaping the Future*. Geneva: World Health Organization. Available: http://www.who.int/whr/2003/en/whr03_en.pdf.

Williamson J (2004). *The Washington Consensus as Policy Prescription for Development*. World Bank Practitioners for Development lecture. Washington, DC: World Bank, January. Available: http://www.iie.com/publications/papers/williamson0204.pdf.

Woodward D (2003). *Trading Health for Profit: the Implications of the GATS and Trade in Health Services for Health in Developing Countries*. London: UK Partnership for Global Health. Available: http://www.ukglobalhealth.org/content/Text/GATS_Woodward.pdf.

Woodward D, Drager N, Beaglehole R, and Lipson D (2001). Globalization and health: a framework for analysis and action. *Bulletin of the World Health Organization* 79: 875–881.

Woodward D, and Smith R (2003). Global public goods and health: concepts and issues. In: Smith R, Beaglehole R, Woodward D, and Drager N, eds., *Global Public Goods for Health: Health Economic and Public Health Perspectives*. Oxford: Oxford University Press, pp. 3–29.

World Bank (1993). *World Development Report 1993: Investing in Health*. New York: Oxford University Press.

World Bank (1995). *World Development Report 1995: Workers in an Integrating World*. New York: Oxford University Press.

World Bank (2001a). *Global Economic Prospects and the Developing Countries 2001*. Washington, DC: World Bank.

World Bank (2001b). *Global Economic Prospects and the Developing Countries 2002*. Washington, DC: World Bank.

World Bank (2001c). *World Development Report 2000/2001: Attacking Poverty*. New York: World Bank and Oxford University Press.

World Bank (2002). *World Development Indicators 2002*. Washington, DC: World Bank.

World Bank (2003a). Briefing Note to the Board: Costing the Service Delivery MDGs: Primary Education, Health and Water Supply and Sanitation. Washington, DC: World Bank. Available: http://www-wds.worldbank.org/servlet/WDSContentServer/WDSP/IB/2003/04/25/000094946_03041604014621/Rendered/PDF/multi0page.pdf.

World Bank (2003b). *Annual Report 2003*. Vol. 1: *Year in Review*. Washington, DC: World Bank.

World Bank (2004). *World Development Indicators 2004*. Washington, DC: World Bank.

World Commission on Environment and Development (1987). *Our Common Future*. New York: Oxford University Press.

Wroughton L (2005). World Bank report calls for changes to G8 debt plan. London: Reuters, August 3. Available: http://today.reuters.com/news/newsArticleSearch.aspx?storyID=68045+03-Aug-2005+RTRS&srch=lesley+wroughton

WTO (2001). *Declaration on the TRIPS Agreement and Public Health*. Geneva: World Trade Organization. Available: http://www.wto.org/english/thewto_e/minist_e/min01_e/mindecl_trips_e.pdf.

WTO (2003). *Implementation of paragraph 6 of the Doha Declaration on the TRIPS Agreement and Public Health*. Decision of the General Council, August 30, 2003. Geneva: World Trade Organization. Available: http://www.wto.org/english/tratop_e/trips_e/implem_para6_e.htm.

WTO (2004). *Doha Work Programme*. Decision adopted by the General Council August 1, 2004, WT/L/579. Geneva: World Trade Organization. Available: http://www.wto.org/english/tratop_e/dda_e/ddadraft_31ju104_e.pdf.

Chapter 18

Military Spending: Global Health Threat or Global Public Good?

Raymond R. Hyatt, Jr.

Globalization is taking place on several fronts, economic, political, and social, each involving the behaviors of a rather diverse set of global actors. Economic globalization is occurring, for example, in the growing influence of multinational corporations in both the developed and the developing world that are credited with spreading both jobs and obesity within the global community (Amin 2000). Political globalization is played out in the actions of nation-states and international organizations as leadership, power, and dominance are negotiated among official state delegations and thus woven into the fabric of the global community (Meyer et al. 2004). And, the emergence of an international civil society is taking place within the networks of nongovernmental organizations that create, change, and recreate social and cultural norms and behaviors in such diverse contexts as the United Kingdom and Malaysia (Boli and Thomas 2004). Each aspect of globalization has an impact on the individuals of the world in terms of

opportunities for employment and education, family structure, social networks, and perhaps most important, health.

Regardless of the specific lens we choose to focus on globalization, however, one common aspect is apparent: there is a tug between the individuality and sovereignty of the nation-state and the growing convergence and importance of the collective global community. Nowhere is this tug more evident than in the tradeoff of nation-state actions to provide for the security of the state and its population and state actions to improve the welfare of its citizens.

Through the perspective of world systems theory, we see this tug in terms of a national focus on materialism and power that takes precedence over many of the emerging community issues of the global neighborhood (Wallerstein 2004; Baylis and Smith 1997; Epsing-Anderson 1990). This focus has become particularly evident in the United States and other Western countries since the events of September 11, 2001, and can be seen in many unilateral sovereign state actions to ensure security that are now seemingly justified by the threat of potential terrorist activities.

Within the scope of the world systems perspective, we expect nation-states to behave as sovereign individuals in the global community. States construct their actions in a manner consistent with national priorities and the perceived ability to implement action that will accomplish the goals of assured control over the flow of resources and protection of their relative power. One central challenge to the nation-state involves the tradeoff around the acquisition and distribution of resources necessary to provide for the welfare of the homeland population versus alternative assignment of resources in order to maintain a strong posture to potential enemies. Along this path, states become Janus-faced with respect to long-term stability (Skocpol and Rueschemeyer 1996), where one face looks over the well-being of citizens and the development of the welfare state, while the other is focused on threats to the order and survival of the state.

Large-scale development projects such as public sanitation, clean water supply, food production, and distribution are essential to the welfare of a population. In order to accomplish such tasks, the costs of such goods must be shared, and thus, the state takes ownership and distributes the cost across the population via a broadly defined revenue mechanism such as taxation. National security is also a public good where costs are supported via the broad-based financial mechanisms of the state.

In a system of finite resources (as national budgets are in the short term), decisions to allocate resources broadly involve tradeoffs between security demands and projects that further social welfare (the zero-sum game, Thurow 2001). Given the assumption that resources are finite, we can measure the magnitude of security–welfare tradeoff in the percentage of state resources allocated to military programs. The remaining percentage is that which is available for welfare projects and thus becomes respectively smaller or larger as military commitments either grow or shrink.

Security from external threats (and increasingly from internal threats) at the state level is the primary benefit of military allocations of resources. The benefits of social welfare expenditures may be more difficult to measure. Amartya Sen (1999) points out that ultimately an operationalization of the concept of freedom is the most basic aspect of any definition of well-being. This concept is rooted in ability of the

individual to make social choices and that the underlying mechanism of choice is opportunity. Thus, a key factor in choice is being alive to have the opportunity to make choices. However, Sen's opportunity horizon is unequally distributed among nation-states. Some citizens may have this opportunity for over seventy-five years (e.g., Sweden, Japan, the United States), while those in less fortunate countries may face an opportunity frontier that is present for less than forty-five years (e.g., Afghanistan). Research suggests that mortality measures may be the most useful operationalizations of well-being at the ecological level. We must attempt, then, to understand state action in the global community not only as it affects economic outcomes but also in light of the impact on the well-being of populations (Coburn 2000; Nathanson 1996).

The analysis presented in this chapter assesses the effects of this duality of state focus by examining the specific tradeoff between military spending and social welfare spending (the well-known guns vs. butter tradeoff) and the effects of expenditures in military budgets for recently expanding peacekeeping operations. The methodology of this study provides a cross-national statistical test of the following three hypotheses using multiple-source data covering the period between 1963 and 2001.

The first hypothesis (H_1) is that increased allocation of government resources to military expenditure results in a higher infant mortality rate (IMR). IMR is an operationalization of well-being that is particularly sensitive to short-term changes in social, economic, family, and educational resources. H_2 is that increased allocation of government resources to military expenditure leads to a lower measure of life expectancy at birth (LEB). LEB, in contrast to IMR, is a longer term measure of population well-being and is likely to be sensitive to longer terms trends in resource availability within a particular context. H_3 is that recent increases in military expenditures for peacekeeping missions have had a mitigating affect on the relationship between military expenditures and health outcomes.

MILITARY SPENDING AND ECONOMIC GROWTH

Research on the tradeoff of state allocations between security and welfare has focused mainly on the economic consequences of military spending (Chan 1992; Mintz and Stevenson 1995). Modernization theory argues that military spending, though it does drain domestic investment, results in a mobilization of resources and advancement of skills particularly within developing countries (Chan 1992). This approach suggests that increased military spending improves economic performance in developing countries due to a positive stimulus effect on the private sector economy. According to this model, developing countries may experience gross domestic product (GDP) growth from the stimulation of industrial activity and the higher productive output of a more highly skilled labor force motivated by competition for projects funded from increases in state spending on military programs.

The capital formation model stresses the role of private, versus public, investment as a determinant of economic growth. Proponents of this model argue that the negative effects of military expenditures on savings (and investment) outweigh the positive modernization and technological effects (Deger and Smith 1983; Smith 1980). To the extent that military spending dampens capital formation, erodes the investment base of the economy, and thus eventually slows economic growth, it is a major contributing cause of the hegemonic power's decline in global influence over time (Smith 1977). Research in this area is focused on how capital formation is retarded by shifts in capital away from the private sector related to increases in military spending and whether or not hegemony is eventually reduced when increased levels of military spending result in slower economic growth.

A third perspective on the impact of military spending on economic performance, the balance of payment or export-led model, argues that military spending tends to deprive resources to the most dynamic sectors of the economy, in fact, the very sectors that tend to be most heavily involved in exports. States that are the most adept in expanding exports, and thus creating a positive flow of resources into the country, have tended to grow fastest economically (Rothschild 1973). This concept provides links among military spending, resource dependency, and economic performance: as military spending increases, the balance of trade worsens, resource dependency expands, and resources are taken away from the domestic economic sectors that have the most promise for development.

The application of this theory may be limited for countries that export a large volume of military goods. In 1999, for example, the list of the fifteen largest arms-exporting countries included the United States (the number 1 arms exporter in 1999), the United Kingdom (2), France (4), Germany (5), Sweden (6), and Canada (9) (U.S. Department of State 2003). All are countries with relatively high LEBs and low IMRs. This is in line with thinking that arms-exporting countries may become richer and achieve higher levels of population health as a result of the production and export of military goods (Krug 1999). For many of these countries, the military goods that are exported are likely to be expendable items such as artillery shells, land mines, and surface-to-air missiles, rather than state-of-the-art versions of equipment such as tanks, airplanes, and helicopters (U.S. Department of State 2003). Thus, there is a repeat market for these goods, and the list of high-volume arms exporters remains relatively stable over time (SIPRI 2003).

However, the top fifteen arms-exporting countries in 1999 also included Russia (3), Ukraine (10), Mainland China (12), Belarus (13), Bulgaria (14), and North Korea (15), countries that do not have claim to high levels of aggregate population health (U.S. Department of State 2003). It is worth noting that differences between the two groups of countries above include the level of economic development and the development of social welfare supports. Rich, more developed countries may be able to export large volumes of arms and also have high levels of population health. This does not appear to be true for poor countries. It is also notable that the country with the highest LEB and lowest IMR, Japan, does not appear in the list of top arms exporters and is still limited in arms production and arms exports by post-World War II agreements.

The fourth theoretical approach is the technological displacement model. This theory argues that, by drawing scientific and engineering talents from the civilian sector to military research and development, defense spending tends to hamper innovation in the civilian society and therefore dampen the growth of the private economy (Dumas 1977; Russett 1970). Focusing on a developing country, Deger and Sen (1983) argue that military spending has negatively affected the technological advance of civilian industries in India, which has one of the largest armament industries in the third world.

Though very different in their approach to military spending and economic development, each of the four models agrees on one basic principle—that there is competition between resources garnered for military programs and those available for economic growth. Since economic growth is the basic mechanism by which resources become available within the state for the development of a social welfare structure, poorer economic performance translates into fewer social supports. Thus, the negative effects of lowered economic growth extend to state sponsored programs for education, income support, and public health, all of which have strong effects on population health outcomes (Kawachi and Kennedy 2002; Price-Smith 2002).

This security–welfare substitution effect of the resource allocation problem is examined more closely in three primary perspectives that describe the mechanisms that link state allocations for security versus allocations to welfare.

The guns-versus-butter tradeoff (Domke et al. 1983; Russett 1982) posits a direct negative effect to a population as a result of the shift in state resources from welfare to warfare. The underlying assumption of the zero-sum game in national budgets is that there is a finite amount of resources to be allocated, and thus, allocations to military projects take away resources that could be allocated to social welfare and public health programs. While some analysts question the zero-sum assumption and suggest that modernization may play a role in the creation of additional resources as a result of the allocations to the military, research shows that this tradeoff is a reasonable model of resource allocation effects in many contexts (Chan 1992; Russett 1982). However, military spending may have differential effects in states, depending on the level of economic development and the extent to which social welfare programs have been developed, a question that deserves more research.

The basic needs approach provides another perspective on security–welfare substitution effects (Davis and Chan 1990; Dixon and Moon 1986; Moon and Dixon 1985) that is focused on the impact of military service on the bottom line of the physical quality of life. In a cross-sectional study of less developed countries, Dixon and Moon (1986) found that military participation (active duty) is positively correlated with physical well-being. In the same study, they also found that increased military spending is negatively correlated with well-being. The initial association implies that a high level of sociopolitical mobilization and military recruitment may constitute an investment in human resources (particularly in poor countries where unemployment rates are high), which in turn results in a higher quality of life. They also suggest that spending on these programs incurs a penalty to the population in terms of lost investment in social welfare programs. Importantly, they do not take into account the war status of countries in their analysis when military participation may not be positively correlated with well-being.

The third line of inquiry into this tradeoff has focused on the impact of the military cost burden on the size distribution of income, that is, the question of whether military expenditures tend to exacerbate social and economic inequality (Bollen 1985). Cross-national evidence suggests that military manpower (but not military spending) is positively correlated with income inequality (Chan 1989; Weede 1980b, 1983b; Weede and Tiefenbach 1981). Income inequality, according to some views, is related to poor health outcomes and, in particular, to increased mortality (Wilkinson 1996; see also chapter 7). This potential link between military spending and mortality has not received very much attention to date, most likely because the data needed to assess this affect, such as within-country measures of income inequality (GINI coefficients), are not available for a sufficient number of countries over a large enough span of time to support cross-sectional time-series comparisons. An analysis of income inequality is not included is this analysis for these reasons, though it is a question in need of further research.

MILITARY SPENDING AND MORTALITY

At the turn of the twentieth century, LEB in Japan was similar to that in England/Wales and Italy (Johansson and Mosk 1987). For example, in 1908, LEB in Japan was forty-three years, the same as it was for Italy and only two years less than that in England/Wales. Japan had made strides in public health both in providing better sanitation for the population and in fighting infectious disease. At the time, with an LEB at or close to the leading Western European countries, Japan was the recognized leader among the Asian countries with respect to public health. This trend scarcely continued into the 1930s, when improvement in the LEB for the Japanese population stalled. In 1933, the LEB in Japan was only forty-three years, versus fifty-three and fifty-eight, respectively, for Italy and England/Wales.

During the 1940s LEB in Japan fell to only twenty-six years for males, largely due to the effects of World War II on the mortality rates of Japanese men. Following the war, however, Japan returned to the remarkable progress in controlling mortality and expanding the LEB for its population that it enjoyed in the early part of the century. By 1947, LEB was already back up to fifty-two years and then to sixty-one years by 1951. From 1951 to 1996, LEB continued to rise in Japan at a rate of about five years per decade (Wilmoth 1998). By 1996, Japan had again become a leading country in the world with an LEB for males, at seventy-seven years and for females at eighty-four years. In fact, by the mid-1990s, Japan had surpassed all of the western countries including Sweden, which had boasted the largest LEB in the world for most of the 1900s.

But what caused the improvements LEB to disappear in the early 1930s? It is certainly understandable during the late 1930s and early 1940s when Japan was engaged in war with the United States and China that the LEB for males and for the overall population might fall.

Johansson and Mosk (1987) forward the view that Japan's focus in the first half of the twentieth century (1910–1940) had shifted from social welfare development, particularly focused on public health, to making itself a world military power. As this focus became a framework, resources were allocated and policy formed in order to build up the military. The reasons for this shift in focus are contextual and better left to the historians; however, it is clear that where the focus had previously been on internal development, the shift in resource allocation toward external conquests resulted in a penalty on the level of well-being of Japanese citizens.

Mortality trends in the United States in the latter half of the twentieth century bear some similarity to the example in Japan. LEB in the United States was at sixty-three years in 1950 and had expanded to seventy-seven years in 1996. While the United States enjoyed a forefront position in LEB for many years (though not the world leader), there was a stall in the expansion of LEB in the early 1980s. Correspondingly, there was also a marked slowdown in the

decline in IMR in the United States: while other countries continued a long-term trend of improvement, improvements IMR in the United States stalled (National Center for Health Statistics 2004).

Increasing income inequality in the United States during the 1980s may have been a factor in the slowdown in mortality improvements (Deaton 1999; Deaton and Paxson 1999; Daly et al. 1998; Kawachi et al. 1997; Wilkinson 1996). Deaton and Paxson (1999) have found that income inequality rose dramatically during the 1980s coincident with the stall in the overall LEB. Importantly, though, the first half of the 1980s was also marked by substantial reductions in government-sponsored social programs, including the cancellation of some social security benefits and the closing of many federally supported hospitals and mental health facilities. This period also featured a virtually unprecedented peacetime buildup in military arms, resulting in a new arms race with the Soviet Union. Like Japan, the U.S. focus had turned sharply to preoccupation with the military buildup. As a result, government funding for programs including both Social Security Insurance and Social Security Disability Insurance were dramatically reduced. Many disabled Americans were forced to fend for themselves as a result of the discontinuation of benefits by the federal government. During this period, several state-level mental health hospitals were closed due to federal cutbacks, and programs that were in place to help low-income and poor families obtain food for newborns and their siblings and mothers (e.g., Women, Infants and Children nutrition program) and subsidies for prenatal and postnatal care were either discontinued or severely reduced. The focus on arms and the resulting arms race with the former Soviet Union would eventually bankrupt the Soviet Union, dramatically expand the U.S. national debt, and weaken the Soviet Union enough to lead to the breakup of the Eastern European communist block. The outcome of this was the severe mortality crisis that the newly constituted sovereign state of Russia experienced in the 1990s, when LEB in Russia fell below sixty years, putting Russia on a par with some third-world countries (Rose 2000; Bloom and Malaney 1998; Kennedy et al. 1998a).

Johansson and Mosk (1987) suggest that, above a certain fairly minimum threshold standard of living, the "right" to live to old age can be secured for the average citizen even in low-income developing countries if the government is dedicated to the efficient exploitation of existing public health technology and the population is educated and cooperative. Sen (1999) suggests that this right to live to old age is the most basic aspect of social choice and also the most basic element of the concept of freedom. While income, education, medical advances, and the public all play important roles in the early stages of mortality improvements in populations, a key ingredient to improved mortality experience as societies develop is a state focus on improving the well-being of its citizens that is not conflicted by external preoccupations.

Woolhandler and Himmelstein (1985) examined the relationship between the level of state resources allocated to militarism and the impact on mortality. Controlling for economic, health, and social indicators, they examined military expenditures to explain differentials in IMR for 141 countries for 1979. They estimated a cross-sectional model with four control variables to measure the relationship of military expenditure to IMR. Their model included gross national product (GNP)[1] per capita, the number of teachers per capita, caloric consumption per capita, and the percentage of the population with access to clean water. Adjusting for these covariates, military expenditure as a percentage of GNP was found to be a significant predictor of IMR. They estimate that 3.29 infant deaths per 1,000 live births are associated with each 1% of GNP devoted to military spending. They estimate that as many as 2 million infant deaths were associated spending for armaments in 1979. The Woolhandler and Himmelstein study suggests that there is a significant link between mortality and the amount of state resources allocated to the military.

The Woolhandler and Himmelstein study is also important in that they suggest factors that may be useful in assessing cross-national differences in mortality. Their choice of variables reflects their public health perspective of mortality and rightfully identifies four important covariates in addition to military spending.

The analysis presented here borrows from both the Woolhandler and Himmelstein (1985) study and the studies of military spending and economic growth. However, the choice to expand extant analyses to include both cross sections and time series limits the choice of some measures that are not available for a sufficient number of countries over the time period included in this study. For example, measures of sanitation and the availability of clean water do not exist in the cross-sectional time-series context. Remedies and adjustments to these data issues such as the use of alternative and proxy measures are discussed in "Data and Methods."

MILITARY EXPENDITURES FOR PEACEKEEPING MISSIONS

A principal focus of the mission of the United Nations is the maintenance of international peace and security and the economic, social, and political development of the nation-states of the world (Charter of the United Nations 1945). Within this scope, the United Nations assists in many countries providing education, relief services, and population health services and levies various sanctions and penalties on countries that violate United Nations resolutions. The actions of the United Nations are aimed at improving the lives of the citizens of the world. These tasks become more difficult, however, as fears that globalization may spread market dominance, economic inequality, and Western culture exert pressure on nation-states to ensure their own survive and also may exacerbate the risks of conflict in an increasingly complex environment (Tomlinson 2004; Gissinger and Gleditsch 1999).

Kofi Annan, the United Nations Secretary General at the turn of the twenty-first century, has set an agenda for the future of the United Nations centered around three principal themes: freedom from fear, freedom from want, and sustainable development (Annan 2000). The foundation of the first leg of the mission, freedom from fear, is the United Nations' commitment to conflict resolution without warfare. This mission involves careful management and oversight of situations in the world that are known to be conflict ridden as well as the management of conflicts that are emerging. Freedom from want will depend on initiatives to increase development, improve health, and create opportunity for all nations. Sustainable development requires understanding and stewardship of the earth's resources and a forward vision that takes into account how development affects the ecosystem.

A core piece of the United Nations' approach to this triadic mission is humanitarian aid. At the foundation of humanitarian aid are United Nations peacekeeping operations. Though there have been many disappointing peacekeeping missions, Yugoslavia, Somalia, Sierra Leone, for example, the principal underpinnings of peacekeeping as a United Nations mission remain. Negotiation, education, and development struggle to take place in the context of abusive and repressive governments, violations of human rights, predatory economic policy, and the growing economic inequality in the global community. Peacekeeping is a doomed policy in areas where there is no peace to keep.

Peacekeeping missions of the United Nations suffer from a number of limitations. For one, countries with the most resources have more stomach for military operations in the world than they do for peacekeeping. There is a belief among modern militaries that peacekeeping is for "wimps," not for real soldiers, despite the demonstrable dangers and costs of current and past peacekeeping operations (Everts and Isernia 2001). This leaves peacekeeping operations to states that have the political will but that lack the resources, training, and military capability to carry them out. Second, there is little accountability in peacekeeping operations. It is difficult to plan how long troops will be needed and what level of training and force is necessary. Member states fear being held responsible for the failures, many of which seem to be far outside of their control.

Thus, the evaluation of peacekeeping operations, particularly the financial commitments to peacekeeping operations, is of great importance. Only recently have data become available, albeit limited, that can be applied to this task. The analysis presented here examines first the effects of nation-state military spending on the well-being of their populations. This is followed by an analysis of military spending adjusted for expenditures for peacekeeping operations. The key hypothesis (H_3) is that the benefits of peacekeeping operations mitigate some portion of the negative effects of state spending for military purposes.

DATA AND METHODS

Data for this analysis are taken from six sources: the World Bank World Development Indicators (World Bank Data Development Group 2001); the Penn World Tables (1994); the World Bank World Tables of Economic and Social Indicators 1950–1992 (World Bank, International Economics Department 1997); the Stockholm International Peace Research Institute (SIPRI 2003) military expenditure data set; the military expenditure database of the U.S. Arms Control and Disarmament Agency (1975, 1986, 1995); and

the United Nations Department of Peacekeeping Operations. The individual data sets were merged to create a relational database.

The World Bank's World Tables of Economic and Social Indicators contain 118 social and economic indicators measured annually, including such variables as LEB, IMR, and GDP. The data set covers 189 countries in a time-series format from 1950 through 1992. The World Bank's World Development Indicators (World Bank Data Development Group, 2001) provides more than 550 annual time series for 207 countries from 1960 through 2001. The Penn World Tables (1994) provide data on twenty-nine annual measures of economic and social development, including some that are also in the World Bank data set (e.g., measures of GDP and population). The Penn World Tables (1994) cover the same time frame as the World Bank Tables of Economic and Social Indicators (1950–1992) and include 152 countries.

Military expenditure data from the U.S. Arms Control and Disarmament Agency (1975, 1986, 1995) cover three ten-year periods: 1963–1972, 1973–1982, and 1983–1993. The expenditure measures were combined with GNP to create a measure of the percentage GNP spent on the military by country and year. Data for military expenditures was also obtained from the Stockholm International Peace Research Institute (SIPRI 2003), which provides a consistently measured indicator of military expenditure as a percentage of GDP for a large sample of countries from 1988 through 2002. SIPRI also supplied additional military expenditure data for a limited number of countries beginning in 1976.

The peacekeeping data are from the United Nations Department of Peacekeeping Operations and report the annual expenditure for peacekeeping for sixty-three countries from 1998 through 2002. These data were combined with the SIPRI military expenditure measures in the present analysis to adjust the military expenditures of these sixty-three nations from 1998 to 2001. The resulting peacekeeping data set covers ninety-seven countries (including countries with no peacekeeping expenditures) for the period 1988 through 2001.

Due to the different time frames of the military expenditure data, three analysis files were created. Analysis file 1 includes the two World Bank data sets, the Penn World Tables (1994), and the military expenditure measure from the U.S. Arms Control and Disarmament Agency (1975, 1986, 1995). A consistent

TABLE 18.1. Variable Definitions

Description	Name
Well-Being (dependent)	
Life expectancy at birth—WB 2001[a]	LEB
Infant mortality/1,000 births—WB 2001[a]	IMR
Military Expenditure	
Military expenditure as % GNP—ACDA[a]	MIL/ACDA
Military expenditure as % GDP—SIPRI[a]	MIL/SIPRI
Food and Nutrition	
Cereal yield per hectare[a]	CEREAL YIELD
Food production per capita	FOODPROD
Development Indicators	
Gross fixed capital investment—% GDP	FIXED CAPITAL
GDP per capita[a]	CDPPC
Health Resources	
Health expenditures	HEALTHEXP
Hospital beds per 1,000	HOSPBEDS
Physicians per 1,000	PHYSICIANS
Education	
Ideal years to graduate	IDEALYRS
Secondary school—% female	SECFEMALE
Persistence to grade 5—female	GRADE5F
Trade	
Trade (exports-imports)/GDP	TRADE
Population	
Urban population growth—annual %[a]	URBAN GROWTH

ACDA = U.S. Arms Control and Disarmament Agency.

[a] Variables included in final model specifications.

twenty-nine-year time series was formed for eighty-eight countries including 161 indicators. Analysis file 2 was based on the World Bank indicators and the SIPRI military expenditure file. This file covers the period from 1975 through 1991 with up to 100 countries in each year and 157 indicators taken from the World Development Indicators (World Bank Data Development Group 2001). Analysis file 3 has the SIPRI military data, the World Bank's World Development Indicators, and the United Nations Department of Peacekeeping Operations peacekeeping data (United Nations Department of Peacekeeping Operations 2002). Appendix 18.1 contains a full list of the

countries included in each of the six models and the number of observations of the two dependent variables for each country. The short list of variables considered for each analysis, including the dependent variables LEB and IMR and potential covariates, is presented in table 18.1.

Each cross-sectional time-series model is allowed to be unbalanced, that is, have a different *n* for each country (Greene 1997; Judge et al. 1985; StataCorp 2003). Since this investigation is concerned with the aggregate effects of military spending over all time periods and not for specific, individual time-period effects, restriction to the balanced model is unnecessary. If all indicators for a particular state within a given model are specified for at least one year, that state is included in the estimation.

The first set of models (models 1–4, table 18.2) are concerned with overall aggregate mortality outcomes as the dependent variables. Models 1 and 3 are based on the overall country-specific IMR, while models 2 and 4 focus on the overall population LEB.

The cross-sectional time-series model is estimated using Stata (StataCorp 2003). The general form of the linear cross-sectional time-series model is:

$$y_{it} = \alpha + x_{it}\beta + \nu_i + \varepsilon, \qquad (1)$$

where i is a unique numerical identifier for each state, and t is the year of the observation.

In equation (1), y represents the dependent variable, either IMR or LEB; x is the matrix of independent observations; α is the overall constant for all states; and β is the vector of coefficients. The interpretation of $\nu_i + \varepsilon_{it}$ depends on the specification of the model. Since the unit of analysis, the state, is fixed and theoretically important, the fixed-effects estimation method was chosen for the cross-sectional time-series models in this analysis. In the fixed-effects model, the ν_i values are estimated as offsets to the constant α, and the fixed effect for state j is then equal to $\alpha + \nu_j$. Estimation of the ν and ε terms is conditioned on the assumption of independence, and ε is always a normally distributed error term with mean zero and variance σ_0.

As this analysis is concerned only with the overall pooled effects of military expenditure as a percentage of state resources, the estimated fixed effects are not reported.

The U.S. Arms Control and Disarmament Agency analysis (models 1 and 2) is based on a consistent set of eighty-eight countries for the period 1963 through 1991 (29 years). The availability of the covariates in the SIPRI analyses (models 3 and 4) limits the number of years of coverage to a maximum of twenty-two for the IMR analysis and sixteen for the LEB models. The SIPRI data covers a consistent set of 100 countries over the period 1980 through 2001. The peacekeeping models (models 5 and 6) employ the military spending data from SIPRI adjusted by the peacekeeping data from the United Nations Department of Peacekeeping Operations. These models include ninety-seven countries and fourteen years of data.

None of the potential covariates in the health resources or education categories nor the trade variable was a statistically significant correlate of either IMR or LEB. This result may be influenced by the lack of available data for some countries and years.

Indicators of educational opportunities for women were included in the initial model building using three different measures: the percentage of women completing primary education, the percentage completing secondary education, and the percentage of women completing grade 5 or the equivalent. All of these measures suffer from large numbers of missing values. Only the percentage of females that completed grade 5 was a significant correlate in any model. The addition of this variable did not change the magnitude or significance of the coefficients of the other predictors substantially, though the number of cross sections included in the models fell below fifty and the number of total observations fell to less than 200 due to missing values. The reduction in observations and cross sections was deemed unacceptable in the presence of virtually no change in magnitude or significance of the other coefficients. Thus, the effect of women's education, and women's

TABLE 18.2. Models of Military Spending and Well-Being

Model	Dependent Variable and Source[a]	Number of Observations	Number of States	Number of Years (max/average)
1	IMR/ACDA	1,162	88	29/13.2
2	LEB/ACDA	828	88	29/9.4
3	IMR/SIPRI	908	100	22/9.1
4	LEB/SIPRI	762	100	16/7.6
5	IMR/SIPRI Peacekeeping	813	97	14/8.4
6	LEB/SIPRI Peacekeeping	694	97	14/7.2

[a] ACDA = U.S. Arms Control and Disarmament Agency of the U.S. Department of State; Peacekeeping data source: the United Nations Department of Peacekeeping Operations.

320 THE INTERNATIONAL RESPONSES TO GLOBALIZATION

social status more generally, is not directly accounted for in these models, though the differences in women's status between countries, which are likely to change slowly over time, if at all, are accounted for to some extent in the fixed effects.

Other variables that would have been included such as availability of clean water and public sanitation services are not of adequate quality or quantity for inclusion cross-sectional longitudinal models such as those estimated here. Such measures may be available for many countries for a given recent year but do not exist over time for a sufficient number of countries even when considering only the recent past. The same is true for GINI coefficients, though the United Nations World Institute for Development Economics Research (WIDER) project offers hope for this measure in the future.

A parsimonious set of covariates was defined and applied consistently in each of the six models. Covariates include GDP per capita as a measure of the level economic development, percentage urban population growth as a proxy for the position of the nation-state in the population transition from subsistence agriculture to industrialization well as an indicator of the pressure of population change on the nation-state, and the amount of cereal yield per square hectare of land as a proxy for the availability of food in the population. These measures are consistently available for a large number of nation-states and for a substantial time period. They were found to be significant and stable correlates of the two measures of well-being used in the analyses.

The cross-sectional time-series fixed-effects model used in each analysis provides an estimate of the mean or constant value for each of the cross sections, countries, in the sample as an offset to an overall grand mean. These country fixed effects take into account overall differentials between countries that remain mostly fixed over the time period of analysis. Thus, the significance of the fixed effects implies that some of the consistent differences between countries such as position in the world systems order are accounted for in these effects.

RESULTS

Adjusting for the fixed effects of the individual states, availability of food (cereal yield), level of GDP (GDP per capita), and the annual rate of urban population growth (urban growth), military expenditure is found to be a statistically significant correlate of IMR and LEB (table 18.3).

As hypothesized, higher levels of spending on military programs result in higher IMRs (H_1) and lower LEBs (H_2). The coefficient estimates for military expenditure are reasonably similar the across two sets of models. On average, reducing military spending by

TABLE 18.3. The Impact of Military Spending on Well-Being

	Model 1	Model 2	Model 3	Model 4
Dependent	IMR/ACDA	LEB/ACDA	IMR/SIPRI	LEB/SIPRI
R^2	0.3432	0.5371	0.3921	0.3215
Variables (all models)				
Constant	80.865	58.945	42.279	62.996
	(0.001)	(0.001)	(0.001)	(0.001)
Cereal yield	−0.0065	0.0018	−0.0029	0.0004
	(0.001)	(0.001)	(0.001)	(0.044)
GDP per capita	0.00029	0.00008	−0.00009	0.00026
	(0.083)	(0.047)	(0.586)	(0.0001)
Urban growth	1.185	−0.367	0.923	0.3597
	(0.006)	(0.001)	(0.004)	(001)
Military spending	2.536	−0.4597	0.9229	−0.2613
	(0.001)	(0.001)	(0.001)	(0.001)

1% of GNP would reduce IMR by as much as 2.5 deaths per 1,000 per year (model 1).

The models were also estimated using age-five mortality rates as the dependent variable. This option was employed to check how robust these effects are under differing definitions of mortality. Mortality at age five, LEB, and IMR are all correlated. Depending on the country, these correlations range from about 0.30 to 0.97. The models using mortality at age five show the same significant adverse effect of military spending, though these findings are omitted due to the large amount of missing data for age-five mortality measures. Other measures that would be of interest, such as life expectancy at age five, are not available in the current data.

Each of the LEB and IMR models shows a significant effect of population nutrition (cereal yield per hectare) and the population change as measured by the annual percentage of population growth in urban areas. In the IMR models (models 1 and 3), the coefficient of cereal yield is negative, indicating that higher levels of cereal production result in lower IMRs. The coefficient for the LEB models is significant and positive, implying that higher levels of food availability increase LEB. This finding is consistent with theory that nutrition is associated with better health outcomes.

Higher levels of urban population growth are correlated with worse health outcomes in all models except the LEB model using the SIPRI data. Faster rates of growth in urban areas may signal overcrowding, unemployment, and excess burden on public resources such as sanitation, water supply, transportation, and hospitals. The finding for model 4 may well be due to the difference in time periods covered by models 2 and 4, where model 4 includes all of the 1990s, which saw a worldwide economic expansion. The urban population growth during the 1990s may be related to economic expansion rather than a migration to cities to escape the poverty of the rural areas. Model 2 coverage ends in 1991 and is thus not affected by the economic expansion of the 1990s. Additionally, IMR is more sensitive to population changes than to LEB, and the effects of rapid urbanization and overcrowding may appear in a matter of months rather than years.

GDP per capita is a significant correlate of LEB but not of IMR. Though the coefficients are small due to the average magnitude of GDP per capita, higher levels of GDP per capita are correlated with longer LEBs. The logged value of GDP per capita, though producing a larger coefficient, showed no statistically significance different correlation to the mortality measures when compared to the unlogged measure of GDP per capita.

The IMR and LEB models were run separately for those states where GDP per capita is less than $10 per day (poorer states) versus states where GDP per capita is $10 or more per day (richer states). The effect of military spending on mortality in poorer states is uniformly greater for both the LEB models and the IMR models, and this effect is consistent across the two data sets (table 18.4). In terms of the number of infant deaths associated with each additional percentage of GDP allocated to the military, the effect is about three times greater in poorer countries than it is in countries where GDP per capita is 10$ or more per day. This differential between richer and poorer states appears to be even greater when well-being is measured by LEB (table 18.4).

The models were also estimated with military spending adjusted by subtracting the amount allocated to peacekeeping operations and then recalculating the ratio of military spending to GDP (hypothesis H_3). Peacekeeping data are available from 1988 through 2001, and only the SIPRI data set provides annual observations on military spending during this period. Thus, the results in table 18.5 are

TABLE 18.4. Comparison of the Effect of Military Spending in Richer and Poorer States

Data Source/Measure	GDP per Capita ≥ $10 per Day	GDP per Capita < $10 per Day	Ratio of Coefficients
SIPRI/IMR	0.57	1.79	3.14
SIPRI/LEB	−0.125	−0.44	3.52
ACDA/IMR	1.30	5.36	4.12
ACDA/LEB	−0.19	−0.98	5.16

ACDA = U.S. Arms Control and Disarmament Agency.

TABLE 18.5. Military Spending Adjusted for Peace-keeping Expenditures (SIPRI Data Only)

	Model 5	Model 6
Dependent	IMR	LEB
R^2	0.4409	0.2359
Variables (all models)		
Constant	40.4277	63.436
	(0.001)	(0.001)
Cereal yield	−0.00153	−0.0001
	(0.003)	(0.580)
GDP per capita	−0.00024	0.00029
	(0.129)	(0.001)
Urban growth	0.4772	0.4681
	(0.087)	(0.001)
Military spending adjusted for peacekeeping		
(SIPRI/UNDPI)	0.64612	−0.04276
	(0.003)	(0.576)

UNDPI = United Nations Department of Peacekeeping Operations.

for a single model of IMR and LEB each estimated over the period 1988 through 2001 for ninety-seven countries where the military spending measure has been adjusted for peacekeeping.

When peacekeeping efforts are accounted for, the effect of military spending on LEB, though still negative, is not statistically significant. However, the effect of adjusted military spending on IMR is significant ($p = 0.003$) and positive, indicating that military spending adjusted for peacekeeping operations continues to have a detrimental effect on the health of infants.

DISCUSSION

Building on the earlier work reported in Chan and Mintz (1992) and the study by Woolhandler and Himmelstein (1985), the findings of the present analysis confirm the negative relationship between mortality and the allocation of resources to military programs by the state. Citizens in countries with higher allocations to military programs have worse mortality outcomes. Greater percentages of state resources allocated to military programs are associated with higher IMRs and lower overall LEB for the average citizen. As characterized by Sen (1999), the most

basic aspect of freedom—the opportunity to live a life of choice—is restricted as resources are allocated away from domestic programs.

These findings are strengthened in several ways. First, the analysis here includes both a cross-national comparison and a longitudinal perspective. Each of the principal models includes eighty-eight or more countries and averages between seven and thirteen years of observation per cross section. Further, the data are taken from multiple sources, including military expenditure data from the U.S. Arms Control and Disarmament Agency (1975, 1986, 1995) and the Stockholm International Peace Research Institute (SIPRI 2003). The high correspondence in the models and the resultant estimates is encouraging. The quality of cross-national data always deserves scrutiny. However, the consistency of the results of analyses employing two distinct data sources, as demonstrated in this analysis, adds confidence to these findings.

This study shows that when considering a large number of countries in the world over two substantial time periods of the later half of the twentieth century, there is a significant penalty on the infants of the world imposed by resources allocated to militarism. As the world continues to be a dangerous place due to war and terrorism, the direct effects of violence are not the only dangers to our infant children. As many as 2.5 additional infants deaths per 1,000 live births may occur in a given country for each 1% of GNP diverted from domestic welfare programs to military projects.

While some level of security and militarism is necessary for the safety and continuation of the nation-state, this study suggests that these expenditures should be carefully measured against domestic needs. Nation-states do not have unlimited budgets, even those with vast resources. The budget allocation process is a zero-sum game, and allocations for militarism, particularly those that may be expeditionary, take resources away from the needs of the homeland population.

This study also establishes a relationship between military spending and LEB. LEB is reduced by nearly six months for each 1% of GNP spent on military programs (U.S. Arms Control and Disarmament Agency 1975, 1986, 1995). This result is confirmed by the analysis of the SIPRI data where the negative effect of military spending is highly significant and estimated to reduce LEB by about three months for each 1% of GDP increase in military spending. Together, these results are a further indication of the penalty to well-being when resources are diverted from domestic programs to military uses. The mechanism at work here is the guns-versus-butter tradeoff.

There is a positive effect of food availability on mortality as seen in the coefficients of the measure of cereal yield within the state. The negative association of mortality outcomes with urbanization is most likely an indication of overcrowding in cities and increased stress on urban ecological infrastructures such as public sanitation services as well as likely migration to cities in an attempt to leave poverty behind in the rural areas.

The findings in this analysis are also strengthened by the peacekeeping analysis. When military spending is adjusted downward for the amount allocated to peacekeeping operations, the coefficient of the LEB measure is not found to be statistically significant. At the same time, the effect of military spending on IMR is still highly significant, though slightly smaller than it was in the two preceding IMR models (model 1 and 3). This result suggests that the beneficial aspects of peacekeeping operations may accrue differentially in favor of older populations more so than to infants.

One possible mechanism is that peacekeeping forces may lower the level of violent, conflict-related deaths that largely affect older adolescents and adults. However, peacekeeping operations may not initially improve a violent and unstable context enough for social support, health, and educational services to begin operations. While the peacekeepers may lower the level of violent deaths, they may not make the context safe enough for the operation of United Nations and nongovernmental organizations to begin support op-

erations. The persistence of the effect of the resource allocation for military programs on IMR may be a reflection of the serious nature of the social disintegration in areas where United Nations peacekeepers are deployed.

In the end, nation-states must be Janus-faced in order to survive. A balance in the allocation of finite state resources must be struck in order to create the environment within which the state can stabilize and grow, while protecting itself from potential enemies. Historically, the military has played an important role in the formation and growth of states via protection from external threats, control of internal forces, and even, to some extent, the growth and development of the domestic economy (Tilly 1992, 2004). Some level of security is necessary in order to have basic levels of well-being. However, the resource horizon facing states in the expanding political and economic globalization is significantly based in the zero-sum context (Rodrik 1997).

When states divert resources to build military strength, a domestic penalty will accrue. IMRs in the world range from three to five deaths per 1,000 live births per year in Sweden, Finland, and Japan, to well more than 150 per 1,000 in such countries as Mali, Gambia, Afghanistan, Yemen, and Kampuchea. In 1999, Sierra Leone, Zambia, Botswana, Malawi, and Rwanda each had an LEB less than forty years. LEB in Western Europe, Japan, and the United States is approaching or exceeding eighty years for both men and women. In this time of increasingly fast development and globalization, one approach states can use to address this inequity in well-being is to find ways to balance the resource tradeoff identified in this analysis.

APPENDIX 18.1. Tables of Countries and Number of Observations

Country	IMR	LEB	Country	IMR	LEB
Countries and Observations in the U.S. Arms Control and Disarmament Agency Data Set			Malta	16	7
			Mauritania	9	9
Algeria	11	11	Mauritius	9	9
Australia	20	8	Mexico	8	8
Austria	29	11	Mongolia	3	3
Bangladesh	5	5	Morocco	8	8
Belgium	29	11	Nepal	10	11
Bolivia	10	10	Netherlands	29	12
Brazil	11	11	New Zealand	28	11
Bulgaria	3	2	Nicaragua	8	8
Burundi	11	11	Niger	8	8
Cameroon	11	11	Nigeria	9	9
Central African Republic	8	8	Norway	28	12
Sri Lanka	8	8	Pakistan	10	10
Chad	8	8	Paraguay	9	9
Chile	13	9	Peru	9	8
Colombia	9	9	Philippines	8	8
Costa Rica	17	6	Portugal	29	14
Cyprus	8	7	Romania	8	8
Denmark	29	12	Rwanda	8	8
Ecuador	11	11	Saudi Arabia	10	10
El Salvador	8	8	Senegal	11	9
Finland	20	12	Sierra Leone	9	9
France	29	13	South Africa	9	9
Gabon	10	10	Korea, South	8	8
Greece	29	13	Spain	29	14
Guatemala	11	11	Swaziland	7	7
Guinea	1	1	Sweden	29	11
Honduras	6	6	Switzerland	21	8
Hungary	20	7	Syria	11	11
India	18	11	Tanzania	1	1
Indonesia	11	11	Thailand	13	11
Iran	4	4	Togo	10	10
Ireland	29	14	Tunisia	8	8
Israel	29	18	Turkey	10	9
Italy	29	15	Uganda	4	4
Japan	29	20	United Arab Emirates	3	3
Jordan	5	2	United Kingdom	29	16
Kenya	11	11	United States of America	29	29
Kuwait	10	8	Uruguay	11	11
Laos	1	1	Venezuela	11	11
Malawi	10	10	Zambia	9	8
Malaysia	10	11	Total observations	1162	828
Mali	9	9			

Country	IMR	LEB	Country	IMR	LEB
Countries and Observations in the SIPRI Data Set			Israel	10	21
Algeria	6	7	Italy	12	17
Argentina	6	8	Japan	13	13
Australia	12	21	Jordan	8	8
Austria	10	14	Kenya	9	9
Bangladesh	7	9	Kuwait	4	6
Belgium	12	14	Laos	3	3
Bolivia	6	6	Lebanon	6	6
Botswana	7	7	Lesotho	5	5
Brazil	6	7	Malawi	8	8
Bulgaria	11	12	Malaysia	11	8
Burundi	11	11	Mali	10	11
Cambodia	7	7	Malta	8	13
Cameroon	7	7	Mauritania	4	4
Canada	9	12	Mauritius	8	8
Central African Republic	2	3	Mexico	7	7
Sri Lanka	7	10	Mongolia	6	6
Chad	4	4	Morocco	5	5
Chile	6	13	Netherlands	7	12
China, People's Republic	7	7	New Zealand	7	11
Colombia	6	6	Nicaragua	5	5
Costa Rica	4	10	Niger	2	2
Cyprus	8	12	Nigeria	7	7
Denmark	11	14	Norway	13	16
Ecuador	5	5	Pakistan	8	8
El Salvador	6	6	Panama	5	5
Egypt	6	6	Paraguay	6	6
Ethiopia	5	5	Philippines	7	7
Finland	13	16	Poland	12	12
France	16	17	Portugal	12	14
Gabon	2	2	Romania	14	14
Gambia	7	7	Rwanda	9	9
Ghana	9	9	Saudi Arabia	9	9
Greece	12	14	Senegal	10	13
Guatemala	6	8	Sierra Leone	5	5
Guinea	4	4	South Africa	7	7
Guyana	6	6	Korea, South	5	5
Honduras	1	2	Russia	4	4
Hungary	14	14	Spain	12	13
India	11	22	Sudan	1	1
Indonesia	7	7	Swaziland	7	7
Iran	5	6	Sweden	12	21
Ireland	11	14	Switzerland	9	13

Country	IMR	LEB	Country	IMR	LEB
Syria	8	9	Ethiopia	5	5
Tanzania	4	4	Finland	11	13
Thailand	8	10	France	13	14
Togo	3	3	Gambia	7	7
Tunisia	10	14	Ghana	7	7
Turkey	8	13	Greece	12	14
Uganda	9	9	Guatemala	6	8
United Arab Emirates	4	4	Guinea	4	4
United Kingdom	12	13	Guyana	3	3
United States of America	13	14	Hungary	14	14
Uruguay	6	8	India	7	14
Venezuela	7	9	Indonesia	7	7
Germany	9	10	Iran	4	4
Yemen	5	5	Ireland	11	14
Zambia	6	8	Israel	6	13
Total observations	762	908	Italy	9	14
			Japan	13	13
Countries and Observations in the SIPRI Peacekeeping Data Set			Jordan	7	7
			Kenya	7	7
Algeria	6	7	Kuwait	4	6
Argentina	6	8	Laos	4	4
Australia	8	13	Lebanon	6	6
Austria	10	14	Lesotho	6	6
Bangladesh	7	9	Malawi	7	7
Belgium	11	13	Malaysia	11	8
Bolivia	6	6	Mali	6	7
Botswana	7	7	Malta	8	13
Brazil	6	7	Mauritania	5	5
Bulgaria	12	13	Mauritius	8	8
Burundi	7	7	Mexico	6	6
Cambodia	7	7	Mongolia	6	6
Cameroon	7	7	Morocco	7	7
Canada	9	12	Netherlands	6	10
Central African Republic	2	3	New Zealand	7	11
Sri Lanka	7	10	Nicaragua	5	5
Chad	5	5	Niger	4	4
Chile	6	13	Nigeria	7	7
China, People's Republic	7	7	Norway	10	13
Colombia	6	6	Pakistan	7	7
Cyprus	8	12	Panama	5	5
Denmark	11	14	Paraguay	5	5
Ecuador	5	5	Philippines	7	7
El Salvador	6	6	Poland	12	12
Egypt	4	4	Portugal	12	14

Country	IMR	LEB
Romania	14	14
Rwanda	7	7
Saudi Arabia	7	7
Senegal	7	9
Sierra Leone	4	4
South Africa	7	7
Korea, South	5	5
Russia	4	4
Spain	12	13
Sudan	1	1
Swaziland	7	7
Sweden	9	14
Switzerland	9	13
Syria	7	8
Tanzania	4	4
Thailand	7	9
Togo	3	3
Tunisia	8	12
Turkey	7	12
Uganda	7	7
United Arab Emirates	4	4
United Kingdom	12	13
United States of America	12	13
Uruguay	7	9
Venezuela	3	5
Germany	9	10
Yemen	5	5
Zambia	6	8
Total observations	694	813

Note

1. Gross national product (GNP) is equal to gross domestic product (GDP) plus the income earned by resident companies in international markets. GNP is more difficult to measure accurately because it depends on international accounting data.

References

Amin, Samir. 2000. "Economic Globalism and Political Universalism: Conflicting Issues?" Journal of World-Systems Research 6:582–622.

Annan, Kofi. "We the Peoples": The Role of the United Nations in the 21st Century. UN Doc. A/54/2000, March 2000. New York: United Nations.

Baylis, John, and Smith, Steve. 1997. The Globalization of World Politics. Oxford: Oxford University Press.

Bloom, David E., and Malaney, Pia N. 1998. "Macroeconomic Consequences of the Russian Mortality Crisis." Social Science and Medicine 26:2073–2085.

Boli, John, and Thomas, John. 2004. "World Culture in the World Polity: A Century of International Nongovernmental Organizations." In: The Globalization Reader, edited by F. J. Lechner and J. Boli. Malden, MA: Blackwell, pp. 258–264.

Chan, Steve. 1989. "Income Inequality among LDCs: A Comparative Analysis of Alternative Perspectives." International Studies Quarterly 33:45–65.

Chan, Steve. 1992. "Military Burden, Economic Growth, and Income Inequality: The Taiwan Exception." In: Defense, Welfare, and Growth, edited by S. Chan and A. Mintz. London: Rutledge, pp. 163–178.

Chan, Steve, and Mintz, Alex. 1992. Defense, Welfare, and Growth. London: Rutledge.

Coburn, David. 2000. "Income Inequality, Social Cohesion and the Health Status of Populations: The Role of Neo-Liberalism." Social Science and Medicine 52:135–46.

Davis, David R., and Steve Chan. 1990. "The Security-Welfare Relationship: Longitudinal Evidence from Taiwan." Journal of Peace Research 14:145–154.

Deaton, Angus. 1999. "Inequalities in Income and Inequalities in Health." NBER Working Paper 7141. Cambridge, MA: National Bureau of Economic Research.

Deaton, Angus, and Paxson, C. 1999. "Mortality, Education, Income and Inequality Among American Cohorts." NBER Working Paper 7140. Cambridge, MA: National Bureau of Economic Research.

Deger, Saadet, and Sen, Somnath. 1983. "Military Expenditure, Spin-off, and Economic Development." Journal of Developmental Economics 13:67–83.

Deger, Saadet, and Smith, Ron. 1983. "Military Expenditure and Growth in Less Developed Countries." Journal of Conflict Resolution 27:335–353.

Department of Public Information. 1995. "Charter of the United Nations (1945)." In: The United Nations and Human Rights, 1945–1995. New York: Department of Public Information, United Nations.

Dixon, William J., and Moon, Bruce E. 1986. "The Military Burden and Basic Human Needs." Journal of Conflict Resolution 30:660–684.

Domke, William, Eichenberg, Richard, and Kelleher, Catherine. 1983. "The Illusion of Choice: Defense and Welfare in Advanced Industrial Democracies, 1948–1978." American Political Science Review 77:19–35.

Dumas, Lloyd. 1977. "Economic Conversion, Productive Efficiency and Social Welfare." Peace Research Reviews 7:17–52.

Epsing-Anderson, G. 1990. The Three Worlds of Welfare Capitalism. Princeton, NJ: Princeton University Press.

Everts, Philip P., and Isernia, Pierangelo. 2001. Public Opinion and the International Use of Force. London: Routledge.

Gissinger, Ravveig, and Gleditsch, Nils Petter. 1999. "Globalization and Conflict: Welfare, Distribution, and Political Unrest." Journal of World-Systems Research 5:327–365.

Greene, William H. 1997. Econometric Analysis. 3rd ed. Upper Saddle River, NJ: Prentice-Hall.

Johansson, S. Ryan, and Carl Mosk. 1987. "Exposure, Resistance, and Life Expectancy: Disease and Death during the Economic Development of Japan, 1900–1960." Population Studies 41:207–235.

Judge, George G., Griffights, W. E., Hill, R. C., Lutkepohl, H. and Lee, T. C. 1985. The Theory and Practice of Econometrics. 2nd ed. New York: John Wiley and Sons.

Kawachi, Ichiro, and Kennedy, Bruce P. 2002. The Health of Nations: Why Inequality Is Harmful to Your Health. New York: New Press.

Kawachi, Ichiro, Kennedy, B. P., Lochner, K. and Prothrow-Stith, D. 1997. "Social Capital, Income Inequality, and Mortality." American Journal of Public Health 87:1491–1498.

Kennedy, Bruce P., Kawachi, Ichiro and Brainerd, Elizabeth. 1998a. "The Role of Social Capital in the Russian Mortality Crisis." World Development 26:2029–2043.

Krug E. 1999. World Report on Violence and Health. Geneva: World Health Organization, Department of Injuries and Violence Prevention.

Meyer, John W., Boli, John, Thomas, John and Ramirez, Francisco O. 2004. "World Society and the Nation-State." In: The Globalization Reader, edited by F. J. Lechner and J. Boli. Malden, MA: Blackwell, pp. 84–92.

Mintz, Alex, and Stevenson, Randolph T. 1995. "Defense Expenditures, Economic Growth, and the Peace Dividend." Journal of Conflict Resolution 39:282–306.

Moon, Bruce E., and Dixon, William J. 1985. "Politics, the State, and Basic Human Needs: A Cross-National Study." American Journal of Political Science 29:661–694.

Nathanson, Constance A. 1996. "Disease Prevention as Social Change: Toward a Theory of Public Health." Population and Development Review 22:609–637.

National Center for Health Statistics. 2004. Health, United States, 2004, with Chartbook on Trends in the Health of Americans. Hyattsville, MD: National Center for Health Statistics.

Penn World Table Version 5.6. 1999, November. Philadelphia: Center for International Comparisons, University of Pennsylvania.

Price-Smith, Andrew T. 2002. The Health of Nations: Infectious Disease, Environmental Change, and Their Effects on National Security and Development. Cambridge, MA: MIT Press.

Rodrik, Dani. 1997. Has Globalization Gone Too Far? Washington, DC: International Institute for Economics.

Rose, Richard. 2000. "How Much Does Social Capital Add to Individual Health? A Survey Study of Russians." Social Science and Medicine 51:1421–1435.

Rothschild, Kurt W. 1973. "Military Expenditure, Exports and Growth." Kyklos 26:804–814.

Russett, Bruce. 1970. What Price Vigilance? The Burdens of National Defense. New Haven, CT: Yale University Press.

Russett, Bruce. 1982. "Defense Expenditures and National Well-Being." American Political Science Review 76:767–777.

Rutstein, Shea O. 2000. "Factors Associated with Trends in Infant and Child Mortality in Developing Countries during the 1990s." Bulletin of the World Health Organization 78:1256–1270.

Sen, Amartya. 1999. Democracy as Freedom. New York: Alfred A. Knopf.

SIPRI. 2003. Military Expenditure Database 1976 to 2002. Stockholm International Peace Research Institute. http://www.sipri.se.

Skocpol, Theda, and Rueschemeyer, Dietrich, eds. 1996. States, Social Knowledge, and the Origins of Modern Social Policies. Princeton, NJ: Princeton University Press.

Smith, Ron. 1977. "Military Expenditure and Capitalism." Cambridge Journal of Economics 2:299–304.

Smith, Ron. 1980. "Military Expenditure and Investment in OECD Countries 1954–1973." Journal of Comparative Economics 4:19–32.

StataCorp. 2003. Stata Statistical Software, Release 8.2SE. College Station, TX: StataCorp.

Tomlinson, John. 2004. "Cultural Imperialism." In: The Globalization Reader, edited by F. J. Lechner and J. Boli. Malden, MA: Blackwell, pp. 303–311.

Thurow, Lester C. 2001. The Zero-Sum Society: Distribution and the Possibilities for Economic Change. New York: Basic Books.

Tilly, Charles. 1992. Coercion, Capital, and European States, AD 990–1992. Cambridge, MA: Blackwell.

——— 2004. Contention and Democracy in Europe, 1650–2000. Cambridge: Cambridge University Press.

United Nations Department of Peacekeeping Operations. 2002. Status of Contributions as of 31 December 2002, ST/ADM/SER.B/585. New York: United Nations.

U.S. Arms Control and Disarmament Agency. 1975. World Military Expenditures and Arms Trade, 1963–1973, and Cumulative Arms Trade, 1964–1973 [ICPSR 7454]. Ann Arbor, MI: Inter-University Consortium for Political and Social Research [distributor].

U.S. Arms Control and Disarmament Agency. 1986. World Military Expenditures and Arms Transfers, 1973–1983 [ICPSR 8532]. Ann Arbor, MI: Inter-University Consortium for Political and Social Research [distributor].

U.S. Arms Control and Disarmament Agency. 1995. World Military Expenditures and Arms Transfers, 1983–1993 [ICPSR 6516]. Ann Arbor, MI: Inter-University Consortium for Political and Social Research [distributor].

U.S. Department of State. 2003. World Military Expenditures and Arms Transfers 1999–2000. Washington, DC: U.S. Department of State.

Wallerstein, Immanuel. 2004. "The Rise and Future Demise of the World Capitalist System." In: The Globalization Reader, edited by F. J. Lechner and J. Boli. Malden. MA: Blackwell, pp. 63–69.

Weede, E. 1980a. "Arms Races and Escalation: Some Persisting Doubts." Journal of Conflict Resolution 24:285–287.

Weede, E. 1980b. "Beyond Misspecification in Sociological Analyses of Income Inequality." American Sociological Review 45:497–501.

Weede, E., and Tiefenbach, H. 1981. "Some Recent Explanations of Income Inequality." International Studies Quarterly 25:255–282.

Wilkinson, Richard G. 1996. Unhealthy Societies: The Afflictions of Inequality. London: Routledge.

Wilmoth, John. 1998. "Is the Pace of Japanese Mortality Decline Converging toward International Trends?" Population and Development Review 24: 593–600.

Woolhandler, Steffie, and Himmelstein, D. U. 1985. "Militarism and Mortality. An International Analysis of Arms Spending and Infant Death Rates." Lancet 1:1375–1378.

World Bank Data Development Group. 2001. World Development Indicators CD-ROM. Win*STARS Version 4.2. Washington, DC: World Bank.

World Bank, International Economics Department. 1997. World Tables of Economic and Social Indicators, 1950–1992 [ICPSR 6159]. Ann Arbor, MI: Inter-University Consortium for Political and Social Research [distributor].

Index